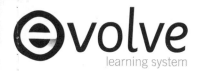

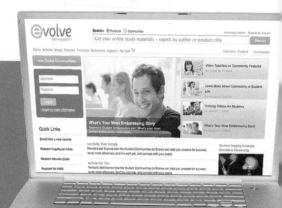

Workbook and Competency Evaluation Review

MOSBY'S TEXTBOOK FOR NURSING ASSISTANTS

Eighth Edition

RELDA T. KELLY, RN, MSN
Professor Emeritus, Kankakee Community College
Kankakee, Illinois;
Parish Nurse, Wesley United Methodist Church
Bradley, Illinois

Procedure checklists by
HELEN CHIGAROS, RN, BS, MSN, CRRN, CNS
Professor Emeritus, Kankakee Community College
Director, Azzarelli Outreach Clinic, St. Teresa Roman Catholic Church
Parish Nurse, St. Teresa Roman Catholic Church
Kankakee, Illinois

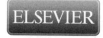

3251 Riverport Lane
St. Louis, Missouri 63043

WORKBOOK AND COMPETENCY EVALUATION REVIEW
MOSBY'S TEXTBOOK FOR NURSING ASSISTANTS, 8E

ISBN: 978-0-323-08157-3

ISBN: 978-0-323-08157-3

Content Strategist: Nancy O'Brien
Senior Content Development Specialist: Maria Broeker
Publishing Services Manager: Jeff Patterson
Project Manager: Tracey Schriefer

Printed in the United States of America

Last digit is the print number: 9 8 7 6 5 4 3 2 1

REVIEWERS

Stephanie Johnson, BA, ADN, RN
Nurse Educator
The Villages of North Branch
North Branch, Minnesota

Juanita Schueler, BSN, RN
Nursing Instructor
Clovis Community College
Clovis, New Mexico

PREFACE

This *Workbook* is written to be used with the Sorrentino and Remmert *Mosby's Textbook for Nursing Assistants*, Eighth Edition. You will not need other resources to complete the exercises in this *Workbook*.

This *Workbook* is designed to help you apply what you have learned in each chapter of the textbook. You are encouraged to use this book as a study guide. Each chapter is thoroughly covered in the multiple-choice questions, which will help prepare you to take the NAACEP test. In addition, other exercises such as fill-in-the-blank, matching, labeling, and crossword puzzles are used in many chapters. The section titled **Optional Learning Activities** may be used as an alternative exercise to give you more practice in studying the materials. **Independent Learning Activities** at the end of each chapter may be used to apply the information you will learn in a practical setting.

In addition, **Procedure Checklists** that correspond with the procedures of the textbook are provided. These checklists are designed to help you become skilled at performing procedures that affect quality of care. In addition to NNAAP® skills being identified for you, icons indicate skills that are (1) on the textbook companion CD, (2) in Mosby's Nursing Assistant Video Skills 3.0, and (3) on the EVOLVE Student Learning Resources website (video clips).

The **Competency Evaluation Review** includes a general review section and two practice exams with answers to help you prepare for the written certification exam. It also features a skills evaluation review to help you practice procedures required for certification.

Assistive personnel are important members of the health team. Completing the exercises in this *Workbook* will increase your knowledge and skills. The goal is to prepare you to provide the best possible care and to encourage pride in a job well done.

Relda T. Kelly

1 Introduction to Health Care Agencies

Fill in the Blank: Key Terms

Acute illness
Assisted living residence (ALR)
Case management
Chronic illness
Functional nursing
Health team
Hospice
Licensed practical nurse (LPN)
Licensed vocational nurse (LVN)
Nursing assistant
Nursing team
Patient-focused care
Primary nursing
Registered nurse (RN)
Team nursing
Terminal illness

1. _Primary Nursing_ is a nursing care pattern where the RN is responsible for the person's total care.

2. A person who performs delegated nursing tasks under the supervision of an RN or LPN/LVN is a _Nursing Assistant_.

3. When an illness or injury has no reasonable expectation of recovery for the person, it is a _Terminal Illness_ illness.

4. A nurse who has completed a 1-year nursing program and has passed a licensing test is a _Licensed Practical nurse_.

5. The _nursing team_ are those who provide nursing care—RNs, LPNs/LVNs, and nursing assistants.

6. A sudden illness from which the person is expected to recover is an _acute illness_.

7. When a nursing care pattern focuses on tasks and jobs, and each nursing team member has certain tasks and jobs to do, it is called _Functional Nursing_.

8. An _Assisted living residence_ provides housing, personal care, support services, health care, and social activities in a homelike setting to persons needing help with daily activities.

9. When an illness or injury is ongoing, is slow or gradual in onset, and has no known cure, it is a _Chronic Illness_ illness.

10. _Hospice_ is a health care agency or program for persons who are dying.

11. LPNs are sometimes called _Licensed vocational nurse_.

12. _Case management_ is a nursing care pattern in which a case manager (an RN) coordinates a person's care from admission through discharge and into the home setting.

13. A _registered nurse_ is a nurse who has completed a 2-, 3-, or 4-year nursing program and has passed a licensing test.

14. The many health care workers whose skills and knowledge focus on the person's total care are called the _health team_.

15. _team nursing_ is a nursing care pattern in which a team of nursing staff is led by an RN who decides the amount and kind of care each person needs.

16. When services are moved from departments to the bedside, this is a nursing care pattern called _Patient-focused care_.

Circle the Best Answer

17. When health care agencies offer services, the focus of care is always
    A. To cure illness
    B. To give daily personal care
    C. The person
    D. To provide care after surgery or injury

18. Health promotion includes
    A. Immunizations against infectious diseases
    B. Respiratory, physical, and occupational therapies
    C. Learning skills needed to live, work, and enjoy life
    D. Receiving teaching and counseling about healthy living

19. Diagnostic tests, physical exams, surgery, emergency care, and drugs are used in
    A. Health promotion
    B. Detection and treatment of disease
    C. Rehabilitation and restorative care
    D. Disease prevention

20. The goal of rehabilitation and restorative care is
    A. To teach the person about healthy living
    B. To return persons to their highest possible level of physical and psychological functioning
    C. To return the person completely to normal functioning
    D. To treat the illness with diet, exercise, and medications

21. A person with an acute illness will probably be treated in
    A. A hospital
    B. A long-term care center
    C. An assisted living facility
    D. A rehabilitation agency

22. Subacute care is needed when the person needs
    A. Minor surgery
    B. Care that falls between hospital care and long-term care
    C. Help with personal care and drugs
    D. Care at the end of life when the person is dying

23. Persons in a long-term care center
    A. Need hospital care
    B. Are acutely ill
    C. May be older with chronic diseases, poor nutrition, or poor health
    D. Never are able to return home

24. Skilled nursing facilities
    A. Provide nursing care needed until death
    B. Provide more complex care than do nursing centers
    C. Provide care in the person's home
    D. Provide outpatient care

25. A person may have an apartment and receive help with personal care when living in
    A. A long-term care center
    B. An assisted living facility
    C. A rehabilitation care agency
    D. A skilled nursing facility

26. Persons who have problems dealing with life events may be treated in a
    A. Mental health center   C. Long-term care center
    B. Skilled care facility   D. Hospice

27. Home care agencies provide
    A. Health teaching and supervision
    B. Bedside nursing care
    C. Physical therapy, rehabilitation, and food services
    D. All of the above

28. Hospices
    A. Provide short-term care until the person recovers
    B. Give care only in the home
    C. Provide care to persons who no longer respond to treatments aimed at cures
    D. Only provide care to meet the person's physical needs

29. Health care systems are
    A. Agencies that join together as one provider of care
    B. Members of the health team that give bedside care
    C. Members of the health team that work in a hospital
    D. The hospitals in a community

30. All of these are members of the health team *except*
    A. Occupational therapist
    B. Janitor
    C. Social worker
    D. Cleric

31. The person responsible for nursing service is
    A. A medical doctor
    B. An RN with a bachelor's or master's degree (DON)
    C. A person with many years experience in giving nursing care
    D. The board of trustees

32. Nursing education staff may teach all of these *except*
    A. Basic nursing skills needed to begin employment as a nurse
    B. How to use new equipment
    C. New employee orientation programs
    D. New and changing information for the nursing team

33. A registered nurse who completes a university program will be in school for
    A. 2 years   C. 3 years
    B. 1 year   D. 4 years

34. An RN
    A. Assesses, makes nursing diagnoses, plans, implements, and evaluates nursing care
    B. Is supervised by licensed doctors and licensed dentists
    C. Only gives care when the person's condition is stable and care is simple
    D. Always is able to diagnose diseases or illnesses

35. An LPN/LVN
    A. Must pass a licensing test to work
    B. Assists RNs in caring for acutely ill person and with complex procedures
    C. Has fewer responsibilities and functions than RNs
    D. All of the above

36. When a team leader delegates the care of certain persons to other nurses, the nursing care pattern is called
    A. Patient-focused care
    B. Team nursing
    C. Functional nursing
    D. Primary nursing

37. An example of functional nursing is
    A. An RN coordinates a person's care from admission through discharge
    B. Nursing tasks and procedures are delegated to nursing assistants
    C. One nurse gives all treatments
    D. Services are moved from departments to the bedside

38. When the number of people caring for each person is reduced, this nursing care pattern is
    A. Functional nursing
    B. Case management
    C. Patient-focused care
    D. Team nursing

39. Medicare
    A. Is bought by individuals and families from an insurance company
    B. Helps to pay medical costs for low income families
    C. May be provided by an employer
    D. Is a federal health insurance program for persons 65 years and older

40. A system that limits the amounts paid by insurers, Medicare, and Medicaid by determining the amount paid before care is called
    A. Prospective payment   C. Managed care
    B. Medicaid   D. Group insurance

41. In a Preferred Provider Organization (PPO)
    A. The patient may choose any doctor in the PPO
    B. The focus is on preventing disease and maintaining health
    C. The cost of services is paid by a prepaid fee
    D. Doctors or hospitals may charge whatever is necessary

42. When a health care agency is accredited
    A. It is voluntary and signals quality and excellence
    B. The agency is licensed by the state to operate and provide care
    C. It allows the agency to receive Medicare and Medicaid funds
    D. The agency meets standards set by the federal and state governments

43. If a deficiency is found during a survey of a health care agency, the agency
    A. Usually is given 60 days to correct it
    B. Will be closed immediately
    C. Can decide whether or not to correct the deficiency
    D. Can sue the survey team

44. When you are asked questions by a surveyor, you should
    A. Explain that you are not allowed to answer any questions
    B. Answer the questions honestly and as thoroughly as you can
    C. Tell the surveyor you are busy and cannot talk now
    D. Tell the surveyor you do not know the answer and he or she will have to ask someone else

Matching

Match the type of health care agency with the service provided.

A. Hospital
B. Rehabilitation agency
C. Long-term care center
D. Mental health center
E. Home care agency
F. Hospice
G. Skilled nursing facility
H. Assisted living residence

45. __F__ Serves people who are dying
46. __G__ Provides complex care while the person recovers from illness or surgery before returning home
47. __C__ Provides services to persons who do not need hospital care but cannot care for themselves at home
48. __A__ Serves people of all ages for acute, chronic, or terminal illnesses
49. __D__ Treats people who may have difficulty dealing with events in life
50. __H__ Provides housing, personal care, and other services in a homelike setting
51. __B__ Serves people who do not need hospital care, but need complex equipment and care measures
52. __E__ Provides care to persons at home

Fill in the Blank

53. Write out the abbreviations
    A. DON _____
    B. HMO _____
    C. LPN _____
    D. LVN _____
    E. PPO _____
    F. RN _____
    G. SNF _____

Write the name of the health team member described in questions 54–65.

54. _____ Supervises LPN/LVNs and assistive personnel
55. _____ Diagnoses and treats diseases and injuries
56. _____ Collects samples and performs laboratory tests on blood, urine, and other body fluids and secretions
57. _____ Takes x-rays and processes film for viewing
58. _____ Gives respiratory treatments and therapies
59. _____ Assesses and plans for nutritional needs
60. _____ Assists persons with musculoskeletal problems
61. _____ Assists persons to learn or retain skills needed to perform activities of daily living
62. _____ Treats persons with speech, voice, hearing, communication, and swallowing disorders
63. _____ Assists persons with their spiritual needs
64. _____ Helps patients and families with social, emotional, and environmental issues affecting illness and recovery
65. _____ Tests hearing and prescribes hearing aids

Use Focus on PRIDE in the Textbook to complete questions 66–71.

66. You can have a great impact on the quality of care each person receives when you remember to show
    _____, _____,
    _____, and _____.

67. When you are asked to fill out a survey about how you feel about your job, you have the right to
    _____.

68. When filling out a survey, you should
    A. _____
    B. _____
    C. _____

69. When you help promote feelings of improvement and success, this helps the person take pride in working to _____.

70. When you offer to help team members, it shows that you are _____ and you value _____.

71. To protect yourself and others, you should know the limits of _____ in your state and agency.

Labeling

72. Fill in members of the Nursing service on the organizational chart.

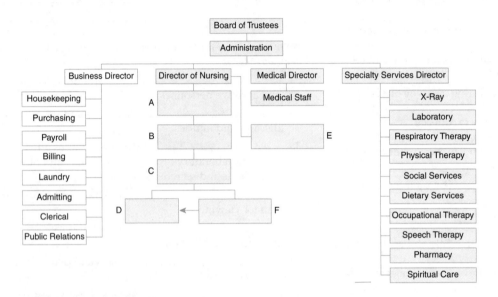

73. Refer to the previous organizational chart. The nursing assistant reports to two groups of nursing service. They are

    A. _____

    B. _____

Optional Learning Exercises

Name the member of the Health Team who provides the service described in questions 74–85.

74. Mr. Williams needs assistance to regain skills to dress, shave, and feed himself (ADLs). He is assisted by the _____

75. The nurse has a concern about a drug action, so he calls the _____.

76. Mrs. Young needs the corns on her feet treated. The nurse notifies the _____.

77. Ms. Stewart has the responsibility of doing physical examinations, health assessments, and health education for the center where she works. She is a _____

78. Mr. Gomez keeps turning up the volume of his TV. His hearing is tested by the _____.

79. The _____ meets with a new resident and his family to discuss his nutritional needs.

80. Mr. Fox had a stroke and has weakness on his left side. The _____ assists him by developing a plan that focuses on restoring function and preventing disability from his illness.

81. The doctor orders x-rays after Mr. Jackson falls. The x-rays are done by the _____.

82. Mr. Ling has chronic lung disease and needs respiratory treatments. These are given by the _____

83. Ms. Walker plans the recreational needs of a nursing center. She is an _____.

84. After a stroke, Mr. Stubbs has difficulty swallowing. He is evaluated by the _____.

85. When the doctor orders blood tests, the samples are collected by the _____.

Name the Nursing Care Pattern described in questions 86–90.

86. Ms. Hines works with Dr. Hogan. When his patient, Harry Forbes, is admitted to the hospital, Ms. Hines coordinates his care from admission to discharge. She also communicates with the insurance company and community agencies involved in Mr. Forbes' care. This is an example of _____.

87. When Mr. Holcomb reports for work as a nursing assistant, he is assigned to make all the beds on the unit. The RN gives all the drugs, and the LPN gives all the treatments. This nursing care pattern is _____

88. Ms. Conroy works on the same nursing unit each day. She has a group of patients and she gives total care to each of them. She teaches and counsels the person and family, and she plans for home care or long-term care when needed. This is an example of

_____

89. Ms. Ryan is a nursing assistant. She gives care that is delegated by an RN. The RN leads a team of nursing staff members and she decides the amount and kind of care each person needs. This is _____.

90. Mrs. Young receives her care and physical therapy on the nursing unit. She does *not* have to go to different departments to receive treatments and care. This care is provided by the nursing team instead of by other health team members. This is called

_____

Independent Learning Activities

Gather the following information about health care agencies in your area.

- How many hospitals are located in your area? Choose one hospital and answer the following questions.
  - What services are provided by this hospital?
  - How many beds are available for patients?
  - How many staff members work there?
  - How many staff members are RNs? LPNs? Nursing assistants?
  - What care is provided by nursing assistants?
  - Does the hospital have a skilled nursing facility? What types of patients are admitted to this unit?
  - Does the hospital have a rehabilitation or subacute unit? What care is provided on this unit?
  - What services are provided for person who needs care at home after discharge?
- How many long-term nursing centers are located in your area? Choose one center and answer the following questions.
  - What types of residents are accepted in the center? (For example, does the center consider level of care needed, the resident's disease, or method of payment?)

- What rehabilitation services are given?
- How many residents live in the center?
- How many staff members work there?
- How many staff members are RNs? LPNs? Nursing assistants?
- What care is provided by nursing assistants?
- How many nursing centers in your area provide skilled nursing care? Choose one center and answer these questions.
  - How many residents live in the center?
  - How many staff members work there?
  - How many staff members are RNs? LPNs? Nursing assistants?
  - What care is provided by nursing assistants?
- How many assisted living facilities are located in your area? Choose one center and answer the following questions.
  - Is this facility independent or part of a long-term care center?
  - How many residents live in the facility?
  - What kind of living quarters do the residents have? (For example, does each resident have an apartment or studio? Do they share kitchen facilities or does each person have a kitchen?)
  - How many staff members work there?
  - How many staff members are RNs? LPNs? Nursing assistants?
  - What care is provided by nursing assistants?
- What agency provides care for persons with mental illnesses?
  - What type of care is provided?
- Does your area have a hospice program? If so, answer the following questions about the program?
  - Is this program located within a center or does it provide care in the person's facility?
  - What type of care is provided?
  - What special training is given to the staff? What duties can be performed by a nursing assistant?

2 The Person's Rights

Fill in the Blank: Key Terms

Involuntary seclusion   Ombudsman   Representative   Treatment

1. A ___representative___ is any person who has the legal right to act on the resident's behalf when he or she cannot do so for himself or herself.

2. Separating a person from others against his or her will, keeping the person to a certain area, or keeping the person away from his or her room without consent is ___involuntary seclusion___.

3. The care provided to maintain or restore health, improve function, or relieve symptoms is ___treatment___.

4. An ___ombudsman___ is someone who supports or promotes the needs and interests of another person.

Circle the Best Answer

5. Which of these is a part of the Patient Care Partnership?
   A. The person must follow all recommended treatments or plans of care.
   B. The doctor does not need to share all of the information about his or her treatments.
   C. The person should know when students or other trainees are involved in his or her care.
   D. Hospital charges are not given to the person, only to the insurance companies.

6. Resident rights include all of the following rights *except*
   A. The right to have a private room in which to live
   B. The right to have personal choice to choose what to wear and how to spend their time
   C. The right to personal privacy
   D. The right to refuse treatment

7. Under OBRA, if a resident is incompetent (not able) to exercise the rights, who can exercise these rights for the person?
   A. The doctor
   B. A responsible party such as a partner, adult child, or court appointed guardian
   C. The charge nurse
   D. A neighbor

8. If a resident refuses treatment what should you do?
   A. Avoid giving any care to the person and go on to other duties
   B. Report the refusal to the nurse
   C. Tell the resident the treatment must be done and continue to carry out the treatment
   D. Tell his family so they can make him take the treatment

9. A student wants to observe a treatment, but the resident does *not* want her to be present. What is the correct action?
   A. The student cannot watch as this violates the resident's right to privacy.
   B. The student may observe from the doorway where the resident cannot see her.
   C. The staff nurse tells the resident he must allow the student to watch.
   D. The nurse calls the resident's wife to get her permission.

10. The resident should be given personal choice whenever it
    A. Is safely possible
    B. Does not interfere with scheduled activities
    C. Is approved by the director of nursing
    D. Is ordered by the doctor

11. If a resident voices concerns about care and the center promptly tries to correct the situation, this action meets the resident's right to
    A. Participate in a resident group
    B. Voice a dispute or grievance
    C. Personal choice
    D. Freedom from abuse, mistreatment, and neglect

12. A resident volunteers to take care of houseplants at the center. This is an acceptable part of the following *except*
    A. The care plan
    B. A requirement to receive care or care items
    C. The resident's regular activity
    D. Rehabilitation

13. When residents and their families plan activities together, this meets the resident's right to
    A. Privacy
    B. Freedom from restraint
    C. Freedom from mistreatment
    D. Participate in resident and family groups

14. The resident you are caring for has many old holiday decorations covering her nightstand. If you throw away these items without her permission you are denying her right to
    A. Privacy
    B. Work
    C. Keep and use personal items
    D. Freedom from abuse

15. A staff member tells a resident he cannot leave his room because he talks too much. This action denies the resident
    A. Freedom from abuse, mistreatment, and neglect (involuntary seclusion)
    B. Freedom from restraint
    C. Care and security of personal possessions
    D. Personal choice

16. When a resident is given certain drugs that affect his mood, behavior, or mental function, it may deny his right to
    A. Freedom from abuse, mistreatment, and neglect
    B. Personal choice
    C. Privacy
    D. Freedom from restraint

17. Which of these actions will promote courteous and dignified care?
    A. Calling the resident by a nickname he does not choose
    B. Assist with dressing him in clothing appropriate to the time of day
    C. Changing the resident's hairstyle without her permission
    D. Leaving the bathroom door open so you can see the person

18. You ask a resident if you may touch him. This is an example of
    A. Courteous and dignified interaction
    B. Courteous and dignified care.
    C. Providing privacy and self-determination
    D. Maintaining personal choice and independence

19. Assisting a resident to ambulate without interfering with his independence is an example of
    A. Courteous and dignified interaction
    B. Courteous and dignified care
    C. Providing privacy and self-determination
    D. Maintaining personal choice and independence

20. You provide privacy and self-determination for a resident when you
    A. Knock on the door before entering and wait to be asked in
    B. Allow the resident to smoke in designated areas
    C. Listen with interest to what the person is saying
    D. Groom his beard as he wishes

21. You allow the resident to maintain personal choice and independence when you
    A. Obtain her attention before interacting with her
    B. Provide extra clothing for warmth such as a sweater or lap robe
    C. Assist the resident to take part in activities according to his interests
    D. Use curtains or screens during personal care and procedures

22. Which of these activities would be carried out by an ombudsman?
    A. Organize activities for a group of residents
    B. Accompany residents to a religious service at a house of worship
    C. Investigate and resolve complaints made by a resident
    D. Assist the resident to choose friends

Fill in the Blank

Write out the meaning of the abbreviations in questions 23–24.

23. AHA _____

24. OBRA _____

25. According to the Patient Care Partnership, in order for the patient to make informed decisions with his or her doctor, the person needs to understand
    A. _____
    _____
    B. _____
    _____
    C. _____
    _____
    D. _____
    _____
    E. _____
    _____

26. According to the Resident's Rights, what should the nursing center do if a resident refuses treatment?
    A. _____
    B. _____
    C. _____
    D. _____
    _____

Use Focus on PRIDE in the Textbook to complete questions 27–30.

27. You are responsible for the care you give. To provide quality care, you should
    A. _____
    B. _____
    C. _____
    D. _____
    E. _____
    F. _____

28. When a person refuses treatment, the health team offers _____.

29. You can encourage social interaction by telling the person about _____ and offering _____ activities.

30. You help to keep a person's personal information private when you only discuss the person's treatment with staff _____ _____.

Optional Learning Exercises

OBRA-Required Actions to Promote Dignity and Privacy (Box 2-3)

Match the action to promote dignity and privacy with the example given in questions 31–39.

    A. Courteous and dignified interaction
    B. Courteous and dignified care
    C. Privacy and self-determination
    D. Maintain personal choice and independence

31. _____ File fingernails and apply polish as resident requests.

32. _____ Cover the resident with a blanket during a bath.

33. _____ You gain the person's attention before giving care.

34. _____ Show interest when a resident tells stories about his past.

35. _____ Open containers and arrange food at mealtimes to assist the resident.

36. _____ Close the door when the person asks for privacy.

37. _____ Allow a resident to smoke in a designated area.

38. _____ Make sure the resident is wearing his dentures when he goes to the dining room.

39. _____ You take the resident to his weekly card game.

Independent Learning Activities

Visit a nursing center and ask for a copy of the Persons Rights.

- Compare it to the information in this chapter. What is the same? What is different?
- Ask if they have an ombudsman. If so, ask for an appointment to meet with this person. Ask the ombudsman the following questions:
   - What are the primary responsibilities he or she has in the center?
   - How often does he or she meet with persons?
   - What problems has he or she helped to resolve?

3 The Nursing Assistant

Fill in the Blank: Key Terms

Accountable   Delegate   Job Description   Nursing task   Responsibility

1. To _delegate_ means to authorize another person to perform a nursing task in a certain situation.

2. A _nursing task_ is nursing care or a nursing procedure, activity, or work that can be delegated to nursing assistants when it does *not* require an RN's professional knowledge or judgment.

3. Being responsible for one's actions and the actions of others who perform delegated tasks is being _accountable_.

4. _Responsibility_ is the duty or obligation to perform some act or function.

5. A _job description_ is a document that describes what the agency expects you to do.

Circle the Best Answer

6. Until the 1980s, nursing assistants
   A. Attended nursing assistant classes approved by the state
   B. Were not used to provide basic nursing care
   C. Received on-the-job training from nurses
   D. Only worked in hospitals

7. Efforts to reduce health care costs include
   A. Nursing shortages
   B. Changes made by the Omnibus Budget Reconciliation Act (OBRA) of 1987
   C. Hospital closings and mergers
   D. Changes in the nurse practice acts

8. When staff members are given training to perform basic skills that are provided by other health team members, it is called
   A. Staff mixing
   B. Cross-training
   C. Managed care
   D. Scope of practice

9. An example of cross-training would be
   A. A nursing assistant is delegated to give basic care to a patient
   B. Blood is drawn by a medical technician sent from the laboratory
   C. An RN gives medications to a group of patients
   D. A member of the nursing team draws blood when the order is given

10. Nurse Practice Acts
    A. Only affect RNS and LPNs/LVNs
    B. Teach classes for nurses and nursing assistants
    C. Define RNs, LPNs/LVNs and sometimes also regulate nursing assistants
    D. Are exactly the same in every state

11. _____ decides what nursing assistants can do
    A. Joint Commission of Hospital Accreditation
    B. The nurse practice act
    C. The state medical society
    D. The hospital board of directors

12. If you do something beyond the legal limits of your role, you could be
    A. Protected by the nurse practice act
    B. Practicing nursing without a license
    C. Protected by the nurse who supervises your work
    D. Accused of a criminal act

13. Nursing assistants can have their certification, license, or registration denied, revoked, or suspended for
    A. Violating the privacy of a patient or resident
    B. Failing to maintain the confidentiality of patient or resident information
    C. Abusing a patient or resident
    D. All of the above

14. OBRA requires that the nursing assistant training and competency evaluation program have at least _____ hours of instruction
    A. 16   C. 120
    B. 75   D. 200

15. Which of these areas of study is *not* included in a training program for nursing assistants?
    A. Communication
    B. Elimination procedures
    C. Resident rights
    D. Phlebotomy (drawing blood)

16. The competency evaluation for nursing assistants has two parts. They are a
    A. Written test and a skills test
    B. Multiple-choice test and a true-false test
    C. Skills test and a complete bed bath demonstration
    D. Written test and an oral question-and-answer test

17. If you fail the competency evaluation the first time it is taken, you
    A. May retest a second time
    B. Can retest two more times for a total of three times
    C. Must repeat your training program
    D. Can retest as often as necessary, free of charge

18. All of the following information is contained in the nursing assistant registry *except*
    A. Information about findings of abuse or neglect and of dishonest use of property
    B. Date of birth
    C. Number of dependents
    D. Date the competency test was passed

19. OBRA requires that retraining and a new competency evaluation test must be taken if you have *not* worked as a certified nursing assistant for
    A. 2 consecutive years
    B. 5 years
    C. 1 year
    D. 6 months
20. If you want to work in another state, the state agency will require all of these *except*
    A. Proof of full-time employment within the last month
    B. Proof of successfully completing a NATCEP
    C. Written registry verification from the state in which you are currently certified
    D. Fingerprints
21. Your work as a nursing assistant is supervised by
    A. A licensed nurse
    B. A doctor or dentist
    C. The director of nursing
    D. A nursing assistant with more experience
22. As a nursing assistant, you never give medications unless
    A. The nurse is busy and asks you to give the medications
    B. The person is in the shower and the nurse leaves the medications at the bedside
    C. You have completed a state-approved medication assistant training program
    D. You are feeding the person and the nurse asks you to mix the medications with the food
23. You are alone in the nurses' station and you answer the phone. Dr. Smith begins to give verbal orders to you. You should
    A. Hang up the phone
    B. Politely give her your name and title, and ask her to wait while you get the nurse
    C. Quickly write down the orders, and give them to the nurse
    D. Politely give her your name and title, and tell her to call back later when the nurse is there
24. The nurse asks you to assist him as he changes sterile dressings. You should
    A. Assist him as needed
    B. Tell him you cannot assist to perform any sterile procedures
    C. Tell him you will change the dressings yourself, so that he can carry out duties
    D. Report his request to the director of nursing
25. Who can tell the person or family a diagnosis or prescribe treatments?
    A. Director of nursing
    B. RN
    C. Doctor
    D. Experienced nursing assistant
26. The nurse asks you carry out a task that you do *not* know how to do. You should
    A. Ignore the order because it would not be safe for you to carry out the task
    B. Promptly explain to the nurse why you cannot carry out the task
    C. Perform the task as well as you can
    D. Ask another nursing assistant to show you how to carry out the task

27. The nurse knows you are an EMT in addition to being a CNA. She is very busy and asks if you will start an IV on a patient. You should
    A. Politely tell her that you cannot start an IV as a CNA
    B. Start the IV since you start IVs routinely as an EMT
    C. Ask her to spend a few minutes supervising you as you start the IV
    D. Report her to the State Board of Nursing
28. If you are giving care in a home, you may be expected to
    A. Give medications
    B. Provide personal care and prepare meals
    C. Move heavy furniture
    D. Drive the person's car so the person can shop or run errands
29. When you read a job description, you should *not* take a job if it requires you to
    A. Carry out duties you do not like to do
    B. Function beyond your training limits
    C. Maintain required certification
    D. Attend in-service training
30. Which of the following is *not* acceptable?
    A. An RN delegates a task to an LPN/LVN
    B. An RN delegates a task to a nursing assistant
    C. An LPN/LVN delegates a task to a nursing assistant
    D. A nursing assistant delegates a task to another nursing assistant
31. When a nurse decides how to delegate tasks, the decision depends on
    A. What is best for the person at the time
    B. How well the nurse likes the nursing assistant
    C. How busy the nurse is that day
    D. Whether the nurse likes the person receiving the care
32. You have been caring for Mr. Watson for several weeks. The nurse tells you that she will give his care today. Her delegation decision is based on
    A. How well you gave his care in the past
    B. Changes in Mr. Watson's condition today
    C. How well she knows you
    D. How much supervision you need
33. At which step of the delegation process would you tell the nurse you have *not* performed a task before or often?
    A. Assess and plan
    B. Communication
    C. Surveillance and supervision
    D. Evaluation and feedback
34. When the nurse supervises the nursing assistant, she
    A. Tells the nursing assistant how to perform and complete the task
    B. Determines what knowledge and skills are needed to safely perform the nursing task
    C. Observes the care that the nursing assistant gives
    D. Decides whether the care plan needs to change
35. Which of the following is *not* a right of delegation?
    A. The right task
    B. The right time
    C. The right person
    D. The right supervision

36. You may refuse to carry out a task for all of these reasons *except*
    A. The task is not in your job description
    B. You do not know how to use the supplies or equipment
    C. You are too busy
    D. The task could harm the person

Fill in the Blank

37. Write out the abbreviations
    A. CNA _____
    B. LNA _____
    C. LPN _____
    D. LVN _____
    E. OBRA _____
    F. NATCEP _____
    G. NCSBN _____
    H. RN _____
    I. RNA _____

38. When hospitals make an effort to reduce costs with a staffing mix, nursing care is given by a mix of
    A. _____
    B. _____
    C. _____

39. A Nurse Practice Act
    A. Defines _____
    _____
    B. Describes the scope and _____
    _____
    C. Describes the education and _____
    _____
    D. Protects the public from _____
    _____

40. The Nursing Assistant Registry has this information about each nursing assistant:
    A. _____
    B. _____
    C. _____
    D. _____
    E. _____
    F. _____
    G. _____

41. Why does OBRA require 12 hours of educational programs and performance reviews each year for every nursing assistant? _____
    _____

Use the Focus on PRIDE in the Textbook to complete questions 42–45.

42. Continuing to learn new skills and new knowledge as a nursing assistant is personal and
    _____.

43. If a patient refuses to have a student care for him, you should _____ the person's rights to choose who is involved in his care.

44. As a nursing assistant, it is important to make sure your action and conversations are _____. This shows good _____.

45. When delegated several tasks, it is important for the nursing team to work _____ to provide care.

Optional Learning Exercises

OBRA Requirements Related to the Nursing Assistant

46. OBRA requires _____ hours of instruction. _____ hours must be supervised practical training. Where can the practical training take place? _____ or _____

47. OBRA requires 15 areas of study. Write the area of study where you learn the skill used in each example.
    A. You make a bed.
    _____
    B. You close Mr. Smith's door to give him privacy.
    _____
    C. You tell Mrs. Forbes the time of day and the day of the week frequently.
    _____
    D. You apply lotion to a resident's skin.
    _____
    E. You assist a person to put on his shirt.
    _____
    F. When assigned to a new unit, you check the location of the fire alarm.
    _____
    G. You practice hand hygiene before and after giving care.
    _____
    H. You get help to move a person from his bed to the chair.
    _____
    I. When speaking to Mr. Jackson, you maintain good eye contact.
    _____
    J. The nurse tells you to exercise a person's extremities (limbs).
    _____

K. You shave Mr. Stewart.

_____

L. You position a urinal for a resident in bed.

_____

M. You assist Mrs. Young to walk in the hall.

_____

N. You notice that Mrs. Peck has an elevated temperature and her skin is warm.

_____

O. You cut up the meat on Mr. Sanyo's plate before helping him to eat.

_____

The National Nurse Aide Assessment Program (NNAAP®) (See Appendix A)

48. The NNAAP® written test has _____ questions.

List the percent of questions in each area.

A. _____ ADL

B. _____ Basic nursing skills

C. _____ Restorative skills

D. _____ Emotional and mental health needs

E. _____ Spiritual and cultural needs

F. _____ Communications

G. _____ Client rights

H. _____ Legal and ethical behavior

I. _____ Member of the health team

49. List the skills that may be tested on the NNAAP®.

A. _____
B. _____
C. _____
D. _____
E. _____
F. _____
G. _____
H. _____
I. _____
J. _____
K. _____
L. _____
M. _____
N. _____
O. _____
P. _____
Q. _____
R. _____

S. _____
T. _____
U. _____
V. _____
W. _____
X. _____
Y. _____

Working in Another State

50. To work in another state, you must meet that state's

_____.

51. To find the state agency responsible for NATCEPs and the nursing assistant registry, you will

A. _____
B. _____

52. When the state determines that you may work in that state as a nursing assistant, the state may use these terms:

A. _____
B. _____
C. _____

53. When you apply to work in another state, expect to

A. _____
B. _____
C. _____
D. _____
E. _____

_____

Position Description (Figure 3-2)

54. The nursing assistant assists with assessing when he recognizes abnormal _____ and reports them to _____.

55. When the nursing assistant consistently strives to use time effectively, he or she is assisting with

_____

56. When a nursing assistant reviews basic care provided to patients and reports when changes are needed, this assists with _____.

57. The nursing assistant assists with teaching and learning information when he or she serves as a resource person for _____.

58. When a nursing assistant practices hand hygiene before and after each patient contact, this meets the job description criterion that maintains

_____

59. Nursing assistants are expected to attend and participate actively in unit meetings _____ of the time.

Independent Learning Activities

Role-play this situation with a classmate acting as the nurse.
The nurse asks you to perform a task you have only done once before. You tell her you do not feel comfortable doing this task. She says she is sure you will do a fine job of carrying out the task.

- What is your reaction when asked? How would you explain your feelings?
- What suggestions do you offer to make sure the task is done?

The nurse continues to insist that you can carry out the task and becomes angry and tells you that you can be fired for refusing her delegation.

- How would you handle her request if you feel frightened by her reaction?
- What could happen if you accept the assignment and cannot perform the task safely?
- What would happen if you accept the assignment and do not carry it out?

4 Ethics and Laws

Fill in the Blank: Key Terms

Abuse
Assault
Battery
Boundary
  crossing
Boundary sign
Boundary violation

Civil law
Crime
Criminal law
Defamation
Elder abuse
Ethics
False imprisonment

Fraud
Invasion of
  privacy
Law
Libel
Malpractice
Neglect

Negligence
Professional
  boundary
Professional sexual
  misconduct
Protected health
  information

Self-neglect
Slander
Standard of care
Tort
Vulnerable adult
Will

1. Any knowing, intentional, or negligent act by a caregiver or any other person to an older adult is _elder abuse_.

2. A rule of conduct made by a government body is a _Law_.

3. _Defamation_ is injuring a person's name and reputation by making false statements to a third person.

4. An act, behavior, or comment that is sexual in nature is _professional sexual misconduct_.

5. Touching a person's body without his or her consent is _battery_.

6. _Criminal law_ are laws concerned with offenses against the public and society in general.

7. Failure to provide the person with the goods or services needed to avoid physical harm, mental anguish, or mental illness is _neglect_.

8. An act, behavior, or thought that warns of a boundary crossing or violation is a _boundary sign_.

9. _Standard of care_ is the skills, care, and judgments required by a health team member under similar conditions.

10. A _will_ is a legal document of how a person wants property distributed after death.

11. _Fraud_ is saying or doing something to trick, fool, or deceive a person.

12. The intentional mistreatment or harm of another person is _abuse_.

13. An unintentional wrong in which a person did *not* act in a reasonable and careful manner and causes harm to a person or to the person's property is _negligence_.

14. _Self-neglect_ is a person's behavior that puts him or her at high risk for harm, health and safety are threatened.

15. A wrong committed against a person or the person's property is a _tort_.

16. _Boundary crossing_ is a brief act or behavior outside of the helpful zone.

17. Making false statements in print, writing, or through pictures or drawings is _libel_.

18. A _crime_ is an act that violates a criminal law.

19. _Ethics_ is knowledge of what is right conduct and wrong conduct.

20. Violating a person's right *not* to have his or her name, photo, or private affairs exposed or made public without giving consent is an _invasion of privacy_.

21. Identifying information and information about the person's health care is _protected health information_.

22. A _vulnerable adult_ is a person 18 years old or older who has a disability or condition that makes him or her at risk to be wounded, attacked, or damaged.

23. A _boundary violation_ is an act or behavior that meets your needs, not the person's.

24. Negligence by a professional person is _malpractice_.

25. Making false statements orally is _slander_.

26. _Civil law_ are laws concerned with relationships between people.

27. _Professional boundary_ is that which separates helpful behaviors from behaviors that are *not* helpful.

28. Unlawful restraint or restriction of a person's freedom of movement is _false imprisonment_.

29. _Assault_ is intentionally attempting or threatening to touch a person's body without the person's consent.

Circle the Best Answer

30. Which situation is unethical behavior for a nursing assistant?
    A. A person of another race is given personal care as delegated by the nurse.
    B. The nursing assistant avoids giving care to a person with body piercings.
    C. The nursing assistant reports that an elderly patient says her son sometimes hits her.
    D. The nursing assistant gives good care to a man who does *not* want life-saving measures, even though the nursing assistant disagrees with his decision.

31. What should the nursing assistant do if he finds a co-worker drinking alcohol at work?
    A. Report this behavior to the nurse
    B. Tell the co-worker that he will report this behavior unless the person pays him not to
    C. Give the co-worker information about a program for alcoholics
    D. Ignore the behavior to be loyal to his co-worker

32. Which code of conduct for nursing assistants is followed when you schedule your lunch to finish giving personal care to a person?
    A. Perform no act that will cause the person harm
    B. Know the limits of your role and knowledge
    C. Consider the person's needs to be more important than your own
    D. Protect the person's privacy

33. An example of boundary crossing would be all of these *except*
    A. Telling a person you are caring for details about your family
    B. Hugging the person each time you see him
    C. Comforting the person with a hug when you find her crying one day
    D. Accepting cash from the person

34. You may be accused of negligence when giving care if you
    A. Tell the nurse that you know the person you are assigned to care for
    B. Assist a person to the bathroom and make sure the signal light is available for her to call you
    C. Give the wrong care to the wrong person because they both have the same name
    D. Report to the nurse that the person is complaining of chest pain

35. You tell another nursing assistant that you think the housekeeper is stealing money from the staff. This is an example of
    A. Defamation   C. Invasion of privacy
    B. Boundary crossing   D. Libel

36. In the cafeteria, you overhear two nursing assistants talking about a person they are caring for. This is an example of
    A. Defamation   C. Boundary crossing
    B. Libel   D. Invasion of privacy

37. If you begin to give care to a person without asking permission, you may be guilty of
    A. Battery   C. Invasion of privacy
    B. Assault   D. Defamation

38. A person *cannot* give consent for treatment or care if
    A. He or she is over legal age (usually over 18 years of age)
    B. He or she clearly understands what will be done
    C. The person is sedated
    D. The person is mentally competent

39. If a person you are caring for asks you to witness the signing of a will, you
    A. Must know the agency policy on whether you may do this
    B. Should always refuse as it is not legal to do this
    C. Cannot ethically or legally witness a will
    D. Cannot refuse as it is part of your responsibility

40. If you are convicted of abuse, neglect, or mistreatment, this information will be
    A. In your nursing assistant registry information
    B. In the nurse's notes
    C. Only in the court records
    D. Destroyed as soon as the abused person leaves the agency

41. You notice a home care patient has no food in the house and the water has been turned off. This could be a sign of
    A. Self-neglect   C. Involuntary seclusion
    B. Physical abuse   D. Emotional abuse

42. If you suspect an elderly person is being abused, you should
    A. Ask the person to tell you who is abusing him or her
    B. Discuss the abuse with the caregiver
    C. Call the police
    D. Discuss the matter and your observations with the nurse

43. Child abuse and neglect may occur when
    A. Caregivers have little education
    B. Children have birth defects or chronic illness
    C. The abuser has a history of being abused
    D. All of the above

44. A child who shows great affection to others may be a victim of
    A. Physical abuse
    B. Neglect
    C. Sexual abuse
    D. Emotional abuse

45. If you suspect a child is being abused
    A. Ask the child whether he is being abused
    B. Share your concerns with the nurse
    C. Call the local child welfare agency
    D. Talk to the parents

Matching
Match the statements to the correct topic.

46. _____ Keep the person's information confidential.
47. _____ You borrow money from a patient's family.
48. _____ Do *not* date a current patient or resident or family members of a current patient or resident.
49. _____ You believe you are the only person who understands the person and his needs.
50. _____ You hug a person because he or she is crying.
51. _____ You tell a person about your personal relationships or problems.
52. _____ You select what you report and record. You do not give complete information.
53. _____ You trade assignments with other nursing assistants so you can provide the person's care.

A. Rules for maintaining professional boundaries
B. Boundary signs
C. Boundary crossing
D. Boundary violation

Fill in the Blank

54. HIPAA is the abbreviation for _____
    _____ .

55. When you judge a person based on your values and standards, you are not using _____
    _____ behavior.

56. It violates rules _____
    _____ if you accept a gift from a patient, resident, or his or her family.

57. If you cause harm to a person because you did not act in reasonable and careful manner, you may be found
    _____ .

58. When giving care, you must follow standards of care. Standards of care are found in
    A. _____
    B. _____
    C. _____
    D. _____
    E. _____
    F. _____
    G. _____

59. If you injure a person's name and reputation by making false statements to a third person, you can be accused of _____. Explain the difference between two forms of this offense.
    A. Libel _____
    _____
    B. Slander _____
    _____

60. When you get a person's consent to give him or her a shower, you protect yourself from being accused of _____ and
    _____

61. As a nursing assistant, you are never responsible for obtaining written _____ .

62. What problems would cause a person to be considered a vulnerable adult?
    A. _____
    B. _____
    C. _____

63. If an elderly person is deprived of a basic need, such as food or clothing, this would be _____
    abuse and _____ .

64. Name the type of child abuse described in the examples.
    A. The child is injured mentally. _____
    B. The child was left in circumstances where the child suffers serious harm. _____
    C. The child has been kicked, burned, or bitten.
    _____
    D. The child has engaged in sexual activity with a family member. _____
    E. Drug activity has taken place when the child is present. _____

65. What kinds of abuse are considered domestic abuse or domestic violence?
    A. _____
    B. _____
    C. _____
    D. _____
    E. _____

66. When a domestic partner controls friendships and other relationships of the other person, this is
    _____ abuse.

Use Focus on PRIDE in the Textbook to complete questions 67–70.

67. If you make an error, it must be reported because you are _____ for your actions.

68. If you suspect a person is being abused, tell
    _____ .

69. To maintain professional boundaries, you can
    A. Follow the _____
    _____
    B. Obey the _____
    _____
    C. Monitor for _____
    D. Ask the _____
    _____

70. Accepting a task beyond the legal limits of your role can lead to _____.

Optional Learning Exercises
Write the rule in the Code of Conduct for Nursing Assistants that applies to the situations in questions 71–75.

71. A nursing assistant has back pain and takes her mother's medication to treat it.
    _____

72. A nursing assistant is caring for a person her sister knows. The sister asks for information about the person. _____

73. A nursing assistant changes her lunchtime because her assigned patient needs unexpected care.
    _____

74. The nursing assistant tells the nurse that he recorded information on the wrong patient.
    _____

75. The nursing assistant knows that she is not allowed to carry out sterile procedures by herself.
    _____

76. If a nursing assistant causes unintentional harm to a person, it is called _____. If a nurse or other professional person causes unintentional harm, it is called _____.

77. If you are giving care in a home and you notice the person is not taking needed drugs, you think this is a sign of _____. What should you do about this situation? _____

78. When you are working in a long-term care center, you notice another nursing assistant forcing food into a 90-year-old person's mouth. When you ask about her actions, she laughs and says, "That's the only way I can get done with my assignments, so I can go to lunch." This is an example of _____. What should you do? _____
_____

Independent Learning Activities
Make a list of your values and standards that might influence how you react to decisions made by another person.
- How would you deal with these differences when caring for a person?
- How would you react if these differences occurred between you and another employee?
- What would you do if you are assigned to give care and find that you must carry out tasks that oppose your values and standards?
  ○ What would be the ethical way to deal with this?

Role-play a situation in which you are asked to perform one of the tasks you identified in the previous exercise. Have one student play the person asking you to perform the task. Have a second student observe and answer these questions:
- What was your reaction when asked?
- In what ways did you communicate your discomfort?
- What suggestions did you offer to make sure the task was done?

Identify agencies in your community that help victims of abuse (elder, child, domestic). Visit one of the agencies and ask these questions:
- How do you find out about the victim? How can a victim contact you?
- What services do you offer? What happens to the victim after you identify the problem? What plan is available to protect the victim from future abuse?

5 Work Ethics

Fill in the Blank: Key Terms

Confidentiality   Harassment   Priority   Stress   Teamwork
Courtesy   Mentor   Professionalism   Stressor   Work Ethics
Gossip   Preceptor

1. Another word that means "preceptor" is
   mentor.

2. A staff member who guides is a
   preceptor.

3. Following laws, being ethical, having good work ethics, and having the skills to do your work is
   professionalism.

4. A _stressor_ is the event or factor that causes stress.

5. The most important thing at the time is the
   priority.

6. Trusting others with personal and private information is _confidentiality_.

7. _Work ethics_ is behavior in the workplace.

8. _Gossip_ is to spread rumors or talk about the private matters of others.

9. The response or change in the body caused by any emotional, physical, social, or economic factor is
   stress.

10. _Courtesy_ is a polite, considerate, or helpful comment or act.

11. _Harassment_ means to trouble, torment, offend, or worry a person by one's behavior or comments.

12. When staff members work together as a group it is called _teamwork_.

Circle the Best Answer

13. Work ethics involve
    A. How well you do your skills
    B. What religion you practice
    C. How you treat others and work with others
    D. Cultural beliefs and attitudes

14. Your diet will maintain your weight if
    A. You avoid salty and sweet foods
    B. You take in fewer calories than your energy needs require
    C. It includes foods with fats and oils
    D. You balance the number of calories taken in with your energy needs

15. Adults need about _____ hours of sleep daily.
    A. 7   C. 4
    B. 10   D. 12

16. Exercise is needed for
    A. Rest and sleep
    B. Muscle tone and circulation
    C. Good body mechanics
    D. Good nutrition

17. Smoking odors
    A. Disappear quickly when the person finishes smoking
    B. Can be covered up by chewing gum
    C. Are only noticed by the smoker
    D. Stay on the person's breath, hands, clothing, and hair

18. The most important reason a person should *not* work under the influence of alcohol or drugs is that it
    A. Affects the person's safety
    B. Causes the person to be disorganized
    C. Makes co-workers angry
    D. Is not allowed by your nursing center

19. Which of these is *not* part of good personal hygiene for work?
    A. Bathe daily and use a deodorant
    B. Practice good hand washing
    C. Cut toenails straight across
    D. Keep fingernails long and polished

20. Tattoos should be covered when working because they
    A. May offend persons you care for, their families, and co-workers
    B. Can become infected
    C. May confuse persons
    D. Increase the risk of skin injuries

21. When working the nursing assistant may wear
    A. Jewelry in pierced eyebrow, nose, lips or tongue
    B. Wedding and engagement rings
    C. Multiple earrings in each ear
    D. Nail polish

22. When working the nursing assistant should *not* wear
    A. A beard or mustache that is clean and trimmed
    B. Hair that is off the collar and away from the face
    C. Perfume, cologne, or aftershave
    D. A wristwatch with a second hand

23. Displaying good work ethics at your clinical experience site may help you find a job because
    A. You will pass the course
    B. It will show you care
    C. You will get better grades
    D. The staff always looks at students as future employees

24. You should be well-groomed when looking for a job because it
    A. Shows you are cooperative
    B. Makes a good first impression
    C. Shows you are respectful
    D. Shows you have values and attitudes that fit with the center

25. How does an employer know you can perform required job skills?
    A. They will request proof of training and will check your record in the state nursing assistant registry.
    B. They will have you give a demonstration of your skills.
    C. You will be asked many questions about performing certain skills.
    D. You will be required to take a written test.

26. Which of these is *not* an OBRA requirement to work in long-term care?
    A. You must complete a state-approved training and competency evaluation program.
    B. You must have 3 references from former employers.
    C. The employer checks your record in the state nursing assistant registry.
    D. The nursing center cannot hire persons who were convicted of abusing, neglecting, or mistreating a person.

27. You can get a job application from
    A. The personnel office or the human resources office
    B. A friend who works at the center
    C. From the director of nursing
    D. The receptionist in the lobby of the center

28. You should take a dry run to a job interview to
    A. Show you follow directions well
    B. Show you listen well
    C. Know how long it takes to get from your home to the personnel office
    D. Look over the center to see if you want to work there

29. When you are interviewing it is correct to
    A. Have a glass of wine before going
    B. Look directly at the interviewer
    C. Wear a sweat suit and athletic shoes
    D. Shake hands very gently

30. What is a good way to share your list of skills with the interviewer?
    A. Tell the person verbally what you can do
    B. Ask for a list of skills and check the ones you know
    C. Bring a list of your skills and give it to the interviewer
    D. Tell the interviewer you will send a list as soon as possible

31. It is important for you to ask questions at the end of the interview because it
    A. Will show the interviewer you are interested in the job
    B. Will help you to decide if the job is right for you
    C. Shows you have good communication skills
    D. Shows you are dependable

32. After an interview, it is advised that you
    A. Send a thank you note within 24 hours of the interview
    B. Call the interviewer every day to see if you are being hired
    C. Wait for the employer to contact you
    D. Call 1 week after the interview to thank the person for the interview

33. When a preceptor is assigned to a nursing assistant, the preceptor may be
    A. A registered nurse
    B. A nursing assistant
    C. An LPN/LVN
    D. Any of the above

34. When you have a job, it is most important to plan good childcare and transportation in advance because it will
    A. Prevent absences and tardiness
    B. Show you are a responsible person
    C. Prevent stress
    D. Show you are a good parent

35. What is a common reason for losing a job?
    A. Not knowing how to perform a task
    B. Absences and tardiness
    C. Being disorganized
    D. Lacking self-confidence

36. When you are scheduled to begin work at 3 PM, you should
    A. Plan to arrive by 2:30 PM
    B. Arrive at exactly 3 PM
    C. Plan to arrive at few minutes early and be ready to work at 3 PM
    D. Arrive within a few minutes before or after 3 PM

37. Which of these statements would signal you have a good attitude?
    A. "I will do that right away."
    B. "It's not my turn. I did that yesterday."
    C. "That's not my patient."
    D. "It's not my fault."

38. You can avoid being part of gossip by
    A. Remaining quiet when you are in a group where gossip is occurring
    B. Only talking about persons and family members to co-workers
    C. Only repeating comments in writing
    D. Removing yourself from a group or situation where gossip is occurring

39. The person's information can be shared
    A. With the person's family
    B. Only among health care team members involved in his or her care
    C. With your family
    D. With friends who know the person

40. When you are working, you should *not* wear
    A. A wristwatch with a second hand
    B. Tight or revealing clothing
    C. A shirt with the top button open.
    D. White socks.
41. Slang or swearing should *not* be used at work because
    A. Words used with family and friends may offend persons and family members
    B. The person may not understand you
    C. The person may have difficulty hearing
    D. Co-workers may overhear it
42. You should say "please" and "thank you" to others because
    A. Courtesies mean so much to people; it can brighten someone's day
    B. It shows respect to the person
    C. It is required by your job
    D. It shows you like the person
43. It is acceptable at work if you
    A. Take a pen to use at home
    B. Sell cookies for your child's school project
    C. Use a pay phone or wireless phone on your break to call your child
    D. Make a copy of a letter on the copier in the nurse's station
44. When you leave and return to the unit for breaks or lunch you should
    A. Tell each person
    B. Tell any family members present
    C. Tell the nurse
    D. All of the above
45. Safety practices are important to follow because
    A. They help you to be more organized
    B. Negligent behavior affects the safety of others
    C. They save the center money
    D. You will get promoted more quickly

46. Which of these would *not* be a good safety practice?
    A. Know the contents and policies in personnel and procedure manuals
    B. Question unclear instructions and things you do understand
    C. Do not tell anyone when you make a mistake
    D. Ask for any training that you might need
47. Care should be planned around
    A. Your break and lunch time
    B. The person's mealtimes, visiting hours, activities, and therapies
    C. Co-workers' schedules
    D. The time scheduled by the nurse
48. Stress occurs
    A. Only when you have unpleasant situations in your life
    B. Because you do not handle your problems well
    C. Because you are in the wrong job
    D. Every minute of every day and in everything you do
49. What physical effects of stress can be life-threatening?
    A. High blood pressure, heart attack, strokes, ulcers
    B. Increased heart rate, faster and deeper breathing
    C. Anxiety, fear, anger, depression
    D. Headaches, insomnia, muscle tension
50. Which of these actions is harassment?
    A. Offending others with gestures or remarks
    B. Offending others with jokes or pictures
    C. Making a sexual advance or requesting sexual favors
    D. All of the above
51. If you resign from a job, it is good practice to give
    A. One week's notice   C. Four weeks notice
    B. Two weeks notice   D. No notice

Matching

Match the qualities and characteristics of good work ethics with the examples.

52. __E__ While working with Mr. Smith, you try to understand and feel what it must be like to be paralyzed on one side.
53. __M__ You realize you are very good at giving basic care. You know you need to improve your communication skills.
54. __A__ When caring for elderly residents you try to do small things to make them happy or to find ways to ease their pain.
55. __H__ You thank co-workers when they help you and remember to wish residents happy birthday as appropriate.
56. __C__ When Mrs. Gibson is upset and angry, you remember to respect her feelings and to be kind.
57. __J__ You report the blood pressure and temperature readings accurately to the nurse.
58. __L__ You realize giving care to residents is important and you are excited about your work.
59. __B__ Your supervisor tells you she knows she can count on you because you are always on time and perform delegated tasks as assigned.
60. __G__ Even though Mr. Acevado has different cultural and religious views than yours, you value his feelings and beliefs.
61. __D__ Before you left home today you had an argument with your child. When you get to work you make every effort to put that aside and be pleasant and happy.

A. Caring
B. Dependable
C. Considerate
D. Cheerful
E. Empathetic
F. Trustworthy
G. Respectful
H. Courteous
I. Conscientious
J. Honest
K. Cooperative
L. Enthusiastic
M. Self-aware

62. __F__ The nurse discusses a resident's problem with you and states she knows you will keep the information confidential.

63. __I__ When you are assigned to give care to a resident, you make sure his care is done thoroughly and exactly as instructed.

64. __k__ Your co-worker says she needs help to turn her resident and you cheerfully offer to help.

Fill in the Blank

65. Write out the meaning of the abbreviations.

    A. NATCEP _____

    B. OBRA _____

66. Work ethics involves

    A. _____

    B. _____

    C. _____

    D. _____

    E. _____

67. Personal health is important when you are on the job and caring for other persons. Name a part of your health that is described in these examples.

    A. _____ Hand washing and good personal hygiene are needed to remove odors on your breath, hands, clothing, and hair.

    B. _____ If you have fatigue, a lack of energy, and irritability it may mean you need more of this.

    C. _____ You will feel better physically and mentally if you walk, run, swim, or bike regularly.

    D. _____ Some of these affect thinking, feeling, behavior, and function. This may affect the person's safety.

    E. _____ Avoid foods from the fats, oils, and sweets groups. Also avoid salty foods and crash diets.

    F. _____ You may not be able to read instructions and take measurements accurately, if you do not have these checked.

    G. _____ Practice this when you bend, carry heavy objects, and lift, move, and turn persons.

    H. _____ This substance depresses the brain and affects thinking, balance, coordination, and mental alertness.

68. List 8 places you can find out about jobs.

    A. _____

    B. _____

    C. _____

    D. _____

    E. _____

    F. _____

    G. _____

    H. _____

69. When an employer requests proof of required training, give the person these items.

    A. _____

    B. _____

    C. _____

70. If a job application asks you to print in black ink, why is it a poor idea to use blue ink? _____ _____

71. Your writing on a job application should be readable so the agency can _____ _____.

72. When a section on a job application does not apply to you, you should _____.

73. When you provide information about employment gaps, it gives the employer a good impression about your _____.

74. When filling out an application, you should be prepared to provide

    A. _____

    B. _____

    C. _____

    D. _____

75. If you lie on a job application it is _____. If you do this, what can happen? _____

76. When you fill out a job application, it is easier to complete if you have a file that contains

    A. _____

    B. _____

    C. _____

    D. _____

    E. _____

    F. _____

    G. _____

    H. _____

    I. _____

        a. _____

        b. _____

        c. _____

        d. _____

    J. _____

77. You should ask questions at the end of an interview because the agency wants to hire someone who

   _____

   _____ .

78. If you're assigned to a preceptor, this person should

   A. _____

   B. _____

   C. _____

   D. _____

   E. _____

79. What should you do if you will be late or cannot

   work? _____ and follow

   the _____ .

80. How can you promote teamwork and manage your time when someone is late or does *not* show up for work?

   A. _____

   B. _____

   C. _____

81. You hear a co-worker say, "It's not my turn. I did it yesterday." This is an example of having

   a _____ .

82. If you make or repeat any comment that you do *not* know to be true, or a comment that can hurt a person, or family member, you are

   _____ .

83. You are caring for a friend of your mother and your mother asks for information about her friend's illness and care. If you repeat this information to your mother, you will violate the person's

   _____ and

84. You should *not* wear perfume, cologne, or after-shave lotion when working because the scents

   _____

   _____ .

85. If your friends or family need to visit with you when you are working, they must meet you

   _____ .

86. Setting priorities involves deciding

   A. _____

   B. _____

   C. _____

   D. _____

   E. _____

   F. _____

   G. _____

   H. _____

87. What physical symptoms may occur when a person has stress?

   A. _____

   B. _____

   C. _____

   D. _____

   E. _____

Use Focus on PRIDE in the Textbook to complete questions 88–90.

88. Patients, residents, families, visitors, and co-workers depend on you to give safe and effective care. They trust that you will

   A. _____

   B. _____

   C. _____

   D. _____

   E. _____

   F. _____

89. When you smile and greet patients and residents and politely introduce yourself, you are displaying good

   social _____ .

90. When you offer to help others, ask the nurse if you can help others, and return from breaks on time you are displaying actions that help build a strong

   _____

Optional Learning Exercises

Applying for a Job in Home Care

91. When the RN is *not* at the bedside to help you if problems occur, you are expected to be able to

   _____

92. When you arrive at homes on time, you are using

   _____

   What temptations should be avoided when you are giving home care?

   _____

   _____

93. When you shop for a person, you should accurately report to the person or family the _____

   _____ .

   When you do these things you are displaying your

   _____

94. You should read the manufacturer's instructions before using any appliance. This shows

   _____ for the person's property.

95. What questions should you ask if you are interviewing for a job in home care?

   A. _____

   B. _____

   C. _____

   D. _____

   E. _____

     _____

   F. _____

   _____

96. When you are in the home, what should you do if a conflict or problem occurs?

   A. Make every effort _____.

   B. Explain the problem to _____.

   C. Do *not* _____.

   This would be very _____ behavior. It is also _____ and a _____.

Independent Learning Activities

How well do you take care of your own health? What can you do to improve your health practices?

- Do you maintain a healthy weight by eating calories adequate for your energy needs? What can you do to improve your diet?
- How much sleep do you get each night?
- How do you practice good body mechanics at all times—not just at work?
- How many hours do you exercise each week? What type of exercise do you do?
- When did you last have your eyes checked? Do you wear glasses if they were prescribed?
- Do you smoke? How much? Have you considered any smoking cessation programs?
- Are you taking any drugs that affect your thinking, feeling, behavior, and function? Did a doctor prescribe them or are you self-medicating? Have you talked with your doctor about the effect of any drugs you are taking?
- Do you drink alcohol? How much? Have you been told it affects your behavior? Have you considered finding a program to help you to quit drinking alcohol?

Have you ever applied for a job? How did you feel when you were being interviewed?

- After reading this chapter, how would you handle a future interview?

Role-play a job interview with a classmate. Take turns playing the interviewer and the job applicant.

- Use the lists in this chapter to ask questions.
- Practice answers that you can use in a real interview.

Think of three people you could use as references when applying for a job. Ask their permission to use them as references.

- If they agree, make a list of the people and their titles, addresses, and telephone numbers to use when you apply for a job.

6 Communicating With the Health Team

Fill in the Blank: Key Terms

Abbreviation	Conflict	Lateral	Progress note	Suffix
Anterior	Distal	Medial	Proximal	Ventral
Chart	Dorsal	Medical record	Recording	Word element
Clinical record	End-of-shift report	Posterior	Reporting	
Communication	Kardex	Prefix	Root	

1. Another term for medical record is _clinical records_.

2. At or toward the front of the body or body part is ventral or _anterior_.

3. A _suffix_ is a word element placed after a root; it changes the meaning of the word.

4. At the side of the body or body part is _lateral_.

5. A clash between opposing interests or ideas is _conflict_.

6. An _abbreviation_ is a shortened form of a word or phrase.

7. A part of a word is a _word element_.

8. A _kardex_ is a type of card file that summarizes information found in the medical record.

9. The medical record is also called the _chart_.

10. The part nearest to the center or the point of origin is _proximal_.

11. _Communication_ is the exchange of information — a message sent is received and interpreted by the intended person.

12. Another term for anterior is _ventral_.

13. A written account of a person's condition and response to treatment and care is the chart or _medical records_.

14. _Dorsal_ is at or toward the back of the body or body part; posterior.

15. The oral account of care and observations is _reporting_.

16. _Distal_ is the part farthest from the center or from the point of attachment.

17. A word element placed before a root is the _prefix_. It changes the meaning of the word.

18. A word element containing the basic meaning of the word is the _root_.

19. Another word for dorsal is _posterior_.

20. _Recording_ is the written account of care and observations.

21. _Medial_ is at or near the middle or midline of the body or body part.

22. _Progress note_ describes the care given and the person's response and progress.

23. An _End-of-shift report_ is a report that the nurse gives at the end of the shift to the on-coming shift.

Circle the Best Answer

24. When health team members communicate, they share all of this information *except*
    A. Gossip about the person and his family
    B. What was done for the person
    C. What needs to be done for the person
    D. The person's response to treatment

25. A nursing assistant tells the nurse that Mr. Jones ate a small amount of his lunch. The nurse
    A. Knows this means Mr. Jones ate one half of his meal
    B. Thinks Mr. Jones ate two or three bites of food
    C. Thinks Mr. Jones ate only 25% of his meal
    D. Asks for further information because words may have different meanings to different people

26. When giving information to another health team member
    A. Be brief and concise to reduce omitting important details
    B. Use terms that may or may not be familiar to others
    C. Give many details and information that is unrelated to the information
    D. Use general terms, instead of facts

27. The medical record or chart is
    A. A temporary record of the person
    B. Discarded when the person leaves the agency
    C. A permanent legal document
    D. Given to the person when he or she is discharged

28. Which of these is *not* included in the person's chart?
    A. The daily menu   C. Special consents
    B. X-ray reports   D. Health history

29. A nursing assistant
    A. May read the charts in all health care agencies
    B. Are never allowed to read the person's charts
    C. Must know the agency policy before reading the chart
    D. Is allowed to tell the person what is recorded in the chart

30. If a person asks to see his or her record, the nursing assistant
    A. Reports the request to the nurse
    B. Checks the agency policy to see if this is allowed
    C. Gives the chart to the person's legal representative
    D. Gives the chart to the person
31. The admission record contains
    A. Doctors orders
    B. The name, birth date, age, and gender of the person
    C. Test results
    D. Special diet information
32. The health history is completed
    A. When the person is discharged
    B. When the person is admitted
    C. By the doctor
    D. By the nursing assistant
33. The nurse records the person's reason for seeking health care in the
    A. Health history
    B. Graphic sheet
    C. Progress notes
    D. Kardex
34. Vital signs taken every shift are recorded in the
    A. Health history
    B. Graphic sheet
    C. Flow sheet
    D. Progress notes
35. In long-term care, OBRA requires a written summary of the person
    A. Each shift
    B. Each day
    C. Every month
    D. Every 3 months
36. A weekly care record that has boxes for each day of the week is used in
    A. Home care
    B. Hospitals
    C. Long-term care
    D. Special care units
37. The Kardex is
    A. Used to record visits by health team members
    B. A sheet used to record vital signs taken every 15 minutes
    C. A record of the person's family history
    D. A quick, easy source of information about the person
38. The nursing assistant reports information about the person
    A. At the end of the shift
    B. When there is a change in the person's condition
    C. Each time care is given
    D. Only in writing
39. During the end-of-shift report, signal lights, care, and routine tasks are done
    A. After the report is finished
    B. By the staff going off duty
    C. By the staff coming on duty
    D. By the person assigned by the charge nurse to carry out the task
40. The general rules for recording include all of these *except*
    A. Include the date and time for every recording
    B. Use ditto marks if needed
    C. Sign all entries with your name and title as required by the agency
    D. Record only what you observed and did yourself

41. If you are recording using the 24-hour clock, which of these is correct?
    A. 8 AM
    B. 1 PM
    C. 1300
    D. 5:30 PM

Choose the correct spelling of medical terms in questions 42–46.

42. Slow heart rate
    A. Bradecardia
    B. Bradycardia
    C. Bradacordia
    D. Bradicardia
43. Difficulty in urinating
    A. Dysuria
    B. Dysurya
    C. Dysuira
    D. Disuria
44. Blue color or condition
    A. Cyonosis
    B. Cyinosis
    C. Cyanosis
    D. Cianosys
45. Rapid breathing
    A. Tachepnea
    B. Tachypinea
    C. Tachypnea
    D. Tachypnia
46. An opening into the trachea is a
    A. Tracheastomy
    B. Trachiostomy
    C. Tracheostome
    D. Tracheostomy
47. If a person points to the left side of his body below the umbilicus and tells you he has pain, you will tell the nurse he has pain in the
    A. Right upper quadrant
    B. Left lower quadrant
    C. Left upper quadrant
    D. Right lower quadrant
48. When describing the position of body parts, the hands and fingers are
    A. Medial
    B. Distal
    C. Proximal
    D. Posterior
49. When you are given a computer password you
    A. Must never change it
    B. Can share it with a co-worker
    C. Should never tell anyone your password
    D. Can use another person's password when entering the computer
50. The agency computers should *not* be used to
    A. Send messages and reports to the nursing unit
    B. Store resident records and care plans
    C. Send e-mails that require immediate reporting
    D. Monitor blood pressures, temperatures, and heart rates
51. Privacy is protected when you
    A. Log off after making an entry
    B. Prevent others from seeing what is on the screen
    C. Destroy or shred computer-printed worksheets
    D. All of the above
52. When you answer the telephone, do *not* put the caller on hold if
    A. The person has an emergency
    B. The caller is a doctor
    C. The call needs to be transferred to another unit
    D. You are too busy to find the nurse
53. When you answer a phone when giving home care, you should
    A. Give your name, title, and location
    B. Simply answer with "Hello"
    C. Explain that you are there to give care to the person who lives in the home
    D. Not speak to the caller. Hand the receiver to the person in the home

54. If you have a conflict with a co-worker you should
    A. Ask the nurse in charge to schedule you at different times
    B. Ignore the person
    C. Work out the problem to avoid unkind words or actions
    D. Talk to other co-workers to explain your side of the story
55. When a conflict occurs, what is the first step you should take?
    A. Talk with co-workers to see if they have a conflict with the person also
    B. Confront the person and demand that the person meet with you
    C. Define the problem
    D. Assume the conflict will resolve itself if you ignore it

Matching

Match the word with the correct definition.

A. Arthroscope	I. Gastrostomy
B. Bronchoscope	J. Gastritis
C. Cholecystectomy	K. Glossitis
D. Colostomy	L. Nephritis
E. Cyanotic	M. Neuralgia
F. Dermatology	N. Oophorectomy
G. Dysuria	O. Proctoscopy
H. Enteritis	

56. ___G___ Difficulty urinating
57. ___L___ Inflammation of kidneys
58. ___E___ Pertaining to blue coloration
59. ___A___ Joint examination with a scope
60. ___F___ Study of the skin
61. ___D___ Incision into large intestine
62. ___B___ Instrument used to examine bronchi
63. ___K___ Inflammation of the tongue
64. ___M___ Nerve pain
65. ___O___ Examination of rectum with instrument
66. ___C___ Excision of gallbladder
67. ___N___ Excision of ovary
68. ___I___ Incision into stomach
69. ___J___ Inflammation of stomach
70. ___H___ Inflammation of intestine

Fill in the Blank

71. Write out the meaning of the abbreviations.
    A. ADL _____
    B. EPHI; ePHI _____
    C. OBRA _____
    D. PHI _____

72. Next to each time, write the 24-hour clock time.
    A. _____ 11:00 AM
    B. _____ 8:00 AM
    C. _____ 4:00 PM
    D. _____ 7:30 AM
    E. _____ 6:45 PM
    F. _____ 12 NOON
    G. _____ 3:00 AM
    H. _____ 4:50 AM
    I. _____ 5:30 PM
    J. _____ 10:45 PM
    K. _____ 11:55 PM
    L. _____ 9:15 PM

Write the definition of each prefix for questions 73–81.

73. auto- _____
75. brady- _____
75. dys- _____
76. ecto- _____
77. leuk- _____
78. macro- _____
79. neo- _____
80. supra- _____
81. uni- _____

Write the definition of each root word for questions 82–90.

82. adeno _____
83. angio _____
84. broncho _____
85. cranio _____
86. duodeno _____
87. entero _____
88. gyneco _____
89. masto _____
90. pyo _____

Write the definition of each suffix for questions 91–99.

91. -asis _____
92. -genic _____
93. -oma _____
94. -phasia _____
95. -ptosis _____
96. -plegia _____
97. -megaly _____
98. -scopy _____
99. -stasis _____

Write the correct abbreviations for questions 100–107.

100. Before meals _____

101. After meals _____

102. With _____

103. Cancer _____

104. Intake and output _____

105. Lower left quadrant _____

106. Temperature, pulse, respiration _____

107. Range-of-motion _____

Use Focus on PRIDE in the Textbook to complete questions 108–111.

108. If your agency allows nursing assistants to chart, you have a professional responsibility to

 A. _____

 B. _____

 C. _____

 D. _____

109. When conflict among workers occurs, those involved should focus on the _____ and the _____.

110. When the delegating nurse asks what was done and what was not done, you can show you are accountable by

 A. _____

 B. _____

 C. _____

 D. _____

111. If charting is *not* truthful, _____ can be taken against the person who records false information.

Labeling

For questions 112–121 convert the times from military to standard time or from standard to military time. Use figure as a guide.

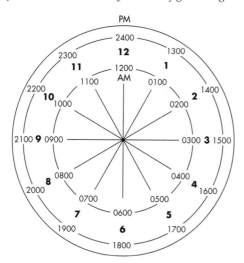

112. 2:00 AM = *0200*

113. 10:30 AM = *1030*

114. 5:00 AM = *0500*

115. 9:30 AM = *0930*

116. 5:45 PM = *1745*

117. 10:45 PM = *2245*

118. 0600 hrs = *6:00 AM* _____ AM/PM

119. 1145 hrs = *11:45 AM* _____ AM/PM

120. 1800 hrs = *6:00 PM* _____ AM/PM

121. 2200 hrs = *10:00 PM* _____ AM/PM

122. Name the 4 abdominal regions. Use RUQ, LUQ, RLQ, LLQ to name.

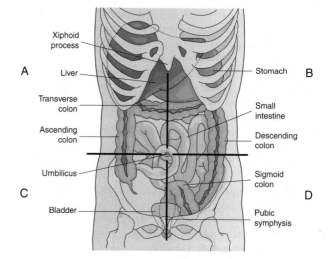

 A. *RUQ*

 B. *LUQ*

 C. *RLQ*

 D. *LLQ*

Optional Learning Exercises

Class Experiment

It is often difficult to describe fluids in a clear and precise manner. Set up the following examples that imitate situations where you need to describe intake, output, or drainage. Describe as accurately as possible what you see in terms of amounts, colors, and textures. Compare your notes with classmates to see if you are using words that all have the same meaning. What words were used that were clear to understand? What words were used that had more than one meaning?

1. Bloody drainage: Mix a teaspoon of ketchup and a teaspoon of water. Pour onto the center of a paper napkin.

2. Urine: Pour a tablespoon of tea into the center of a paper towel.

3. Bleeding: Smear a teaspoon of red jelly in the center of a paper towel.

4. Broth: Pour 4 ounces of tea into a bowl.

Class Experiment	
Substance	Observations
Bloody drainage	
Urine	
Bleeding	
Broth	

Case Study

Mr. Larsen was admitted to a subacute care center after his abdominal surgery 1 week ago. This morning the nursing assistant gave Mr. Larsen a shower and assisted him to sit in a comfortable chair. The nursing assistant noticed that he sat there very still and held his arms across his abdomen. He asked for a pillow and held it tightly against his abdomen.

Imagine you are the patient and answer these questions.

- What would you like the nursing assistant to ask you?
- How would you communicate your feelings to the nursing assistant?
- How could you let the nursing assistant know that you had pain without telling her?

Imagine you are the nursing assistant and answer these questions.

- As the nursing assistant, what observations would be important to make about Mr. Larsen?
- What questions could you ask Mr. Larsen?
- What nonverbal communication would give you information about Mr. Larsen?

Case Study

Mrs. Miller was admitted to the health care center since you worked 3 days ago. You have just started your shift and have been assigned to Mrs. Miller.

- What information would you need to know before giving care? Why?
- What information would be important to provide to the oncoming shift?
- What methods would you use to communicate this information?

Independent Learning Activities

Answer these questions about situations in which you may need to communicate with others.

- When have you had a problem with communicating? Why was it difficult? How did you handle this?
- Think about a time when you felt you communicated well. What made the communication successful? How could you use a similar technique in caring for others?
- How would you communicate with a person who speaks a language that you do not speak or understand? What methods could you use to explain what you are going to do?
- How would you communicate with a person from a different culture?

Make flash cards of the prefixes, suffixes, and root words in the Textbook chapter.

- Put the meaning of each one on the back of the appropriate card. Work alone or with a partner, and by looking at the cards, practice identifying the correct meaning of each term.

The next time you or a member of your family visit the doctor and are instructed to fill a prescription, look at what the doctor has written.

- Do you see any abbreviations that you learned in this chapter? What do they mean?
- How did this chapter help you to understand what was written?

7 Assisting With the Nursing Process

Fill in the Blank: Key Terms

Assessment
Evaluation
Goal

Implementation
Medical diagnosis
Nursing care plan

Nursing diagnosis
Nursing intervention
Nursing process

Objective data
Observation
Planning

Signs
Subjective data
Symptoms

1. _Subjective data_ are things a person tells you about that you cannot observe through your senses; symptoms.

2. _Implementation_ is to perform or carry out measures in the care plan; a step in the nursing process.

3. The method RNs use to plan and deliver nursing care is the _nursing process_.

4. Another name for subjective data is _symptoms_.

5. A written guide about the person's care is the _nursing care plan_.

6. _Assessment_ is collecting information about the person; a step in the nursing process.

7. Another name for objective data is _signs_.

8. The _nursing diagnosis_ describes a health problem that can be treated by nursing measure; a step in the nursing process.

9. Information that is seen, heard, felt, or smelled is _objective data_ or signs.

10. A step in the nursing process that is used to measure if goals in the planning step were met is called _evaluation_.

11. _Planning_ is setting priorities and goals; a step in the nursing process.

12. A _nursing intervention_ is an action or measure taken by the nursing team to help the person reach a goal.

13. A _goal_ is that which is desired in or by the person as a result of nursing care.

14. Using the senses of sight, hearing, touch, and smell to collect information is _observations_.

15. The identification of a disease or condition by a doctor is a _medical diagnosis_.

Circle the Best Answer

16. Which of these is *not* a step in the nursing process?
    A. Assessment
    B. Objective data
    C. Planning
    D. Evaluation

17. The nursing process focuses on
    A. The doctor's orders
    B. The person's nursing needs
    C. Tasks and procedures that are needed
    D. Reducing the cost of health care

18. The nursing process
    A. Stays the same from admission to discharge
    B. Is used in all health care settings
    C. Cannot be used in home care
    D. Can only be used for adults

19. When you observe by using your senses, you assist the nurse to
    A. Assess the person
    B. Plan for care
    C. Implement care for the person
    D. Evaluate the person

20. Which of these is an example of objective data you can collect?
    A. Mrs. Hewitt complains of pain and nausea
    B. Mr. Stewart tells you he has a dull ache in his stomach
    C. You are taking Mrs. Jensen's blood pressure and you notice her skin is hot and moist
    D. Mrs. Murano tells you she is tired because she could not sleep last night

21. When you take Mr. Young's blood pressure, you notice it is 50 points higher than when you took it in the morning. You
    A. Chart the results on the graphic sheet
    B. Tell the nurse when you report off at the end of your shift
    C. Tell the nurse at once
    D. Call the doctor

22. A minimum data set (MDS) is used
    A. In long-term care centers
    B. In all health care settings
    C. In acute care settings
    D. In home care

23. The MDS is updated
    A. Only once a year
    B. Every month
    C. Before each care conference
    D. Once every 2 months

24. A nursing diagnosis
    A. Identifies a disease or condition
    B. Helps to identify drugs or therapies used by the doctor
    C. Describes a health problem that can be treated by nursing measures
    D. Identifies only physical problems
25. When a nurse uses the nursing process, the person is given
    A. Only one nursing diagnosis
    B. No more than 5 nursing diagnoses
    C. As many nursing diagnoses as are needed
    D. Nursing diagnoses that involve only physical needs
26. Planning involves all of these *except*
    A. Setting priorities and goals
    B. Choosing nursing actions to help the person meet goals
    C. Writing the nursing care plan
    D. Measuring whether all goals are met
27. A problem-focused conference is held
    A. Once a month for each person
    B. To meet agency guidelines
    C. When one problem affects the person's care
    D. To implement the care plan
28. OBRA requires a comprehensive care plan. It is a
    A. Conference held to update care plan
    B. Written guide about the person's care
    C. Conference held when one problem affect a person's care
    D. Conference held regularly to review and update care plans
29. What part of the nursing process is being carried out when you give personal care to a person?
    A. Assessing   C. Implementation
    B. Planning   D. Evaluation
30. Nurses will measure if goals in the planning steps are met during
    A. Assessing   C. Implementation
    B. Planning   D. Evaluation

Fill in the Blank

31. Write out the meaning of the abbreviations.
    A. ADL _____
    B. CAA _____
    C. IDCP _____
    D. MDS _____
    E. NANDA-I _____
    F. OASIS _____
    G. RN _____
32. When you make observations while you give care, what senses are used?
    A. _____
    B. _____
    C. _____
    D. _____

33. Name the body system or other area you are observing in each of these examples (*from Box 7-2, Basic Observations*)
    A. Is the abdomen firm or soft?
    _____
    B. Is the person sensitive to bright lights?
    _____
    C. Are sores or reddened areas present?
    _____
    D. What is the frequency of the person's cough?
    _____
    E. Can the person bathe without help?
    _____
    F. Can the person swallow food and fluids?
    _____
    G. What is the position of comfort?
    _____
    H. Does the person answer questions correctly?
    _____
    I. Does the person complain of stiff or painful joints?
    _____
34. An assessment and screening tool completed when the person is admitted to long-term care is called
    _____.
    A. The form is updated before each
    _____.
    B. A new form is completed _____ and whenever _____.
35. When planning care, needs that are required for life and survival must be met before _____.
36. Name the two resident care conferences used in long-term care.
    A. The _____ is held regularly to develop, review, and update care plans.
    B. _____ are held when one problem affects a person's care.
37. The assignment sheet tells you about
    A. _____
    B. _____
    C. _____
38. You have a key role in the nursing process. How do you assist the nurse?
    A. The nurse uses your observation for
    _____ and _____.
    B. You may help develop the _____.
    C. In the _____ step, you perform nursing actions and measures.
    D. Your observations are used for the _____ step.

Use Focus on PRIDE in the Textbook to complete questions 39–41.

39. When you learn skills and practice until you are comfortable performing the skills, it shows you take _____ in learning to do your job well.

40. To encourage independence and to help the person feel involved in his or her care, you can

    A. _____

    B. _____

    C. _____
    _____

41. When you keep your assignment sheets with you at all times and place them in the waste basket for shredding at the end of your shift, it shows that you take pride in protecting the _____
    _____.

Optional Learning Exercises

List at least three nursing interventions for each of these Nursing Diagnoses and Goals

42. Nursing Diagnosis: Feeding Self-Care Deficit related to weakness in right arm

    Goal: Patient will eat 75% of each meal by 2/1

    Interventions:

    A. _____

    B. _____

    C. _____

43. Nursing Diagnosis: Hygiene Self-Care Deficit related to forgetfulness

    Goal: Patient will be assisted to maintain good hygiene throughout hospital stay

    Nursing interventions:

    A. _____

    B. _____

    C. _____

Independent Learning Activities

Ask permission to look at the nursing care plans used at the agency where you have your clinical experience. Answer these questions about the nursing care plans.

- How do the nurses develop the plans? What resources do they use?
- How often are the plans reviewed and revised?
- How are the plans used by the nursing assistants?
- How do nursing assistants help to develop and revise the interventions?
- How do the nurses communicate the information on the nursing care plan?

8 Understanding the Person

Fill in the Blank: Key Terms

Bariatrics
Body language
Comatose
Culture
Disability

Esteem
Geriatrics
Holism
Morbid
  obesity

Need
Nonverbal
  communication
Obesity
Obstetrics

Optimal level of
  functioning
Paraphrasing
Pediatrics
Psychiatry

Religion
Self-actualization
Self-esteem
Verbal communication

1. When a person's weight is 20% or more above what is considered normal for that person's height and age, he or she has _Obesity_.

2. _Culture_ is the characteristics of a group of people—language, values, beliefs, habits, likes, dislikes, customs—passed from one generation to the next.

3. Communication that uses written or spoken word is _Verbal Communication_.

4. _Paraphrasing_ is restating the person's message in your own words.

5. The branch of medicine concerned with the problems and diseases of old age and older persons is _Geriatrics_.

6. Messages sent through facial expressions, gestures, posture, hand and body movements, gait, eye contact, and appearance is _body language_.

7. The field of medicine focused on the treatment and control of obesity is _bariatrics_.

8. The worth, value, or opinion one has of a person is _Esteem_.

9. _Nonverbal Communication_ is communications that does not use words.

10. The branch of medicine concerned with mental health problems is _pyschiatry_.

11. Thinking well of oneself and seeing oneself as useful and having value is _self-esteem_.

12. _Holism_ is a concept that considers the whole person—physical, social, psychological, and spiritual parts are woven together and cannot be separated.

13. A lost, absent, or impaired physical or mental function is a _disability_.

14. The branch of medicine concerned with the care of women during pregnancy, labor, and childbirth, and the 6 to 8 weeks after birth is _Obstetrics_.

15. _Self-actualization_ is experiencing one's potential.

16. _Pediatrics_ is the branch of medicine concerned with the growth, development, and care of children who range in age from newborn to teenagers.

17. A _need_ is something necessary or desired for maintaining life and well being.

18. _Religion_ is spiritual beliefs, needs, and practices.

19. Being unable to respond to verbal stimuli is called a _Comatose_.

20. _Optimal level of functioning_ is a person's highest potential for mental and physical performance.

21. The person has _Morbid obesity_ when he or she weighs 100 pounds or more over his or her normal weight.

Circle the Best Answer

22. Who is the most important person in the health care agency?
    A. The patient or resident
    B. The doctor
    C. The director of nursing
    D. The administrator

23. When you are caring for a person, you should
    A. Consider only the physical problems the person has
    B. Treat the physical, social, psychological, and spiritual parts separately
    C. Ignore the person's experiences, life style, culture, joys, sorrows, and needs
    D. Consider the whole person—physical, social, psychological, and spiritual parts

24. You can show you see the person as a whole person by which of these statements?
    A. "I need to give a bath to the gallbladder in 205."
    B. "The old guy in 220 needs something for pain."
    C. "Mrs. Jones is complaining of a lot of pain in her leg this morning."
    D. "Room 235 needs something for pain."

25. The lowest level basic needs are
    A. Physiological or physical needs
    B. Safety and security needs
    C. Love and belonging needs
    D. Self-esteem needs

26. Oxygen, food, water, elimination, rest, and shelter needs
    A. Relate to feeling safe from harm, danger, and fear
    B. Are needed to survive
    C. Relate to love, closeness, and affection
    D. Relate to the worth, value, or opinion one has of a person

27. It is important to tell a person why a procedure is needed because it
    A. Helps the person feel more safe and secure
    B. Makes the person feel loved
    C. Is required by law
    D. Increases the person's self-esteem

28. You may need to repeat information many times to a person admitted to a long-term care nursing center, because the person
    A. May be scared and confused
    B. Is not in a secure home setting
    C. Is in a strange place with strange routines
    D. All of the above

29. Meeting love and belonging needs is important because
    A. It helps a person to think well of oneself
    B. Some people become weaker or die from the lack of love and belonging
    C. The person will feel more safe and secure
    D. It helps the person experience his or her potential

30. A need that is rarely, if ever, totally met is
    A. Safety and security   C. Self-actualization
    B. Love and belonging   D. Self-esteem

31. When you are caring for a person from a different culture or religion than your own you must
    A. Judge the person's behavior according to your own practices
    B. Assume that the person's behavior will not be influenced by culture or religion
    C. Give needed care and do not worry about culture or religious beliefs
    D. Respect and accept the person's culture and religion

32. A culture that believes hot and cold imbalances cause disease is from
    A. Mexico   C. America
    B. England   D. Russia

33. If a person wants to visit with a spiritual leader while you are giving care you should
    A. Tell the spiritual leader that you must complete care first
    B. Provide privacy during the visit
    C. Stay with the person during the visit
    D. Tell the person this is not allowed while in the nursing facility

34. When a person does not follow all beliefs and practices of his or her religion, you
    A. Assume the person is not religious
    B. Know each person is unique
    C. Can call a spiritual leader to help the person follow the beliefs
    D. Should not be concerned about the person's religion when giving care

35. You are caring for Mrs. Kim, who is foreign speaking, and she nods "yes" to all of your questions. This may mean that
    A. Mrs. Kim is a very cooperative patient
    B. She does not understand what you are saying and is pretending to understand
    C. In her culture, that is the polite thing to do
    D. She is concealing negative emotions

36. When people are ill, they
    A. Feel angry, upset, and useless
    B. May fear death, disability, chronic illness, and loss of function
    C. Fear being laughed at for being afraid
    D. All of the above

37. A person who is having the appendix removed is
    A. An adult with medical problems
    B. A person having surgery
    C. A person with mental health problems
    D. A person needing subacute care or rehabilitation

38. Which of these persons would need the care of a branch of medicine called pediatrics?
    A. A woman who had a new baby today
    B. An older person with problems and diseases of old age
    C. A 7-year-old child with pneumonia
    D. A person receiving kidney dialysis

39. A person who weighs 600 pounds would need
    A. Subacute care
    B. Bariatric care
    C. Care in a special care unit
    D. Geriatric care

40. Which of these persons would *not* receive care in a long-term care center?
    A. A man who is recovering from minor surgery
    B. An alert person with a chronic illness who requires help with personal care
    C. A 25-year-old who is unable to care for himself due to injuries
    D. A person with a terminal illness

41. Which of these would *not* help effective communication?
    A. Use words that have the same meaning to both you and the person
    B. Communicate in a logical and orderly manner
    C. Give specific and factual information
    D. Use medical terminology when talking to the person

42. When using verbal communication, a rule to follow is
    A. Ask one question at a time
    B. Speak in a loud voice so the person can hear you
    C. Ask several questions at a time and then wait for answers
    D. Use slang words to make the person comfortable

43. Mrs. Stevens cannot speak. How does she use verbal communication?
    A. She may use touch.
    B. Her body language sends messages.
    C. She can use gestures to communicate.
    D. She may write messages on a paper pad.

44. When you use touch to communicate, it is important to
    A. Be aware of the person's culture and practices about touch
    B. Make sure the person likes to be touched
    C. Follow the person's care plan
    D. All of the above

45. Which of these would be a sign that Mrs. Green is not happy or is not feeling well?
    A. Her hair is well groomed.
    B. She has a slumped posture.
    C. She smiles when you come in the room.
    D. She has applied her makeup.

46. All of these would show you listen effectively *except* when you
    A. Face the resident and have good eye contact
    B. Lean back and cross your arms
    C. Respond to the resident by asking questions
    D. Use words the person can understand

47. Which of these is paraphrasing?
    A. "You don't know how long you will be here."
    B. "Do you want to take a tub bath or a shower?"
    C. "Tell me about living on a farm."
    D. "Can you explain what you mean?"

48. When you say, "Mr. Davis, have you taken a shower this morning?" you are
    A. Paraphrasing his thoughts
    B. Asking a direct question
    C. Focusing his thoughts
    D. Asking an open-ended question

49. Responses to open-ended questions generally are
    A. Longer and give more information than direct questions
    B. Yes or no answers
    C. Able to make sure you understand the message
    D. Focused on dealing with a certain topic

50. When you do not understand the message, you may
    A. Ask the person an open-ended question
    B. Make a statement to clarify what he is saying
    C. Use nonverbal communication
    D. Use silence to show you do not understand

51. Mr. Parker often rambles and tells long stories where his thoughts wander. You need to know if he had a bowel movement today, so you will
    A. Make a clarifying statement
    B. Ask an open-ended question
    C. Ask a focusing question
    D. Paraphrase his thoughts

52. What is best if the person takes long pauses between statements?
    A. Just being there shows you care.
    B. Try to cheer the person up by talking.
    C. Leave the room.
    D. Find another resident to talk with him.

53. A barrier to communication would be
    A. Asking a clarifying question
    B. Giving your opinion
    C. Remaining silent when the person is silent
    D. Paraphrasing the person's message

54. When you care for a person who is comatose, you
    A. Explain what you are going to do
    B. Remain silent so you do not disturb the person
    C. Enter the room quietly so you do not startle the person
    D. Do all of the above

55. Mrs. Duke has visitors and you need to give care. What would you do?
    A. Give the care while visitors are present
    B. Politely ask the visitors to leave the room until you are finished
    C. Ask the visitors to give the care
    D. Tell the visitors that they must leave the nursing center

56. When a person is admitted to a nursing center for respite care it means
    A. The person needs complex care
    B. The caregivers need a break from giving care
    C. The family no longer wants the person to live with them
    D. The person is dying and needs terminal care

57. When you are caring for a person who becomes angry, you should
    A. Avoid answering signal lights
    B. Tell the person what you are going to do and when
    C. Explain to the person why he or she should not be angry
    D. Tell the person to stop being angry

58. If a person hits, pinches, or bites you when you are giving care, you should
    A. Protect the person, others, and yourself from harm
    B. Stop giving care to the person
    C. Firmly tell the person to stop acting like that
    D. Refuse to care for the person when he or she is assigned to you

Fill in the Blank

59. What are the parts of the person you consider when you use the concept of holism?

    A. _____

    B. _____

    C. _____

    D. _____

60. List the basic needs in order, starting with the lowest level.
    A. _____
    B. _____
    C. _____
    D. _____
    E. _____

61. Name the culture or country that may follow the listed belief or custom.
    A. _____ Food and medicine is given to restore the hot-cold balance.
    B. _____ Folk healers called *yerbero* uses herbs and spices to prevent or cure disease.
    C. In Vietnam or _____ men shake hands with other men, but do *not* shake hands with women,
    D. _____ Eyes are rolled upward to express disapproval.
    E. _____ Facial expressions may mean the opposite of what the person is feeling. Negative emotions may be concealed with a smile.
    F. In _____ and Asian cultures, eye contact is impolite and an invasion of privacy.
    G. In some _____ cultures, silence is a sign of respect, particularly to an older person.
    H. In _____, all family members are involved in the person's care.

62. When you use verbal communication, words are _____ or _____.

63. Written words are used when a person cannot _____ or _____.

64. If a person can hear but cannot speak or read, ask questions that have _____.

65. Nonverbal communication messages more accurately reflect a person's _____ than words do.

66. Body language is nonverbal communication that is shown with
    A. _____
    B. _____
    C. _____
    D. _____
    E. _____
    F. _____
    G. _____

67. When you listen, you follow these guidelines.
    A. _____
    B. _____
    C. _____
    D. _____
    E. _____

68. When you fail to listen, you can miss complaints of _____.

Use Focus on PRIDE in the Textbook to complete questions 69–70.

69. To promote a sense of identity, worth, and belonging when communicating you should
    A. _____
    B. _____
    C. _____
    D. _____
    E. _____
    F. _____
    G. _____

70. When you care for person's with different ideas, values, and lifestyles, it is not ethical to
    A. _____
    B. _____
    C. _____

Crossword

Fill in the following crossword by answering the clues with the words from this list:

Clarifying	Direct	Holism	Paraphrasing	Silence
Comatose	Esteem	Need	Touch	Verbal
Culture	Focusing	Nonverbal		

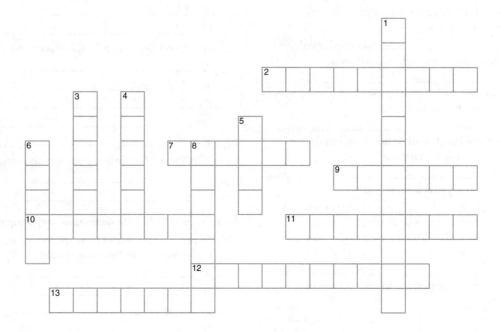

Across

2. Communication expressed with gestures, facial expressions, posture, body movements, touch, and smell
7. The worth, value, or opinion one has of a person
9. Communication in which the words are spoken or written
10. An unconscious person who cannot respond to others
11. A communication method that is useful when a person rambles or wanders in thought
12. A communication method in which you can ask the person to repeat the message, say you do not understand, or restate the message
13. The characteristics of a group of people—language, values, beliefs, habits, likes, dislikes, customs—passed from one generation to another

Down

1. Restating the person's message in your own words
3. A concept that considers the whole person—physical, social, psychological, and spiritual parts
4. A question that focuses on certain information and may require a "yes" or "no" answer or more information
5. Something necessary or desired for maintaining life and mental well-being
6. Nonverbal communication that conveys comfort, caring, loving, affection, interest, concern, and reassurance
8. Communicating by not saying anything

Optional Learning Exercises

Basic Needs

Physical Needs

71. What are the six physical needs required for survival?

    A. _____

    B. _____

    C. _____

    D. _____

    E. _____

    F. _____

72. The physical needs must be met before the
    _____ needs.

Safety and Security

73. Safety and security needs relate to protection from

    A. _____

    B. _____

    C. _____

74. When a person is in a health care agency, you can help meet safety and security needs when you explain what for every task

    A. _____

    B. _____

    C. _____

    D. _____

Love and Belonging

75. The need for love and belonging relates to

    A. _____

    B. _____

    C. _____

Self-Esteem

76. Self-esteem means to

    A. Think _____

    B. See _____

    C. See oneself as having _____

77. Why is it important to encourage residents to do as much as possible for themselves?

    _____

Self-Actualization

78. What does self-actualization involve?

    A. _____

    B. _____

    C. _____

79. Self-actualization is the highest

    _____

Culture and Religion Practices

Religion

80. How can you help a resident to observe religious practices if services are held in the nursing center?

    _____

81. If the resident wants a spiritual leader or advisor to visit in the room you should tell the nurse and

    A. _____

    B. _____

    C. _____

Cultural Health Care Beliefs

82. People from Mexico or Vietnam believe when hot and cold imbalances occur, it causes

    _____.

Cultural Sick Practices

83. How do Vietnamese folk practices treat these illnesses?

    A. Common cold _____

    B. Headache and sore throat _____

84. What illnesses do these Russian folk practices treat?

    A. Placing an ointment behind the ears and temples, and also the back of the neck

    _____

    B. Placing a dough made of dark rye flour and honey on the spinal column _____

Cultural Touch Practices

85. What is the meaning of touch to some people from Mexico? _____

    _____

86. If you are caring for a resident from India, what might you notice about his practice of shaking hands?

    _____

87. Residents from some countries might not like to be touched. Name two of these countries.

    _____

Eye Contact Practices

88. Why would you avoid making direct eye contact with a resident from Mexico?

    _____

89. If a resident from Vietnam blinks when you explain a procedure, it probably means that the message

    _____.

90. Eye contact in the American culture signals

    _____

Family Roles in Sick Care

91. You are caring for a resident from China. You might expect the family members to _____,
    _____, and _____ the person.

92. A man from Pakistan is a resident and his daughter says she must go home at night. This may be because in Pakistan, members of the opposite sex are not

    _____.

Using Communication Methods

You have completed your duties for the morning and have some free time. Mr. Harry Donal is a resident in nursing center. He rarely has visitors and you try to spend time with him when you can. Answer questions 93–101 about communication techniques you use when you visit with Mr. Donal.

93. You sit in a chair next to Mr. Donal so you can see each other. This position will help you to have better

    _____

94. You should lean _____ Mr. Donal to show interest.

95. Mr. Donal says, "I know this is the best place for me, but I miss my flower garden at home." You respond, "You miss your home." This is an example of

    _____

96. You ask Mr. Donal, "You told me you did not sleep well last night. Can you tell me why?" He replies, "There was a lot of noise in the hall." This is an example of a

    _____

97. You say to Mr. Donal, "Tell me about your flower garden at home." This is an _____ question.

98. When you say, "Can you explain what that means," you are asking a person to _____ .

99. Mr. Donal says he "hurts all over" and then begins to talk about the weather. You say, "Tell me more about where you hurt. You said you hurt all over." This statement helps in _____ the topic.

100. Mr. Donal begins to cry when he talks about his flower garden. How can you show caring and respect for his situation and feelings?

    _____

101. When Mr. Donal begins to cry, you quickly begin to talk about the activities planned this morning. Changing the subject is a

    _____

Independent Learning Activities

Use the Basic Needs content in the Textbook chapter to answer these questions about how well you are meeting your own needs. The answers may be shared in a discussion group or answered privately to help you to understand yourself better.

- Do you smoke? What need may be affected by smoking?
- What kinds of foods and fluids do you eat? Is your diet meeting your basic needs for food and water?
- How much rest and sleep do you get each day? How much do you need to feel well rested?
- How safe do you feel at home? At school? In your community? How do your feelings affect your ability to hold a job or attend school?
- Who are the people who make you feel loved? Who helps you when you have problems?
- What are you doing that helps you meet the need for self-actualization?

Answer these questions about your personal health care practices.

- What health care practices are followed in your family? How are these practices related to your cultural or religious beliefs?
- How often do you go to the doctor? For regular checkups? Only when ill?
- When do you go to the dentist? Once or twice a year for cleaning and checkups? Only when you have a toothache?
- When a family member is in a health care center, how does your family respond? Does someone stay with the person and do all of the care? Or do family members visit for brief periods and let health care workers provide all care? Is the family response related to any cultural or religious practices?

Look at your answers to the two previous sets of questions and answer the following questions.

- How well are you meeting your basic needs? How could you improve in meeting needs? What changes would be the most beneficial?
- How much influence on your practices comes from cultural or religious traditions in your family? Are these influences helping you or hindering you to meet needs?

9 Body Structure and Function

Fill in the Blank: Key Terms

Artery	Digestion	Immunity	Organ	System
Capillary	Hemoglobin	Menstruation	Peristalsis	Tissue
Cell	Hormone	Metabolism	Respiration	Vein

1. The substance in red blood cells that carries oxygen and gives blood its color is _____.

2. _____ is protection against a disease or condition.

3. The process of supplying the cells with oxygen and removing carbon dioxide from them is

    _____.

4. The process of physically and chemically breaking down food so that it can be absorbed for use by the

    cells is _____.

5. _____ is the burning of food for heat and energy by the cells.

6. A blood vessel that carries blood away from the heart

    is an _____.

7. _____ is the involuntary muscle contractions in the digestive system that move food through the alimentary canal.

8. Organs that work together to perform special

    functions form a _____.

9. The basic unit of body structure is a

    _____.

10. Groups of tissues with the same function form an

    _____.

11. A _____ is a tiny blood vessel.

12. A group of cells with similar function is

    _____.

13. _____ is the process in which the lining of the uterus breaks up and is discharged from the body through the vagina.

14. A chemical substance secreted by the glands into the

    bloodstream is a _____.

15. A _____ is a blood vessel that carries blood back to the heart.

Circle the Best Answer

16. A cell is
    A. Only found in muscles
    B. The basic unit of body structure
    C. Can live without oxygen
    D. A group of tissues

17. The control center of a cell is the
    A. Membrane   C. Cytoplasm
    B. Protoplasm   D. Nucleus

18. Genes control
    A. Cell division
    B. Tissues
    C. Physical and chemical traits inherited by children
    D. Organs

19. Connective tissue
    A. Covers internal and external body surface
    B. Receives and carries impulses to the brain and back to body parts
    C. Anchors, connects, and supports other body tissues
    D. Allows the body to move by stretching and contracting

20. Living cells of the epidermis contain
    A. Blood vessels and many nerves
    B. Sweat and oil glands
    C. Pigment that gives skin color
    D. Hair roots

21. Sweat glands help
    A. The body regulate temperature
    B. To keep the hair and skin soft and shiny
    C. Protect the nose from dust, insects, and other foreign objects
    D. The skin sense pleasant and unpleasant sensations

22. Long bones
    A. Allow skill and ease in movement
    B. Bear the weight of the body
    C. Protect organs
    D. Allow various degrees of movement and flexion

23. Blood cells are manufactured in
    A. The heart   C. Blood vessels
    B. The liver   D. Bone marrow

24. Joints move smoothly because of
    A. Cartilage   C. Muscle
    B. Synovial fluid   D. Ligaments

25. A joint that moves in all directions is a
    A. Ball-and-socket   C. Pivot
    B. Hinge   D. All of the above

26. Voluntary muscles are
    A. Found in the stomach and intestines
    B. Attached to bones
    C. Cardiac muscle
    D. Tendons

27. Muscles produce heat by
    A. Contracting
    B. Relaxing
    C. Maintaining posture
    D. Working automatically
28. The central nervous system consists of
    A. A myelin sheath
    B. Nerves throughout the body
    C. The brain and spinal column
    D. Cranial nerves
29. The medulla controls
    A. Muscle contraction and relaxation
    B. Heart rate, breathing, blood vessel size, and swallowing
    C. Reasoning, memory, and consciousness
    D. Hearing and vision
30. Cerebrospinal fluid
    A. Cushions shocks that could injure structure of the brain and spinal cord
    B. Controls voluntary muscles
    C. Lubricates movement
    D. Controls involuntary muscles
31. Cranial nerves conduct impulses between the
    A. Brain and the head, neck, chest, and abdomen
    B. Brain and the skin and extremities
    C. Brain and internal body structure
    D. Spinal cord and lower extremities
32. When you are frightened the _____ nervous system is stimulated.
    A. Sympathetic
    B. Parasympathetic
    C. Central
    D. Cranial
33. Receptors for vision and nerve fibers of the optic nerve are found in the
    A. Sclera
    B. Choroids
    C. Retina
    D. Cornea
34. What structure of the ear is involved in balance?
    A. Malleus
    B. Auditory canal
    C. Tympanic membranes
    D. Semicircular canals
35. Hemoglobin in red blood cells gives blood its red color and carries _____ to the cells.
    A. Oxygen
    B. Food
    C. Waste products
    D. Water
36. Red blood cells live for
    A. About 9 days
    B. 3 or 4 months
    C. 4 days
    D. A year
37. White blood cells or leukocytes
    A. Protect the body against infection
    B. Are necessary for blood clotting
    C. Carries food, hormone, chemicals, and waste products
    D. Pick up carbon dioxide
38. The left atrium of the heart
    A. Receives blood from the lungs
    B. Receives blood from the body tissues
    C. Pumps blood to the lungs
    D. Pumps blood to all parts of the body
39. Arteries
    A. Return blood to the heart
    B. Pass food, oxygen, and other substances into the cells
    C. Pick up waste products including carbon dioxide from the cells
    D. Carry blood away from the heart

40. In the lungs, oxygen and carbon dioxide are exchanged
    A. In the epiglottis
    B. Between the right bronchus and the left bronchus
    C. By the bronchioles
    D. Between the alveoli and capillaries
41. The lungs are protected by
    A. The diaphragm
    B. The pleura
    C. A bony framework of the ribs, sternum, and vertebrae
    D. The lobes
42. Food is moved through the alimentary canal (GI tract) by
    A. Chyme
    B. Peristalsis
    C. Swallowing
    D. Bile
43. Water is absorbed from chyme in the
    A. Small intestine
    B. Stomach
    C. Esophagus
    D. Large intestine
44. Digested food is absorbed through tiny projections called
    A. Jejunum
    B. Ileum
    C. Villi
    D. Colon
45. A function of the urinary system is to
    A. Remove waste products from the blood
    B. Rid the body of solid waste
    C. Rid the body of carbon dioxide
    D. Burn food for energy
46. A person feels the need to urinate when the bladder contains about
    A. 1000 mL of urine
    B. 500 mL of urine
    C. 250 mL of urine
    D. 125 mL of urine
47. Testosterone is needed for
    A. Male secondary sex characteristics
    B. Female secondary sex characteristics
    C. Sperm to be produced
    D. Ova to be produced
48. The prostate gland lies
    A. In the scrotum
    B. In the testes
    C. Just below the bladder
    D. In the penis
49. The ovaries secrete progesterone and
    A. Estrogen
    B. Testosterone
    C. Ova
    D. Semen
50. When an ovum is released from an ovary it travels first through the
    A. Uterus
    B. Fallopian tubes
    C. Endometrium
    D. Vagina
51. Menstruation occurs when
    A. The hymen is ruptured
    B. The ovary releases an ovum
    C. The endometrium breaks up
    D. Fertilization occurs
52. A fertilized cell implants in the
    A. Ovary
    B. Fallopian tubes
    C. Endometrium
    D. Vagina
53. The master gland is the
    A. Thyroid gland
    B. Parathyroid gland
    C. Adrenal gland
    D. Pituitary gland

54. Thyroid hormone regulates
    A. Growth
    B. Metabolism
    C. Proper functioning of nerves and muscles
    D. Energy produced during energy
55. If too little insulin is produced by the pancreas, the person has
    A. Tetany
    B. Slow growth
    C. Diabetes mellitus
    D. Slowed metabolism
56. When antigens enter the body, they are attacked and destroyed by
    A. Antibodies
    B. Lymphocytes
    C. B cells
    D. T cells

Fill in the Blank

57. Write out these abbreviations.
    A. CNS _____
    B. GI _____
    C. mL _____
    D. RBC _____
    E. WBC _____

Use Focus on PRIDE in the Textbook to complete questions 58–59.

58. To care for others, you need a strong and healthy body. You can stay healthy by
    A. Seeing your doctor at least
    _____
    B. Keeping your _____ up to date
    C. Protecting your bones and muscles from injury by
    _____
    D. Practicing good hand
    _____

59. You can help a person maintain their optimal level of function when you
    A. _____
    B. _____
    C. _____
    D. _____
    E. _____

Matching

Match the terms with the description.
Musculoskeletal

A. Periosteum   D. Synovial fluid   G. Cardiac muscle
B. Joint   E. Striated muscle   H. Tendons
C. Cartilage   F. Smooth muscle

60. ___C___ Connective tissue at end of long bones
61. ___E___ Skeletal muscle
62. ___A___ Membrane that covers bone
63. ___H___ Connects muscle to bone
64. ___B___ Point at which two or more bones meet
65. ___G___ Heart muscle
66. ___F___ Involuntary muscle
67. ___D___ Acts as a lubricant so the joint can move smoothly

Nervous System

A. Sclera   F. Inner ear   I. Autonomic
B. Cornea   G. Brainstem   nervous system
C. Retina   H. Cerebral   J. Peripheral
D. Cerumen   cortex   nervous
E. Middle ear   system

68. ___E___ Contains eustachian tubes and ossicles
69. ___J___ Has 12 pairs of cranial nerves and 31 pairs of spinal nerves
70. ___A___ White of the eye
71. ___H___ Outside of cerebrum; controls highest function of brain
72. ___C___ Inner layer of eye; receptors for vision are contained here
73. ___I___ Controls involuntary muscles, heartbeat, blood pressure, and other functions
74. ___B___ Light enters eye through this structure
75. ___G___ Contain midbrain, pons, and medulla
76. ___D___ Waxy substance secreted in auditory canal
77. ___F___ Contains semicircular canal and cochlea

Circulatory System

A. Plasma   E. Thrombocytes   I. Arteries
B. Erythrocytes F. Pericardium   J. Veins
C. Hemoglobin   G. Myocardium   K. Capillaries
D. Leukocytes   H. Endocardium

78. ___A___ Liquid part of blood
79. ___F___ Thin sac covering the heart
80. ___K___ Very tiny blood vessels
81. ___C___ Substance in blood that picks up oxygen
82. ___J___ Carry blood away from heart
83. ___D___ White blood cells
84. ___J___ Carry blood toward heart
85. ___A___ Red blood cells
86. ___G___ Thick muscular portion of heart
87. ___E___ Platelets; necessary for clotting
88. ___H___ Membrane lining inner surface of heart

Respiratory System

A. Epiglottis   D. Trachea   F. Diaphragm
B. Larynx   E. Alveoli   G. Pleura
C. Bronchiole

89. ___D___ Air passes from larynx into this structure
90. ___G___ A two-layered sac that covers the lungs
91. ___A___ Piece of cartilage that acts like a lid over the larynx
92. ___F___ Separates lungs from the abdominal cavity
93. ___B___ The voice box
94. ___C___ Several small branches that divide from the bronchus
95. ___E___ Tiny one-celled air sacs

Digestive System

A. Liver	D. Duodenum	G. Pancreas
B. Chyme	E. Jejunum	H. Gallbladder
C. Colon	F. Saliva	

96. ___G___ Structure that adds more digestive juices to chyme
97. ___B___ Semiliquid food mixture formed in stomach
98. ___E___ Portion of GI tract that absorbs food
99. ___H___ Stores bile
100. ___C___ Portion of GI tract that absorbs water
101. ___A___ Produces bile
102. ___F___ Moistens food particles in the mouth
103. ___D___ Produces digestive juices

Urinary System

A. Bladder	D. Meatus	G. Ureter
B. Glomerulus	E. Nephrons	H. Urethra
C. Kidney	F. Tubules	

104. ___E___ Basic working unit of the kidney
105. ___C___ Bean-shaped structure that produces urine
106. ___B___ A cluster of capillaries in Bowman capsule
107. ___H___ Structure that allows urine to pass from the bladder
108. ___G___ A tube attached to the renal pelvis of the kidney
109. ___A___ Hollow muscular sac that stores urine
110. ___D___ Opening at the end of the urethra
111. ___F___ Fluid and waste products form urine in this structure

Reproductive System

A. Scrotum	D. Gonads	G. Labia
B. Testes	E. Fallopian	H. Vulva
C. Seminal	tubes	
vesicle	F. Endometrium	

112. ___D___ Male or female sex organs
113. ___G___ Two folds of tissue on each side of the vagina
114. ___A___ Sac between thighs that contains testes
115. ___H___ External genitalia of female
116. ___B___ Testicles; sperm produced here
117. ___E___ Attached to the uterus; ovum travels through this structure
118. ___C___ Stores sperm and produces semen
119. ___F___ Tissue lining the uterus

Endocrine System

A. Epinephrine	C. Insulin	E. Testosterone
B. Estrogen	D. Parathormone	F. Thyroxine

120. ___C___ Released by pancreas; regulates sugar in blood
121. ___E___ Sex hormone secreted by testes
122. ___B___ Sex hormone secreted by ovaries
123. ___F___ Regulates metabolism
124. ___D___ Regulates calcium levels in the body
125. ___A___ Stimulates to produce energy during emergencies

Immune System

A. Antibodies	C. Phagocytes	E. B cells
B. Antigens	D. Lymphocytes	F. T cells

126. ___A___ Normal body substances that recognize abnormal or unwanted substances
127. ___F___ Type of cell that destroys invading cells
128. ___C___ Type of white blood cell that digests and destroys microorganisms
129. ___E___ Type of cell that causes production of antibodies
130. ___B___ An abnormal or unwanted substance
131. ___D___ Types of white blood cells that produce antibodies

Labeling

132. Name the parts of the cell in the figure.

A. _____

B. _____

C. _____

133. Name each type of joint in the figures.

A. _____

B. _____

C. _____

134. Name the parts of the brain in the figure.

A. _____

B. _____

C. _____

A ————

C

B ————

135. Name the four chambers of the heart in the figure.

A. _____

B. _____

C. _____

D. _____

C

D

A

B

136. Name the structures of the respiratory system in the figure.

A. _____

B. _____

C. _____

D. _____

E. _____

F. _____

G. _____

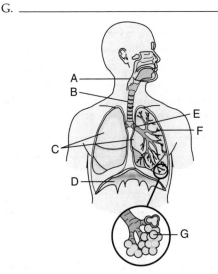

137. Name the structures of the digestive system in the figure.

A. _____

B. _____

C. _____

D. _____

E. _____

F. _____

G. _____

H. _____

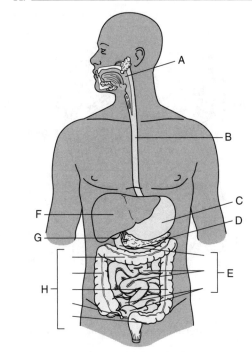

138. Name the structures of the urinary system in the figure.

A. _____

B. _____

C. _____

D. _____

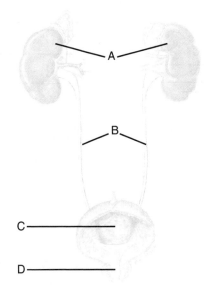

139. Name the structures of the male reproductive system in the figure.

A. _____

B. _____

C. _____

D. _____

E. _____

F. _____

G. _____

H. _____

140. Name the external female genitalia in the figure.

A. _____

B. _____

C. _____

D. _____

E. _____

F. _____

Optional Learning Exercises

141. Explain the function of each part of the cell.

A. Cell membrane _____

B. Nucleus _____

C. Cytoplasm _____

D. Protoplasm _____

E. Chromosomes _____

F. Genes _____

142. List what structures are contained in the two skin layers.

A. Epidermis _____

B. Dermis _____

143. Explain the function of the types of bone.

A. Long bones _____

B. Short bones _____

C. Flat bones _____

D. Irregular bones _____

144. Describe how each type of joint moves and give an example of each type.

A. Ball-and-socket _____

Example: _____

B. Hinge _____

Example: _____

C. Pivot _____

Example: _____

145. Explain what happens when muscles contract.

_____

_____

_____

146. Explain the function of the three main parts of the brain. Include the function of the cerebral cortex and the midbrain, pons, and medulla.

A. Cerebrum _____

1. Cerebral cortex _____

_____

B. Cerebellum _____

_____

C. Brainstem _____

1. Midbrain and pons _____

2. Medulla _____

_____

147. Explain how the sympathetic and parasympathetic nervous systems balance each other.

_____

_____

_____

_____

_____

148. Explain what happens to each of these structures when light enters the eye.
    A. Choroid _____
    B. Cornea _____
    C. Lens _____
    D. Retina _____

149. Explain how each of these structure help to carry sound in the ear.
    A. Ossicles _____
    _____
    B. Cochlea _____
    _____
    C. Acoustic nerve _____

150. Where are red blood cells destroyed as they wear out? _____

151. When an infection occurs, what do white blood cells do? _____
    _____

152. Explain the function of the four atria of the heart.
    A. Right atrium _____
    B. Left atrium _____
    C. Right ventricle _____
    D. Left ventricle _____

153. Explain where each of these veins carries blood.
    A. Inferior vena cava _____
    _____
    B. Superior vena cava _____

154. Explain what happens in the alveoli. _____
    _____
    _____
    _____
    _____

155. After food is swallowed, explain what happens in each of these parts of the digestive tract.
    A. Stomach _____
    _____
    B. Duodenum _____
    C. Jejunum and ileum _____
    D. Colon _____
    E. Rectum _____
    _____
    F. Anus _____

156. Explain what happens in these structures of the kidney.
    A. Glomerulus _____
    B. Collecting tubules _____
    C. Ureters _____
    D. Urethra _____
    E. Meatus _____

157. Sperm is produced in the testicles. What happens to the sperm in each of these structures?
    A. Testes _____
    B. Vas deferens _____
    C. Seminal vesicle _____
    D. Ejaculatory duct _____
    E. Prostate gland _____
    F. Urethra _____

158. What is the function of the endometrium?
    _____
    _____

159. Menstruation occurs about every _____ days. Ovulation usually occurs on or about day _____ of the cycle.

160. What is the function of each of these pituitary hormones?
    A. Growth hormone _____
    _____
    B. Thyroid-stimulating hormone _____
    C. Adrenocorticotropic hormone _____
    D. Antidiuretic hormone _____
    _____
    E. Oxytocin _____
    _____

161. What is the function of insulin? _____
    _____
    What happens if too little insulin is produced?
    _____
    _____

162. What happens when the body senses an antigen?
    _____

Independent Learning Activities

Using your own body, move joints of each type to see how they move.

- What joint is a ball-and-socket? How many ways were you able to move it?
- What joint moves like a hinge? How does it work differently than the ball-and-socket?
- What joint is a pivot joint? Compare its movement to the other two joints.

Listen to a friend's chest with a stethoscope.

- What sounds do you hear?
- What body systems are making the sounds?
- Are you able to count any of the sounds you hear? What are you counting?

Listen to your lower abdomen with a stethoscope.

- What sounds can you hear?
- What causes sound in the abdomen? What body system is involved in this activity?
- What is occurring when you hear your "stomach growl"? What is the term for this activity that you learned in this chapter?

Look at a friend's eyes in a dimly lit area and observe the size of the pupils.

- What size are the pupils? Are they both the same?
- Shine a flashlight in the eye. What happens to the pupil?
- What happens when you move the light away? If you see a change, how quickly does it occur?

10 Growth and Development

Fill in the Blank: Key Terms

Adolescence   Ejaculation   Menarche   Primary caregiver   Reflex

Development   Growth   Menopause   Puberty   Sexual orientation

Developmental task   Infancy   Peer

1. The first menstruation and the start of menstrual cycles is _____.

2. _____ is the time between puberty and adulthood; a time of rapid growth and physical and social maturity.

3. The release of semen is _____.

4. The period when reproductive organs begin to function and secondary sex characteristics appear is _____.

5. _____ is the first year of life.

6. Changes in mental, emotional, and social function is _____.

7. An involuntary movement is a _____.

8. _____ is the physical changes that can be measured and that occur in a steady, orderly manner.

9. The person mainly responsible for providing or assisting with the child's basic needs is the _____.

10. A skill that must be completed during a stage of development is a _____.

11. _____ is the time when menstruation stops and menstrual cycles end.

12. A person of the same age group and background is a _____.

13. _____ refers to sexual arousal or romantic attraction to persons of the other gender, the same gender, or both genders.

Circle the Best Answer

14. Growth is measured all of these ways *except*
    A. The ways a person behaves and thinks
    B. In height and weight
    C. By changes in appearance
    D. By changes in body functions

15. Growth and development begin
    A. At fertilization
    B. At birth
    C. When the baby sits up
    D. When children have growth spurts

16. The process of growth and development
    A. Occurs in a random order or pattern
    B. Progresses at a steady pace in each stage
    C. Occurs from the center of the body outward
    D. From the foot to the head

17. Movements in the newborn are uncoordinated and lack purpose because
    A. The baby has not been taught to move in a pattern
    B. The central nervous system is not well developed
    C. The baby moves only with reflexes
    D. The baby has skipped a developmental task

18. The birth weight of a newborn
    A. Doubles in the first year
    B. Triples in the first year
    C. Doubles in the first 3 months
    D. Triples in the first 6 months

19. Reflexes present in newborns
    A. Are learned behaviors
    B. Remain active through the first year
    C. Are an abnormal developmental task
    D. Decline and then disappear as the central nervous system develops

20. Infants can play peek-a-boo by
    A. 2-3 months   C. 8-9 months
    B. 4-5 months   D. The first birthday

21. Toddlerhood is called the "terrible twos" because the child
    A. Needs to assert independence
    B. Is more dependent on the primary caregiver
    C. Begins to walk
    D. Is not yet toilet trained

22. A major task for toddlers is
    A. Learning to walk
    B. Learning to feed themselves
    C. Learning to share toys with others
    D. Toilet training

23. Toddlers learn to feel secure when
    A. Primary caregivers are consistently present
    B. Long periods of separation from primary caregivers are planned
    C. Needs are not met quickly
    D. They are allowed to be alone for long periods of time

24. Three-year-olds are able to
    A. Play simple games and learn simple rules
    B. Use a pencil well to print letters, numbers, and their first names
    C. Hop, skip, and throw and catch a ball
    D. Be more responsible and truthful

25. During the preschool years, children grow
    A. Much more rapidly than during infancy
    B. 2-3 inches per year and gain about 5 pounds per year
    C. Very slowly, if at all
    D. 6-7 inches per year and gain about 10 pounds per year
26. Baby teeth are lost and permanent teeth erupt at about
    A. 2 years of age
    B. The end of the first year
    C. Around age 6 years
    D. At 9 or 10 years of age
27. Reading, writing, grammar, and math skills develop during
    A. Toddlerhood   C. School age
    B. Preschool years   D. Late childhood
28. Girls have a growth spurt during
    A. School-age   C. Adolescence
    B. Late childhood   D. Young adulthood
29. During late childhood, children
    A. Do not accept adult standards and rules without question
    B. Increase math and language skills
    C. Need factual sex education
    D. All of the above
30. Girls reach puberty
    A. When menarche occurs
    B. Between the ages of 12 and 16 years
    C. When they stop growing
    D. Later than boys
31. Coordination and graceful movements develop in adolescence as
    A. Growth spurts occur
    B. Puberty is reached
    C. When all growth stops
    D. As muscle and bone growth even out
32. Adolescents need guidance and discipline because
    A. They need to remain dependent on parents
    B. Judgment and reasoning are not always sound
    C. They are just learning right from wrong
    D. All of the above
33. Teens usually do *not* understand why parents worry about sexual activities, pregnancy, and sexually transmitted diseases because
    A. They are emotionally unstable at this stage
    B. Independence from adults is important
    C. They may have trouble controlling sexual urges and considering the consequences of sexual activity
    D. They do not have a sense of right and wrong, or good and bad
34. Development ends
    A. When puberty occurs
    B. When all physical growth is complete
    C. At young adulthood
    D. At death
35. Young adulthood includes all of these tasks *except*
    A. Adjusting to physical changes
    B. Learning to live with a partner
    C. Developing a satisfactory sex life
    D. Choosing education and a career
36. A developmental task of middle adulthood is
    A. Developing leisure time activities
    B. Coping with a partner's death
    C. Preparing for one's own death
    D. Learning to live with a partner

Fill in the Blank
Use Focus on PRIDE in the Textbook to complete questions 37–40.

37. When caring for 1-year-old, you can gain the child's trust when you are checking the pulse when you
    A. Ask _____
    B. Show _____
    C. Let _____
    D. Talk _____
38. You show respect for different family situations when you
    A. Do not _____
    B. Treat them as _____
    C. Take pride in not allowing _____
39. When a child becomes an emancipated minor, it means he or she is able to make his or her _____
40. A child can become emancipated by
    A. _____
    B. _____
    C. _____
    D. In some states, _____

Matching
Match the correct reflex of a newborn with the descriptions in questions 41–45.
    A. Moro (startle) reflex   D. Grasp (palmar) reflex
    B. Rooting reflex   E. Step reflex
    C. Sucking reflex
41. ___A___ Legs extend and then flex
42. ___E___ Occurs when baby is held upright and the feet touch a surface
43. ___D___ Guides baby's mouth to the nipple
44. ___C___ Occurs when lips are touched
45. ___D___ Fingers close firmly around the object

Match the correct age group with the developmental tasks in questions 46–65.
    A. Infancy (birth-1 year)
    B. Toddler (1-3 years)
    C. Preschooler (3-6 years)
    D. School age (6-9 or 10 years)
    E. Late childhood (9 or 10 to 12 years)
    G. Young adulthood (18-40 years)
    H. Middle adulthood (40-65 years)
    I. Late adulthood (65 years and older)
46. _____ Accepting changes in body and appearance
47. _____ Developing leisure time activities
48. _____ Gaining control of bowel and bladder functions
49. _____ Becoming independent from parents and adults
50. _____ Learning to eat solid foods
51. _____ Adjust to decreased strength and loss of health
52. _____ Learning how to study
53. _____ Learning how to get along with peers

54. _____ Increasing ability to communicate and understand others
55. _____ Tolerating separation from primary caregiver
56. _____ Learning to live with a partner
57. _____ Developing moral or ethical behavior
58. _____ Learning basic reading, writing, and arithmetic skills
59. _____ Developing stable sleep and feeding patterns

60. _____ Performing self-care
61. _____ Using words to communicate with others
62. _____ Adjusting to aging parents
63. _____ Accepting male or female role appropriate for one's age
64. _____ Beginning to talk and communicate with others
65. _____ Choosing education and a career

Crossword

Fill in the following crossword by answering the clues with the words from this list:

Development
Grasp
Growth

Menopause
Moro

Neonatal
Preadolescence

Puberty
Rooting

Step
Sucking

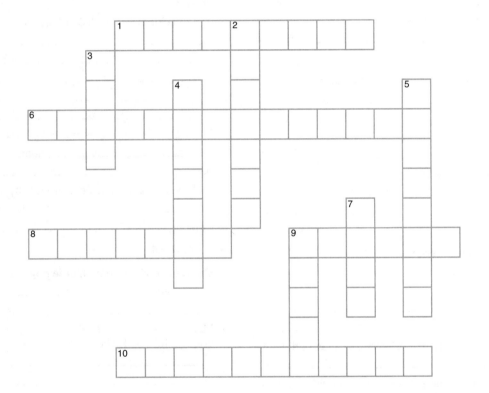

Across

1. Event that occurs to women between ages 40 and 55
6. Time between childhood and adolescence (late childhood)
8. Reflex that occurs when the lips are touched
9. Physical changes that can be measured and that occur in a steady, orderly manner
10. Changes in mental, emotional, and social function

Down

2. Period between ages 9 and 15 years that girls reach; period between ages 12 and 16 years that boys reach
3. Reflex in which the feet move up and down as in stepping motions
4. Reflex that occurs when the cheek is touched near the mouth
5. Period of infancy from birth to 1 month of age
7. Reflex that occurs when a loud noise, a sudden movement, or the head falling back startles the baby
9. Reflex that occurs when the palm is stroked

Optional Learning Exercises

Infancy

66. You are observing a newborn. You know the neonate

    A. Sleeps _____ a day

    B. Can turn the head from _____

67. When an infant is between 1 month and 1 year old,

    A. It has tears and can follow objects with the eyes at _____ months

    B. The Moro, rooting, and grasp reflexes disappear by _____ months

    C. The baby can roll from front to back by _____ months

    D. It can learn to drink from a cup with handles by _____ months

    E. Walking skills increase by _____ months

Toddlerhood

68. During toddlerhood, the developmental tasks are

    A. _____

    B. _____

    C. _____

    D. _____

69. At 18 months, a toddler knows only _____ words. By age 2 years, the child knows about _____ words.

Preschool

70. What personal skills can be done by 3-year-olds?

    A. Put on _____

    B. Manage _____

    C. Wash _____

    D. Brush _____

71. Four-year-olds prefer the primary caregiver of the _____ sex.

72. Communication skills increase in a 5-year-old. They can

    A. Speak in _____

    B. Questions have more _____

    C. The child wants words _____

School-Age

73. Play in school-age children has a _____

    A. They like household tasks such as _____

    B. Rewards are important such as _____

Late Childhood

74. The developmental tasks of late childhood are like those for _____ _____. Preadolescents show more _____ and _____ in achieving the tasks. The tasks are

    A. _____

    B. _____

    C. _____

    D. _____

    E. _____

    F. _____

Adolescence

75. The developmental task of adolescence are

    A. _____

    B. _____

    C. _____

    D. _____

    E. _____

76. During adolescence girls and boys need about _____ hours of sleep at night because of _____.

77. Girls usually complete development by age _____. Boys usually stop growing between _____ years.

Young Adulthood

78. During young adulthood, little physical growth occurs, but _____ _____ development continues.

79. Many factors affect the selection of a partner during young adulthood. They include

    A. _____

    B. _____

    C. _____

    D. _____

    E. _____

    F. _____

    G. _____

Middle Adulthood

80. During middle adulthood, weight control becomes a problem because _____

81. People in middle adulthood may have parents

    who are _____ and

    _____. Many also deal with the

    _____ of parents.

Late Adulthood

82. The developmental tasks of late adulthood are

    A. _____

    B. _____

    C. _____

    D. _____

    E. _____

Independent Learning Activities

Ask permission to observe a group of children either at home or in a day-care setting. After observing them, answer these questions.

- How many children did you observe? What stages did you see?
- List the developmental tasks you could observe in each age group.
- How many children in each age group were meeting all of the developmental tasks? How many children did you see that were *not* meeting any developmental tasks for the age group?
- How much difference did you see in physical sizes of children in the same age groups? How did physical size relate to development? For example, did the biggest children seem more or less advanced in developmental tasks?

Look at the information in the Textbook that relates to your own age and answer these questions.

- How many developmental tasks have been met? Were these tasks met during the stage you are in or at an earlier stage?
- How many developmental tasks have *not* been met? Are these tasks that you are working toward now? What steps are you taking to meet these tasks?

11 Care of the Older Person

Fill in the Blank: Key Terms

Atrophy   Geriatrics   Gerontology

1. _____ is the care of aging people.
2. Another word for shrink is _____.
3. The study of the aging process is _____.

Circle the Best Answer

4. In 2010, how many people were 65 years and older?
   A. 15,400,000
   B. 4,200,000
   C. 40,000,000
   D. 20,600,000
5. Most older people live
   A. In a nursing center
   B. Alone
   C. In a family setting
   D. With non-relatives
6. The oldest-old are
   A. 65-74 years
   B. 75-84 years
   C. 60-65 years
   D. 85 years and older
7. As aging occurs
   A. Disability always results
   B. Changes are slow
   C. Most people adapt poorly
   D. All of the above
8. A myth about aging is
   A. Many older people enjoy a fulfilling sex life
   B. Mental function declines with age
   C. Many older persons have jobs
   D. Most older persons have frequent contact with their children
9. Social changes of aging include
   A. Graying hair
   B. Disabilities
   C. Retirement and deaths of loved ones
   D. Decreased physical strength
10. All of these are benefits of retiring except
    A. The person can do whatever he or she wants
    B. Travel and leisure time activities are possible
    C. The person can relax and enjoy life
    D. The person may have poor health and medical bills
11. Money problems can result with retirement because
    A. Income is reduced
    B. Expenses increase
    C. The person is unable to work
    D. The person planned for retirement
12. Reduced income may force lifestyle changes such as
    A. Buying cheaper food
    B. Avoiding buying needed drugs
    C. Relying on family for money
    D. All of the above

13. Loneliness may be a bigger problem for foreign-born persons because
    A. Families from other cultures do not care about older persons
    B. The person is not accepted by native-born persons
    C. They may not have anyone to talk to in their native language
    D. They have more chronic illnesses
14. An older person can adjust to social relationship changes by doing all of these *except*
    A. Staying at home alone to save money
    B. Finding new friends
    C. Developing hobbies; church and community activities
    D. Having regular contact with family
15. A benefit when children care for older parents may be that
    A. The older person may feel unwanted and useless
    B. The older person may feel more secure
    C. Tension may develop among the children and the family
    D. Parents and children change roles
16. When a partner dies, the older person
    A. Accepts this as part of life
    B. May develop serious physical and mental problems
    C. Forms new friendships easily
    D. Usually has prepared for this change
17. What causes wrinkles to appear on an older person?
    A. Decreases in oil and sweat gland secretions
    B. Fewer nerve endings
    C. Loss of elasticity, strength, and fatty tissue layer
    D. Poor circulation
18. Healing in older people is delayed because of
    A. Poor nutrition
    B. Fragile blood vessels in the skin
    C. Fewer nerve endings
    D. Loss of fatty tissue
19. Hot water bottles and heating pads are *not* used with older persons because
    A. They generally complain of being too warm
    B. The skin is dry
    C. Burns are a risk because of decreased sensing of heat and cold
    D. Blood vessels decrease in number
20. Older persons can prevent bone loss and loss of muscle strength by
    A. Activity, exercise, and diet
    B. Taking hormones
    C. Resting with feet elevated
    D. Taking vitamins

21. Bones may break easily because
    A. Joints become stiff and painful
    B. Joints become slightly flexed
    C. Bones lose strength and become brittle
    D. Vertebrae shorten
22. Dizziness may increase in older people because
    A. They have difficulty sleeping
    B. Blood flow to the brain is reduced
    C. Nerve cells are lost
    D. Brain cells are lost
23. Older persons
    A. Have longer memories
    B. Often remember events from long ago better than recent events
    C. May remember more recent events better than events of long ago
    D. Always become confused as aging progresses
24. Painful injuries and disease may go unnoticed because
    A. The person is confused
    B. Touch and sensitivity to pain are reduced
    C. Memory is shorter
    D. The blood flow is reduced
25. Older people often complain that food has no taste because
    A. Of memory loss
    B. The appetite decreases
    C. Taste buds decrease in number
    D. They cannot sense heat and cold
26. Eyes become irritated easily because
    A. The lens yellows
    B. The eye takes longer to adjust to changes in light
    C. Tear secretion is less
    D. The person becomes farsighted
27. An older person may have difficulty in hearing
    A. Loud music   C. High-pitched sounds
    B. Low-pitched sounds D. All sounds
28. When severe circulatory changes occur, the person
    A. May be encouraged to walk long distances
    B. May need rest periods during the day
    C. May not do any kind of exercise
    D. Should only exercise once a week
29. When a person has difficulty breathing, it is easier to breathe when
    A. Lying flat in bed
    B. Covered with heavy bed linens
    C. Allowed to be on bedrest
    D. Resting in the semi-Fowler position
30. Dulled taste and smell decreases
    A. Peristalsis   C. Saliva
    B. Appetite   D. Swallowing
31. Older persons need
    A. Fewer calories   C. More calories
    B. Less fluids   D. Low protein diets
32. Many older persons have to urinate several times during the night because
    A. Bladder infections are common
    B. Urine is more concentrated
    C. The bladder stores less urine
    D. Urinary incontinence may occur

33. An older woman may find intercourse uncomfortable or painful because
    A. Her partner does not achieve an erection easily
    B. There is vaginal dryness
    C. Arousal takes longer
    D. Orgasm is less intense
34. All of these are advantages of an older person living with family *except*
    A. It provides companionship
    B. The family can provide care
    C. They can share living expenses
    D. Sleeping plans may need to change
35. Adult day-care centers
    A. Provide meals, supervision, and activities for older persons
    B. Only accept self-care persons and those who can walk without help
    C. Provide complete care
    D. Provide respite care
36. Living in an apartment allows persons to
    A. Remain independent
    B. Share common meals with others
    C. Enjoy gardening and yard work
    D. Repair appliances and maintain the property
37. Residential hotels may offer
    A. Private rooms or apartments
    B. Recreational activities
    C. A location close to shopping, places of worship, and civic services
    D. All of the above
38. A housing option that is a group of apartments designed to meet the needs of older persons is
    A. An accessory apartment
    B. Congregate housing
    C. Home-sharing
    D. Assisted living
39. Senior citizen housing is available to
    A. Only those who can afford the rent
    B. Those who have no disabilities
    C. Older and disabled persons
    D. Families who live with an older person
40. Home-sharing is a way to
    A. Avoid living alone
    B. Paying rent
    C. Doing housework or yard work
    D. Avoid disabilities
41. Assisted living facilities provide the following *except*
    A. Nursing care
    B. Help with meals
    C. Health care
    D. Social contact with other residents
42. Continuing care retirement communities (CCRC)
    A. Have independent living units
    B. Have food service and help nearby
    C. Add services, as the person's needs change
    D. All of the above
43. Nursing centers are housing options for older persons who
    A. Need only companionship
    B. Cannot care for themselves
    C. Need care during the daytime while family works
    D. Are developmentally disabled

44. A quality nursing center must meet OBRA and CMS requirements to
    A. Be approved by the medical society
    B. Receive Medicare and Medicaid funds
    C. Give care
    D. Be licensed by the local health department
45. A quality nursing center would *not* be required to have
    A. An activity area for resident's use
    B. Halls wide enough so two wheelchairs can pass with ease
    C. Toilet facilities that allow wheelchair use
    D. An area where residents may have a private garden
46. A feature of a quality nursing center is
    A. Hand rails are provided in hallways
    B. Each resident must have a private bathroom
    C. Residents are expected to provide furniture for their rooms
    D. Tablecloths and cloth napkins are used in the dining room

Matching

Match physical changes during the aging process with the body system affected.

   A. Integumentary   E. Respiratory
   B. Musculoskeletal   F. Digestive
   C. Nervous   G. Urinary
   D. Circulatory

47. _____ Reduced blood flow to kidneys
48. _____ Arteries narrow and are less elastic
49. _____ Forgetfulness
50. _____ Gradual loss of height
51. _____ Decreased strength for coughing
52. _____ Decreased secretion of oil and sweat glands
53. _____ Difficulty digesting fried and fatty foods
54. _____ Heart pumps with less force
55. _____ Bladder muscles weaken
56. _____ Difficulty seeing green and blue colors
57. _____ Difficulty swallowing
58. _____ Lung tissue less elastic
59. _____ Bone mass decreases
60. _____ Facial hair in some women

Fill in the Blank

61. Write out the meaning of the abbreviations
    A. ADU _____
    B. CCRC _____
    C. CMS _____
    D. OBRA _____
62. What changes can be made in the home to make it safer for a person with poor eyesight?
    A. _____
    B. _____
    C. _____

D. _____
E. _____
F. _____
G. _____

63. What changes can be made in the home to make it safer for a person with a hearing loss?
    A. _____
    B. _____
    C. _____
    D. _____
    E. _____
    F. _____

64. Name the housing options described in each of the following:
    A. A small portable home can be placed in the yard of a single-family home. _____
    B. Provides meals, supervision, activities, and sometimes rehabilitation to elderly during daytime. _____
    C. The elderly person lives with older brothers, sisters, or cousins for companionship or to share living expenses. _____
    D. The elderly person pays rent and utility bills, but does not need to do maintenance, yard work, or snow removal. _____
    E. The elderly who needs help with activities of daily living, but does not need nursing care may live in a
    _____.
    F. A _____ meets the changing needs of older persons. Services change as the person's needs change.

Use Focus on PRIDE in the Textbook to complete questions 65–67.

65. It is your responsibility to avoid believing myths about aging. These myths are
    A. _____
    B. _____
    C. _____
    D. _____
    E. _____
    F. _____
    G. _____
66. You can promote social interaction when caring for an older person when you
    A. Encourage _____
    B. Ask _____
    C. Use _____
    D. Take _____

67. If you are asked questions during a survey, you should answer survey questions _____ _____. You should also act _____ and use _____.

Optional Learning Exercises

68. When bathing an older person, what kind of soap should be used? _____ Often no soap is used on the _____ _____.

69. What can happen if a nick or cut occurs on the feet? _____

   Why can this happen? _____

70. When bone mass decreases why is it important to turn an older person carefully? _____

71. Why does an older person often have a gradual loss of height? _____

72. What types of exercise help prevent bone loss and loss of muscle strength? _____

73. Older people have changes in the nervous system. When the changes listed happen, what can happen?

   A. Nerve conduction and reflexes are slower _____

   B. Blood flow to brain is reduced _____

   C. Progressive loss of brain cells _____

74. When you are eating with an older person, you notice she puts salt on vegetables that taste fine to you. What may be a reason she does this? _____

75. A female nurse has a high-pitched voice and several residents seem to have difficulty hearing her. They do not complain about hearing the male charge nurse. What may be a reason for the difference? _____

76. What exercises will help a person with circulation changes who must stay in bed? _____

77. What can the nursing assistant do to prevent respiratory complications from bedrest? _____

78. The stomach and colon empty slower, and flatulence and constipation are common in the older person. What causes these problems? _____

79. How will good oral hygiene and denture care improve food intake? _____

80. How can a nursing assistant help to prevent urinary tract infections in an older person? _____

81. Why should you plan to give most fluids to the older person before 1700 (5:00 PM)? _____

Independent Learning Activities

Interview an older person who lives independently. Use these questions to find what concerns the person has about remaining independent.
- What physical problems does the person have, if any?
- What activities are more difficult than they were when the person was younger?
- What does the person use to provide safety? (walkers, canes, alarms, daily phone calls, etc.)
- What comfort measures are needed to decrease pain or help the person sleep?
- What are transportation needs? Does the person drive? How does the person shop for groceries? Visit with family and friends? Attend social functions?
- How are social needs met? How often does the person go to socialize? How often does the person have visitors?

Interview an older person and talk about life when the person was young.
- Observe facial expression and tone of voice when the person talks about events remembered. What changes do you see?
- Compare how well the person remembers events of long ago with what happened more recently.
- How do you feel differently about the person after hearing about the person's youth?

12 Safety

Fill in the Blank: Key Terms

Coma
Dementia
Disaster
Electrical shock

Ground
Hazard
Hazardous substance
Hemiplegia

Incident
Paralysis
Paraplegia
Poison

Quadriplegia
Suffocation
Tetraplegia
Workplace violence

1. The loss of cognitive and social function caused by changes in the brain is _____.

2. _____ are violent acts (including assault or threat of assault) directed toward persons at work or while on duty.

3. Paralysis from the neck down is _____.

4. _____ is any chemical that presents a physical hazard or a health hazard in the workplace.

5. A _____ is a sudden catastrophic event in which many people are injured and killed and property is destroyed.

6. _____ occurs when breathing stops from the lack of oxygen.

7. Paralysis on one side of the body is

_____.

8. A _____ is a state of being unaware of one's surroundings and being unable to react or respond to people, places, or things.

9. That which carries leaking electricity to the earth and away from an electrical appliance is a

_____.

10. _____ is paralysis from the waist down.

11. _____ occurs when electrical current passes through the body.

12. Any event that has harmed or could harm a patient, resident, visitor, or staff member is an

_____.

13. _____ means loss of muscle function, loss of sensation, or loss of both of muscle function and sensation.

14. _____ is any substance harmful to the body when ingested, inhaled, injected, or absorbed through the skin.

15. Another term for quadriplegia is

_____.

16. Anything in the person's setting that may cause injury or illness is a_____.

Circle the Best Answer

17. Safety measures needed by a person can be found
    A. In the doctor's orders
    B. In the person's care plan
    C. By talking to the family
    D. Asking the person

18. Older persons are at risk for accidents because
    A. Some are unsteady
    B. They may have decreased strength and move slowly
    C. They often have poor vision, hearing problems, or a dulled sense of smell
    D. All of the above

19. A reason drugs can be an accident risk factor is because they
    A. Affect hearing
    B. Reduce ability to sense heat and cold
    C. Can cause loss of balance or lack of coordination
    D. Can cause hemiplegia

20. Children are at risk of injury because they
    A. Have not learned the difference between safety and danger
    B. Have not learned right from wrong
    C. Have problems sensing heat and cold
    D. Have poor vision

21. All of these are safety measures to use with young children *except*
    A. Prop the baby bottle on a rolled towel or blanket to feed a baby
    B. Children between 4 and 8 years of age should use booster seats with lap and shoulder belts in a vehicle
    C. Remove drawstrings from jackets, coats, sweaters, and other clothing
    D. Do not let children play with toys that make loud, sharp, or shrill noises

22. When an older person has impaired smell and touch, he or she is at risk for burns because he or she
    A. May not detect smoke or gas odors
    B. Knows there is danger, but cannot move away
    C. Does not move out of the way to safety
    D. Is more sensitive to hazardous materials

23. Identifying persons is most important because
    A. Life and health are threatened if the wrong care is given
    B. Visitors may ask your help to find someone
    C. You need to call the person by the right name
    D. You will have to give care to two people if you give it to the wrong person first
24. Which of these is *not* a reliable way to identify the person?
    A. Check the identification bracelet
    B. Use the person's picture to compare with the person
    C. If person is alert and oriented, follow the center policy to identify
    D. Just call the person by name
25. When a child is lying on a scale, bed, table, or other surface
    A. Place a chair or other object against the surface
    B. Make sure another person is present to assist
    C. Always keep one hand on the child
    D. Cover the child with a blanket to prevent movement
26. When children are in the kitchen
    A. Use the stove's back burners
    B. Turn pot and pan handles so they point outward
    C. Let children help you cook at the stove
    D. Leave cooking utensils in pots and pans
27. Burns can be avoided if oven mitts and pot holders are kept dry because
    A. They conduct heat better
    B. Water conducts heat and can cause burns
    C. Moisture allows bacteria to move through the cloth
    D. All of the above
28. Accidental poisoning of children can occur when
    A. Harmful products are kept in their original containers
    B. Harmful substances are labeled and stored in high, locked areas
    C. Drugs are carried in purses, back packs, and briefcases
    D. Safety latches are used on kitchen, bathroom, garage, basement, and workshop cabinets
29. Poison warning stickers should be placed on common poisons such as
    A. Drugs and vitamins
    B. Detergents, sprays, window cleaners, and paint thinner
    C. Fertilizers, insecticides, and bug sprays
    D. All of the above
30. Children are at risk for lead poisoning between the ages of
    A. Birth and 3 months   C. 6 years to 9 years
    B. 6 months to 6 years   D. 12 years to 18 years
31. How can you prevent exposure to lead-based plumbing?
    A. Use only bottled water
    B. Run the water until it is hot before drinking
    C. Boil all water used in cooking
    D. Let cold water run 1 to 2 minutes before using for cooking or coffee

32. A gas that can cause suffocation is
    A. Oxygen   C. Carbon monoxide
    B. Carbon dioxide   D. Nitrogen
33. You can be poisoned by carbon monoxide from
    A. Furnaces
    B. Automobiles, especially if one is running in a garage
    C. Gas stoves or space heaters
    D. All of the above
34. A choking hazard for older persons can be
    A. Loose teeth or dentures
    B. Sitting up in a wheelchair to eat
    C. Food that is cut into small, bite-sized pieces
    D. Making sure the person is positioned properly in bed
35. Which of these would prevent choking in children?
    A. Position infants on their stomachs for sleep
    B. Use Mylar balloons instead of latex ones
    C. Give the child food such as hot dogs, peanuts, or popcorn
    D. Place an infant on a soft pillow or comforter to sleep
36. The universal sign of choking is when the
    A. Person begins to cough forcefully
    B. Conscious person clutches at the throat
    C. Person tells you he is choking
    D. Person becomes unconscious
37. Abdominal thrusts given for choking can be used on
    A. Pregnant women
    B. Obese people
    C. Infants
    D. Other adults or children over 1 year of age
38. When giving abdominal thrusts, the correct procedure is to
    A. Make a fist, place the thumb side against the abdomen, and quickly thrust upward
    B. Press your fist against the abdomen and slowly push straight down
    C. Gently thrust upward with the fist
    D. Lay the hands flat on the abdomen and push down
39. If you see a foreign object in the mouth of an unconscious person, you should
    A. Turn the head to one side
    B. Leave the object in place
    C. Grasp and remove the object if it is within reach
    D. Ask the person to cough out the object
40. If an infant is choking, you should
    A. Take the infant to the emergency room
    B. Give abdominal thrusts
    C. Hold the infant face down over your forearm and give 5 forceful back slaps between the shoulder blades
    D. Reach in the mouth and try to retrieve the object
41. If a choking person becomes unresponsive, you should
    A. Make sure EMS or RRT was called
    B. Begin abdominal thrusts
    C. Begin chest thrusts
    D. Do a finger sweep for foreign objects in the mouth

42. If you find a piece of equipment that is damaged, take it to the
    A. Nurse
    B. Maintenance department
    C. Fire department
    D. Director of nursing
43. When using electrical items, you
    A. Should always use a three-pronged plug
    B. May touch the equipment even if you are wet
    C. Should unplug the equipment before turning it off
    D. May use water to put out an electrical fire
44. An electrical shock is especially dangerous because it can
    A. Start a fire
    B. Damage equipment
    C. Affect the heart and cause death
    D. Violate OBRA regulations
45. If you are shocked by electric equipment, you should
    A. Report the shock at once
    B. Try to see what is wrong with the equipment
    C. Make sure it has a ground prong
    D. Test the equipment in a different outlet
46. Lock both wheels on wheelchairs
    A. To keep the equipment properly positioned
    B. To prevent the person from moving about
    C. Before you transfer the person
    D. To keep your body in alignment
47. When moving a person on a stretcher, all of these practices are correct *except*
    A. Use safety straps only when the person is confused.
    B. Lock the stretcher before transferring the person.
    C. Do not leave the person alone.
    D. Stand at the head of the stretcher; your co-worker stands at the foot
48. _____ requires that health care employees understand the risks of hazardous substances and how to handle them safely.
    A. Omnibus Budget Reconciliation Act of 1987 (OBRA)
    B. Occupational Safety and Health Administration (OSHA)
    C. Joint Commission on Accreditation of Healthcare Organization (JCAHO)
    D. Material Safety Data Sheets (MSDS)
49. Warning labels may include all of these *except*
    A. Physical hazards and health hazards
    B. What protective equipment to wear
    C. The phone number of the local emergency system
    D. Storage and disposal information
50. Where would you find the Material Safety Data Sheets (MSDS) for hazardous materials?
    A. Attached to the substance
    B. In the administrator's office
    C. In a place on your nursing unit where employees have ready access
    D. On the Internet
51. All of these things are needed for a fire *except*
    A. Spark or flame
    B. Electrical equipment
    C. Materials that will burn
    D. Oxygen

52. When a person is receiving oxygen, which of these is allowed in the room?
    A. Visitors may smoke, but the person receiving oxygen may not
    B. Wool blankets and fabrics that may cause static electricity
    C. Electrical items that are in good working order
    D. Oil, grease, alcohol, and nail polish remover
53. If a fire occurs, what should you do first?
    A. Rescue people in immediate danger
    B. Sound the nearest fire alarm and call the switchboard operator
    C. Close doors and windows to confine the fire
    D. Use a fire extinguisher on a small fire that has not spread to a larger area
54. If evacuation is necessary, persons who are
    A. Closest to the outside door are rescued first
    B. Able to walk are rescued last
    C. Closest to the fire are evacuated first
    D. Are helpless are rescued last
55. If a space heater is used in a home, a safety practice is
    A. Place the heater in doorways or on stairs
    B. Keep heater 3 feet away from curtains, drapes, furniture
    C. Store fuel nearby the heater
    D. Fill the heater when it is hot or running
56. If there is a disaster, you
    A. Are expected to go to your agency immediately
    B. May be called into work if you are off duty
    C. Should stay away or leave to get out of the way
    D. May go home to check on your family
57. Why do more assaults occur in health care settings than in other industries?
    A. Patients may be someone who is arrested or convicted of crimes.
    B. Acutely disturbed and violent persons may seek health care.
    C. Agency pharmacies are a source of drugs and therefore a target for robberies.
    D. All of the above
58. Which of these would *not* be effective to prevent or control workplace violence?
    A. Stand away from the person.
    B. Know where to find panic buttons, call bells, and alarms.
    C. Sit quietly with the person in his room. Hold his hand to calm him.
    D. Tell the person you will get a nurse to speak to him or her.
59. You can help prevent workplace violence by doing all of these *except*
    A. Wearing long hair up and off the collar
    B. Making sure shoes have good soles that do not slip
    C. Wearing necklaces, bracelets, and earrings
    D. Wearing uniforms that fit well
60. If you are uncomfortable or threatened in a home setting, you should
    A. Report the matter to the nurse
    B. Stay at the home and try to resolve the matter
    C. Confront the person who is making you uncomfortable
    D. Ignore the situation and continue to give care

61. The intent of risk management is to
    A. Prevent accidents and fires
    B. Prevent workplace violence
    C. Protect patients, residents, visitors, and staff
    D. All of the above
62. A yellow color-coded wristband may indicate that the person
    A. Has allergies
    B. Has an order for "do not resuscitate"
    C. Has a restricted diet
    D. Is at risk for falling

Matching

Match each safety measure to the risk it prevents.

    A. Burns   D. Equipment accident
    B. Poisoning   E. Hazardous substances
    C. Suffocation   F. Fire

63. _____ Do *not* allow the person to sleep with a heating pad
64. _____ Supervise persons who smoke
65. _____ Keep child-resistant caps on all harmful products
66. _____ Wear PPE to clean spills and leaks
67. _____ Report loose teeth or dentures to the nurse
68. _____ Do *not* touch a person who is experiencing an electrical shock
69. _____ Move all persons from the area if you smell gas or smoke
70. _____ Have water heaters set at 120° F or less
71. _____ Never call drugs or vitamins "candy"
72. _____ Store fuel and flammable liquids outside

Fill in the Blank

73. Write out the meaning of the abbreviations
    A. AED _____
    B. CDC _____
    C. CO _____
    D. CPR _____
    E. EMS _____
    F. FBAO _____
    G. MSDS _____
    H. OSHA _____
    I. PASS _____
    J. RRT _____
74. As part of the team, you can help provide a safe setting by correcting something that is unsafe. What could you do if
    A. You see a water spill _____
    B. You see a person sliding out of a wheelchair
       _____

C. A person is having problems holding a cup of coffee _____
D. Food is left unattended in a microwave
   _____

E. A grab bar is loose in the bathroom
   _____

75. A person who is agitated or aggressive may be at risk for injuries. What can cause these behaviors?
    A. _____
    B. _____
    C. _____
    D. _____
76. What health hazards can be caused by hazardous substances?
    A. _____
    B. _____
    C. _____
       _____
    D. _____
77. When a fire occurs, what action is taken for each of the steps?
    A. R _____
       _____
    B. A _____
       _____
    C. C _____
       _____
    D. E _____
       _____
78. The word PASS is used to remember how to use a
    _____.
    What action is taken for each step?
    A. P _____
       _____
    B. A _____
       _____
    C. S _____
       _____
    D. S _____
       _____
79. If a disaster occurs, the agency usually has a plan that generally provides for
    A. _____
    B. _____
    C. _____
    D. _____

Use Focus on PRIDE in Textbook to complete questions 80-81.

80. If you make a mistake, you show personal and professional responsibility when you

A. _____

B. _____

C. _____

81. You work as a team when you ensure the safety of all staff arriving and leaving the agency when you

A. _____

B. _____

C. _____
_____

D. _____
_____

E. _____
_____

Optional Learning Exercises

Write the safety measure for infants and children that is being followed in questions 82–92. (Box 12-1)

82. The babysitter makes sure she can see the child when she goes to answer the phone.

_____
_____

83. You replace the bottle cap on the floor cleaner after you use it.

_____
_____

84. The 5-year-old sleeps in the bottom bunk and the 8-year-old sleeps in the top bunk.

_____

85. The primary caregiver keeps the hair dryer in the bedroom, *not* in the bathroom.

_____

86. The furniture in the living room is arranged so that no furniture is under the window.

_____

87. A mother is holding her 2-year-old's hand when walking up a flight of stairs.

_____

88. When you finish cleaning the floor, you empty the bucket and turn it upside down for storage.

_____
_____

89. Parents decide to get a new car safety seat for an infant instead of using the seat they used for their 11-year-old.

_____
_____

90. The mother takes away her necklace from the child, even though it makes the child cry.

_____
_____

91. When the mother buys a kids' meal at a fast food restaurant, she reads the toy package before giving it to her 3-year-old. _____

_____

92. When you are helping the primary caregiver set the table for dinner, she tells you not to use the place mats. _____

_____

Write the safety measure to prevent burns that is being followed in questions 93–98. (Box 12-2)

93. You keep matches on the top shelf of the cupboard.

_____
_____

94. When you get ready to cook, you take off your bulky sweater. _____

_____

95. Before picking up her baby, the mother sets her coffee cup on the table. _____

96. Before putting a young child in the bathtub, the primary caregiver reaches in and stirs the water.

97. The nursing assistant takes the heating pad out of the bed before the person goes to bed for the night.

_____

98. The nursing assistant sits with the confused person while he smokes. _____

Write the safety measure to prevent poisoning that is being followed in questions 99–102. (Boxes 12-3, 12-4)

99. You check the labels on harmful products in your home. _____

_____

100. You ask a visitor to your home to put her purse on a shelf. _____

101. You scrape loose paint on a windowsill.

_____

102. You discard a can of food when you notice it was canned in Mexico. _____

Write the safety measure to prevent equipment accidents being followed in questions 103–111. (Boxes 12-8, 12-9)

103. The nursing assistant tells the person his shower will be delayed until the storm passes.

_____

104. The nursing assistant tells the nurse she has never used the portable footbath before.

_____

105. The nursing assistant dries her hands carefully before plugging in a razor. _____

_____

106. An electric fan will not work and the staff member follows the correct procedure to have it repaired.

_____

107. The nursing assistant moves an electrical cord that is lying across a heat vent. _____

108. The nursing assistant makes sure the person has both feet on the wheelchair footplates before moving the wheelchair. _____

_____

109. The nursing assistant notices one wheel is flat on a wheelchair and reports it to the nurse.

_____

_____

110. The nursing assistant locks the wheelchair when the person is being transferred to his bed.

_____

_____

111. You ask a co-worker to stay with a patient lying on a stretcher while you get another pillow.

_____

Write what you should do when handling hazardous materials in the situations in questions 112–115. (Box 12-10)

112. When cleaning up a hazardous material, how do you know what equipment to wear?

_____

_____

113. When a spill occurs, what is the correct way to wipe it up? _____

_____

114. The nurse tells the nursing assistant the person is having an x-ray done in her room.

_____

_____

115. The nurse tells you to open the windows in a room where you are cleaning up a hazardous material.

_____

Write the fire prevention measure that is being practiced in questions 116–118. (Box 12-11)

116. When you go to the kitchen to heat food for the person, you blow out the candle in the living room. _____

_____

117. When cleaning a smoking area, the staff uses a metal can partially filled with sand.

_____

_____

118. When heating food for a person, the nursing assistant remains in the kitchen. _____

Write the measures to prevent or control workplace violence that should be used in questions 119–123. (Box 12-12)

119. What types of jewelry can serve as a weapon?

_____

_____

120. Why is long hair worn up? _____

_____

121. Why are pictures, vases, and other items removed from certain areas? _____

122. What type of glass protects nurses' stations, reception areas, and admitting areas?

_____

123. What clothing items should be worn by staff to assist the ability to run? _____

Write personal safety practices that apply in questions 124–131. (Box 12-13)

124. What safety practices should be used when parking your car in a parking garage?

_____

_____

125. What items should you keep in the car for safety?

_____

_____

126. Why is a "dry run" important?

_____

_____

127. If you think someone is following you, what should you do? _____

_____

128. If someone wants your wallet or purse, what should you do? _____

_____

129. How can you use your car keys as a weapon?

_____

_____

_____

130. How can you use your thumbs as a weapon?

_____

_____

131. What part of the body can you attack on either a man or woman? _____

_____

Independent Learning Activities

Safety is important to everyone and needs to be practiced at all times. Check the following items or areas in your own home to determine how safe it is.

- What areas are adequately lighted for safety? What areas need improved lighting?
- Check electrical cords and plugs on appliances and lamps. How many have frayed cords? Ungrounded plugs? Other problems that make them unsafe to use?
- How many smoke detectors do you have in your home? When were batteries last replaced? How can you check the smoke detector to make sure it is working correctly?

- Where are hazardous materials (medications, cleaning solutions, painting supplies, etc.) stored? Which of these could be reached by children? What could be done to store them more safely?
- Make a list of good safety practices in your home. Make a list of safety practices that could be improved.

Develop a plan for your home and family that helps everyone know how to escape if a fire occurs.

- Make sure every person knows at least two escape routes from the sleeping area.
- Practice how to check a door for heat before opening.
- Arrange a place to meet once you are outside the building.

13 Preventing Falls

Fill in the Blank: Key Terms

Bed rail   Gait belt   Transfer belt

1. A device used to support a person who is unsteady or disabled is a _____

_____.

2. A _____ is a device that serves as a guard or barrier along the side of the bed.

3. Another name for a transfer belt is a

_____.

Circle the Best Answer

4. Most falls occur
   A. In hallways
   B. In resident rooms and bathrooms
   C. Outside
   D. In dining areas

5. Falls are more likely to occur
   A. After midnight
   B. During shift changes
   C. At mealtime
   D. In the morning, after breakfast

6. Which of these would help to prevent falls?
   A. Answer call light promptly
   B. Take the person to the bathroom once a shift
   C. Always keep side rails up
   D. Have the person wear socks to walk in room

7. A safety measure that can help prevent falls would be
   A. Have the person wear reading glasses when walking
   B. Assist the person to the bathroom at regular times and whenever requested
   C. Rearrange the furniture in the room often
   D. Turn off lights and night-lights at night

8. Which of these physical problems can cause falls?
   A. Low blood pressure
   B. Joint pain and stiffness
   C. Incontinence
   D. All of the above

9. Bed rails
   A. Are used for all older persons
   B. Are considered restraints by OBRA and CMS in certain situations
   C. Prevent falls
   D. Are never used when giving care

10. Information about whether to raise bed rails for a particular person can be found in the
    A. Care plan   C. Agency policies
    B. Doctor's orders D. Procedure book

11. When giving bedside care, the bed wheels are
    A. Unlocked
    B. Locked
    C. Unlocked on the side of the bed where you are working
    D. Locked when moving the bed

12. A transfer belt is
    A. Applied over clothing
    B. Applied with the buckle in the front
    C. Applied very loosely
    D. Always applied next to the skin

13. A transfer belt is usually *not* used when a person
    A. Is unsteady when moving from a chair to the bed
    B. When a person needs helps to walk
    C. Has an abdominal wound, incision, or drainage tube
    D. When helping a person to stand up

14. If a person begins to fall, you should
    A. Try to prevent the fall
    B. Call for help and hold the person up
    C. Ease the person to the floor
    D. Stand back and let the person fall

15. If a bariatric person starts to fall, you should
    A. Try to prevent the fall
    B. Ease the person to the floor
    C. Move any items out of the way that could cause injury
    D. Call for help and hold the person up

Fill in the Blank

16. Most falls occur between _____ and

_____.

17. You may calm an agitated person by giving the person

a _____, _____,

or a _____.

18. Tubs and showers may be made safer if they have

_____ surfaces.

19. The need for bed rails is noted in the person's

_____ and _____.

20. You raise the bed to give care. If the person uses bed rails, and you are working alone, what do you do with the side rails?

A. _____

B. _____

21. After you are done giving care, how is the bed positioned? _____

_____.

22. Hand rails in hallways and stairways give support to persons who are _____
_____.

23. When a transfer belt is applied, you should be able to slide _____ under the belt.

24. When a person starts to fall, you can protect the person's _____ as you ease the person to the floor.

25. What information is recorded on an incident report when a person falls?
    A. _____
    B. _____
    C. _____
    D. _____
    E. _____

Use Focus on PRIDE in the Textbook to complete questions 26–28.

26. You support the person's right to safety and security when you promote comfort using good
    _____

27. You show personal and professional responsibility when you do not take short cuts and take time to
    A. _____
    B. _____
    C. _____
    D. _____
    E. _____

28. When assisting a co-worker with a transfer, what information do you need?
    A. _____
    B. _____
    C. _____
    D. _____
    E. _____
    F. _____

Optional Learning Exercises

29. Why are falls more likely to happen during shift changes? Staff _____
    _____. Confusion
    _____.

30. What kinds of equipment help to make bathrooms and showers safer?
    A. _____
    B. _____
    C. _____
    D. _____

31. Why should floor coverings be one color in areas where older persons are living? _____
_____

32. How are falls prevented when the person's phone, lamp, and personal belongings are at the bedside?
_____

33. What kind of footwear and clothing will help to prevent falls?
    A. Footwear _____
    _____
    B. Clothing _____
    _____

34. Why is it important to answer signal lights promptly?
_____
_____

35. If a person needs bed rails, keep them up at all times except _____.

36. For a person who uses bed rails, always raise the far bed rail if you _____.

37. If a person does not use bed rails and you are giving care, how do you protect them from falling?
_____
_____

38. Wheels are locked at all times except when
_____

39. If a person starts to fall, you _____.
    This lets you control _____.

Independent Learning Activities

Look at the nursing center where you are assigned to answer these questions about safety.
- How quickly are signal lights answered? How does the staff know who should answer each light?
- If you are there during shift change, how does the staff make sure residents do not fall?
- What safety measures do you see being used? (Use Box 13-2 as a guide to check for these measures.)
- How many residents use bed rails? What are the reasons these residents need bed rails?

Practice easing a falling person to the floor with a classmate.
- How did you support the person?
- How did using the transfer/gait belt help to control the fall?
- What was easy and what was difficult about this practice?
- How did this practice help you to feel more confident about helping a falling person?

14 Restraint Alternatives and Safe Restraint Use

Fill in the Blank: Key Terms

Chemical restraint
Enabler
Freedom of movement
Medical symptom
Physical restraint
Remove easily

1. Any manual method or physical or mechanical device, material, or equipment attached to or near the person's body that he or she cannot remove easily is a

   _____.

2. _____ is a term used when a manual method device, material, or equipment can be removed intentionally by the person in the same manner it was applied by the staff.

3. A device that limits freedom of movement but is used to promote independence is an

   _____.

4. Any change in place or position for the body that the person is physically able to control is called

   _____.

5. An indication or characteristic of a physical or psychological condition is a

   _____.

6. A _____ is any drug used for discipline or convenience and *not* required to treat medical symptoms.

Circle the Best Answer

7. Restraints are used
   A. Whenever the nurse feels they are necessary.
   B. Only to treat a medical symptom or for the immediate physical safety of the person or others
   C. To make sure the person does not fall
   D. To decrease work for the staff

8. When restraints are needed, their use is determined by
   A. Using the nursing process
   B. The person's behavior
   C. Family requests
   D. Nursing assistants who provide care

9. Research shows that restraints
   A. Prevent falls
   B. Cause falls
   C. Are used whenever the nurse decides
   D. Are not effective

10. A person's harmful behaviors may be caused by
    A. Being afraid of a new setting
    B. Being too hot or too cold
    C. Being hungry or thirsty
    D. All of the above

11. Guidelines about using restraints are part of the resident rights in
    A. CDC regulations
    B. OSHA rules
    C. OBRA, FDA, and CMS regulations
    D. JCAHO recommendations

12. Restraints are *not* used to
    A. Prevent harm to the person
    B. Control the person's behaviors
    C. Prevent a person from pulling at a wound or dressing
    D. Keep an IV from being pulled out

13. Which of these is a type of restraint?
    A. A soft chair with a footstool to elevate the feet
    B. A bed without bed rails
    C. A chair with a tray that prevents the person from rising
    D. A drug that helps a person function at his or her highest level

14. The most serious risk from restraints is
    A. Cuts, bruises, and fractures
    B. Death from strangulation
    C. Falls
    D. Depression, anger, and agitation

15. Using a restraint requires informed consent. This consent is obtained by
    A. The person's legal representative
    B. The doctor or nurse
    C. The person
    D. The nursing assistant

16. All of these are legal aspects of restraint use *except*
    A. Unnecessary restraint use is false imprisonment
    B. Nurses can decide when to use restraints, what type of restraints to use, and how long to use the restraints
    C. The least restrictive method is used
    D. Restraints must protect the person

17. Restraints may increase
    A. Rest and sleep
    B. Confusion and agitation
    C. Calmness and alertness
    D. Cooperation with care and procedures

18. After receiving instructions about safely applying a restraint you should
    A. Ask for help to apply it to a person
    B. Demonstrate correct application back to the nurse
    C. Watch someone else apply it to a person
    D. Apply it to the person independently

19. Which of these is physical restraint?
    A. Vest   C. Wedge cushion
    B. Bed rail   D. Pillow

20. When restraining a combative and agitated person, it should be done
    A. Slowly by only one person
    B. Only after explaining to the person what will be done
    C. With enough staff to complete the task safely and quickly
    D. In a public area so the person is distracted
21. The person who is restrained must be observed every
    A. 5 minutes   C. Hour
    B. 15 minutes   D. 2 hours
22. When a person is restrained, at least every 2 hours you should
    A. Check the person
    B. Remove the restraints, reposition the person, and meet basic needs
    C. Make sure the restraints are secure
    D. Remove the restraints until the next shift
23. Wrist restraints are used when a person
    A. Tries to get out of bed
    B. Moves his wheelchair without permission
    C. Pulls at tubes used in medical treatments
    D. Slides out of a chair easily
24. A roll belt restraint
    A. Is more restrictive than other restraints
    B. Allows the person to turn from side to side
    C. Must be released by the staff
    D. Can only be used in bed
25. The straps of vest and jacket restraints
    A. Always cross in the front
    B. Are applied next to the skin under clothing
    C. Must be secured very tightly to be safe
    D. May cross in the back
26. Elbow restraints are used
    A. To prevent older persons from pulling at tubes
    B. For children to limit movements and prevent scratching and touching incisions
    C. On only one arm at a time
    D. To prevent injury to the staff by a confused person
27. When applying wrist restraints
    A. Tie the straps to the bed rail
    B. Tie firm knots in the straps
    C. Place the restraints over clothing
    D. Place the soft part toward the skin
28. If you are using padded mitts restraints you should
    A. Give the person a hand roll to hold
    B. Pad the mitt with soft material
    C. Make sure the person's hands are clean and dry
    D. Tie the straps to the bed rails
29. A belt restraint should be
    A. Used only when the person is in a chair or wheelchair
    B. Secured tightly with no slack in the straps
    C. Checked to make sure the person is comfortable and in good body alignment
    D. Applied next to the skin
30. When using a vest restraint in bed
    s are secured to the bed frame out of the
    's reach
    s are secured to the bed rail
    st crosses in the back
    erson can turn over

31. When you check a person in a vest, jacket, or belt restraint, report at once if
    A. The skin is slightly reddened under the restraint
    B. The person needs to urinate
    C. The person is not breathing or is having difficulty breathing
    D. You need to reposition the person

Matching

Match the legal aspects and safety guidelines with the correct example.
    A. Restraints must protect the person.
    B. Restraints require a written doctor's order.
    C. The least restrictive method of restraint is used.
    D. Restraints are used only after other methods fail to protect the person.
    E. Unnecessary restraint is false imprisonment.
    F. Informed consent is required for restraint use.
    G. The manufacturer's instructions are followed.
    H. Restraints are applied with enough help to protect the person and staff from injury.
    I. Restraints can increase a person's confusion and agitation.
    J. Quality of life must be protected.
    K. The person is observed at least every 15 minutes or more often as required by the care plan.
    L. The restraint is removed, the person repositioned, and basic needs met at least every 2 hours.

32. _____ Injuries and deaths have occurred from improper restraint and poor observation.
33. _____ A restraint is used only when it is the best safety precaution for the person.
34. _____ The nurse gives you the manufacturer's instructions about applying and securing the restraint safely.
35. _____ Restrained persons need repeated explanations and reassurance.
36. _____ The doctor gives the reason for the restraint, what to use, and how long to use the restraint.
37. _____ Persons in immediate danger of harming themselves or others are restrained quickly.
38. _____ Because they are the least restrictive, passive physical restraints should be used when possible.
39. _____ Restraints are used for as short a time as possible and needs are met with as little restraint as possible
40. _____ If told to apply a restraint, you must clearly understand the need for restraints and the risks.
41. _____ When the restraint is removed, range-of-motion exercises are done or the person is ambulated.
42. _____ The care plan must include measures to protect the person and to prevent the person from harming others.
43. _____ The person must understand the reason for the restraints.

Fill in the Blank

44. When using restraints, what information is reported and recorded?

A. _____

B. _____

C. _____

D. _____

E. _____

F. _____

G. _____

H. _____

I. _____

J. _____

K. _____

L. _____

M. _____

45. When you check the restrained person's circulation every 15 minutes, tell the nurse at once if you observe these signs or symptoms.

A. _____

B. _____

C. _____

D. _____

46. When you remove the restraints every 2 hours, what are the basic needs that should be met?

A. _____

B. _____

C. _____

D. _____

E. _____

F. _____

G. _____

47. Persons restrained in a supine position must be monitored constantly because they are a great risk for

_____.

48. You should carry scissors with you because in an

emergency _____

_____.

49. When you are delegated to apply restraints, what information do you need from the nurse and the care plan?

A. _____

B. _____

C. _____

D. _____

E. _____

F. _____

G. _____

H. _____

I. _____

J. _____

K. _____

L. _____

M. _____

N. _____

Use Focus on PRIDE in the Textbook to complete questions 50–51.

50. When a person has restraints in place, your professional responsibilities mean you must

A. _____

B. _____

C. _____

D. _____

E. _____

F. _____

51. When you practice ethical behavior, you would treat a person like _____ with

_____.

Labeling

52. Explain what is being done.

_____

_____

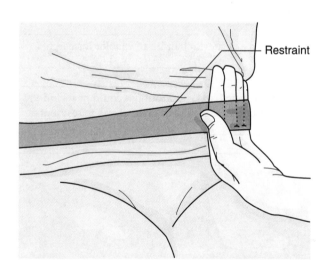

Restraint

53. Draw a belt restraint applied correctly on the person. What is the correct angle for this belt?

_____

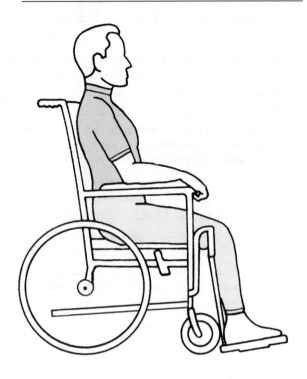

Optional Learning Exercises

54. Drugs or drug dosages are restraints if they
    A. _____
    B. _____

55. How can a geriatric chair be an enabler instead of a restraint? _____
    _____

56. What lifelong habits and routines could be included in the nursing care plan as alternatives to restraints?

    _____
    _____

57. Why would a person in restraints be at risk for dehydration? _____
    _____

58. Why would videotapes of family and friends or visiting with family be good alternatives to restraints?

    _____
    _____

59. What is the purpose of padded hip protectors and floor cushions? _____.

Independent Learning Activities

Role-play that one person is a nursing assistant and one is a person who is restrained. An active physical restraint is applied as the person sits in a chair or wheelchair. When the restraint is in place, the nursing assistant leaves and does not return for 15 minutes. Discuss the following questions with each other after the experiment.

- How did the person feel when the restraints were applied? What did the nursing assistant tell the person about the restraints?
- Did the nursing assistant ask the person if toileting was needed? If the person was thirsty?
- Was the chair comfortable? Was there any padding? Did the nursing assistant check for wrinkles? Could the person move around to reposition the body for comfort?
- How was the person able to get help during the 15 minutes of being alone?
- What diversions were offered while the person was restrained? TV or radio? Reading materials? A window with a pleasant view? If any of these were provided, who chose the channel, station, book, or view?
- Was the person told someone would return in 15 minutes? Was a clock or watch available to see the time? How long did it seem?
- What was learned from this experience by both people?

15 Preventing Infection

Fill in the Blank: Key Terms

Antibiotic
Asepsis
Biohazardous waste
Carrier
Clean technique
Communicable
  disease

Contagious disease
Contamination
Disinfection
Healthcare-associated
  infection (HAI)
Immunity

Infection
Infection control
Medical asepsis
Microbe
Microorganism
Non-pathogen
Normal flora

Pathogen
Reservoir
Spore
Sterile
Sterile field
Sterile technique
Sterilization

Surgical asepsis
Vaccination
Vaccine
Vector
Vehicle

1. A carrier (animal, insect) that transmits disease is a _____.

2. A _____ is a small living plant or animal seen only with a microscope; a microbe.

3. A human or animal that is a reservoir for microbes but does *not* have signs and symptoms of infection is a _____.

4. Protection against a certain disease is _____.

5. A preparation containing dead or weakened microbes is a _____.

6. A work area free of all pathogens and nonpathogens is a _____.

7. _____ are items contaminated with blood, body fluids, secretions, and excretions that may be harmful to others.

8. _____ are the practices used to remove or destroy pathogens and to prevent their spread from one person or place to another person or place; clean technique.

9. A communicable disease is also called a _____.

10. An _____ is a disease state resulting from the invasion and growth of microorganisms in the body.

11. _____ is the practices that keep equipment and supplies free of all microbes; sterile technique.

12. A _____ is a disease caused by pathogens that spread easily; contagious disease.

13. The process of destroying pathogens is _____.

14. A _____ is an infection that develops in a person cared for in any setting where health care is given.

15. _____ is being free of disease-producing microbes.

16. Another name for a microorganism is a _____.

17. The environment in which microbes live and grow is a _____.

18. Medical asepsis is also called _____.

19. The process of becoming unclean is _____.

20. The absence of all microbes is _____.

21. Surgical asepsis is also called _____.

22. A bacterium protected by a hard shell is a _____.

23. _____ are microbes that usually live and grow in a certain area.

24. A microbe that does *not* usually cause an infection is a _____.

25. _____ is the process of destroying all microbes.

26. A microbe that is harmful and can cause an infection is a _____.

27. The administration of a vaccine to produce immunity against an infectious disease is _____.

28. Practices and procedures that prevent the spread of disease is _____.

29. An _____ is a drug that kills microbes that cause infections.

30. Any substance that transmits microbes is a _____.

Circle the Best Answer

31. Germs are another name for a type of microbe called
    A. Protozoa
    B. Fungi
    C. Viruses
    D. Bacteria
32. Rickettsiae are transmitted to humans by
    A. Plants
    B. Other humans
    C. Insect bites
    D. One-celled animals
33. In order to live and grow, all microbes require
    A. Oxygen
    B. A reservoir
    C. A hot environment
    D. Plenty of light
34. Normal flora
    A. Are always pathogens
    B. Are always nonpathogens
    C. Become pathogens when transmitted from its natural site to another site
    D. Cause signs and symptoms of an infection
35. Multidrug-resistant organisms are organisms that
    A. Can be destroyed by certain antibiotics
    B. Can resist the effects of antibiotics
    C. Are viruses that cause influenza and colds
    D. Are spread by insects
36. Which of these is *not* a sign or symptom of infection?
    A. Rash
    B. Fatigue and loss of energy
    C. Constipation
    D. Sores on mucous membranes
37. An older person may not show the signs or symptoms of an infection because of changes in
    A. Diet
    B. The immune system
    C. Mobility of the person
    D. Confusion and delirium
38. The source of infection is
    A. A break in the skin
    B. A human or animal
    C. Nutritional status
    D. A pathogen
39. In the chain of infection, a portal of exit can be
    A. Blood
    B. Human and animals
    C. General health
    D. A carrier
40. Healthcare-associated infections often occur when
    A. Insects are present
    B. Hand washing is poor
    C. Medical asepsis is used correctly
    D. A person is in isolation
41. The practice that keeps equipment and supplies free of *all* microbes is
    A. Medical asepsis
    B. Clean technique
    C. Contamination
    D. Surgical asepsis
42. What is the easiest and most important way to prevent the spread of infection?
    A. Sterilize all equipment.
    B. Use only disposable equipment.
    C. Keep all residents in isolation.
    D. Practice good hand washing.
43. When washing hands you should
    A. Use hot water
    B. Keep hands lower than the elbows
    C. Turn off faucets after lathering
    D. Keep hands higher than elbows

44. Clean under the fingernails by rubbing your fingers against your palms
    A. Each time you wash your hands
    B. If you have long nails
    C. Only for the first hand washing of the day
    D. For at least 10 seconds
45. To avoid contaminating your hands, turn off the faucets
    A. After soap is applied
    B. Before drying hands
    C. With clean paper towels
    D. With your elbows
46. An alcohol-based hand rub may be used to decontaminate your hands
    A. When the hands are visibly dirty or soiled with blood, body fluids, or secretions and excretions
    B. After using the restroom
    C. After contact with the intact skin
    D. Before eating
47. You can prevent the spread of microbes in the home by
    A. Thawing frozen foods at room temperature
    B. Using a disinfectant to clean surfaces in the bathroom every day
    C. Refreezing food items that have partially thawed
    D. Wiping cutting boards with a dry paper towel after use
48. Older persons with dementia rely on others to protect them from infection because they
    A. Do not understand aseptic practices
    B. Are more resistant to infection
    C. Resist hand washing and other aseptic practices
    D. Never learned good hygiene practices
49. When cleaning contaminated equipment
    A. Wear personal protective equipment (PPE)
    B. Rinse in hot water first
    C. Use the clean utility room.
    D. Remove any organic materials with a paper towel.
50. Reusable items are disinfected with
    A. Soap and water
    B. An autoclave
    C. Chemical disinfectants
    D. High temperatures
51. A good, cheap disinfectant to use in the home is
    A. Chlorine bleach
    B. Ammonia
    C. White vinegar solution
    D. Soap and water
52. If you use boiling water to sterilize items in the home, you should
    A. Pour the water over the items in a sink
    B. Boil the items for 5 to 15 minutes
    C. Boil the items for 30 to 45 minutes
    D. Place the items in the water, bring the water to a boil, and turn it off

53. Isolation precautions are used for
    A. All persons
    B. Any person who has had surgery
    C. All older persons
    D. As a method to prevent spreading communicable diseases
54. When a person is in isolation, you can help the person by
    A. Restricting all visitors
    B. Keeping the door open so the person can see into the hallway
    C. Saying "hello" from the doorway often
    D. Avoiding going into the room
55. Standard precautions are used:
    A. For a person with a respiratory infection
    B. For a person with a wound infection
    C. For a person with tuberculosis
    D. For all persons whenever care is given
56. Gloves worn in standard precautions
    A. Do not need to be changed when performing several tasks for the same person
    B. Can be worn until they tear or are punctured
    C. Must be removed before going to another person
    D. Only are worn if the person has an infection
57. When you are working in a room with isolation precautions, you use paper towels to
    A. Handle contaminated items
    B. Turn faucets on and off
    C. Open the door to the person's room
    D. All of the above
58. Practice hand hygiene
    A. After removing gloves
    B. Only when you leave the isolation area
    C. Only when moving between residents
    D. Only if gloves were not worn
59. If you are allergic to latex gloves, you should
    A. Wash your hands each time you remove the gloves
    B. Make sure the gloves have powder inside
    C. Wear latex-free gloves
    D. Never wear any gloves
60. When you wear a gown for isolation precautions, the contaminated areas are
    A. The ties at the neck and waist
    B. The gown front and sleeves
    C. The gown back and sleeves
    D. Only the areas that touch the patient
61. When you remove gown and gloves worn for isolation precautions, what step is done first?
    A. Untie the neck and waist strings
    B. Remove and discard your gloves
    C. Turn the gown inside out as it is removed
    D. Pull the gown down from each shoulder toward the same hand
62. A gown is worn when entering a room
    A. Isolated for airborne precautions
    B. Isolated for droplet precautions
    C. Isolated for standard precautions
    D. Depending on what tasks, procedures, and care measures you will do

63. Which of these statements about wearing gloves is *true*?
    A. The inside of the glove is contaminated.
    B. Slightly used gloves can be saved and reused.
    C. You may need more than one pair of gloves for a task.
    D. Gloves are easier to put on when hands are damp.
64. When removing gloves
    A. Make sure that glove touches only glove
    B. Pull the gloves off by the fingers
    C. Reach inside the glove with the gloved hand to pull it off
    D. Hold the discarded gloves tightly in your ungloved hand.
65. When removing a mask, only the ties or elastic bands are touched because
    A. The front of the mask is contaminated
    B. The front of the mask is sterile
    C. Your gloves are contaminated
    D. Your hands are contaminated
66. When donning a gown which of these is done first?
    A. Tie the strings at the back of the neck
    B. Tie the waist strings at the back
    C. Put on the gloves
    D. It doesn't matter
67. When removing protective apparel which of these is done first?
    A. Remove the face mask
    B. Remove and discard the gloves
    C. Remove the gown
    D. Untie the waist strings of the gown
68. If you wear reusable eyewear and it is contaminated
    A. It should be discarded
    B. It should be autoclaved
    C. Wash it with soap and water and then a disinfectant
    D. Rinse it in cool running water
69. How are contaminated items identified when sent to the laundry or trash collection?
    A. Bags are transparent so materials are visible
    B. Labeled as "contaminated"
    C. Always are double-bagged
    D. Labeled with BIOHAZARD symbol
70. How are specimens collected in a contaminated room handled?
    A. Place specimen container in a BIOHAZARD specimen bag
    B. It depends on center policy
    C. Testing must be done in the room
    D. Special containers are needed
71. If a resident in isolation precautions must be transported to another area, all of these would be done *except*
    A. The person wears a mask as required by the Transmission-Based Precautions used
    B. The staff wears gown, mask, and gloves as required
    C. The staff is the receiving area is alerted so they can wear protective equipment as needed
    D. The wheelchair or stretcher is disinfected after use

72. When a child is in isolation, it may be helpful if
    A. Favorite toys or blankets are brought from home
    B. Personal protective equipment is put on before entering the room
    C. The child is given a mask, eyewear, and a gown to touch and play with
    D. You avoid the room so you do not upset the child
73. You can help a person with poor vision, confusion, or dementia to tolerate isolation by
    A. Putting on personal protective equipment outside the room
    B. Keeping the door open so they can see people in the hall
    C. Letting the person see your face and state your name and what you are doing.
    D. Not wearing a mask when in the room
74. A person placed in Airborne Precautions may have
    A. Meningitis, pneumonia, or influenza
    B. A wound infection.
    C. Mumps, rubella, or pertussis
    D. Measles, chickenpox, or tuberculosis
75. When the person has Airborne Precautions, you do *not* need to wear a mask when
    A. They no longer have skin lesions
    B. You are transporting the person
    C. They are not sneezing or coughing
    D. The skin lesions are covered
76. When contact precautions are being used, gloves are worn when
    A. Entering the room
    B. Touching the person's intact skin
    C. Touching surfaces or items near the person
    D. All of the above
77. What viruses are bloodborne pathogens?
    A. Influenza and pneumococcus
    B. Measles and chickenpox
    C. AIDS (HIV) and hepatitis B (HBV)
    D. Staphylococcus and streptococcus
78. Which of these can transmit bloodborne pathogens?
    A. Body fluid that is visibly contaminated with blood
    B. Dressings soaked with body fluids
    C. Used needles and suction equipment
    D. All of the above
79. How do staff members know what to do if exposed to a bloodborne pathogen?
    A. Training is provided upon employment and yearly by employers
    B. Information is provided on the Internet
    C. They may attend classes offered at colleges or hospitals
    D. The nurse tells them what they need to know
80. The hepatitis B vaccine (HBV)
    A. Only requires 1 vaccination
    B. Must be given every year
    C. Involves 3 injections
    D. Is required by law

81. Which of these is *not* a correct work practice control to reduce exposure risks?
    A. Discard contaminated needles and sharp instruments in containers that are closable, puncture-resistant, and leakproof.
    B. Do not store food or drinks where blood or potential infectious materials are kept.
    C. Break contaminated needles before discarding.
    D. Wash hands after removing gloves.
82. Personal protective equipment
    A. Is free to staff
    B. Is purchased by staff members
    C. Must be worn by all employees instead of regular uniforms
    D. Is paid for by deducting the cost from the employee's paycheck
83. Broken glass is cleaned up by
    A. Picking it up carefully with gloved hands
    B. Using a brush and dustpan or tongs
    C. A person especially trained to remove biohazardous materials
    D. Wiping it up with wet paper towels
84. When discarding regulated waste, the containers are
    A. Plastic bags that are specially labeled
    B. Labeled as "contaminated" in red letters
    C. Melt-away bags
    D. Closable, puncture-resistant, leak-proof and labeled with the BIOHAZARD symbol
85. If you are working in a home and need to dispose of sharps, you may need to
    A. Place needles, syringes, and other sharp items into hard plastic containers
    B. Take them with you at the end of each shift
    C. Place them in a plastic bag labeled with the BIOHAZARD symbol
    D. Discard with the regular trash each day
86. If an exposure incident occurs
    A. Report it at once
    B. You can have free medical evaluation and follow-up
    C. You will receive a written opinion of the medical evaluation
    D. All of the above.
87. If a sterile item touches a clean item
    A. It can still be used
    B. It is contaminated
    C. It should be handled with sterile gloves
    D. It can be placed on the sterile field
88. When working with a sterile field you should
    A. Always wear a mask
    B. Keep items within your vision and above your waist
    C. Keep the door open
    D. Wear clean gloves

89. When arranging the inner package of sterile gloves
    A. Have the right glove on the left and left glove on the right
    B. Have the fingers pointing toward you
    C. Have the right glove on the right and left glove on the left
    D. Straighten the gloves to remove the cuff
90. When picking up the first glove
    A. Grasp it by the cuff only touching the inside
    B. Reach under the cuff with your fingers
    C. Grasp the edge of the cuff with your hand
    D. Slide your hand into the glove without touching it with the other hand

Matching

Match the kind of asepsis being used in questions 91–97.
    A. Medical asepsis (clean technique)
    B. Surgical asepsis (sterile technique)

91. _____ An item is placed in an autoclave.
92. _____ Each person has his or her own toothbrush, towel, washcloth, and other personal care items.
93. _____ Hands are washed before preparing food.
94. _____ Contaminated items are boiled in water for 15 minutes.
95. _____ Single-use or multi-use disposable items reduce the spread of infection.
96. _____ Liquid or gas chemicals are used to destroy microbes.
97. _____ Hands are washed every time you use the bathroom.

Match the aseptic measures used to control the related chain of infection with the step in the chain in questions 98–110.
    A. Reservoir (host)   D. Portal of entry
    B. Portal of exit   E. Susceptible host
    C. Method of transmission

98. _____ Provide the person with tissues to use when coughing or sneezing.
99. _____ Make sure linens are dry and wrinkle-free to protect the skin.
100. _____ Use leakproof plastic bags for soiled tissues, linens, and other materials.
101. _____ Wear personal protective equipment.
102. _____ Hold equipment and linens away from your uniform.
103. _____ Assist with cleaning or clean the genital area after elimination.
104. _____ Clean from cleanest area to the dirtiest.
105. _____ Label bottles with person's name and date it was opened.
106. _____ Follow the care plan to meet the person's nutritional and fluid needs.
107. _____ Make sure drainage tubes are properly connected.
108. _____ Do not use items that are on the floor.
109. _____ Assist the person with cough and deep breathing exercises as directed.
110. _____ Avoid sitting on a person's bed. You will pick up microorganisms and transfer them.

Match the practices with the correct principles for surgical asepsis in questions 111–119.
    A. A sterile item can only touch another sterile item.
    B. Sterile items or a sterile field are always kept within your vision and above your waist.
    C. Airborne microbes can contaminate sterile items or a sterile field.
    D. Fluid flows down, in the direction of gravity.
    E. The sterile field is kept dry, unless the area below it is sterile.
    F. The edges of a sterile field are contaminated.
    G. Honesty is essential to sterile technique.

111. _____ Consider any item as contaminated if it touches a clean item.
112. _____ Wear a mask if you need to talk during the procedure.
113. _____ Place all sterile items inside the 1-inch margin of the sterile field.
114. _____ Do not turn your back on a sterile field.
115. _____ Prevent drafts by closing the door and avoiding extra movements.
116. _____ Avoid spilling and splashing when pouring sterile fluids into sterile containers.
117. _____ If you cannot see an item, it is contaminated.
118. _____ You report to the nurse that you contaminated an item or a field.
119. _____ Hold wet items down.

Fill in the Blank

120. Write out the meaning of the abbreviations.
    A. AIDS _____
    B. AIIR _____
    C. CDC _____
    D. EPA _____
    E. HAI _____
    F. HBV _____
    G. HIV _____
    H. MDRO _____
    I. MSDS _____
    J. MRSA _____
    K. OPIM _____
    L. OSHA _____
    M. PPE _____
    N. SARS _____
    O. TB _____
    P. VRE _____

Use Focus on PRIDE in the Textbook to complete questions 121–122.

121. You show personal and professional responsibility when you prevent infections by

A. Practicing good hand hygiene _____ and _____ giving care

B. Removing items that become _____

C. Not using a _____

D. Being honest with _____

122. If delegated care of a person at increased risk for infection, you must

A. _____

B. _____

C. _____

D. _____

E. _____

F. _____

G. _____

H. _____

I. _____

J. _____

Labeling

123. The figure shows how to remove gloves. List the steps of the procedure shown in each drawing.

A.

(1) _____

(2) _____

B.

(1) _____

C.

(1) _____

(2) _____

D.

(1) _____

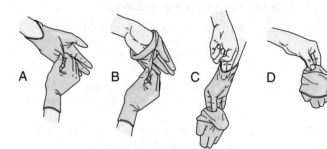

A   B   C   D

Crossword

Fill in the following crossword by answering the clues with the words from this list:

Asepsis	Fungi	Isolation	PPE	Sharps
Autoclave	HBV	OPIM	Protozoa	Sterilize
Bacteria	HIV	Parenteral	Rickettsiae	Viruses

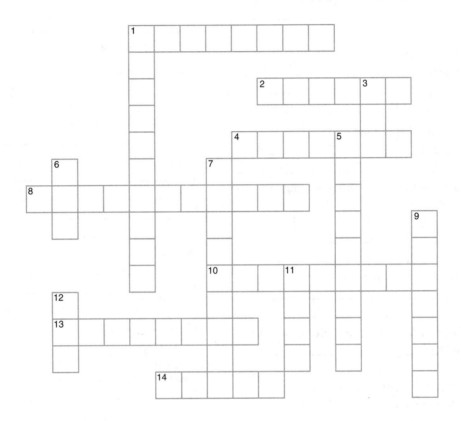

Across

1. One-celled animals; can infect the blood, brain, intestines, and other body areas
2. Any object, such as needles, scalpels, broken glass, and broken capillary tubes, that can penetrate the skin
4. Grows in living cells; causes many diseases such as the common cold, herpes, and hepatitis
8. Found in fleas, lice, ticks, and other insects; spread to humans by insect bites
10. A pressure-steam sterilizer
13. Plant life that multiplies rapidly; germs
14. Plants that live on other plants or animals; can infect the mouth, vagina, skin, feet, and other body areas

Down

1. Piercing mucous membranes or the skin barrier through such events as needle-sticks, human bites, cuts, and abrasions
3. Clothing or equipment worn by an employee for protection against a hazard
5. The use of physical or chemical procedure designed to destroy all microbial life, including highly resistant bacterial spores
6. Human immunodeficiency virus
7. Barriers that prevent the escape of pathogens to other areas; usually this area is the person's room
9. Being free of disease-producing microbes
11. Other potentially infectious materials; human body fluids, any tissue or organ from a human, HIV-containing cell or tissue cultures
12. Hepatitis B virus

Optional Learning Exercises

124. Compare medical asepsis to surgical asepsis.

A. Medical asepsis is _____

_____

_____.

B. Surgical asepsis is _____.

_____

_____

125. Why are hands and forearms kept lower than elbows in hand washing? _____

_____

_____

126. Why is lotion applied after hand washing?

_____

_____

_____

127. When are the following worn when practicing Standard Precautions

A. Gloves

_____

_____

B. Masks, eye protections, and face shields

_____

_____

128. If a person has measles and you are susceptible, what should you do? _____

_____

129. If a person is in Airborne Precautions and must leave the room, the person must wear a

_____

130. When you wear gloves, you protect yourself and the person.

A. They protect you from _____

_____

B. They protect the person from _____.

131. Why is the gown turned inside out as you remove it?

_____

_____

132. Why is a moist mask or gown changed?

_____

_____

133. What basic needs may not be met when a person is in isolation? _____

_____

134. What information is included in training about Bloodborne Pathogens?

A. _____

B. _____

C. _____

D. _____

E. _____

F. _____

G. _____

H. _____

I. _____

J. _____

135. OSHA requires these measures for safely handling and using personal protective equipment.

A. _____

_____

B. _____

_____

C. _____

_____

D. _____

_____

E. _____

_____

F. _____

_____

G. _____

_____

H. _____

_____

136. If you are asked to assist with a sterile procedure, what information do you need before beginning?

A. _____

B. _____

C. _____

D. _____

E. _____

F. _____

Independent Learning Activities

Hand washing practices are important to use wherever you are to prevent the spread of infection. Use this exercise to make yourself aware of your own habits.

- Make a list of when you washed your hands for one day.
  - How did you wash your hands? Did you use the method taught in the chapter?
  - How many times did you wash your hands at work? At home?
  - How many times did you realize you had forgotten to wash your hands? What was the reason you forgot?
- How can you improve your hand washing practices? What will you change after studying this chapter?

16 Body Mechanics

Fill in the Blank: Key Terms

Base of support
Body alignment
Body mechanics

Dorsal recumbent
   position
Ergonomics

Fowler's position
Lateral position
Posture

Prone position
Semi-prone side
   position

Side-lying position
Sims' position
Supine position

1. Another name for the lateral position is

   _____.

2. The way in which the head, trunk, arms, and legs are aligned with one another is _____ or posture.

3. The _____ is also called the side-lying position.

4. The _____ is the same as the back-lying or supine position.

5. The area on which an object rests is the

   _____.

6. _____ is a left side-lying position in which the upper leg is sharply flexed so that it is not on the lower leg and the lower arm is behind the person.

7. A semi-sitting position with the head of the bed elevated 45 to 60 degrees is

   _____.

8. Lying on the abdomen with the head turned to one side is _____

9. _____ is using the body in an efficient and careful way.

10. The back-lying or dorsal recumbent position is also called the _____

11. _____ or body alignment is the way in which body parts are aligned with one another.

12. _____ is the science of designing the job to fit the worker.

13. Another name for the Sims' position is

   _____.

Circle the Best Answer

14. Using good body mechanics will
    A. Prevent good posture
    B. Cause back injuries
    C. Reduce the risk of injury
    D. Cause muscle injury

15. For a wider base of support and balance
    A. Keep your feet close together
    B. The head, trunk, arms, and legs are aligned with one another
    C. Stand with your feet apart
    D. Make sure you are in good physical condition

16. When you bend your knees and squat to lift a heavy object, you are
    A. Using good body alignment
    B. In danger of injury
    C. Likely to strain your back
    D. Using good body mechanics

17. If you need to move a heavy object
    A. Push, slide, or pull the object
    B. Get help from a co-worker
    C. Bend your hips and knees to lift from the floor
    D. All of the above

18. Work-related musculoskeletal disorders (MSDs) are a risk
    A. When the worker does not exercise regularly
    B. When the worker is small and weak
    C. When force or repeating action is used when moving persons
    D. Only when the staff member is using poor body mechanics

19. If you have pain when standing or rising from a seated position you
    A. May have a back injury
    B. Are using poor body mechanics
    C. Have worked too many hours
    D. Should exercise more

20. According to the Occupational Safety and Health Administration (OSHA), which of these is *not* a factor that can lead to back disorders?
    A. Reaching while lifting
    B. Getting help when lifting or moving heavy objects
    C. Bending while lifting
    D. Lifting with forceful movement

21. Which of these activities will help to prevent back injury?
    A. Reach across the bed to give care
    B. Bend at the waist to pick up an object from the floor
    C. Lift an object above your shoulder
    D. Keep objects close to your body when you lift, move, or carry

22. Regular position changes and good alignment
    A. Cause pressure ulcers and contractures
    B. Promote comfort and well-being
    C. Interrupt rest and sleep
    D. Decrease circulation
23. A resident who depends on the nursing team for position changes needs to be positioned
    A. At least every 2 hours
    B. Once an hour
    C. Every 15 minutes
    D. Once a shift
24. Linens need to be clean, dry, and wrinkle-free to help prevent
    A. Pressure ulcers
    B. Contractures
    C. Breathing problems
    D. Frequent repositioning
25. Persons with heart and respiratory disorders usually can breathe more easily in the
    A. Fowler's position
    B. Semi-Fowler's position
    C. Supine position
    D. Prone position
26. Most older persons have limited range of motion in their necks and so do *not* tolerate
    A. Lateral position
    B. Sims' position
    C. Fowler's position
    D. Prone position
27. When positioning a person in the supine position, the nurse may ask you to place a pillow under the person's lower legs to
    A. Improve the circulation
    B. Assist the person to breathe easier
    C. Prevent the heels from rubbing on the sheets
    D. To prevent swelling of the legs and feet
28. A small pillow is positioned against the person's back in the
    A. Lateral position
    B. Prone position position
    C. Supine position
    D. Semi-Fowler's
29. When a person cannot keep their upper bodies erect in a chair,
    A. A vest restraint may be used
    B. Postural supports help keep them in good alignment
    C. A geriatric chair with a tray will be used
    D. A belt restraint can be applied
30. In the chair position, a pillow is *not* used
    A. To position paralyzed arms
    B. To support the feet
    C. Under the upper arm and hand
    D. Behind the back if restraints are used

Fill in the Blank

31. Write out the abbreviations
    A. MSD _____
    B. OSHA _____
32. Where are strong, large muscles located that are used to lift and move heavy objects?
    A. _____
    B. _____
    C. _____
    D. _____

33. Back injuries are a major risk when lifting. For good body mechanics you should
    A. Bend _____
    B. Hold _____
34. Describe these risk factors for musculoskeletal disorders (MSDs) in nursing centers
    A. Force _____
    B. Repeating action _____
    C. Awkward postures _____
    D. Heavy lifting _____
35. Early signs and symptoms of MSDs are
    _____
    _____
36. What nursing tasks are known to be high risk for MSDs?
    A. _____
    B. _____
    C. _____
    D. _____
    E. _____
    F. _____
    G. _____
    H. _____
    I. _____
    J. _____
    K. _____
    L. _____
    M. _____
    N. _____
    O. _____
    P. _____
    Q. _____
37. Instructions to reposition a person are received from the _____ and the _____
    _____.
38. If you are delegated the task to position the person, what information do you need?
    A. _____
    B. _____
    C. _____
    D. _____
    E. _____
    F. _____
    G. _____
    H. _____
    I. _____
    J. _____
    K. _____

List the measures needed for good alignment for each position in questions 39–44.

39. What measures are needed for good alignment when the person is in Fowler's position?

    A. _____
    B. _____
    C. _____

40. For supine position?

    A. _____
    B. _____
    C. _____

41. For prone position?

    A. _____
    B. _____
    C. _____

42. For lateral position?

    A. _____
    B. _____
    C. _____
    D. _____
    E. _____
    F. _____

43. For Sims' position?

    A. _____
    B. _____
    C. _____
    D. _____

44. For chair position?

    A. _____
    B. _____
    C. _____

Use Focus on PRIDE in the Textbook to complete questions 45–46.

45. You take responsibility for protecting yourself from harm when moving patients. Some risks for injury are

    A. _____
    B. _____
    C. _____
    D. _____
    E. _____
    F. _____
    G. _____
    H. _____

46. How can you promote comfort, independence and social interaction for a person you are caring for?

    A. _____
    B. _____
    C. _____
    D. _____

Labeling

47. Label the positions in each of the drawings.

A. _____

B. _____

C. _____

D. _____

E. _____

F. _____

Optional Learning Exercises

48. According to OSHA, certain activities can lead to back injuries. Read the examples and list the activity that could cause a back injury in each one. *(listed in Textbook)*

   A. The nursing assistant does not raise the level of the bed when changing linens. _____

   B. While you are walking with Mr. Smith he slips and starts to fall. _____

   C. Mrs. Tippett slides down in bed and looks uncomfortable. _____

   _____

   D. You assist Mrs. Miller to use the toilet in her small bathroom. _____

   E. Mr. Thomas is confused and often hits you when being moved. _____

   F. You lean across the bed to hold the person while the nurse washes his back. _____

   _____

49. Regular position changes and good alignment promote

   A. _____

   B. _____

   C. _____

   D. _____

   It prevents

   E. _____

   F. _____

50. _____, _____, and _____ help prevent contractures.

Independent Learning Activities

After learning about using good body mechanics in this chapter, think about how well you practice body mechanics in your daily life and answer these questions.

- How much do the books you carry with you each day weigh? How do you carry them? When carrying them, where is your base of support? Is your body in good alignment?
- Do you have small children that you pick up? How do you lift them? What methods listed in the chapter do you use?
- When carrying groceries into the house, do you carry them held close to the body? How well are you using good body mechanics?
- At the end of the day, how do you feel? How could using good body mechanics help you to avoid any discomfort?

17 Safely Moving and Transferring the Person

Fill in the Blank: Key Terms

Friction   Shearing
Logrolling   Transfer

1. _____ occurs when skin sticks to a surface and muscles slide in the direction the body is moving.

2. Moving a person from one place to another is a _____.

3. The rubbing of one surface against another is _____

4. Turning the person as a unit, in alignment, with one motion is _____.

Circle the Best Answer

5. To prevent injuries when moving older persons
   A. Move the person without help
   B. Grab the person under the arms
   C. Allow the person to move himself or herself
   D. Move the person carefully to prevent injury or pain

6. When moving a person up in bed, prevent hitting the head-board with the head by
   A. Keeping the person in good body alignment
   B. Placing the pillow upright against the headboard
   C. Placing your hand on the person's head
   D. Asking the person to bend his or her neck forward

7. When moving residents it is best if you move the person
   A. By yourself
   B. With at least 2 staff members
   C. Using a mechanical lift
   D. Only with staff members that you like

8. To prevent work-related injuries, OSHA recommends that
   A. Manual lifting be minimized or eliminated when possible
   B. Manual lifting be used at all times
   C. Never lift any person or object alone
   D. Always use mechanical lifts for any lifting

9. Which of these would *not* be correct when you are using manual lifting?
   A. Try to keep what you are moving close to you
   B. Stand with your feet close together
   C. Lift on the "count of 3" when working with others
   D. Move the person toward you, not away from you

10. To make lateral transfers safe for the staff members
    A. Make sure bed rails are up
    B. Never use drawsheets, turning pads, or other devices to assist in the move
    C. Adjust surfaces so they are at about waist height
    D. Reach across the bed or stretcher to transfer the person

11. When the person can bear some weight, can sit up with help, and may be able to pivot to transfer, you know that the person's level of dependence is
    A. Code 4   C. Code 2
    B. Code 3   D. Code 1

12. Why are beds raised to move persons in bed?
    A. It prevents the person from falling out of bed
    B. It reduces friction and shearing
    C. It prevents pulling on drainage tubes
    D. It reduces bending and reaching for staff members

13. How can you reduce friction and shearing?
    A. Raise the head of the bed to a sitting position before moving the person
    B. Roll or lift the person to reposition
    C. Pull the person up in bed by grasping under the arms
    D. Massage the skin

14. If a person with dementia resists being moved, you should
    A. Move the person by yourself
    B. Proceed slowly and use a calm, pleasant voice
    C. Let the person alone and do not reposition him
    D. Tell the person firmly that he must cooperate to be moved

15. When you are delegated to move a person in bed, you need to know all of these *except*
    A. What equipment is needed
    B. Whether the person is awake
    C. How many workers are needed to safely move the person
    D. Any limits in the person's ability to move or be repositioned

16. When raising a person's head and shoulders
    A. It is best to have help with an older person to prevent pain and injury
    B. A mechanical lift should be used
    C. You can always do this alone
    D. A transfer belt will be needed

17. In order to correctly raise the head and shoulders
    A. Both of your hands are placed under the person's back
    B. The person puts his near arm under your near arm and behind your shoulder
    C. Use a lift sheet to raise the person up
    D. Your free arm rests on the edge of the bed
18. You may move a person up in bed alone if the
    A. Person can assist using a trapeze
    B. Rest of the staff is busy and cannot help
    C. Nurse tells you to use a lift sheet or slide sheet
    D. Nurse tells you have to move the person alone
19. What is the position of the bed when you are moving a person up in bed?
    A. Fowler's
    B. Flat
    C. As flat as possible for the person's condition
    D. Semi-Fowler's
20. The person is moved
    A. On the "count of 3"
    B. On the "count of 2"
    C. When the person says he is ready
    D. As soon as the workers are all in position
21. An assist device such as a lift sheet is used for
    A. A person who weighs less than 200 pounds
    B. A person who weighs more than 200 pounds
    C. A person with a dependence level of Code 4: Total Dependence
    D. All of the above
22. Where is the lift sheet positioned?
    A. Under the head and shoulders
    B. Under the buttocks
    C. From the head to above the knees or lower
    D. From the hips to below the knees
23. When using a lift sheet as an assist device, the workers should
    A. Roll the sheet up close to the person
    B. Grasp the sheet at the edges
    C. Move one side of the sheet at a time
    D. Grasp the sheet only at the top edge
24. A person is moved to the side of the bed before turning because
    A. Otherwise, after turning, the person lies on the side of the bed
    B. It makes it easier to turn the person
    C. It prevents injury to the person
    D. It prevents friction and shearing
25. When you move a person in segments, which of these is *incorrect*?
    A. First place your arms under the person's neck and shoulders and grasp the far shoulder
    B. First move the hips and legs
    C. Move the center part of the body by placing one arm under the waist and one under the thighs
    D. Rock backward and shift your weight to your rear leg when moving the upper part of the body
26. When using a drawsheet to move a person to the side of the bed, support the person's
    A. Back   C. Head
    B. Knees   D. Hips

27. After the person is turned,
    A. Give the person good personal care
    B. Position him or her in good body alignment
    C. Elevate the head of the bed
    D. Elevate the bed to its highest position
28. When delegated to turn a person, you need all of this information from the nurse and care plan *except*
    A. How much help the person needs
    B. Which procedure to use
    C. Whether the doctor has ordered turning
    D. What supportive devices are needed for positioning
29. When you have completed turning a person in bed, he or she should
    A. Have the back against the bed rail
    B. Have his or her face near the bed rail
    C. Be positioned in good body alignment
    D. Lay flat on the mattress without any supportive pillows
30. When a person is turned, musculoskeletal injuries, skin breakdown, and pressure ulcers could occur if a person is *not* in
    A. A special bed
    B. Good body alignment
    C. Good body mechanics
    D. The middle of the bed
31. How do you decide whether to turn the person toward you or away from you?
    A. Check the doctor's order
    B. It depends on the person's condition and the situation
    C. Use the method you like best
    D. Ask the person which way is best
32. Why do you need 2 or 3 staff members to logroll a person?
    A. A person who is being logrolled is usually in pain
    B. It is important to keep the spine straight and in alignment
    C. The person is probably a Code 4 level of dependence and needs extra help
    D. No assistive devices are used when you logroll
33. When preparing to logroll a person, place a pillow
    A. At the head of the bed
    B. Between the knees
    C. Under the head
    D. Under the shoulders
34. What information do you need before dangling a person?
    A. The person's diagnosis
    B. When the person ate last
    C. The person's dependence level
    D. Whether the person likes to dangle
35. What should you do if a person who is dangling becomes faint or dizzy?
    A. Lay the person down
    B. Go and report this to the nurse
    C. Tell the person to take deep breaths
    D. Have the person move his or her legs back and forth in circles

36. When preparing to dangle a person, the head of the bed should be
    A. Flat
    B. Slightly raised
    C. In a sitting position
    D. At a comfortable height for the person
37. When preparing to transfer a person, you should
    A. Arrange the room so there is enough space for a safe transfer
    B. Keep furniture in the position the resident likes
    C. Remove all furniture from the room
    D. Ask the person how to arrange the furniture
38. The person being transferred should wear non-skid footwear to
    A. Protect the person from falls
    B. Allow the person to bend the feet more easily
    C. Promote comfort for the person
    D. Keep the feet warm
39. Lock the bed, wheelchair, or assist device wheels when transferring to
    A. Help the staff use good body mechanics
    B. Prevent damage to the equipment being used
    C. Prevent the bed and the device from moving during the transfer
    D. Make sure the person is kept in good body alignment
40. When a person is transferring to a chair or wheelchair help the person of out of bed on
    A. The right side of the bed
    B. His or her strong side
    C. His or her weak side
    D. The side of the bed that is most convenient for the staff
41. If *not* using a mechanical lift, which of these is the preferred method for chair or wheelchair transfers?
    A. Use a gait/transfer belt
    B. Have the person put his or her arms around your neck
    C. Put your arms around the person and the grasp the shoulder blades
    D. Have the person use a trapeze
42. When a person is seated in a wheelchair, you can increase the person's comfort by
    A. Placing pillows around the person
    B. Making sure nothing covers the vinyl seat and back
    C. Cover the back and seat with a folded bath blanket
    D. Removing any cushions or positioning devices
43. When you transfer a person, the nurse may ask you to take and report the _____ before and after the transfer.
    A. Blood pressure   C. Respirations
    B. Pulse rate   D. Temperature
44. When using a transfer belt you can prevent the person from sliding or falling by
    A. Bracing your knees against the person's knees
    B. Use the knee and foot of one leg to block the person's weak leg or foot
    C. Straddle your legs around the person's weak leg
    D. All of the above

45. A transfer belt must be used for a transfer *unless*
    A. The doctor has written an order that states no belt is needed
    B. You are directed by the nurse and care plan to transfer without a belt
    C. The person asks you not to use the belt
    D. You feel safer moving the person without the belt
46. When you are transferring a person back to bed from a chair or wheelchair, the person should be positioned
    A. With the weak side near the bed
    B. With the strong side near the bed
    C. With the chair in the same position as it was when the person got out of bed
    D. Where you have the most space to work
47. A mechanical sling is used
    A. For all persons regardless of the level of dependence
    B. For persons who are too heavy for the staff to transfer
    C. When staff members prefer to use them instead of manually lifting
    D. Only when ordered by the doctor
48. When you are delegated to use a mechanical lift, you need to know
    A. The person's dependency level
    B. What sling to use
    C. How many staff members are needed to perform the task safely
    D. All of the above
49. As a person is lifted in the sling of the mechanical lift, the person
    A. May hold the swivel bar
    B. May hold the straps or chains
    C. Crosses the arms across the chest
    D. Should keep the legs outstretched
50. When transferring a person from a wheelchair to the toilet
    A. The toilet should have a raised seat
    B. The toilet seat should be removed
    C. Always position the wheelchair next to the toilet
    D. Unlock the wheelchair to allow movement during the transfer
51. A sliding board may be used to transfer a person from a wheelchair to a toilet if
    A. The person can stand and pivot
    B. There is enough room to position the wheelchair next to the toilet
    C. The staff member does not want to use a transfer belt
    D. The person has lower body strength
52. When moving a person who weighs more than 200 pounds to a stretcher, OSHA recommends
    A. Use a lateral sliding aid and 2 staff members
    B. Use a lateral sliding aid and 3 staff members
    C. Use a lateral sliding aid or a friction-reducing device and 2 staff members
    D. Use a drawsheet, turning pad, or a large incontinence underpad

53. During transport on the stretcher, the person is moved feet first so
    A. The staff member at the foot can clear the pathway
    B. The staff member at the head can watch the person's breathing and color
    C. The person can see where he or she is going
    D. The person does not become disoriented

54. It is important to reposition a person sitting in a chair or wheelchair
    A. For good alignment and safety
    B. To make sure the back and buttocks are against the back of the chair
    C. Because some persons cannot move and reposition him or herself
    D. All of the above

Fill in the Blank

55. To prevent injuries in older persons with fragile bones and joints, what safety measures need to be used?
    A. _____
    B. _____
    C. _____
    D. _____
    E. _____
    F. _____

56. To promote mental comfort when handling, moving, or transferring the person, you should
    A. _____
    _____
    B. _____
    _____

57. To promote physical comfort when handling, moving, or transferring the person, you should
    A. _____
    _____
    B. _____
    _____
    C. _____
    _____
    D. _____

58. When manual lifting, you use good body mechanics when you
    A. _____
    B. _____
    C. _____
    D. _____
    E. _____

59. To prevent work-related injuries when handling, moving, and transferring, the nurse and health team determine
    A. _____
    B. _____
    C. _____
    D. _____

60. Explain how a person is lifted and transferred for each level of dependence
    A. Code 4: Total Dependence _____
    _____
    _____
    B. Code 3: Extensive Assistance _____
    _____
    _____
    C. Code 2: Limited Assistance _____
    _____
    _____
    D. Code 1: Supervision _____
    _____
    _____
    E. Code 0: Independent _____
    _____
    _____

61. When you move a person in bed, report and record
    A. _____
    B. _____
    C. _____
    D. _____
    E. _____

62. Friction and shearing can be reduced when moving a person in bed by
    A. _____
    B. _____

63. You can sometimes move a person up in bed alone if the person can use a _____.

64. When moving a person up in bed and the person can assist, ask the person to
    A. Grasp the _____
    B. Flex _____
    C. Move on the count of _____

65. What assist devices, other than mechanical lifts, are used to move persons to the side of the bed?
    _____
    _____

66. Why are assist devices used when moving a person to the side of the bed?

    A. Prevent _____ and _____ damage

    B. Prevents injury to the _____

    _____.

67. Before turning and repositioning a person, what information do you need from the nurse and care plan?

    A. _____

    B. _____

    C. _____

    D. _____

    E. _____

    F. _____

    G. _____

    H. _____

    I. _____

      • _____

      • _____

      • _____

      • _____

      • _____

    J. _____

    K. _____

68. After turning and repositioning a person, it is common to place a small pillow under the

    _____.

69. When a person is logrolled, the spine is

    _____.

70. Logrolling is used to turn these persons.

    A. _____

    B. _____

    C. _____

    D. _____

71. When a person is dangling, the circulation can be stimulated by having the person move _____.

72. What observations should be reported and recorded after dangling a person?

    A. _____

    B. _____

    C. _____

    D. _____

    E. _____

    F. _____

    G. _____

    H. _____

73. While a person is dangling, check the person's condition by

    A. Asking _____

    B. Checking _____

    C. Checking _____

    D. Noting _____

74. A person can transfer from the bed to the chair with a stand and pivot transfer if the

    A. _____

    _____

    B. _____

    _____

    C. _____

    _____

75. During a chair or wheelchair transfer, the person must *not* put his or her arms around you neck, because _____

    _____

    _____.

76. Locked wheelchairs may be considered to be restraints if the person _____

    _____

77. When using a transfer belt to transfer a person to a chair or wheelchair, grasp the belt at _____ and from _____

    _____

78. If you transfer a person to a chair without a transfer belt, place your hands _____ and around the person's _____.

79. In what situations would you use the slings listed?

    A. Standard full sling _____

    _____

    B. Extended length sling _____

    _____

    C. Bathing sling _____

    _____

    D. Toileting sling _____

    _____

    E. Amputee sling _____

    _____

    F. Bariatric sling _____

    _____

80. What information do you need when you are delegated to use a mechanical lift?

    A. _____

    B. _____

    C. _____

    D. _____

    E. _____

    F. _____

    G. _____

81. To promote mental comfort when using a mechanical lift, you should explain _____ and show the person _____.

82. A sliding board can be used when transferring a person to and from a toilet if

A. _____

B. _____

C. _____

D. _____

83. If a person weighs more than 200 pounds and is being moved to a stretcher, OSHA recommends the use of one of the following

A. _____

_____

B. _____

_____

C. _____

_____

84. When moving a person with bariatric needs to a stretcher, the nurse and care plan may direct the staff to

A. _____

_____

B. _____

_____

C. _____

_____

D. _____

_____

E. _____

_____

Use Focus on PRIDE in the Textbook to complete questions 85–87.

85. When moving or transferring a person, remember to respect his or her privacy by _____.

86. You provide for safety during transfers when you

A. Use a _____

B. Avoid _____

87. To promote pride and independence while handling, moving, and transferring the person, you should

A. _____

B. _____

C. _____

D. _____

Optional Learning Exercises

88. When planning to move a person, why is it important to know the person's height and weight, dependence level, physical abilities, and medical condition?

_____

_____

89. If you need to move a person with dementia, he or she may resist because he or she may *not*

_____

What measures in the care plan will help you give safe care?

A. _____

B. _____

C. _____

90. It is safe to move a person up in bed alone only if

A. _____

B. _____

C. _____

D. _____

E. _____

F. _____

G. _____

91. What types of pads are *not* strong enough to be used during a lift? _____

_____

For a safe lift, the underpad must

A. _____

B. _____

C. _____

92. How does moving a person to the side of the bed avoid work-related injuries for you?

_____

93. When you are delegated to turn a person, how will you know whether to turn them alone, with help, or by using logrolling? _____

94. When you turn a person and reposition them, what must be done to the bed level before you leave the room? _____

95. When two staff members are logrolling a person without a turning sheet, where does each person place the hands? (Use Figure 17-15A)

A. Staff at head _____

B. Staff at legs _____

96. Why should a person dangle for 1 to 5 minutes before walking or transferring? _____

_____

97. What simple hygiene measures can be performed while the person is dangling? _____

_____

In addition to refreshing the person, what is another benefit this activity will provide?

_____

98. After you are finished using a mechanical lift, what should you do with it that will help teamwork and time management?

A. _____

B. _____

99. If a person cannot assist with the transfer, what method would be safe to use in a bed to chair transfer? _____

_____

100. Why should you know the person's weight before using a mechanical lift? _____

_____

101. What should you do if the mechanical lift available is different than one you have used before?

_____

_____

_____

Independent Learning Activities

Work with classmates and practice the following activities. Each of you should take a turn as the resident.

- Practice moving a person up in bed with and without assist devices. Answer these questions after you have completed this exercise
  - Which method was easier for the worker? For the person being moved?
  - How did you feel when you were being moved? Did anyone explain what was being done?
- Practice transferring a person who is weak on one side to a chair from the bed and then return the person to the bed. Answer the questions after you complete the exercise.
  - As the worker: How did you position the chair? How did the chair position change when you returned the person to bed?
  - As the person: How safe did you feel during the transfer? What could the worker have done to help you feel safe? What else could the staff have done to make you more comfortable?
- Practice logrolling a person with and without a turning sheet. Answer the questions after you have completed the exercise
  - As the worker: How many workers were used to logroll the person? Which method was easier—with or without the turning sheet? How well do you think the workers did with the turns? Did the spine stay straight?
  - As the person: How did you feel—did you understand what was being done? Was the turn smooth or did you feel as if your spine twisted?
- Ask your instructor if you can use a mechanical lift to practice with each other. If the instructor approves this exercise, answer these questions.
  - As the worker: What did you do before beginning the lift? What questions did you ask? What other information should you have gathered before starting?
  - As the person: How did you feel when you were lifted? Did you feel as if you understood what was happening? What other information would have helped make you more comfortable?
- Overall, how will these practices help you as you move residents? What would you do differently now that you have practiced these exercises?

18 The Person's Unit

Fill in the Blank: Key Terms

Fowler's position
Full visual privacy
High Fowler's position

Reverse Trendelenburg's position

Semi-Fowler's position

Trendelenburg's position

1. In _____, the head of the bed is raised 30 degrees, and the knee portion is raised 15 degrees; or the head of the bed is raised 30 degrees.

2. _____ is a semi-sitting position; the head of the bed is raised 45 to 60 degrees.

3. The head of the bed is raised, and the foot of the bed is lowered in _____.

4. In _____, the head of the bed is lowered, and the foot of the bed is raised.

5. The person has the means to be completely free from public view while in bed when they have

_____.

6. _____ is a semi-sitting position with the head of the bed raised 60 to 90 degrees.

Circle the Best Answer

7. When people share a room
   - A. You may rearrange items and furniture in the room as needed
   - B. A resident cannot take or use another person's space
   - C. They may use each other's belongings
   - D. They generally share furniture such as a dresser

8. OBRA and CMS requires that nursing centers maintain a temperature range of
   - A. 68° F to 74° F
   - B. 61° F to 71° F
   - C. 71° F to 81° F
   - D. 78° F to 85° F

9. Older persons and those who are ill
   - A. Need cooler room temperatures
   - B. Need higher room temperatures
   - C. Are insensitive to room temperature changes
   - D. Need a warmer room at night

10. The nursing staff cannot control which factor that affects comfort?
    - A. Illness
    - B. Temperature
    - C. Noise
    - D. Odors

11. You may best protect a person who is sensitive to drafts by
    - A. Putting the person to bed.
    - B. Giving the person a hot shower or bath.
    - C. Offering a lap robe or making sure the person is wearing enough clothing.
    - D. Pulling the privacy curtain around the person.

12. Older persons are sensitive to cold because they
    - A. Have poor circulation and less fatty tissue
    - B. Are often confused about their surroundings
    - C. Are more active
    - D. Are used to wearing heavier clothes

13. If unpleasant odors occur, do all of these *except*
    - A. Use spray deodorizers in all rooms where odors are present
    - B. Provide good personal hygiene for persons
    - C. Change and dispose of soiled linens and clothing
    - D. Empty and clean bedpans, commodes, urinals, and kidney basins promptly

14. Noises in a health care agency may keep a person from meeting the need for
    - A. Love and belonging
    - B. Self-esteem
    - C. Rest
    - D. Safety and security

15. Which of these measures will *not* reduce noises in a health care agency?
    - A. Have drapes in rooms
    - B. Use metal equipment
    - C. Answer telephone promptly
    - D. Keep equipment in good working order

16. Bright lighting is helpful for all of these *except*
    - A. Persons with poor vision
    - B. Helping the staff to perform procedures
    - C. Making the room more cheerful
    - D. Helping persons to rest and relax

17. Beds are kept at the lowest horizontal position to
    - A. Give care
    - B. Let the person get out of bed with ease
    - C. Transfer persons to a stretcher
    - D. Maintain good body alignment

18. Cranks on manual beds are kept down when not in use to
    - A. Prevent persons from operating the bed.
    - B. Prevent anyone walking past the crank from bumping into it
    - C. Keep the bed in the correct position
    - D. Make sure they are ready to use at all times

19. How can the staff prevent a person from adjusting an electric bed to unsafe positions?
    - A. Lock the bed into a position.
    - B. Unplug the bed.
    - C. Put the person in a bed that cannot be repositioned.
    - D. Keep reminding the person not to change the position.
20. What bed position raises the head of the bed and the knee portion?
    - A. Fowler's
    - B. Semi-Fowler's
    - C. Trendelenburg's
    - D. Reverse Trendelenburg's
21. The bed wheels are locked
    - A. Only when giving care
    - B. When the person is not using bed rails
    - C. At all times except when moving the bed
    - D. When the person requests it
22. Hospital bed entrapment can occur with persons who are
    - A. Alert and oriented
    - B. Able to move easily in bed independently
    - C. Older, frail, and confused
    - D. Are large in size
23. A person who weighs 600 pounds will need
    - A. An electric bed
    - B. A manual bed
    - C. A bariatric bed
    - D. Bedrails
24. Hospital bed entrapment zone 4 is between
    - A. The top of the compressed mattress and the bottom of the bed rail and at the end of the bed rail
    - B. The split bed rails
    - C. The top of the compressed mattress and the bottom of the bed rail and between the rail supports
    - D. The bed rail and the mattress
25. A child can become entrapped in a crib if the
    - A. Mattress is larger than the crib
    - B. Mattress is smaller than the crib
    - C. Mattress is too soft
    - D. Bumper pad does not fit correctly
26. What items are never placed on the overbed table?
    - A. Meals
    - B. Personal care items
    - C. Writing and reading materials
    - D. Bedpans, urinals, and soiled linens
27. Where are the bedpan and urinal kept in the bedside stand?
    - A. Wherever the person wants
    - B. On the top shelf
    - C. On the bottom shelf or in the lower drawer
    - D. In the top drawer
28. Why are privacy curtains used?
    - A. To block sounds and voices from others in the room
    - B. To provide privacy for the person
    - C. To confine the person
    - D. To keep the area sterile

29. Full visual privacy as required by OBRA and CMS can be achieved by
    - A. Closing a privacy curtain
    - B. Placing a moveable screen around the person
    - C. Closing the door in a private room
    - D. All of the above
30. Personal care items
    - A. May be supplied by the agency
    - B. Must be supplied by the person
    - C. Are supplied when ordered by the doctor
    - D. Cannot be brought into the agency by the person
31. When the person is weak on the left side, the signal light is
    - A. Placed on the left side
    - B. Removed from the room
    - C. Placed on the right side
    - D. Replaced by an intercom
32. If a confused person cannot use a signal light
    - A. Explain often how to use the signal light
    - B. Use an intercom instead
    - C. Remove the signal light
    - D. Check the person often to make sure needs are met
33. When a person turns on a signal light, who should answer it?
    - A. Only the person assigned to give care to the person
    - B. Any nursing team member who is available should answer and assist the person as needed
    - C. The charge nurse
    - D. Another team member may answer, but is not expected to give any care
34. Elevated toilet seats
    - A. Help persons with joint problems
    - B. Make wheelchair transfers more difficult
    - C. Help if you transfer the person with a mechanical lift
    - D. Are used if the person is very tall
35. When a person uses a bathroom signal light
    - A. It flashes above the room door and at the nurse's station
    - B. It makes the same sound as the room signal light
    - C. It activates the intercom
    - D. Flashes a different color than the room signal light
36. Closet and drawer space
    - A. Is shared by persons in a room with more than one person.
    - B. Can be cleaned out by a staff member.
    - C. Can be searched without the person's permission.
    - D. Must give the person free access to the closet and drawers
37. Which of these is *not* a responsibility when maintaining the person's unit?
    - A. Throw away extra papers and other items that may clutter the room.
    - B. Arrange personal items as the person prefers.
    - C. Empty the wastebasket as least once a day.
    - D. Explain the causes of strange noises.

Fill in the Blank

38. Write out the abbreviations.
    A. CMS _____
    B. CNA _____
    C. F _____
    D. FDA _____
    E. IV _____
    F. OBRA _____

39. If you smoke, before giving care, you should
    A. _____
    B. _____
    C. _____

40. According to the CMS, a "comfortable" sound level
    A. _____
    B. _____
    C. _____

41. According to CMS, comfortable lighting
    A. _____
    B. _____
    _____ .
    C. _____
    _____

42. Describe each hospital bed system entrapment zone.
    A. Zone 1 _____
    B. Zone 2 _____
    _____
    C. Zone 3 _____
    D. Zone 4 _____
    _____
    E. Zone 5 _____
    F. Zone 6 _____
    _____
    G. Zone 7 _____

Use Focus on PRIDE in the Textbook to complete questions 43–44.

43. You help to protect the rights of the person and respect the person when you allow personal choice when arranging items. Make sure the person's choices
    A. _____
    B. _____
    C. _____

44. The location of items in the person's unit can prevent injuries when you help the person to
    A. _____
    B. _____
    C. _____

Labeling

45. A. What is the bed position called?
    _____
    B. What is the angle of the head of the bed?
    _____

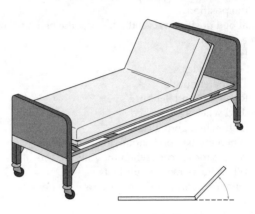

46. A. What is the bed position called?
    _____
    B. What is the angle of the head of the bed?
    _____
    C. What is the angle of the foot of the bed?
    _____

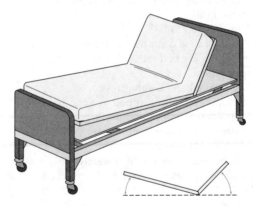

47. A. What is the bed position called?
    _____
    B. What is the angle of the head of the bed?
    _____

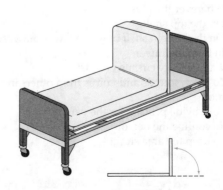

48. A. What is the bed position called?

    _____

    B. What is the position of the head of the bed and the foot of the bed?

    _____

    C. Who decides when this position is to be used?

    _____

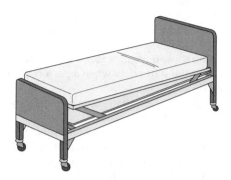

49. A. What is the bed position called?

    _____

    B. What is the position of the head of the bed and the foot of the bed?

    _____

    C. Who decides when this position is to be used?

    _____

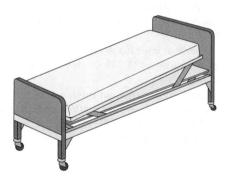

Optional Learning Exercises

50. Comfort is affected by three factors that cannot be controlled. These factors are

    A. _____

    B. _____

    C. _____

51. What factors can be controlled that affect comfort?

    A. _____

    B. _____

    C. _____

    D. _____

    E. _____

52. In these situations, how would you protect a person from drafts?

    A. The person is dressing for the day. _____

    _____

    B. The person is sitting in a wheelchair.

    _____

    _____

    C. You are assisting a person who is going to bed for the night. _____

    _____

    D. You are giving personal care to the person. _____

    _____

53. How can you help to eliminate odors in these situations?

    A. You are caring for a person who is frequently incontinent. _____

    _____

    B. The person is vomiting and has wound drainage. _____

    _____

    C. The person changes his own ostomy drainage bag in his bathroom. _____

    D. The person keeps a urinal at his bedside and uses it himself during the day.

    _____

54. When the staff talks loudly and laughs in hallways, some persons may think that

    _____.

55. How can the staff reduce noises and increase person comfort?

    A. Control _____

    B. Handle _____

    C. Keep _____

    D. Answer _____

56. What are 2 times when bright lights are helpful for a person with poor vision?

    A. _____

    B. _____

57. What does OBRA require for furniture and equipment listed?

    A. Closet space _____

    _____

    B. Bedding _____

    C. Chair _____

    D. Temperature _____

    E. Toilet seat _____

    F. Number of persons in a room _____

    G. Windows _____

H. Call system _____

_____

I. Lighting _____

J. Hand rails _____

58. The bed in the flat position is used when sleeping and for

A. _____

B. _____

59. Semi-Fowler's has 2 different definitions. They are

A. _____

B. _____

60. How do you know which of the ways to position the bed when semi-Fowler's position is ordered?

_____

61. What two methods are used to raise the foot of the bed with Trendelenburg's position?

A. _____

B. _____

62. How can you place a person in Fowler's or semi-Fowler's position if the person has a regular bed?

_____

_____

63. When the nursing team uses the overbed table as a work area, what are the only items that can be placed on it? _____

64. What are your responsibilities in these situations regarding the signal light?

A. The person is sitting in a chair next to the bed. _____

_____

B. The person is weak on the right side. _____

_____

C. The person calls out instead of using the signal light. _____

_____

D. The person is embarrassed because she soiled the bed after signaling for assistance.

_____

E. The signal light in a bathroom rings while you are busy in another room. _____

Independent Learning Activities

When you are in the health care center as a student, find an empty room and practice using the equipment. Answer these questions about the equipment.

- Where are the controls for the bed?
  - How do you operate the head of the bed?
  - How do you operate the knee control of the bed?
  - How do you adjust the height of the bed?
- Where is the call bell located?
- Where are controls for the television and radio?
- Does the center have an intercom system? How is it used?
- Ask the staff these questions about the call bells.
  - How does the staff know when a person turns on the call bell?
  - When a person uses a bathroom call bell, how does the staff know the difference?

Think about what temperature is comfortable for you and answer these questions. This exercise will help you to understand the importance of individual preferences for persons in the health care center.

- What is the usual temperature of your home?
- Who decides what the temperature will be in your home? Partner, spouse, roommate, children?
- Would the temperature you prefer be comfortable for an infant? An older person? Why or why not?

Think about the noises in your home and how they affect you. This exercise will help you to understand why noise levels in the nursing center can affect the persons.

- When you study, do you turn on the TV or radio? Listen to music? Prefer complete silence?
- What noises do you like when going to sleep? TV? Radio? Soft music?
- Does everyone in your household agree on how loud or soft to play a radio or TV? How are conflicts about noise levels resolved?
- If you are in a noisy surrounding that is unacceptable, how do you react? How does it affect your ability to think? To rest? To study? How does it affect your relationship with others?

19 Bedmaking

Fill in the Blank: Key Terms

Drawsheet   Cotton drawsheet   Waterproof drawsheet

1. A drawsheet placed between the bottom sheet and cotton drawsheet to keep the mattress and bottom linens clean and dry is a ___Waterproof drawsheet___
_____.

2. A ___Drawsheet___ is a small sheet placed over the middle of the bottom sheet.

3. A drawsheet made of cotton that helps keep the mattress and bottom linens clean is a
___Cotton drawsheet___.

Circle the Best Answer

4. Beds are made
   A. Only when the linens are wet or soiled.
   B. Every day.
   C. On the person's bath or shower day.
   D. Twice a week.

5. Making the bed every day
   A. Promotes comfort
   B. Prevents skin breakdown
   C. Prevents pressure ulcers
   D. All of the above

6. A closed bed is
   A. Not in use
   B. Made with the top linens fan-folded back to make it easier for the person to get in to bed
   C. Made with the person in it
   D. Made to transfer a person from a stretcher to the bed

7. An open bed is
   A. Made with the person in it
   B. In use; the top linens are folded back so that the person can get into bed
   C. Not in use until bedtime; the top linens are not folded back
   D. Made to transfer a person from a stretcher to the bed

8. When making a bed, medical asepsis is practiced by
   A. Putting clean or dirty linens on the floor
   B. Shaking the lines as you place them on the bed
   C. Raising the bed to a comfortable height to prevent injury to the nursing assistant
   D. Holding the linens away from your uniform

9. If extra clean linens are brought to a person's room, you should
   A. Return the unused linens to the linen room
   B. Use the linens for the person's roommate
   C. Put the unused linens in the laundry because they are contaminated
   D. Use the linens for a person in the next room

10. Which of these linens will be collected first when making a bed?
    A. Bath towel
    B. Bath blanket
    C. Mattress pad
    D. Top sheet

11. When you remove dirty linens, which of these actions is *incorrect*?
    A. Gather all the dirty linens in one large roll.
    B. Roll each piece away from you.
    C. Top and bottom sheets, drawsheets, and pillowcases are always changed.
    D. The blanket and bedspread may be reused for the same person.

12. You allow the person the right of personal choice when you
    A. Allow the person to choose the time when you make the bed
    B. Decide which linens will look best in the room
    C. Tell the person you will make the bed at 9 AM.
    D. Choose the pillows and blanket the person needs for comfort

13. When caring for a person in the home, the linens are usually changed
    A. Once a day
    B. Twice a week
    C. Only if the person gives you permission
    D. Weekly or more often if the person asks you to do so

14. A waterproof drawsheet can
    A. Retain heat
    B. Be hard to keep tight and wrinkle-free
    C. Protect the mattress and bottom linens from dampness and soiling
    D. All of the above

15. When caring for a person at home, the mattress and linens may be protected with all of these *except*
    A. A flat sheet folded in half
    B. A plastic trash bag
    C. A cotton drawsheet
    D. A plastic mattress protector

16. When you are delegated to make a bed, why do you need to know the person's schedule for treatments, therapies, and activities?
    A. You need to make sure the bed is flat.
    B. It is best to change linens after the treatment or when the person is out of the room.
    C. You need to unlock beds that have been locked in a certain position.
    D. You will know what type of bed to make.

17. When making a bed in the home, you should
    A. Always follow the person's wishes
    B. Only make the bed as stated in the care plan
    C. Follow the person's wishes unless they ask you to do something unsafe
    D. Use your own methods to make the bed

18. When making beds for children, it is important to
    A. Make sure if bumper pads are used that they fit snugly against the slats
    B. Check to make sure the mattress is at least 26 inches lower than the top of the crib rails
    C. Tell the nurse if there is any gap between the mattress and crib sides
    D. All of the above

19. When making a bed, you are using good body mechanics when you
    A. Bend from the waist to remove and replace linens
    B. Stretch across the bed to smooth linens
    C. Raise the bed to a comfortable height to work
    D. Lock the wheels

20. When a person is discharged, what is done in addition to changing the bed?
    A. New pillows are placed on the bed.
    B. The bed frame and mattress are cleaned according to center policy.
    C. The bed is sterilized.
    D. The bedspread and blanket may be reused.

21. When making a bed, position the bottom flat sheet with
    A. The lower edge even with the top of the mattress
    B. The hem stitching facing downward, away from the person
    C. The large hem at the bottom and the small hem at the top
    D. The crease crosswise on the bed

22. When the top sheet, blanket, bedspread are in place on the bed
    A. Each one is tucked under the mattress separately
    B. The sheet and blanket are tucked together and the bedspread is allowed to hang loose over them
    C. All top linens are tucked together under the foot of the bed and the corners are mitered
    D. All three are allowed to hang loose over the foot of the bed

23. The pillow is placed on the bed
    A. So the open end is away from the door
    B. The seam of the pillowcase is toward the foot of the bed
    C. Leaning against the head of the bed
    D. So the open end is toward the door

24. An open bed is made
    A. With the linens fan-folded to one side
    B. The same as a closed bed with the top linens folded back
    C. With the person in the bed
    D. When the room is unoccupied

25. When you change the linens for a comatose person, it is important to
    A. Keep the bed in the low position
    B. Unlock the wheels
    C. Use special linens
    D. Explain each step of the procedure to the person before it is done

26. When making an occupied bed, a bath blanket is used to
    A. Protect the person while he is being bathed
    B. Cover the person for warmth and privacy
    C. Protect the bed linens
    D. To protect the person from dirty linens

27. When making an occupied bed for a person who does *not* use bed rails, you should
    A. Have a co-worker work on the other side of the bed
    B. Push the bed against the wall
    C. Always keep one hand on the person while you are making the bed
    D. Only change linens when the person is out of the bed for tests or therapies

28. When making an occupied bed
    A. Remove all the dirty linens from the bed first
    B. Have the person roll from side to side for each piece of the bottom linens
    C. Tuck the dirty bottom linens and the clean bottom linens under the person
    D. Ask the person to raise the hips so you can push the linens under the buttocks

29. Which of these steps is *not* done when making a surgical bed?
    A. Tuck all top linens under the mattress together and make a mitered corner.
    B. Remove all linens from the bed.
    C. Put the mattress pad on the mattress.
    D. Place the bottom flat sheet with the lower edge even with the bottom of the mattress.

Fill in the Blank

30. Number this list from 1–13 in the order you would collect the linens to make a bed.

    _____ Pillowcase(s)

    _____ Top sheet

    _____ Gown

    _____ Bottom sheet (flat or fitted)

    _____ Mattress pad (if needed)

    _____ Bedspread

    _____ Plastic drawsheet, waterproof drawsheet, or waterproof pad if needed

    _____ Bath blanket

    _____ Hand towel

    _____ Cotton drawsheet (if needed)

    _____ Bath towel(s)

    _____ Blanket

    _____ Washcloth

31. Beds are made every day to
    A. Promote _____
    B. Prevent _____
    C. Prevent _____.

32. When doing home care, what guidelines should you follow when doing laundry?

    A. _____

    _____

    B. _____

    _____

    C. _____

    _____

33. How will you be able to tell the difference between a closed bed and an open bed _____

    _____

    _____

34. When you make a surgical bed fan-fold linens

    _____

    from the door.

Use Focus on PRIDE in the Textbook to complete this question.

35. When handling dirty linens, it is important as a team member that you

    A. Do not _____

    B. Linens must not _____

    If you see a full cart, _____

    C. If you fill a cart, _____

    If you place an item in a cart that will cause an odor, _____

    D. Place dirty linen _____

    E. Follow agency policy for _____

Optional Learning Exercises

36. Compare how linen changes in a hospital and nursing center.

    A. How often is a complete linen change made in a nursing center? _____

    _____

    B. How often are linens changed in a hospital?

    _____

    _____

    C. Why are linen changes done less often in a nursing center? _____

    _____

37. Even when a complete linen change is *not* scheduled, you should do the following to keep beds neat and clean.

    A. _____

    B. _____

    C. _____

    D. _____

    _____

    E. _____

    _____

    F. _____

    _____

38. The mattress pad, waterproof drawsheet, blanket, and bedspread are reused when making a bed unless they are _____.

39. If you were making a bed in a home, how would you use a twin sheet for a drawsheet? _____

40. When giving care in a home, what should you tell a family member who suggests using a plastic trash bag to protect the linens and mattress?

    A. _____

    B. _____

    C. _____

41. Explain the safety concern with each of these examples

    A. A soft crib mattress _____

    _____

    B. A crib mattress is smaller than the crib _____

    _____

    C. The mattress is 20 inches below the top of the crib rails _____

    _____

    D. Bumper pads do not fit snugly against the slats

    _____

    _____

Independent Learning Activities

When you make beds at home this week, practice the methods you learned in this chapter.

- What linens did you collect? What was the order of the linens?
- Did you remember to make as much of one side of the bed as possible before moving to the other side?
- What step could *not* be carried out at home that would have helped you to use good body mechanics?
- Think about the methods you used to change your bed before reading this chapter. How did you change your bedmaking practices now that you studied this chapter?

Practice with a classmate and take turns as a resident who must have an occupied bed made. Ask these questions about your feelings.

- In what ways was your privacy protected?
- Did the caregiver offer you any choices before making your bed? What were these choices?
- Did you feel safe at all times? If not, what made you feel unsafe?
- What was uncomfortable during the bed change?
- How were you positioned after the bed was made?

It is sometimes difficult for a new nursing assistant to remember the order in which to collect linens. If you have difficulty with this, make a list in a pocket notebook or on a 3 × 5 index card so you can carry it with you when you are working.

20 Personal Hygiene

Fill in the Blank: Key Terms

AM care	Diaphoresis	Morning care	Perineal care	PM care
Aspiration	Early morning care	Oral hygiene	Plaque	Tartar
Denture	Evening care	Pericare		

1. Care given at bedtime or PM care is
   Evening care.

2. _Perineal care_ is cleaning
   the genital and anal areas; pericare.

3. Sometimes evening care is called
   PM Care.

4. Sometimes early morning care is called
   AM Care.

5. _Oral hygiene_ is mouth care.

6. Hardened plaque on teeth is
   Tartar.

7. _Aspiration_ occurs
   when breathing fluid, food, vomitus, or an object into
   the lungs.

8. Care given after breakfast is called
   Morning care.
   Hygiene measures are more thorough at this time.

9. Another name for perineal care is
   pericare.

10. _Plaque_ is a thin film
    that sticks to the teeth. It contains saliva, microbes,
    and other substances.

11. Another name for AM care is
    early morning care.

12. An artificial tooth or a set of artificial teeth is a
    denture.

13. Profuse sweating is
    diaphoresis.

Circle the Best Answer

14. If a person needs help with personal hygiene, you
    can find out what needs they have by
    A. Following the nurse's directions and the
       care plan
    B. Asking the family
    C. Asking other staff members
    D. Making your own decisions

15. You should assist a person with personal hygiene
    A. Only when the person asks
    B. Only in the morning
    C. Whenever help is needed
    D. Only when it is your assignment

16. When giving personal hygiene, you need to
    remember to protect the person's right to
    A. Privacy and personal choice
    B. Care and security of personal possessions
    C. Activities
    D. Environment

17. Which of these hygiene measures is *not* done before
    breakfast?
    A. Assisting with elimination
    B. Straightening resident units, including
       making beds
    C. Assisting with activity by providing range-of-
       motion exercises
    D. Assisting with oral hygiene

18. Which of these is done every time you assist with
    hygiene measures throughout the day?
    A. Assist with dressing and hair care
    B. Face and hand washing, oral hygiene
    C. Assist with activity
    D. Helping person change into sleepwear

19. If good oral hygiene is not done regularly, the person
    may develop tartar which will lead to
    A. A dry mouth
    B. Periodontal disease
    C. A bad taste in the mouth
    D. Plaque

20. All of these health team members may assess the
    person's need for mouth care *except* the
    A. Speech/language pathologist
    B. Physical therapist
    C. Nurse
    D. Dietician

21. Teeth are flossed to
    A. Remove plaque from the teeth
    B. Remove tartar from the teeth
    C. Remove food from between the teeth
    D. All of the above

22. Sponge swabs are used for
    A. Persons with sore, tender mouths and for
       unconscious persons
    B. Cleaning dentures
    C. Oral care on children
    D. Oral care on all residents

23. You follow Standard Precautions and the Bloodborne Pathogen Standard when giving oral hygiene because
    A. You will not spread bacteria to the person
    B. It will help you avoid bad breath odors from the person
    C. Gums may bleed during mouth care
    D. You will avoid any loose teeth or rough dentures

24. When the person is able to perform oral hygiene in bed, you arrange the items on
    A. The overbed table   C. The sink counter
    B. The bedside table   D. The bed

25. When you are brushing the person's teeth, which of these steps would be incorrect?
    A. Let the person rinse the mouth with water.
    B. Only use a sponge swab to clean the teeth.
    C. Brush the person's tongue gently, if needed.
    D. Floss the person's teeth.

26. Which of these steps is incorrect to do when flossing the teeth?
    A. Start at the lower back tooth on the right side.
    B. Hold the floss between the middle fingers.
    C. Move the floss gently up and down between the teeth.
    D. Move to a new section of floss after every second tooth.

27. When providing mouth care for an unconscious person, position the person on one side with the head turned well to the side to
    A. Make it easier to brush the teeth
    B. Make the person more comfortable
    C. Prevent or reduce the risk of aspiration
    D. Make is easier for the person to breathe

28. When giving oral hygiene to an unconscious person who wears dentures you should
    A. Remove the dentures, clean them, and replace them in the mouth
    B. Dentures are not worn when the person is unconscious
    C. Clean the dentures in the mouth without removing them
    D. Place a padded tongue blade in the mouth to prevent biting

29. Mouth care is given to an unconscious person
    A. After each meal
    B. When AM and PM care is given
    C. At least every 2 hours
    D. Once a day

30. A padded tongue blade is used when giving oral hygiene to an unconscious person to
    A. Keep the mouth open   C. Clean the tongue
    B. Clean the teeth   D. Prevent aspiration

31. When cleaning dentures at a sink, line the sink with a towel to
    A. Prevent infections
    B. Prevent damage to the dentures if they are dropped
    C. Dry the dentures
    D. Clean the dentures

32. If dentures are not worn after cleaning, store them in
    A. Cool water   C. A soft towel
    B. Hot water   D. Soft tissues or a napkin

33. If the person cannot remove the dentures, you can use _____ to get a good grip on the slippery dentures.
    A. Gloves   C. Gauze squares
    B. Washcloth   D. Bare hands

34. Older persons usually need a complete bath or shower only twice a week because
    A. They are less active
    B. They are often ill
    C. They have increased perspiration
    D. Dry skin often occurs with aging

35. If a person has dry skin, which of these will help keep it soft?
    A. Soaps
    B. Lotions and oils
    C. Powders
    D. Deodorants and antiperspirants

36. If a person with dementia resists bathing, you may
    A. Hurry through the bath
    B. Speak firmly in a loud voice
    C. Try giving the bath during time of day when the person is calmer
    D. Use restraints so the person will not harm you

37. When choosing skin care products for bathing, you should use
    A. Soap
    B. Products the person prefers whenever possible
    C. Bath oils
    D. Creams and lotions

38. The water temperature for a complete bed bath is usually between 110° F and 115° F (43.3° C and 46.1° C) for adults. For older persons, the temperature
    A. Should be between 110° F and 115° F (43.3° C and 46.1° C)
    B. May need to be lower
    C. Should be whatever you feel is comfortable
    D. May need to be warmer

39. When applying powder
    A. Shake or sprinkle the powder directly on the person
    B. Sprinkle a small amount of powder onto your hands or a cloth
    C. Apply a thick layer of powder
    D. You should never use powder on any older person

40. The care plan for persons with bariatric needs will probably include
    A. How to dry under skin folds
    B. How to clean under skin folds
    C. What products to place under skin folds
    D. All of the above

41. A complete bed bath is given to persons who
    A. Cannot bathe themselves
    B. Are unconscious or paralyzed
    C. Are weak from illness or surgery
    D. All of the above
42. When you are giving a complete bed bath, the bed is made
    A. Only if needed
    B. Before the bath begins
    C. After the bath is completed
    D. After the person gets out of bed
43. Offering the bedpan, urinal, commode, or bathroom is
    A. Done before the bath begins
    B. Done after the bath ends
    C. Not important in giving a bath
    D. Not needed at all during the bath procedure
44. During the bath, the bath blanket is placed
    A. Over the person after the top linens are removed
    B. Under the top linens
    C. Over the person before top linens are removed
    D. Under the person
45. Do not use soap when washing
    A. The face, ears, and neck
    B. Around the eyes
    C. The abdomen
    D. The perineal area
46. How do you avoid exposing the person when washing the chest?
    A. Keep the bath blanket over the area
    B. Keep the top linens over the chest
    C. Place a towel over the chest crosswise
    D. Make sure the curtains are closed
47. Bath water is changed
    A. Every 5 minutes during the bath
    B. When it becomes cool and soapy
    C. Only once during the bath
    D. After washing the face, ears, and neck
48. A person _____ may respond well to a towel bath.
    A. With dementia
    B. Who has been incontinent
    C. With breaks in the skin
    D. Who needs a partial bath
49. A partial bath involves bathing
    A. The entire body
    B. The face, hands, axillae (underarms), back, buttocks, and perineal area
    C. The arms, legs, and feet
    D. The chest, abdomen, and underarms
50. When giving any type of bath, you should
    A. Wash from the dirtiest to cleanest areas
    B. Allow the skin to air dry to avoid rubbing
    C. Provide for privacy
    D. Decide what is best for the person
51. A tub bath should not last longer than
    A. 10 minutes   C. 20 minutes
    B. 15 minutes   D. 30 minutes

52. If a person is weak or unsteady, a _____ should be used when the person showers.
    A. A shower chair, shower trolley, or shower stall
    B. Transfer belt
    C. A wheelchair
    D. Stretcher
53. Which of these would be good time management when giving a tub bath or shower?
    A. Take the person to the shower room and then collect your equipment.
    B. Ask a co-worker to give the shower for you.
    C. Ask a co-worker to make the person's bed while you give the bath.
    D. Clean and disinfect the tub or shower before returning the person to his or her room.
54. When assisting with a tub bath or shower, which of these steps is first?
    A. Help the person undress and remove footwear.
    B. Assist or transport the person to the tub or shower room.
    C. Put the *Occupied* sign on the door.
    D. Place a rubber bath mat in the tub or on the shower floor.
55. The best position for a back massage is
    A. Prone position   C. Side-lying position
    B. Supine position   D. Semi-Fowler's position
56. Back massages are dangerous for persons with all of these problems *except*
    A. Certain heart diseases
    B. Lung disorders
    C. Arthritis
    D. Back injuries or surgeries
57. When giving a back massage, the strokes
    A. Start at the shoulders and go down to the buttocks
    B. Should be light and gentle
    C. Start at the buttocks and go up to the shoulders
    D. Are continued for at least 10 minutes
58. When cleaning the perineal area
    A. You do not need to wear gloves
    B. Work from the anal area to the urethral area (back to front)
    C. Work from the urethral area to the anal area (front to back)
    D. Work from the dirtiest area to the cleanest
59. When gathering equipment for perineal care, you will need
    A. One washcloth   C. At least 3 washcloths
    B. Two washcloths   D. At least 4 washcloths
60. When giving perineal care to a male, you
    A. Retract the foreskin if he is uncircumcised
    B. Wash from the scrotum to the tip of the penis
    C. Use one washcloth for the entire procedure
    D. Leave the foreskin retracted after finishing the care

Matching

In questions 61–68, match the skin care product with the benefits or the problem that may occur if you use the product.

A. Soaps
B. Bath oils
C. Creams and lotions
D. Powders
E. Deodorants and antiperspirants

61. _____ Absorbs moisture and prevents friction
62. _____ Makes showers and tubs slippery
63. _____ Protects skin from the drying effect of air and evaporation
64. _____ Excessive amounts can cause caking and crusts that can irritate the skin
65. _____ Masks and controls body odors or reduces perspiration
66. _____ Tends to dry and irritate skin
67. _____ Keeps skin soft and prevents drying of skin
68. _____ Removes dirt, dead skin, skin oil, some microbes, and perspiration

Fill in the Blank

69. Write out the abbreviations.
   A. C _____
   B. F _____
   C. ID _____

70. The _____ and the _____ of the mouth, genital area, and anus must be intact to prevent microbes from entering the body and causing an _____.

71. The religion of East Indian Hindus requires at least _____ a day.

72. Some Hindus believe that bathing is _____ after a meal.

73. When should you give or offer oral hygiene to a person?
   A. _____
   B. _____
   C. _____
   D. _____

74. When you are delegated to give oral hygiene, what observations should you report?
   A. _____
   B. _____
   C. _____
   D. _____
   E. _____
   F. _____

75. If flossing is done only once a day, the best time to floss is at _____.

76. When giving oral care to an unconscious person, explain what you are doing, because you always assume _____
   _____

77. When following the rules for bathing in Box 20-1, you protect the skin by following these rules.
   A. Rinse _____
   B. Pat _____
   _____
   C. Dry _____
   _____
   D. Bathe _____

78. What methods can be used to measure the water temperature used for a bed bath?
   A. _____
   B. _____

79. When you place a person's hand in the basin during the bed bath, you may have the person _____ the hands and fingers.

80. When assisting with partial baths, most people need help with washing the _____.

81. A tub bath can cause a person to feel _____, especially if the person has been on bedrest.

82. When the shower room has more than one stall or cabinet, you must protect the person's right _____.
   What can you do to protect this right?
   A. _____
   B. _____

83. When giving a tub bath or shower you use safety measures to protect the person from _____, _____, and _____.

84. When giving a back massage, what is the effect of
   A. Fast movements? _____
   B. Slow movements? _____

85. When you are delegated to give a back massage, what observations should you report and record?
   A. _____
   B. _____
   C. _____
   D. _____

86. When you are assisting a person with perineal care, what terms may help the person understand what you are going to do? _____

_____

87. What observations made while assisting with hygiene should be reported at once?

A. _____

B. _____

C. _____

D. _____

E. _____

Use Focus on PRIDE in the Textbook to complete questions 88–89.

88. You show personal and professional responsibility when you focus on the quality of life steps before performing procedures. They are

A. _____

B. _____

C. _____

D. _____

E. _____

89. In order to promote dignity and respect, you protect the right to privacy when you

A. _____

B. _____

C. _____

D. _____

E. _____

Labeling

90. Look at the figure and answer these questions.
   A. Why is the person positioned on his side?

   _____

   B. What is the purpose of the padded tongue blade?

   _____

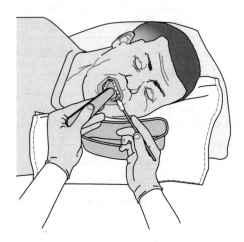

91. In this figure, what is the staff member using to remove the upper denture?

_____

Why? _____

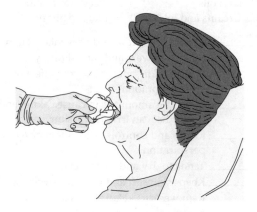

92. In this figure, explain what the staff member is doing.

_____

Why is the towel positioned vertically on the person?

_____.

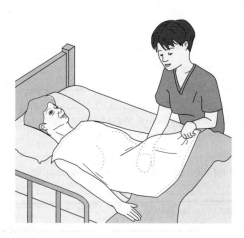

Optional Learning Exercises

93. Hygiene promotes comfort, safety, and health. Answer these questions about hygiene.

   A. Intact skin prevents _____.
   B. What other areas must be clean to maintain intact skin? _____

   _____

   C. Besides, cleansing what are the other benefits of good hygiene?
   1. Prevents _____ and

   _____

   2. It is _____

   3. Increases _____

94. What factors cause mouth dryness for an unconscious person?

    A. _____

    B. _____

    C. _____

95. The factors listed above cause crusting on the

    _____ and _____

    _____.

96. Oral hygiene (mouth care) does the following

    A. _____

    B. _____

    C. _____

    D. _____

    E. _____

97. What are the benefits of bathing?

    A. Cleans _____

    B. Also cleans _____

    C. Removes _____

    D. Bath is _____ and

    _____

    E. Stimulates _____

    F. Exercises _____

    G. You can make _____

    H. You have time _____

98. When you are bathing a person with dementia, what measures are important to help the person through the bath?

    A. _____

    _____

    B. _____

    _____

    C. _____

    D. _____

    E. _____

    _____

    F. _____

    G. _____

    H. _____

    I. _____

    _____

    J. _____

    K. _____

    L. _____

    M. _____

    N. _____

99. You are delegated to give Mrs. Johnson a bath. Before beginning, what information do you need?

    A. _____

    _____

    B. _____

    C. _____

    D. _____

    E. _____

    F. _____

    G. _____

    H. _____

100. As you are bathing Mrs. Johnson, what observations should you make to report and record?

    A. _____

    B. _____

    C. _____

    D. _____

    E. _____

    F. _____

    G. _____

    H. _____

    I. _____

    J. _____

101. You are preparing to give perineal care to Mrs. Johnson. How many washcloths should you gather?

    _____ Why?

    _____

    _____

Independent Learning Activities

Discuss the following questions with several classmates to understand personal preferences about personal hygiene.

- Do you prefer a shower or tub bath?
- What time of day do you usually bathe?
- What skin care products do you use to keep your skin healthy?
- What special measures do you use when brushing your teeth? Special brush? Toothpaste? Do you floss? How often?

As part of your preparation for caring for residents, you may give a classmate a back massage and receive a back massage. Answer these questions about how you felt when you were the "resident."

- How did the lotion feel on your back? Was it warm or cold?
- Which strokes were relaxing? Which were more stimulating?

- How long do you think the back massage lasted? Did you look at the clock to see the actual time?
- What would you like to tell the person giving the back massage that would improve the back massage?
- How will this practice help you when you give a back massage to another person?

As part of your preparation for caring for residents, you may give a classmate oral hygiene. Answer these questions about how you felt when you were the "resident."

- What did the "nursing assistant" tell you before beginning the oral hygiene?
- What choices were offered? Position? Equipment? Products?
- How did it feel to have someone else give you oral hygiene? Flossing your teeth?
- How clean did your teeth feel when the oral hygiene was completed?
- What would you like to tell the person who gave the oral hygiene that would help improve the procedure?
- How will this experience help you when you give oral hygiene to a resident?

21 Grooming

Fill in the Blank: Key Terms

Alopecia   Dandruff   Lice   Pediculosis   Pediculosis corporis

Anticoagulant   Hirsutism Mite   Pediculosis capitis Pediculosis pubis

1. The infestation with lice is _pediculosis_ .

2. A very small spider-like organism is a
   mite .

3. _dandruff_ is an excessive amount of dry, white flakes from the scalp.

4. The infestation of the body with lice is
   pediculosis corporis .

5. Hair loss is _alopecia_ .

6. _Pediculosis pubis_ is the infestation of the pubic hair with lice.

7. Excessive body hair is _hirsutism_ .

8. The infestation of the scalp with wingless insects is
   pediculos capitis .

9. Another description of pediculosis is
   lice .

10. A drug that prevents or slows down blood clotting is
    an _anticoagulant_ .

Circle the Best Answer

11. Hair care, shaving, and nail and foot care are important to many people because these measures affect
    A. Safety and security needs
    B. Love, belonging, and self-esteem needs
    C. Physical needs
    D. Self-actualization needs

12. If you see any signs of lice, you should report it to the nurse because
    A. Lice bites can cause severe infections
    B. Lice are easily spread to other persons through clothing, furniture, bed linens, and sexual contact
    C. It can cause the person's hair to fall out
    D. The lice will cause the hair to mat and tangle

13. If a person has scabies, what signs or symptoms may be present?
    A. You may see lice, which are small and tan to grayish-white in color.
    B. The person has a rash and intense itching between the fingers, around the wrists, and in other areas.
    C. You may see eggs (nits) attached to the hair shaft.
    D. The person has an excessive amount of dry, white flakes on the scalp.

14. Who chooses how you will brush, comb, and style a person's hair?
    A. The person
    B. You decide
    C. The nurse tells you
    D. It is written in the care plan

15. If long hair becomes matted or tangled, you should
    A. Braid the hair.
    B. Cut the hair to remove the tangles and matting
    C. Tell the nurse and ask for directions
    D. Get the family's permission to change the hairstyle

16. If hair is curly, coarse, and dry, which of these would *not* be done?
    A. Braid or cut the hair.
    B. Use a wide-toothed comb.
    C. Work upward, lifting and fluffing hair outward.
    D. Apply a conditioner or petrolatum jelly to make combing easier.

17. When shampooing the person who has small braids
    A. Undo the hair and rebraid each time it is shampooed
    B. The braids are left intact for shampooing
    C. Undo the braids only at night
    D. Comb out the braids once a week

18. If a woman's hair is done by the beautician
    A. Wash her hair only once a week
    B. Shampoo her hair on the day she goes to the beautician
    C. She wears a shower cap during the tub bath or shower
    D. Wash her hair each time she gets a shower or tub bath

19. If a person has limited range of motion in the neck, they are *not* shampooed
    A. At the sink or on a stretcher
    B. In the shower
    C. During a tub bath
    D. In bed

20. Which of these is *not* an observation that is made when shampooing?
    A. Scalp sores
    B. The presence of nits or lice
    C. The amount of hair on the head
    D. Matted or tangled hair

21. If a person receives anticoagulants and needs shaving
    A. Use an electric razor
    B. Use disposable safety razors
    C. It must be done by the nurse or barber
    D. It should only be done during the shower or bath

22. When using safety razors (blade razors)
    A. The same razor can be used for several persons until it becomes dull
    B. Use the resident's own razor as many times as possible
    C. Discard the disposable razor or razor blade into the sharps container
    D. Be careful when shaving a person who takes anticoagulants
23. Why is an electric razor used when shaving a person with dementia?
    A. They usually bleed easily.
    B. They may not understand what you are doing and resist care or move suddenly.
    C. It is faster than using a safety razor.
    D. The skin is tender and sensitive.
24. When shaving a person with a safety razor, wear gloves
    A. To protect the person from infections
    B. To prevent contact with blood
    C. When applying shaving cream
    D. To maintain sterile technique
25. When caring for a mustache and beard, all of these are done *except*
    A. Wash the mustache or beard daily
    B. Combing daily is usually needed
    C. Ask the person how to groom his beard or mustache
    D. Trim a beard or mustache when needed
26. The nursing assistant can cut or trim toenails
    A. Whenever he or she has time
    B. On all persons
    C. If agency policy allows them to trim toenails
    D. If the person agrees to the care
27. When caring for the fingernails or toenails, which of these is *wrong*?
    A. Cut the nails with small scissors
    B. Clean under the nails with an orange stick
    C. Clip the nails straight across with nail clippers
    D. Shape the nails with an emery board or nail file
28. When changing clothing, remove the clothing from
    A. The weak side first
    B. The lower limbs first
    C. The right side last
    D. The strong or "good" side first
29. When you are undressing a person, it is usually done
    A. In the bed in the supine position
    B. With the person sitting in a chair
    C. By having the person stand at the bedside
    D. In the bathroom
30. When you are undressing a person, you use good body mechanics when you
    A. Lower the bed rail on the person's weak side
    B. Position the person in a supine position
    C. Raise the bed to a good working level
    D. Turn the person away from you
31. To provide warmth and privacy when changing clothes, you
    A. Keep the top sheets in place
    B. Cover the person with a bath blanket
    C. Close the curtains
    D. Close the door

32. When changing the gown of a person with an IV
    A. Turn off the IV
    B. Lay the IV bag on the bed and remove the gown
    C. Slide the gathered sleeve over the tubing, hand, arm, and IV site
    D. Disconnect the IV
33. When you have finished changing the gown of a person with an IV, you should
    A. Restart the pump
    B. Reconnect the IV
    C. Ask the nurse to check the flow rate
    D. Check the flow rate

Fill in the Blank
34. Write out the abbreviations.
    A. C _____
    B. F _____
    C. ID _____
    D. IV _____
35. When you are giving care, report these signs and symptoms of lice to the nurse at once.
    A. _____
    B. _____
    C. _____
    D. _____
    E. _____
36. When you brush and comb the hair, you should report and record
    A. _____
    B. _____
    C. _____
    D. _____
    E. _____
    F. _____
    G. _____
    H. _____
37. If you give hair care to a person in bed after a linen change, collect falling hair by _____
    _____.
38. It may help to prevent tangled and matted hair when you brush and comb small sections of the hair, starting at the _____.
39. If hair is curly, coarse, and dry, special measures are needed. You should
    A. Use a _____
    B. Start at _____
    C. Work _____, lift and _____
    D. Wet _____ or apply _____
    _____.
40. You can protect the person's eyes during shampooing by asking the person to hold a _____
    _____.

41. What delegation guidelines do you need when shaving a person?
    A. _____
    B. _____
    C. _____
    D. _____
    E. _____
    F. _____
    G. _____
    H. _____

42. What should be reported *at once* when you are shaving a person?
    A. _____
    B. _____
    C. _____

43. When you are shaving the face and underarms with a safety razor, shave in the direction of the _____.

44. When shaving legs with a safety razor, shave _____.

45. When using an electric shaver, shave _____.

46. When you are delegated to give nail and foot care, report and record
    A. _____
    B. _____
    C. _____
    D. _____
    E. _____
    F. _____

47. Foot care for persons with diabetes or poor circulation is provided by _____ or _____.

48. When undressing the person who cannot raise the head and shoulders
    A. _____
    B. _____
    C. _____
    D. _____
    E. _____

49. When dressing the person who cannot raise the hips off the bed
    A. _____
    B. _____
    C. _____
    D. _____
    E. _____

50. Before changing a person's hospital gown when the person has an IV, what information do you need from the nurse and the care plan?
    A. _____
    B. _____

Use Focus on PRIDE in the Textbook to complete questions 51–55.

51. When a person has clean _____, _____, and _____, it helps mental well-being.

52. It is important for you to be _____ and have a professional _____, because others may question the quality of care you provide if you are not groomed well.

53. When you respect the person's choice of hair styles and personal care products, it shows you respect the person's right to _____.

54. When a person allows family members to assist with giving personal care, this promotes _____

55. If you cut a person's hair or shave a mustache or beard without permission, you have violated the person's right to be free from _____.

Optional Learning Exercises

56. You are caring for a person who is receiving cancer treatments. What effect could this treatment have on the person's hair? _____

57. Dandruff occurs not only on the scalp, but it may also involve the _____.

58. Brushing the hair increases _____ to the scalp. It also brings _____ along the hair shaft.

59. Why do older persons usually have dry hair? _____

60. What water temperature is usually used when shampooing the hair? _____

61. How can the beard be softened before shaving? _____

62. After shaving, why do some people apply aftershave or lotion?
    A. Lotion _____
    B. Aftershave _____

63. Injuries to the feet of a person with poor circulation are serious because poor circulation prolongs _____.

64. When changing clothing or hospital gowns, what rules should be followed?
    A. _____
    B. _____
    C. _____
    D. _____
    E. _____
    F. _____
    G. _____

Independent Learning Activities

Ask another person if you may shave him or her with a safety razor. (Some instructors may be concerned about the liability of this exercise. Make sure that the instructor approves this exercise, especially if you using a classmate as a partner.) Ask the person you shaved to help you answer these questions.

- What did you use for lubricating the skin? Shaving cream? Soap? Water only? How did it feel to the person? What worked best?
- Which technique worked best? When you applied more pressure? Less pressure?
- Shave one side of face with hair growth and one side against the hair growth. Which way was better? Why?
- What way can the person help you shave the face better?
- What area was the most difficult to shave? How did you deal with this area?
- Ask the person you shaved for any tips on how to improve your shaving skills.

Role-play this situation with a classmate. Take turns being the person and the nursing assistant. Remember to keep your left arm and leg limp when you are the person.

Situation: Mr. Olsen is a 58-year-old patient who has weakness on the left side. You are assigned to take off his sleepwear and dress him for the day. You need to remove his pajamas and dress him in a shirt, a pullover sweater, slacks, socks, and shoes.

- How did you provide privacy?
- How was Mr. Olsen positioned for the clothing change?
- What difficulties did you have when you removed his pajamas?
- Which arm did you redress first? What difficulty did you have getting his arms into the shirt?
- How did you put on the sweater? What was most difficult about this?
- What was the most difficult part of putting on the slacks?
- How did you put on the socks and shoes?
- What did you learn from this role-play situation? Did you follow the procedure in the chapter to assist you?
- Discuss with each other how it felt to have someone dress you when you were "Mr. Olsen."

22 Urinary Elimination

Fill in the Blank: Key Terms

Catheter
Catheterization
Dysuria
Foley catheter
Functional incontinence

Hematuria
Indwelling catheter
Micturition
Mixed incontinence
Nocturia

Oliguria
Overflow incontinence
Polyuria
Reflex incontinence
Retention catheter

Straight catheter
Stress incontinence
Transient incontinence
Urge incontinence
Urinary frequency

Urinary incontinence
Urinary urgency
Urination
Voiding

1. The production of abnormally large amounts of urine is _polyuria_.

2. _Mixed incontinence_ is having more than one type of the combination of stress incontinence and urge incontinence.

3. A Foley or indwelling catheter is also called a _Retention catheter_.

4. The process of inserting a catheter is _catheterization_.

5. _Urinary incontinence_ is the loss of bladder control.

6. Frequent urination at night is _nocturia_.

7. A catheter left in the bladder so urine drains constantly into a drainage bag is called a retention, Foley, or _indwelling catheter_.

8. The loss of small amounts of urine that leak from a bladder that is always full is _overflow incontinence_.

9. Another name for urination or voiding is _micturition_.

10. _Functional incontinence_ occurs when the person has bladder control but cannot use the toilet in time.

11. The process of emptying urine from the bladder is micturition, voiding, or _urination_.

12. A _catheter_ is a tube used to drain or inject fluid through a body opening.

13. Blood in the urine is _hematuria_.

14. A catheter that drains the bladder and then is removed is a _straight catheter_.

15. Voiding at frequent intervals is _urinary frequency_.

16. An indwelling or retention catheter is also called a _foley catheter_.

17. When urine leaks during exercise and certain movements that cause pressure on the bladder it is called _stress incontinence_.

18. Another word for urination or micturition is _voiding_.

19. _Urinary urgency_ is the need to void at once.

20. The loss of urine in response to a sudden, urgent need to void is _urge incontinence_.

21. Painful or difficult urination is _dysuria_.

22. The loss of urine at predictable intervals when the bladder is full is _reflex incontinence_.

23. A scant amount of urine, usually less than 500 mL in 24 hours is _oliguria_.

24. _Transient incontinence_ is temporary or occasional incontinence that is reversed when the cause is treated.

Circle the Best Answer

25. Solid wastes are removed from the body by the
    A. Digestive system   C. Blood
    B. Urinary system   D. Integumentary system

26. A healthy adult excretes about _____ of urine a day.
    A. 500 mL   C. 1500 mL
    B. 1000 mL   D. 2000 mL

27. All of these will provide privacy when the person is voiding *except*
    A. Pull drapes or window shades
    B. Always stay in room to give assistance
    C. Pull the curtain around the bed
    D. Close room and bathroom doors

28. If the person has difficulty starting the urine stream it may help to
    A. Play music on the TV
    B. Provide perineal care
    C. Use a stainless steel bedpan
    D. Run water in a nearby sink

29. The urine may be bright yellow if the person eats
    A. Asparagus
    B. Carrots or sweet potatoes
    C. Beets or blackberries
    D. Rhubarb

30. If you are caring for an infant, which of these observations should be report to the nurse at once?
    A. The infant has had a wet diaper 4 times in 3 hours
    B. The infant has not had a wet diaper for several hours
    C. The urine in the diaper is pale yellow
    D. The urine in the diaper has a faint odor

31. When you are getting ready to give a person the bedpan, you should
    A. Raise the head of the bed slightly
    B. Position the person in the Fowler's position
    C. Wash the person's hands
    D. Place the bed in a flat position

32. Urinals are usually placed at the bedside on
    A. Bed rails   C. Bedside stands
    B. Overbed tables   D. The floor

33. If a man is unable to stand and place a urinal to void, you should
    A. Tell the nurse
    B. Ask a male co-worker to help the man
    C. Place and hold the urinal for him
    D. Pad the bed with incontinent pads

34. A commode chair is used when the person
    A. Is unable to walk to the bathroom
    B. Cannot sit up unsupported on the toilet
    C. Needs to be in the normal position for elimination
    D. All of the above

35. When you place a commode over the toilet
    A. Restrain the person
    B. Stay in the room with the person
    C. Lock the wheels
    D. Make sure the container is in place

36. Dribbling of urine that occurs with laughing, sneezing, coughing, lifting, or other activities mean the person has
    A. Urge incontinence
    B. Stress incontinence
    C. Overflow incontinence
    D. Functional incontinence

37. When you do not answer signal lights quickly or do not position the signal light within the person's reach, it can cause
    A. Overflow incontinence
    B. Mixed incontinence
    C. Reflex incontinence
    D. Functional incontinence

38. You are caring for an incontinent person who often wets right after you have changed the clothes and bedding. It would be correct if you
    A. Wait 15 to 30 minutes before changing the person each time
    B. Reuse some of the linens that are only slightly damp
    C. Talk to the nurse at once, if you find yourself becoming impatient
    D. Tell the person that you can only change him once a shift

39. When a person has dementia, what measures may help keep the person clean and dry?
    A. Tell the person to use the signal light when he or she needs to void
    B. Increase fluid intake at bedtime
    C. Observe for signs that the person may need to void, such as pulling at the clothing
    D. Remove any incontinent garments and seat the person on a commode at all times

40. When discussing incontinent products, it may lower a person's self esteem if the products are called
    A. Incontinent briefs   C. Adult diapers
    B. Underwear   D. By the brand name

41. A catheter that is inserted to drain the bladder and is then removed is
    A. An indwelling catheter
    B. A straight catheter
    C. A condom catheter
    D. A Foley catheter

42. A catheter is used for all of these *except*
    A. To keep the bladder empty before, during, and after surgery
    B. When a person is dying
    C. For all persons with incontinence
    D. To protect wounds and pressure ulcers from contact with urine

43. A last resort for incontinence is
    A. Bladder training
    B. Answering signal lights promptly
    C. An indwelling catheter
    D. Adequate fluid intake

44. When cleaning a catheter you should
    A. Wipe four inches up the catheter to the meatus
    B. Disconnect the tubing from the drainage bag
    C. Clean the catheter from the meatus down the catheter about 4 inches
    D. Wash and rinse the catheter by washing up and down the tubing

45. The drainage bag from a catheter should *not* be attached to the
    A. Bed frame   C. Wheelchair
    B. Back of a chair   D. Bed rail

46. If a catheter is accidentally disconnected from the drainage bag, you should tell the nurse at once and then
    A. Quickly reconnect the drainage system
    B. Clamp the catheter to prevent leakage
    C. Wipe the end of the tube and end of the catheter with antiseptic wipes
    D. Discard the drainage bag and get a new bag

47. If a person uses a leg drainage bag it
    A. Is switched to a drainage bag when the person is in bed
    B. Is attached to the clothing with tape or safety pins
    C. Is attached to the bed rail when the person is in bed
    D. Can be worn 24 hours a day

48. A leg bag needs to be emptied more often than a drainage bag because
    A. It holds less than 1000 mL and the drainage bag holds about 2000 mL
    B. It is more likely to leak than the drainage bag
    C. It holds about 250 mL and the drainage bag holds 1000 mL
    D. It interferes with walking if it is full

49. When you empty a drainage bag, you
    A. Disconnect the bag from the tubing
    B. Clamp the catheter to prevent leakage
    C. Open the clamp on the drain and let urine drain into a graduate
    D. Take the bag into the bathroom to empty it
50. When removing an indwelling catheter, a syringe is needed to
    A. Remove water in the balloon
    B. Insert water into the balloon
    C. Flush the catheter with water
    D. Clean the perineal area after removing the catheter
51. When applying a condom catheter
    A. Apply elastic tape in a spiral around the penis
    B. Make sure the catheter tip is touching the head of the penis
    C. Apply adhesive tape securely in a circle entirely around the penis
    D. Remove and reapply every shift
52. The goal of bladder training is
    A. To keep the person dry and clean
    B. Control of urination
    C. Prevention of skin breakdown
    D. Prevention of infection
53. When you are assisting the person with habit training to have normal elimination
    A. Help the person to the bathroom every 15 or 20 minutes
    B. Voiding is scheduled at regular times to match the person's voiding habits
    C. Make sure the person drinks at least 1000 mL each shift
    D. Tell the person he or she can only void once a shift
54. When you assist with bladder training for a person with an indwelling catheter
    A. Empty the drainage bag every hour
    B. At first, clamp the catheter for 1 hour
    C. At first, clamp the catheter for 3 to 4 hours
    D. Give the person 15 to 20 minutes to start voiding

Fill in the Blank
55. Write out the abbreviations.
    A. C _____
    B. CMS _____
    C. F _____
    D. ID _____
    E. IV _____
    F. mL _____
    G. UTI _____
56. What substances increase urine production?
    A. _____
    B. _____
    C. _____
    D. _____

57. A normal position for voiding for women is
    _____.
    For men, a normal position is
    _____.
58. What can you do to mask urination sounds?
    A. _____
    B. _____
    C. _____
59. Fracture pans are used for persons
    A. _____
    B. _____
    C. _____
    D. _____
    E. _____
    F. _____
60. A bariatric bed pan is placed with the
    _____ end under the buttocks.
61. When a person voids in a bedpan or urinal, what observations about the urine are important?
    A. _____
    B. _____
    C. _____
    D. _____
    E. _____
    F. _____
62. When you are handling bedpans, urinals, and commodes and their contents, you should follow
    _____ and
    _____.
63. When you are delegated to provide a urinal, what guidelines should you follow?
    A. _____
    B. _____
    C. _____
    D. _____
    E. _____
    F. _____
    G. _____
    H. _____
64. When you transfer a person to a commode from bed, you must practice safe transfer procedures and use a
    _____ and _____ the wheels.
65. Name 5 causes of urge incontinence.
    A. _____
    B. _____
    C. _____
    D. _____
    E. _____

66. Stress incontinence is common in women because the pelvic muscles weaken from _____ and with _____.

67. Overflow incontinence may occur in men because of an _____.

68. _____ incontinence occurs with nervous system disorders and injuries.

69. Common causes of transient incontinence are

    A. _____
    B. _____
    C. _____
    D. _____
    E. _____
    F. _____

70. When you are delegated to apply incontinence products, you need this information from the nurse and care plan:

    A. _____
    B. _____
    C. _____
    D. _____
    E. _____
    F. _____

71. What observations should you report and record when you are delegated to apply incontinence products?

    A. _____
    B. _____
    C. _____
    D. _____
    E. _____
    F. _____
    G. _____

72. When you provide perineal care after a person is incontinent, remember to

    A. _____
    B. _____
    C. _____
    D. _____
    E. _____
    F. _____

73. When a catheter is inserted after a person voids, it is used to measure how _____.

74. A catheter is secured to the inner thigh or the man's abdomen to prevent _____.

75. When a person has a catheter, what observations should you report and record?

    A. _____
    B. _____
    C. _____
    D. _____
    E. _____
    F. _____
    G. _____
    H. _____

76. When you give catheter care, clean the catheter at least _____ inches. Clean _____ from the meatus with _____ stroke.

77. Is the urinary drainage system sterile or nonsterile?

    _____

78. What happens if a drainage bag is higher than the bladder? _____

    _____

    This can cause _____.

79. If a drainage system is disconnected accidentally, what should you do?

    A. Tell _____
    B. Do not _____
    C. Practice _____
    D. Wipe _____
    E. Wipe _____
    F. Do not _____
    G. Connect _____
    H. Discard _____
    I. Remove _____

80. Before removing a catheter, make sure that

    A. _____
    B. _____
    C. _____
    D. _____
    E. _____

81. Do *not* apply a condom catheter if the penis is _____, and _____, or shows signs of _____.

82. The catheter is clamped for 1 hour at first, and over time, for 3 to 4 hours when _____ is being done.

Use Focus on PRIDE in the Textbook to complete questions 83–84.

83. Your professional responsibility means you need to know what you can and cannot do as regulated by your state _____.

84. What information do you need to know if your state allows you to insert a urinary catheter?

   A. _____

   B. _____

   C. _____

   D. _____

Labeling

85. Mark the places you would secure the catheter. Explain why the catheter is secured this way.

   _____

   _____

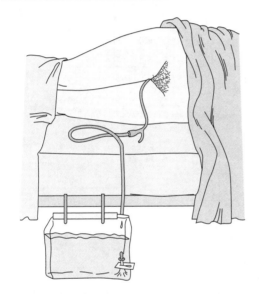

86. Mark the places you would secure the catheter. Explain why the catheter is secured this way.

   _____

   _____

   _____

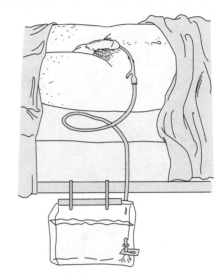

Crossword

Fill in the following crossword by answering the clues with the words from this list:

Dysuria   Hematuria   Nocturia   Polyuria
Frequency   Incontinence Oliguria   Urgency

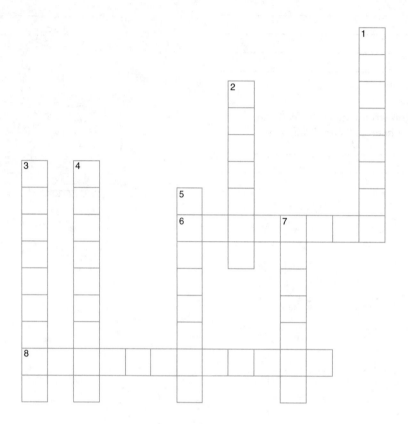

Across

6. Scant amount of urine, usually less than 500 mL in 24 hours
8. Inability to control loss of urine from bladder

Down

1. Production of abnormally large amount of urine
2. Painful or difficult urination
3. Blood in the urine
4. Voiding at frequent intervals
5. Frequent urination at night
7. Need to void immediately

Optional Learning Exercises

87. When a person eats a diet high in salt, it causes the body to _____.
    When this happens, how does it affect urine output?

    _____

    _____

88. You would ask the nurse to observe urine that looks
    or _____.
    You would also report complaints of _____

    _____

89. A fracture pan can be used with older persons who have _____

    _____ or _____

    _____

90. Covering the lap and legs of a person using a commode provides _____ and
    promotes _____.

91. If you are caring for an incontinent person and you become short-tempered and impatient,

    _____

    What right are you protecting when you do this?

    _____

92. When using incontinence products it is important to use the correct size. If the product is too large,

    _____.

    If it is too small, the product will cause

    _____

    _____

93. Even though catheters are a last resort for incontinent persons, they may be used with weak, disabled, or dying persons to

    A. Promote _____

    B. Prevent _____

    C. Protect _____ and

    _____

    D. Allow _____

94. Catheters may have diagnostic reasons for use such as

    A. _____

    B. _____

95. What can happen if microbes enter a closed drainage system? _____

96. What type of tape is used to apply a condom catheter? _____ Why?

    _____

    _____ What can happen if you

    use the wrong tape? _____

    _____

Independent Learning Activities

Role-play the following situation with a classmate. Take turns playing the person using the bedpan and the nursing assistant. Answer the questions about the activity.

Situation: Mrs. Donnelly is a 70-year-old who must use the bedpan. She finds it difficult to move easily and usually does not have enough strength to raise her hips to get on the bedpan. She tells you she will try to help as much as she can.

- As Mrs. Donnelly:
  - When you tried to assist, how easy was it to raise your hips? How did the nursing assistant help you get on the pan?
  - When you were rolled onto the bedpan, how did it feel? How well was the pan positioned under you?
  - How did you feel about sitting on the pan in bed? Did you feel as if this would be an easy or difficult way to void? Explain your feelings.
  - How could the nursing assistant make this procedure better?

- As the nursing assistant:
  - How did you position the bedpan to get ready to slide it under Mrs. Donnelly? Did this method work? How could you improve this?
  - When you rolled Mrs. Donnelly onto the pan, how well positioned was she? What adjustments were necessary?
  - When you rolled her off the pan, what happened? If urine had been in the pan, what would have occurred?
  - How could you change some of your steps to make this procedure better?

23 Bowel Elimination

Fill in the Blank: Key Terms

Colostomy · Diarrhea · Feces · Ostomy · Stool
Constipation · Enema · Flatulence · Peristalsis · Suppository
Defecation · Fecal impaction · Flatus · Stoma
Dehydration · Fecal incontinence · Ileostomy

1. A surgically created opening is a stoma or
   _____ostomy_____.

2. The process of excreting feces from the rectum
   through the anus is a bowel movement or
   _____defecation_____.

3. The excessive formation of gas in the stomach and
   intestines is _____flatulence_____.

4. A _____suppository_____ is a
   cone-shaped solid drug that is inserted into a body
   opening.

5. The frequent passage of liquid stools is
   _____diarrhea_____.

6. _____fecal impaction_____ is the prolonged
   retention and buildup of feces in the rectum.

7. _____dehydration_____ is the excessive
   loss of water from tissues.

8. Gas or air passed through the anus is
   _____flatus_____.

9. The introduction of fluid into the rectum and lower
   colon is an _____enema_____.

10. Excreted feces is _____stool_____.

11. An artificial opening between the colon and
    abdominal wall is a
    _____colostomy_____.

12. _____Peristalsis_____ is the alternating
    contraction and relaxation of intestinal muscles.

13. The passage of a hard, dry stool is
    _____constipation_____.

14. _____fecal incontinence_____ is the inability to
    control the passage of feces and gas through the anus.

15. A surgically created opening is an ostomy or
    _____stoma_____.

16. The semisolid mass of waste products in the colon is
    _____feces_____.

17. An artificial opening between the ileum and
    the abdominal wall is an
    _____ileostomy_____.

Circle the Best Answer

18. People normally have a bowel movement
    A. Every day
    B. Every 2 to 3 days
    C. 2 or 3 times a day
    D. All of these can be normal

19. Bleeding in the stomach and small intestines causes
    stool to be
    A. Brown   C. Red
    B. Black   D. Clay-colored

20. The characteristic odor of stool is caused by
    A. Poor personal hygiene
    B. Poor nutrition
    C. Bacterial action in the intestines
    D. Adequate fluid intake

21. When you observe stool that is abnormal
    A. Ask the nurse to observe the stool
    B. Report your observation and discard the stool
    C. Ask the person if the stool is normal for him
    D. Record your observation when you finish his care

22. Which of these could interfere with defecation?
    A. Being able to relax by reading a book or
       newspaper
    B. Eating a diet with high-fiber foods
    C. Having others present in a semi-private room
    D. Drinking 6 to 8 glasses of water daily

23. A person who must stay in bed most of the time may
    have irregular elimination and constipation because of
    A. Poor diet   C. Inactivity
    B. Poor fluid intake   D. Lack of privacy

24. Which of these would provide safety for the person
    during bowel elimination?
    A. Make sure the bedpan is warm
    B. Place the signal light and toilet tissue within the
       person's reach
    C. Provide perineal care
    D. Allow enough time for defecation

25. Constipation can be relieved by
    A. Giving the person a low-fiber diet
    B. Increasing activity
    C. Decreasing fluids
    D. Ignoring the urge to defecate

26. A person tries several times to have a bowel movement and cannot. Liquid feces seeps from the anus. This may mean he has
    A. Diarrhea
    B. Constipation
    C. A fecal impaction
    D. Fecal incontinence
27. When a fecal impaction is present, it is relieved by
    A. Changing the person's diet
    B. Giving more fluids
    C. Removing the fecal mass with a gloved finger
    D. Increasing the activity of the person
28. If you are delegated to remove a fecal impaction, you should make sure
    A. Your state allows you to perform such procedures
    B. The procedures are in your job description
    C. You have the necessary education and training
    D. All of the above
29. Good skin care is important when a person has diarrhea because
    A. This prevents odors
    B. Skin breakdown and pressure ulcers are risks
    C. It prevents the spread of microbes
    D. It prevents fluid loss
30. Why is diarrhea very serious in older persons?
    A. It causes skin breakdown
    B. It causes odors
    C. It can cause dehydration and death
    D. It increases activity
31. When fecal incontinence occurs, the person may need all of these except
    A. Increased fluid intake
    B. Bowel training
    C. Help with elimination after meals and every 2 to 3 hours
    D. Incontinence products to keep garments and linens clean
32. If flatus is not expelled, the person may complain of
    A. Abdominal cramping or pain
    B. Diarrhea
    C. Fecal incontinence
    D. Nausea
33. Which of these is not a goal of bowel training?
    A. To give laxatives daily to maintain regular bowel movements
    B. To gain control of bowel movements
    C. To develop a regular pattern of elimination
    D. To prevent fecal impaction, constipation, and fecal incontinence
34. When bowel training is planned, which of these is included in the care plan?
    A. The amount of stool the person expels
    B. How many bowel movements the person has each day
    C. The usual time of day the person has a bowel movement
    D. The foods that cause flatus
35. When the nurse delegates you to prepare a soap suds enema, mix
    A. 2 teaspoons of salt in 1000 mL of tap water
    B. 3–5 mL of castile soap in 500–1000 mL of tap water
    C. 2 mL of castile soap in 200 mL of tap water
    D. Mineral oil with sterile water

36. When you give a cleansing enema, it should be given to the person
    A. Within 5 minutes
    B. Over about 30 minutes
    C. Over about 10–15 minutes
    D. Over about 20 minutes
37. The person receiving an enema is usually placed in a
    A. Supine position
    B. Prone position
    C. Semi-Fowler's position
    D. Left side-lying or Sims' position
38. When you prepare and give an enema to an adult, you will do all of these except
    A. Prepare the solution at 110° F
    B. Insert the tubing 2 to 4 inches into the rectum
    C. Hold the solution container about 12 inches above the bed
    D. Lubricate the enema tip before inserting it into the rectum
39. When the doctor orders enemas until clear
    A. Give one enema
    B. Give as many enemas as necessary to return a clear fluid
    C. Ask the nurse how many enemas to give
    D. Give only tap water enemas
40. If you are giving an enema and the person complains of cramping
    A. Tell the person that is normal and continue to give the enema
    B. Clamp the tube until the cramping subsides
    C. Discontinue the enema immediately and tell the nurse
    D. Lower the bag below the level of the bed
41. If you are giving a cleansing enema to a child, which of the following is correct?
    A. Mix 3 mL of castile soap with 500 mL of tap water
    B. A saline enema is used when giving a cleansing enema to a child
    C. Only use a small volume enema
    D. Use room temperature tap water for the solution
42. When giving a small volume enema, do not release pressure on the bottle because
    A. It will cause cramping if pressure is released
    B. The fluid will leak from the rectum
    C. Solution will be drawn back into the bottle
    D. It will cause flatulence
43. When giving a small volume enema
    A. Place the person in the prone position
    B. Insert the enema tip 2 inches into the rectum
    C. Heat the solution to 105° F
    D. Clamp the tubing if cramping occurs
44. An oil-retention enema is given to
    A. Cleanse the bowel to prepare for surgery
    B. Regulate the person who is receiving bowel training
    C. Relieve flatulence
    D. Soften the feces and lubricate the rectum

45. If you feel resistance when you are giving an enema
    A. Lubricate the tube more thoroughly
    B. Push more firmly to insert the tube
    C. Stop tube insertion
    D. Ask the person to take a deep breath and relax
46. When you are caring for a person with an ostomy, you know
    A. All of the stools are solid and formed
    B. The stoma does not have sensation and touching does not cause pain
    C. An ostomy is always temporary and is reconnected after healing
    D. A pouch is worn to protect the stoma
47. Which of these statements is true about an ileostomy?
    A. The stool is solid and formed
    B. The stoma is an opening into the colon
    C. The pouch is changed daily
    D. The skin around the ileostomy can be irritated by the digestive juices in the stool
48. When caring for a person with an ostomy, the pouch is
    A. Changed daily
    B. Changed every 3 to 7 days and when it leaks
    C. Only worn when the person thinks he or she will have a bowel movement
    D. Are changed every time the person has a bowel movement
49. The best time to change the ostomy bag is before breakfast, because
    A. The stoma is less likely to expel feces at this time
    B. The person has more time in the morning
    C. It should be changed before morning care
    D. The person tolerates the procedure better before eating
50. When cleaning the skin around the stoma, you use
    A. Sterile water and sterile gauze pads
    B. Alcohol and sterile cotton
    C. Gauze pads or washcloths and water and soap or cleansing agents as delegated by the nurse
    D. Adhesive remover and sterile cotton balls

Fill in the Blank

51. Write out the abbreviations.
    A. BM _____
    B. C _____
    C. CMS _____
    D. F _____
    E. GI _____
    F. ID _____
    G. IV _____
    H. mL _____
    I. oz _____
    J. SSE _____

52. When observing stool, what should be reported to the nurse?
    A. _____
    B. _____
    C. _____
    D. _____
    E. _____
    F. _____
    G. _____
    H. _____
53. What 3 food groups are high in fiber?
    A. _____
    B. _____
    C. _____
54. Name 6 gas-forming foods
    A. _____
    B. _____
    C. _____
    D. _____
    E. _____
    F. _____
55. Drinking warm fluids such as coffee, tea, hot cider, and warm water will increase
    _____.
56. If you are delegated to remove a fecal impaction, what observations should you report and record?
    A. _____
    B. _____
    C. _____
    D. _____
57. When checking and removing impactions, the vagus nerve may be stimulated. Why is this dangerous?
    _____
58. How will dehydration affect these?
    A. Skin is _____
    B. Urine is _____
    C. Blood pressure _____
    D. Pulse and respirations _____
59. Flatulence may be caused when a tense or anxious person _____ while eating and drinking.
60. When a nurse inserts a suppository, how soon would you expect the person to defecate?
    _____

61. Before giving an enema, make sure that
    A. Your state _____
    B. The procedure _____
    C. You have _____
    D. You review _____
    E. A nurse _____

62. After giving an enema, what should be reported and recorded?
    A. _____
    B. _____
    C. _____
    D. _____
    E. _____
    F. _____
    G. _____

63. Because it is likely you will likely contact stool while giving an enema you should follow

    _____ and

    _____.

64. How can cramping be prevented during an enema?
    A. _____
    B. _____

65. How long does it usually take for a tap water, saline, or soapsuds enema to take effect?

    _____

66. A small volume enema for adults contains

    _____ of solution.

67. A person should retain a small volume enema for

    _____.

68. When you start to insert the tube to give an enema, ask the person to _____.

69. What can you place in the ostomy pouch to prevent odors? _____.

70. Showers and baths are delayed 1 or 2 hours after applying a new pouch to allow

    _____.

Use Focus on PRIDE in the Textbook to complete questions 71–72.

71. If your state allows a nursing assistant to insert suppositories, you may be allowed to insert them in

    persons who _____.
    You are not allowed to give a suppository for

    _____.

72. When the person needs to have a bowel elimination, you can provide comfort and privacy when you
    A. _____
    B. _____
    C. _____
    D. _____
    E. _____
    F. _____
    G. _____

Labeling
Use these figures to answer questions 73–76.

73. Name the four types of colostomies shown
    A. _____
    B. _____
    C. _____
    D. _____
74. Which colostomy will have the most solid and formed
    stool? _____
75. Which colostomy will have the most liquid stool?

    _____

76. Which colostomy is a temporary colostomy?

    _____

Use this figure to answer questions 77–79.

77. What type of ostomy is shown?

    _____

78. What part of the bowel has been removed?
_____

79. Will the stool from the ostomy be liquid or formed?
_____

Optional Learning Exercises

80. You are caring for Mr. Evans who is in a semi-private room. His roommate has a large family and many visitors. Mr. Evans has not had a bowel movement in three days, even though he is eating well and taking medications to assist elimination. What could be a reason he has not had a bowel movement? _____
_____
_____

81. Mrs. Weller usually has a bowel movement after breakfast. What are some activities that may assist her to defecate more easily? _____
_____

82. The nurse tells you to make sure Mr. Johnson eats the high fiber foods in his diet to assist in his elimination. What foods are high in fiber?
_____

83. Mrs. Shaffer tells you she cannot digest fruits and vegetables and she refuses to eat them. What may be added to her cereal and prune juice to provide fiber?
_____

84. You offer Mr. Murphy _____ of water each day to promote normal bowel elimination.

85. Mr. Hernandez has been taking an antibiotic, which is a drug to treat his pneumonia, and he has developed diarrhea. You think he may have diarrhea because
_____.

86. You are caring for 83-year-old Mrs. Chen and you helped her to the bathroom 30 minutes ago, where she had a bowel movement. When you enter her room to make her bed, she tells you she needs to use the bathroom for a bowel movement. You know that older people _____
_____

87. Why can tap water enemas be dangerous? _____
_____
_____ How many tap water enemas can be given? _____
Why? _____
_____

88. Compare small volume enemas and oil retention enemas.
    A. Small volume enemas _____ the rectum. Oil retention enemas are given to
    _____.

    B. Small volume enemas take effect in about
    _____ minutes. Oil retention enemas should be retained for at least
    _____ minutes.

Independent Learning Activities

Think about times when you have had a problem with bowel irregularity. Answer these questions about how you handled the problems.
- What causes you to have irregularity? Foods? Illness? Stress? Inactivity?
- What methods have you used to treat irregularity? Diet? Medication?
- How does irregularity affect you physically? Your appetite? Energy level? Sleep and rest?
- How does irregularity affect your mood? Your daily activities?

Interview a person who has a colostomy or an ileostomy. You may know someone who has an ostomy. Or you may care for someone who has one. Your community may have an ostomy support group that you can contact. Talk to the person and ask these questions.
- How long has the person had the ostomy? Is it permanent or temporary?
- What was the hardest part of learning to live with an ostomy? What was the easiest part?
- How has living with an ostomy affected the person's life? Has the person's work been affected? Were leisure activities affected?
- How has the ostomy affected the person's family? What changes have occurred?
- What equipment works best for the person? How expensive is the equipment? How much time is required each day to care for the ostomy?

24 Nutrition and Fluids

Fill in the Blank: Key Terms

Anorexia
Aspiration
Calorie

Cholesterol
Daily Value (DV)
Dehydration

Dysphagia
Edema
Graduate

Intake
Nutrient

Nutrition
Output

1. ___Intake___ is the amount of fluid taken in.
2. The ___daily value___ is how a serving fits into the daily diet. It is expressed in a percent based on a daily diet of 2000 calories.
3. The loss of appetite is ___anorexia___.
4. The amount of fluid lost is ___output___.
5. A substance that is ingested, digested, absorbed, and used by the body is a ___nutrient___.
6. ___dysphagia___ is difficulty or discomfort in swallowing.
7. The breathing of fluid, food, vomitus, or an object into the lungs is ___aspiration___.
8. The many processes involved in the ingestion, digestion, absorption, and use of food and fluids by the body is ___nutrition___.
9. The amount of energy produced from the burning of food by the body is a ___calorie___.
10. A decrease in the amount of water in body tissues is ___dehydration___.
11. A ___graduate___ is a calibrated container used to measure fluid.
12. ___Edema___ is the swelling of body tissues with water.
13. A soft, waxy substance found in the bloodstream and all body cells is ___cholesterol___.

Circle the Best Answer

14. Which of these occur when the person has a poor diet and poor eating habits?
    A. Decreased risk for infection and chronic diseases
    B. Improved wound healing
    C. Increased risk for accidents and injuries
    D. Decreased risk of acute and chronic infections

15. Body fuel for energy is found in
    A. Vitamins
    B. Minerals
    C. Fats, proteins, and carbohydrates
    D. Water
16. All of the foods are included in MyPlate *except:*
    A. Eating high fat foods
    B. Making half of your plate fruits and vegetables
    C. Increasing the amount of meat and fish in your diet
    D. Drinking water instead of sugary drinks
17. The amount needed from each food group in MyPlate depends on
    A. The ethnic background of the person
    B. The age, sex, and physical activity of the person
    C. The likes and dislikes of the person
    D. The budget available to the person
18. Whole wheat grains in the grain group include
    A. Bulgur, oatmeal, and brown rice
    B. White flour and white rice
    C. Black beans, lentils, and split peas
    D. Potatoes, green bananas, and water chestnuts
19. When choosing from the protein food group, foods that may reduce the risk of heart disease include
    A. Whole eggs
    B. Processed meats
    C. Salmon, trout, and herring
    D. Regular ground beef and chicken with skin
20. All of these are food groups in MyPlate *except*
    A. Grains
    B. Vegetables
    C. Fruits
    D. Oils
21. An example of moderate physical activity in MyPlate would be
    A. Bicycling at less than 10 miles per hour
    B. Freestyle swimming laps
    C. Chopping wood
    D. Running and jogging at 5 miles per hour
22. Which nutrient is needed for tissue growth and repair?
    A. Carbohydrates   C. Vitamins
    B. Fats   D. Protein

23. Which vitamin is needed for the formation of substances that hold tissue together?
    A. Vitamin K   C. Vitamin A
    B. Vitamin C   D. Vitamin B$_{12}$
24. Food labels have all of this information *except*
    A. The serving size
    B. All vitamins and minerals in the food
    C. Total amount of fat and amount of saturated and trans fats
    D. Amount of cholesterol and sodium
25. A cultural group that eats a diet high in sodium is in
    A. The Philippines   C. Poland
    B. China   D. Mexico
26. All pork and pork products are forbidden by
    A. Seventh-Day Adventists
    B. Muslim or Islam
    C. The Church of Jesus Christ of Latter Day Saints
    D. Roman Catholic
27. People with limited incomes often buy
    A. More protein foods
    B. Cheaper carbohydrate foods
    C. Food high in vitamins and minerals
    D. Fatty foods
28. When people buy cheaper foods, the diet may lack
    A. Fats
    B. Starchy foods
    C. Protein and certain vitamins and minerals
    D. Sugars
29. Appetite can be stimulated by
    A. Illness and medications
    B. Decreased senses of taste and smell
    C. Aromas and thoughts of food
    D. Anxiety, pain, and depression
30. Personal choice of foods is influenced by
    A. Foods served in the home
    B. Age and social experience
    C. How food looks and smells
    D. All of the above
31. During illness
    A. Appetite increases
    B. Fewer nutrients are needed
    C. Nutritional needs increase to fight infection and heal tissue
    D. The person will prefer protein foods
32. All of these may occur with aging *except*
    A. Increases in taste and smell
    B. Secretion of digestive juices decreases
    C. Difficulty in chewing
    D. A need for fewer calories than younger people
33. Requirements for food served in nursing centers are made by
    A. MyPlate
    B. OBRA
    C. The nursing center
    D. The public health department
34. All of these are requirements for food served in long-term care centers *except*
    A. The center provides needed adaptive equipment and utensils

B. The person's diet is well-balanced, nourishing, and tastes good
C. All food is served at room temperature
D. Each person must receive at least 3 meals a day and be offered a bedtime snack
35. A general diet
    A. Is ordered for a person with difficulty swallowing
    B. Has no dietary limits or restrictions
    C. May have restricted amounts of sodium
    D. Increase the amount of sugar in the diet
36. The body needs no more than _____ of sodium each day.
    A. 2300 mg   C. 5000 mg
    B. 3000 mg   D. 1000 mg
37. When the body tissues swell with water, what organ has to work harder?
    A. Kidneys   C. Heart
    B. Liver   D. Lungs
38. When you are caring for a person with diabetes, you should do all of these *except*
    A. Serve the person's meals and snacks on time
    B. Tell the nurse what the person did and did not eat
    C. Give the person extra food and snacks whenever it is requested
    D. Provide a between-meal nourishment if all the food was not eaten
39. A person may be given a mechanical soft diet because
    A. The person is overweight
    B. The person has chewing problems
    C. The person has been advanced from a clear-liquid diet
    D. The person has constipation
40. If you are serving a meal to a person on a fiber and residue restricted diet, the meal would *not* include
    A. Raw fruits and vegetables
    B. Strained fruit juices
    C. Canned or cooked fruit without skin or seeds
    D. Plain pasta
41. A person who has serious burns would receive a
    A. Sodium-controlled diet
    B. Fat-controlled diet
    C. High-calorie diet
    D. High-protein diet
42. When a person has dysphagia, the thickness of the food served is chosen by the
    A. Person
    B. Nursing assistant
    C. Family
    D. Speech/language pathologist, occupational therapist, dietician, and doctor or nurse
43. Which of these may be a sign of a swallowing problem (dysphagia)?
    A. Person complains that food will not go down or that food is stuck
    B. Foods that need chewing are avoided
    C. There is excessive drooling of saliva
    D. All of the above

44. When assisting a person who is on aspirations precautions, you can help to prevent aspiration while the person is eating by placing him in
    A. Semi-Fowler's position
    B. Fowler's position
    C. The side-lying position
    D. The supine position
45. If fluid intake exceeds fluid output, the person will
    A. Have edema in the tissues
    B. Be dehydrated
    C. Have vomiting and diarrhea
    D. Have increased urinary output
46. How much fluid is needed every day for normal fluid balance?
    A. 1500 mL   C. 2000–2500 mL
    B. 1000–1500 mL   D. 3000–4000 mL
47. If the person you are caring for has an order for restricted fluids, which of these should you do?
    A. Offer a variety of liquids
    B. Thicken all fluids
    C. Remove the water pitcher or keep it out of sight
    D. Do not allow the person to swallow any liquids during oral hygiene
48. When you are keeping I&O records, you should measure all of these *except*
    A. Milk, water, coffee, and tea
    B. Mashed potatoes and creamed vegetables
    C. Soups and gelatin
    D. Ice cream, custard, and pudding
49. When you are measuring I&O, you need to know that one ounce equals
    A. 10 mL   C. 100 mL
    B. 500 mL   D. 30 mL
50. When you are using the graduate to measure output, you read the amount by
    A. Holding the graduate at waist level and reading the amount
    B. Looking at the graduate while it is held above eye level
    C. Place the graduate at eye level to read
    D. Setting the graduate on the floor and reading it
51. When I&O is ordered, which of the following is *not* included in the measurement?
    A. Urine   C. Drainage from suction
    B. Solid stool   D. Vomitus
52. When residents are served meals in family dining
    A. They serve themselves as at home
    B. The person can eat any time the buffet is open
    C. Mealtime distractions are prevented
    D. Food is served as in a restaurant
53. Which of the following needs to be done before the person is served a meal?
    A. Give complete personal care
    B. Change all linens
    C. Check the person's position
    D. Make sure the person has been shaved or has makeup applied

54. You can provide comfort during meals by
    A. Making sure unpleasant sights, sounds, and odors are removed
    B. Making sure dentures, eyeglasses, or hearing aids are in place
    C. Giving the person good oral care before and after meals
    D. All of the above
55. What should you do if a food tray has not been served within 15 minutes?
    A. Recheck the food temperatures
    B. Serve the tray immediately
    C. Throw the food away
    D. Serve only the cold items on the tray
56. How can you make sure the food tray is complete?
    A. Ask the person being served
    B. Ask the nurse
    C. Call the dietary department
    D. Check items on the tray with the dietary card
57. If you become impatient while feeding a resident with dementia, you should
    A. Refuse to continue caring for the person
    B. Return the person to his or her room
    C. Talk to the nurse
    D. Make the person eat his or her food
58. When you are feeding a person you should
    A. Not allow the person to assist
    B. Give the person a fork and knife to assist with cutting the food
    C. Feed the person in a private area to maintain confidentiality
    D. Use a spoon because it is less likely to cause injury
59. When feeding a person, liquids are given
    A. Only at the start of feeding
    B. During the meal alternating with solid foods
    C. At the end of the meal when all solid have been eaten
    D. Only if the person has difficulty swallowing.
60. When delegated to provide drinking water, what information do you need from the nurse and the care plan?
    A. Whether a person likes water
    B. If a person can have ice
    C. Whether the person can pour water himself
    D. How often to refill the pitcher
61. When reheating cooked foods, it should be heated
    A. To room temperature
    B. To 165° F
    C. To 212° F
    D. To the temperature the person requests
62. When handling food, hand washing should be done before and after
    A. Handling food   C. Handling pets
    B. Using the bathroom   D. All of the above

Fill in the Blank

63. Write out the abbreviations.

    A. CMS _____

    B. DV _____

    C. F _____

    D. GI _____

    E. ID _____

    F. I&O _____

    G. mg _____

    H. mL _____

    I. NPO _____

    J. OBRA _____

    K. oz _____

    L. USDA _____

64. How many calories are in each of these?

    A. 1 gram of fat _____

    B. 1 gram of protein _____

    C. 1 gram of carbohydrate _____

Use the Dietary Guidelines for Americans 2010 to answer questions 65–68.

65. The *Dietary Guidelines for Americans* are for persons

    A. _____

    B. _____

66. Certain diseases are linked to poor diet and lack of physical activity. They are

    A. _____

    B. _____

    C. _____

    D. _____

    E. _____

    F. _____

67. The *Dietary Guidelines* help people

    A. _____

    B. _____

    C. _____

68. The *Dietary Guidelines* focus on

    A. _____

    B. _____

    C. _____

Questions 69 to 72 relate to MyPlate.

69. What are the 5 food groups in MyPlate?

    A. _____

    B. _____

    C. _____

    D. _____

    E. _____

70. When using MyPlate, calories are balanced by

    A. _____

    B. _____

71. When making food choices, which foods are increased in the diet?

    A. _____

    B. _____

    C. _____

72. Which food group or groups has the following health benefits?

    A. Build and maintain bone mass throughout life

    _____

    B. Provides B vitamins and vitamin E

    _____

    C. May prevent constipation

    _____

    D. May reduce risk of kidney stones

    _____

    E. May prevent certain birth defects

    _____

    F. May help lower calorie intake

    _____

    G. Provides nutrients needed for health and body maintenance _____

73. What is the most important nutrient?

    _____

74. If dietary fat is not needed by the body, it is stored as

    _____.

75. What is the function of each of these nutrients?

    A. Protein _____

    B. Carbohydrates _____

    C. Fats _____

    D. Vitamins _____

    E. Minerals _____

    F. Water _____

76. Which vitamins can be stored by the body?

    _____

77. Which vitamins must be ingested daily?

    _____

78. What vitamin is important for these functions? *Forming substances that hold tissues together; healthy blood vessels, skin, gums, bones, and teeth; wound healing; prevention of bleeding; resistance to infection.*

    _____

79. Milk and milk products, liver, green leafy vegetables, eggs, breads, and cereals are good sources of which vitamin? _____

80. What mineral allows red blood cells to carry oxygen?
_____

81. When the diet does not have enough
_____, it may affect nerve
function, muscle contraction, and heart function.

82. Calcium is needed for _____
_____.

83. What information is found on food labels?
A. _____
B. _____
C. _____

84. Those who practice _____ as their
religion eat only fish with scales and fins.

85. Alcohol and coffee are avoided or not allowed by
these religious groups.
A. _____
B. _____
C. _____

86. What religious group may have members that
fast from meats on certain Fridays of the year?
_____

87. Nutritional needs increase during illness when the
body must _____
_____.

88. Older persons need _____
calories than younger people do.

89. Why do the diets of some older people lack protein?
_____

90. What OBRA requirement relates to the temperature
of foods served in long-term
care centers? _____
_____

91. What foods are included in a clear-liquid diet?
_____
_____
_____

92. When the person receives a full-liquid diet, it will
include all of the foods on the clear-liquid diet as
well as these foods _____
_____

93. If a person has poorly fitted dentures and has
chewing problems, the doctor may order a
_____ diet.

94. A person who is constipated and has other GI
disorders may receive a _____
diet. The foods in this diet increase the
_____ to stimulate
_____.

95. If a person is receiving a high-calorie diet, the calorie
intake is _____ daily.

96. What vegetables juices are high in sodium?
_____.

97. When a person is receiving a diabetic diet, the same
amount of _____
_____ are eaten each day.

98. If you are feeding a person a dysphagia diet, what
observations should be reported to the nurse
immediately?
A. _____, _____, or
_____ during or after meal
B. _____ or
_____

99. Why is it important to offer water often to
older persons? _____
_____

100. When you give oral hygiene to a person who is
receiving nothing by mouth, the person must not
_____.

101. List the amount of milliliters in the following
A. 1 ounce equals _____ mL
B. 1 pint equals about _____ mL
C. 1 quart equals about _____ mL

102. What information do you need when you are
delegated to measure intake and output?
A. _____
B. _____
C. _____
D. _____
E. _____

103. What type of dining program may be used with
persons who are quietly confused?
_____

104. What can be done to promote comfort when
preparing residents for meals?
A. _____
B. _____
C. _____
D. _____
E. _____
F. _____

105. If a food tray is not served within 15 minutes, what
should be checked? _____

106. When you are delegated to serve meal trays, what information do you need from the nurse or care plan?

    A. _____

    B. _____

    C. _____

    D. _____

    E. _____

    F. _____

    G. _____

107. When you are serving meal trays, you make sure the right person gets the right tray

    by checking _____

    _____

108. When you are feeding a person the spoon should be

    filled _____

109. Why is it important to sit facing the person when you feed him or her?

    A. _____

    B. _____

    C. _____

110. What should be reported after you have fed a person?

    A. _____

    B. _____

    C. _____

    D. _____

111. If a person is on calorie count, what is recorded?

    _____

    What does the nurse or dietician do with this

    information? _____

112. In order to keep food safe, the USDA recommends that you

    A. Clean: _____

    B. Separate: _____

    C. Cook: _____

    _____

    D. Chill: _____

    _____

113. The safe temperature to keep foods are

    A. Cold foods _____

    B. Hot foods _____

    C. The danger zone for foods is

    _____ for more than

    _____ hours, or

    _____ hour if temperature is

    warmer than 90° F.

    D. Keep the refrigerator at _____

    or below. Keep the freezer at _____

    or below.

Use Focus on PRIDE in the Textbook to complete questions 114–116.

114. When a nursing center uses 24-hour catering or mobile food carts, it allows the residents to have

    freedom and _____.

115. When you respect the person's likes and dislikes of food, or complaints about the food, it meets the right

    to _____.

116. When family members bring food to a resident, it is

    important that you tell _____.
    The food must not interfere with the

    _____.

23. When caring for a person receiving IV therapy, the nursing assistant can
    A. Adjust the flow rate if it is too fast or too slow
    B. Tell the nurse at once if no fluid is dripping
    C. Disconnect the IV to give basic care
    D. Change the IV bag when it is empty
24. You may change a dressing on a peripheral IV if
    A. The nurse asks you to do this
    B. You observe that it is loose and soiled
    C. Your state lets nursing assistants perform the procedure
    D. You think you know how to do this procedure

Fill in the Blank

25. Write out the abbreviations.
    A. GI _____
    B. gtt _____
    C. gtt/min _____
    D. IV _____
    E. mL _____
    F. NG _____
    G. NPO _____
    H. oz _____
    I. PEG _____
    J. TPN _____

26. Naso-gastric and naso-enteral tubes are in place for short-term nutritional support, usually for less than _____.

27. Gastrostomy, jejunostomy, and PEG tubes are used for long-term support, usually longer than _____.

28. Formula is given through a feeding tube at room temperature because cold fluids cause _____.

29. Coughing, sneezing, vomiting, suctioning, and poor positioning can move a tube out of place and are common causes of _____.

30. What can the nursing assistant do to assist the nurse in preventing regurgitation and aspiration?
    A. _____
    B. _____
    C. _____

31. What comfort measures will help a person with a feeding tube who has a dry mouth?
    A. _____
    B. _____
    C. _____

32. The nose and nostrils are cleaned every 4 to 8 hours because a feeding tube can _____ and _____.

33. If you are delegated to give a tube feeding, what should the nurse check first?
    A. RN identifies _____
    B. RN checks _____ and _____

34. How much flushing solution is used before giving a tube feeding to an adult? _____

35. When caring for a person receiving IV therapy, what signs and symptoms of complications may occur at the IV site?
    A. _____
    B. _____
    C. _____
    D. _____
    E. _____
    F. _____

Use Focus on PRIDE in the Textbook to complete question 36.

36. You have a responsibility when a person has an IV. These responsibilities include
    A. When you hear an alarm, _____
    B. If the battery is low, _____
    C. You may help the person to reposition his or her arm for the _____
    D. You do *not* adjust _____ on IV pumps or _____ on IV tubing

Optional Learning Exercises

37. What type of feeding tube would each of these persons probably have in place?
    A. The nurse tells you Mr. S. is expected to have a feeding tube to his stomach for 2–3 weeks. _____
    B. Mrs. G. has had a feeding tube into her stomach for 9 months. _____ or _____
    C. The nurse tells you to observe Mr. H. for irritation of his nose and nostril when you give care. _____ or _____
    D. The nurse tells you that Mrs. K. is at great risk for regurgitation from her feeding tube. _____ or _____

38. You are caring for a person receiving a continuous tube feeding. You note that the formula was hung 7¾ hours ago, so you tell the nurse. Why did you report this to the nurse? _____

    _____

39. Why are older persons more at risk for regurgitation and aspiration?

    A. _____
    B. _____

40. What would you do if a person with a feeding tube asks you for something to eat or drink?

    _____ Why? _____

    _____

41. Mrs. H. has a feeding tube in her nose. Answer these questions about caring for her nose and nostrils.

    A. How often should the nose and nostrils be cleaned? _____

    B. How is the tube secured to the nose?

       _____

    C. Why is the tube secured to the person's garment at the shoulder?

       _____

    D. What are 2 ways the tube can be secured at the shoulder?

       1. _____
       2. _____

42. When giving tube feedings, what answers would you likely get if you asked the nurse these questions?

    A. What feeding method is used?

       _____

    B. What size syringe is used?

       _____

    C. How is the person positioned for the feeding?

       _____

    D. How is the person positioned after the feeding?

       _____

    E. How high is the syringe raised or the feeding bag hung?

       _____

    F. How much fluid is used to flush the tubing?

       _____

    G. How fast is the feeding given if using a syringe?

       _____

43. If a person is receiving TPN, how will you assist the nurse?

    A. _____
    B. _____
    C. _____

44. How can you check the flow rate of an IV?

    _____

45. What would you tell the RN at once when you check the flow rate?

    A. _____
    B. _____
    C. _____

Independent Learning Activities

Have you or anyone you know ever needed enteral nutrition? Either answer these questions or ask the person you know to answer them.
- How long was the tube in place? What type of tube was used?
- What discomfort or pain was felt?
- How did having a feeding tube affect your activity? Your personal care and grooming?

Have you ever had an IV? Answer these questions about the experience.
- What type of IV did you have? Where was it inserted?
- How long was the IV in place?
- How did the IV interfere with your care, grooming, or activity?

You may care for a person who is not receiving any nutritional support or IV therapy. Answer these questions about how you handle this situation.
- How would you feel about caring for a person who is not receiving any nutritional support?
- How would your religious or cultural values affect you in this situation?
- If the situation made you uncomfortable, what would you do?

26 Measuring Vital Signs

Fill in the Blank: Key Terms

Apical-radial pulse   Diastolic pressure   Pulse deficit   Systole
Blood pressure   Fever   Pulse rate   Systolic pressure
Body temperature   Hypertension   Respiration   Tachycardia
Bradycardia   Hypotension   Sphygmomanometer   Thermometer
Diastole   Pulse   Stethoscope   Vital signs

1. A rapid heart rate is _tachycardia_. The heart rate is over 100 beats per minute.

2. The _apical-radial pulse_ is taking the apical and radial pulse at the same time.

3. An instrument used to listen to the sounds produced by the heart, lungs, and other body organs is a _stethoscope_.

4. When the systolic blood pressure is below 90 mm Hg and the diastolic pressure is below 60 mm Hg it is called _hypotension_.

5. The _pulse rate_ is the number of heartbeats or pulses felt in 1 minute.

6. The amount of heat in the body that is a balance between the amount of heat produced and amount lost by the body is the _body temperature_.

7. _Systole_ is the period of heart muscle contraction.

8. _Hypertension_ is when the systolic pressure is 140 mm Hg or higher or diastolic pressure is 90 mm Hg or higher.

9. The cuff and measuring device used to measure blood pressure is a _sphygmomanometer_.

10. The beat of the heart felt at an artery as a wave of blood passes through the artery is the _pulse_.

11. Temperature, pulse, respirations, and blood pressure are _vital signs_.

12. _bradycardia_ is a slow heart rate; the rate is less than 60 beats per minute.

13. The amount of force it takes to pump blood out of the heart into the arterial circulation is the

14. The period of heart muscle relaxation is _diastole_.

15. The difference between the apical and radial pulse rates is the _pulse deficit_.

16. _systolic pressure_ is the amount of force exerted against the walls of an artery by the blood.

17. Breathing air into and out of the lungs is _respiration_.

18. _diastolic pressure_ is the pressure in the arteries when the heart is at rest.

19. Elevated body temperature is _fever_.

20. A _thermometer_ is a device used to measure temperature.

Circle the Best Answer

21. Persons in nursing centers usually have vital signs measured
    A. Once a shift
    B. Every 4 hours
    C. Once a month
    D. Daily, twice a day, or weekly

22. Unless otherwise ordered, take vital signs when the person
    A. Is lying or sitting
    B. Has been walking or exercising
    C. Has just finished eating
    D. Is getting ready to take a shower or tub bath

23. Body temperature is lower in the
    A. Afternoon   C. Evening
    B. Morning   D. Night

24. If you are taking vital signs on a person with dementia, it may be better if
    A. You have a co-worker hold the person so he or she does not move
    B. The vital signs are taken when the person is asleep
    C. You take the pulse and respirations at one time, and the temperature and blood pressure at another time
    D. You ask the nurse to take the vital signs

25. What should you do if a person asks their vital sign measurements?
    A. You can tell the person the measurements if center policy allows
    B. Tell the nurse that the person wants to know the measurements
    C. Tell the person you cannot tell them this information
    D. This information is private and cannot be shared
26. If you take a rectal temperature, the normal range of the temperature would be
    A. 96.6° F to 98.6° F (35.9° C to 37.0° C)
    B. 97.6° F to 99.6° F (36.5° C to 37.5° C)
    C. 98.6° F to 100.6° F (37.0° C to 38.1° C)
    D. 98.6° F (37° C)
27. If you are taking the temperature of an older person, you would expect the temperature to be
    A. Lower than the normal range
    B. Higher than the normal range
    C. About in the middle of the normal range
    D. The same as a younger adult
28. A glass rectal thermometer has
    A. A stubby tip color-coded in red
    B. A long or slender tip
    C. A pear-shaped tip
    D. A blue color-coded end
29. To read a glass thermometer you should hold it at the
    A. Stem above eye level and look up to read it
    B. Bulb end and bring it to eye level
    C. Stem and bring it to eye level to read it
    D. Bulb at waist level and look down to read it
30. If you are preparing to take an oral temperature, ask the person not to
    A. Eat, drink, smoke, or chew gum for at least 15 to 20 minutes
    B. Shower or bathe right before the temperature is taken
    C. Exercise for 30 minutes before
    D. Eat, drink, or smoke for at least 5 to 10 minutes
31. A glass thermometer is inserted into the rectum
    A. 1 inch   C. ½ inch
    B. 2 inch   D. 3 inches
32. When taking a temperature for persons who are confused and resist care, the best choice would be to
    A. Take a rectal temperature
    B. Use a glass oral thermometer
    C. Take an axillary temperature
    D. Use tympanic or temporal artery thermometer
33. Which pulse is most commonly used?
    A. Carotid   C. Radial
    B. Brachial   D. Popliteal
34. A _____ pulse is taken during cardiopulmonary resuscitation (CPR).
    A. Carotid
    B. Temporal
    C. Femoral
    D. Radial

35. When using a stethoscope you can help to prevent infection by
    A. Warming the diaphragm in your hand
    B. Wiping the earpieces and diaphragm with antiseptic wipes before and after use
    C. Placing the diaphragm over the artery
    D. Placing the earpieces in your ears so the bend of the tips point forward
36. When a pulse rate is 120 beats per minute you
    A. Report that the person has bradycardia
    B. Know that this is a normal pulse rate
    C. Report that the person has tachycardia
    D. Report that the pulse is irregular
37. The pulse rate is the number of heartbeats or pulses felt in
    A. 30 seconds   C. 1 minute
    B. 15 seconds   D. 5 minutes
38. You need to feel the pulse to determine the
    A. Force
    B. Rate
    C. Rhythm (whether it is regular or irregular)
    D. Blood pressure
39. When taking the radial pulse, place
    A. The thumb over the pulse site
    B. Two or three fingers on the middle of the wrist
    C. Two or three fingers on the thumb side of the wrist
    D. The stethoscope on the chest wall
40. The apical pulse is taken
    A. For a full minute
    B. On infants and children up to 2 years of age
    C. On persons who have an irregular heartbeat
    D. All of the above
41. An apical pulse of 72 is recorded as
    A. Pulse 72   C. 72Ap
    B. 72 – Apical pulse   D. P 72
42. An apical-radial pulse is taken by
    A. Taking the radial pulse for 1 minute and then taking the apical pulse for 1 minute
    B. Subtracting the apical pulse from the radial pulse
    C. Having one staff member take the apical pulse and second staff member takes the radial pulse at the same time
    D. Having two persons take the apical pulse at the same time
43. A pedal pulse is found
    A. By listening to the heart with a stethoscope
    B. Over a foot bone
    C. On the thumb side of the wrist
    D. At the apex of the heart, just below the left nipple
44. When counting respirations the best way is to
    A. Stand quietly next to the person and watch the chest rise and fall
    B. Keep your fingers or stethoscope over the pulse site so the person thinks you are still counting the pulse
    C. Tell the person to breathe normally so you can count the respirations
    D. Use the stethoscope to hear the respirations clearly and count for 1 minute

45. Each respiration involves
    A. One inhalation (rise of chest)
    B. One exhalation (fall of chest)
    C. One inhalation and one exhalation (rise and fall of chest)
    D. Counting for 30 seconds and multiplying by two
46. The blood pressure may be higher in older persons because
    A. They have orthostatic hypotension
    B. The diet is higher in sodium
    C. Blood pressure increases with age
    D. They are usually overweight
47. The blood pressure should not be taken on an arm
    A. If the person has had breast surgery on that side
    B. With an IV
    C. That has a dialysis access site
    D. All of the above
48. You will find out the size of blood pressure cuff needed
    A. By asking the nurse
    B. By measuring the person's arm
    C. In the doctor's orders
    D. Asking the person
49. When taking the blood pressure, you place the stethoscope diaphragm
    A. Over the radial artery on the thumb side of the wrist
    B. Over the brachial artery at the inner aspect of the elbow
    C. Lightly against the skin
    D. Over the apical pulse site
50. When getting ready to take the blood pressure, position the person's arm
    A. Above the level of the heart
    B. Level with the heart
    C. Below the level of the heart
    D. Abducted from the body
51. The blood pressure cuff is inflated

    _____ beyond the point where you last felt the radial pulse.
    A. 10 mm Hg   C. 30 mm Hg
    B. 20 mm Hg   D. 40 mm Hg

Fill in the Blank
52. Write out the abbreviations.
    A. BP _Blood Pressure_
    B. C _Centigrade_
    C. DUS _Doppler ultrasound Stethoscope_
    D. F _Fahrenheit_
    E. Hg _Mercury_
    F. ID _Identification_
    G. IV _Intravenous_
    H. mm _Millimeter_
    I. mm HG _millimeter of Mercury_
53. Vital signs are taken when the person takes drugs that affect _health_.

54. When vital signs are taken report to the nurse at once if
    A. _Changed from last_
    B. _High_
    C. _Low_
55. Sites for measuring temperature are the
    A. _Oral_
    B. _Rectal_
    C. _Axillary_
    D. _Temporal_
    E. _Tympanic membrane_
56. Which site has the highest normal range temperature?
    Rectal
57. Which site has the lowest baseline temperature?
    Axillary
58. If a glass thermometer breaks
    dispose at once because it may contain _mercury_ which is a _poison_.
59. When you read a Fahrenheit thermometer, the short lines mean _.2 of a degree_.
60. List how long the glass thermometer remains in place for these sites.
    A. Oral _2-3_ or as required by center policy
    B. Rectal _2_ or as required by center policy
    C. Axillary _5-10_ or as required by center policy
61. When taking an oral temperature, place the bulb end of the thermometer
    base of tongue to one side.
62. When taking an axillary temperature, the axilla must be _dry_.
63. Tympanic membrane and temporal artery thermometers are used for confused persons because they are _quick_.
64. When using an electronic thermometer what does the color of the probe mean?
    A. Blue _Oral_
    B. Red _rectal_
65. When you take a rectal temperature, you
    lubricate the tip of the thermometer or the end of the covered probe before inserting it into the rectum.
66. When taking a tympanic membrane temperature on an adult, the ear is pulled
    up and back.
67. The adult pulse rate is between
    _60-100_ per minute.
68. List words used to describe
    A. Forceful pulse _strong, full bounding_
    B. Hard-to-feel pulse _weak, thready, feeble_

69. If a pulse is irregular, count the pulse for
_____1 minute_____.

70. When you take a pulse, what observations should be reported and recorded?
    A. _Rate_
    B. _Observations_
    C. _Abnormal pulse_
    D. _Deficit regularity_
    E. _Strength_

71. Do not use your thumb to take a pulse, because
it has a pulse.

72. When taking an apical pulse, each *lub-dub* sound is counted as _1_.

73. The radial pulse rate is never greater than the
apical pulse.

74. The nurse may mark the skin with an X where the
pulse is found.

75. A healthy adult has _16-18_
respirations per minute.

76. What observations should be reported and recorded when counting respirations?
    A. _None_
    B. _Rate_
    C. _Observations_
    D. _abnormalities_
    E. _____
    F. _____

77. One respiration is counted for each _inhalation_
and exhalation.

78. Respirations are counted for
1 minute if they are
abnormal or irregular.

79. Blood pressure is controlled by
    A. _heart contraction_
    B. _Amount of blood_
    C. _Ease of blood flow_

80. Report blood pressures that have these readings.
    A. Systolic over _140_
       systolic below _90_
    B. Diastolic over _80_
       diastolic below _60_

81. Let the person rest for _10-20_
before taking the blood pressure.

82. When you are taking a blood pressure, the person
should be in a _sitting_
or _lying_ position.
Sometimes the doctor orders blood pressure in the
standing position.

83. When listening to the blood pressure, the first sound
you hear is the _systole_

pressure and the point where the sound disappears
is the _diastolic_ pressure.

Use Focus on PRIDE in the Textbook to complete questions 84–87.

84. Measurements of the vital signs are important because they help the nurse
understand the actual
and _plan_ the person's care.

85. You are responsible for
    A. Knowing _how to measure vital signs_
    B. Reporting _vital signs_

86. You allow the person to have _freedom_
_____ when you use the arm for
blood pressure that the person prefers.

87. If you cannot feel a pulse or hear a blood pressure,
you should never _grow angry_.

Labeling

88. For A-C, identify the type of thermometers shown.
    A. _____

    B. _____

    C. _____

    D. An axillary or oral temperature can be taken
    with _____
    thermometers.
    E. A rectal temperature is taken with a
    _____ thermometer.

89. Fill in the drawings so that the thermometers read correctly.

A   95.8° F

B   98.4° F

C   100.2° F

D   35.5° C

E   36.5° C

F   37° C

90. For A-H, name the pulse sites shown.

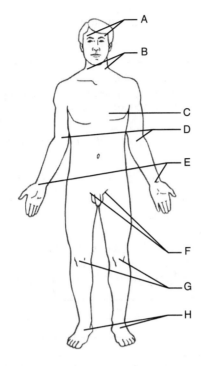

A. _____

B. _____

C. _____

D. _____

E. _____

F. _____

G. _____

H. _____

I. Which pulse is used during cardiopulmonary resuscitation (CPR)?

_____

J. Which pulse is most commonly taken? _____

K. Which pulse is used when taking the blood pressure? _____

L. Which pulse is found with a stethoscope?

_____

91. Fill in the drawings so that the dials show the correct blood pressures.

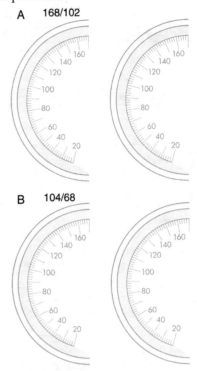

A   168/102

B   104/68

92. Fill in the drawings so the mercury columns show the correct blood pressures.

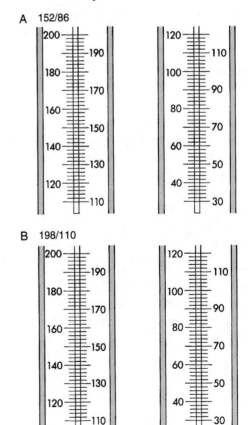

A   152/86

B   198/110

93. Record the readings on the thermometers shown

A _____

B _____

C _____

Optional Learning Exercises

Taking Temperatures

94. You prepare to take Mr. Harrison's temperature with a glass thermometer. When you take the thermometer from the container, it reads 97.8° F. What should you do? _____.

95. If the thermometer registers between two short lines, record the temperature to the

_____.

Taking Pulses and Respirations

96. You are assigned to take Mrs. Sanchez's pulse and respirations. You note that the pulse rate and respirations are regular, so you take each one for _____. When you complete counting the pulse, you keep your _____ and count _____. This is done so that Mrs. Sanchez will _____.

97. When you finish counting Mrs. Sanchez's pulse and respirations, your numbers are pulse 36 and respirations 9. What numbers should be recorded?

Pulse _____ Respirations _____

Why? _____

_____

98. The nurse tells you to take an apical-radial pulse on Mrs. Hellman. Why do you ask a co-worker to help you? _____

99. How long is an apical-radial pulse counted?

_____ After you have taken the apical-radial pulse, how do you find the pulse deficit?

_____

Taking Blood Pressures

100. You are assigned to take Mr. Hardaway's blood pressure. You know that he goes for dialysis 3 times a week. What do need to know before you take his blood pressure? _____

_____

Why? _____

101. When you inflate the cuff, you cannot feel the pulse after you pump the cuff to 130 mm Hg. How high will you inflate the cuff to take his blood pressure?

_____

102. You should deflate the cuff at an even rate of

_____ per second.

Independent Learning Activities

Take turns measuring vital signs on 3 or 4 classmates. If possible, use glass, electronic, and tympanic thermometers for each person to see if they give similar results. Use this table to record the results.

Person	Temperature	Pulse	Respiration	Blood Pressure
#1	Glass Electronic Tympanic	Radial Apical	Rate Rhythm Depth	
#2	Glass Electronic Tympanic	Radial Apical	Rate Rhythm Depth	
#3	Glass Electronic Tympanic	Radial Apical	Rate Rhythm Depth	
#4	Glass Electronic Tympanic	Radial Apical	Rate Rhythm Depth	

Answer these questions about this exercise.

- If you used different thermometers, how did the results compare?
- What differences did you find in finding the radial pulses among your classmates?
- What differences did you find in the rates and rhythms?
- How were you able to measure respirations so that the person did not know you were watching?
- What differences in rhythm and depth of respirations did you find among your classmates?
- What differences did you find in locating the brachial artery in different people?
- How did the sounds of the blood pressure differ among your classmates?
- What difficulties did you have with any of the measurements taken?
- What will you change about measuring vital signs on a resident after this practice?

Practice taking an apical-radial pulse with classmates. Take turns acting as the staff members and the person having the pulses taken. Answer these questions after the exercise is completed.

- How was privacy maintained for the person having the pulse measured?
- How did the "staff members" decide who would begin and end the count?
- What problems did you have in counting for a minute?
- How did the apical and radial counts compare?
- What will you change about measuring the apical-radial pulses on a resident after this experience?

27 Exercise and Activity

Fill in the Blank: Key Terms

Abduction
Adduction
Ambulation
Atrophy
Contracture

Deconditioning
Dorsiflexion
Extension
External rotation
Flexion

Footdrop
Hyperextension
Internal rotation
Orthostatic
  hypotension

Plantar flexion
Postural
  hypotension
Pronation

Range of motion
  (ROM)
Rotation
Supination
Syncope

1. The foot is bent down at the ankle when _plantar flexion_ is present.

2. A brief loss of consciousness or fainting is _syncope_

3. Bending a body part is _flexion_

4. Moving a body part away from the midline of the body is _abduction_.

5. _Range of motion_ is the movement of a joint to the extent possible without causing pain.

6. Turning the joint outward is _external rotation_

7. A drop in blood pressure when the person suddenly stands up is postural hypotension or _orthostatic hypotension_

8. _adduction_ occurs when moving a body part toward the midline of the body.

9. Turning the joint upward is called _supination_.

10. Bending the toes and foot up at the ankle is _dorsiflexion_

11. Excessive straightening of a body part is _hyperextension_

12. A decrease in size or a wasting away of tissue is _atrophy_

13. Turning the joint is _rotation_

14. _Extension_ is straightening of a body part.

15. _Postural Hypotension_ is another name for orthostatic hypotension.

16. _footdrop_ is permanent plantar flexion; the foot falls down at the ankle.

17. The act of walking is _ambulation_

18. _Pronation_ is turning the joint downward.

19. The loss of muscle strength from inactivity is _deconditioning_

20. _Internal rotation_ is turning the joint inward.

21. The lack of joint mobility caused by abnormal shortening of a muscle is a _Contracture_

Circle the Best Answer

22. If a person is on bedrest, he or she
    A. May be allowed to perform some activities of daily living (ADLs)
    B. Can use the bedside commode for elimination needs
    C. May not perform any activities of daily living
    D. Can use the bathroom for elimination needs

23. Complications of bedrest include all of these *except*
    A. Contractures in fingers, wrists, knees, and hips
    B. Muscle atrophy
    C. Increased appetite and improved muscle strength
    D. Orthostatic hypotension and syncope

24. If a contracture develops
    A. It will require extra range-of-motion exercises to correct it
    B. You need to position the person in good body alignment
    C. The person is permanently deformed and disabled
    D. It will be relieved as soon as the person is able to walk and exercise

25. When you are caring for a person who has orthostatic hypotension, you should
    A. Raise the head of the bed slowly to Fowler's position
    B. Have the person get out of bed quickly to prevent weakness
    C. Keep the bed flat when getting the person out of bed
    D. Have the person walk around to decrease weakness and dizziness

26. Nursing care that prevents complications from bedrest include all of these *except*
    A. Positioning in good body alignment
    B. Range-of-motion exercises
    C. Frequent position changes
    D. Deconditioning

27. If a person sitting on the edge of the bed complains of weakness, dizziness, or spots before the eyes, you should
    A. Assist the person to stand
    B. Help the person to sit in a chair or walk around
    C. Help the person to Fowler's position
    D. Tell the person that is a normal response and continue to get the person up
28. Bed boards are used to
    A. Keep the person in alignment by preventing the mattress from sagging
    B. Prevent plantar flexion that can lead to foot drop
    C. Keep the hips abducted
    D. Keep the weight to top linens off the feet
29. Plantar flexion must be prevented to
    A. Keep the feet from bending down at the ankle (footdrop)
    B. Keep the hips from rotating outward
    C. Keep the wrist, thumb, and fingers in normal position
    D. Maintain good body alignment
30. To prevent the hips and legs from turning outward, you can use
    A. Bed cradles   C. Trochanter rolls
    B. Hip abduction wedges D. Splints
31. Exercise occurs when
    A. Activities of daily living (ADLs) are done
    B. The person turns and moves in bed without help
    C. When the person uses a trapeze to lift the trunk off the bed
    D. All of the above
32. When another person moves the joints through their range of motion it is called
    A. Active range-of-motion
    B. Activities of daily living
    C. Active-assistive range-of-motion
    D. Passive range-of-motion
33. A nursing assistant can perform range-of-motion exercises on the _____ only if allowed by center policy
    A. Shoulder   C. Hip
    B. Neck   D. Knee
34. Depending on activity limits, it is best if exercise for children is
    A. Only passive ROM exercises
    B. Active-assistive ROM exercises
    C. Play activities that promote active ROM exercises
    D. Delayed until they are able to get out of bed
35. When exercising the wrist, you will perform all of these motions *except*
    A. Abduction   C. Flexion
    B. Hyperextension   D. Extension
36. Which of these joints can be adducted and abducted?
    A. Neck   C. Forearm
    B. Hip   D. Knee
37. When you help a person to walk you should
    A. Apply a gait (transfer) belt
    B. Help the person lean on furniture to walk around room
    C. Put soft socks on the feet without shoes
    D. Let the person walk without any help

38. When the person is walking with crutches, the person should wear
    A. Soft slippers on the feet   C. Clothes that are loose
    B. Clothes that fit well   D. A gait belt
39. When walking with a cane, it is held
    A. On the strong side of the body
    B. On the weak side of the body
    C. In the right hand
    D. On the left side of the body
40. When a person is using a walker it is
    A. Picked up and moved 3 to 4 inches in front of the person
    B. Moved forward with a rocking motion
    C. Moved first on the left side and then on the right
    D. Pushed and moved 6 to 8 inches in front of his or her feet
41. When you are caring for a person who wears a brace, it is important to report at once
    A. How far the person walks
    B. What care the person can do alone
    C. The amount of mobility in joints when doing range-of-motion exercises
    D. Any redness or signs of skin breakdown when you remove a brace

Fill in the Blank
42. Write out the abbreviations
    A. ADL _____
    B. CMS _____
    C. ID _____
    D. OBRA _____
    E. PT _____
    F. ROM _____
43. Nurses use the nursing process to promote _____ and _____ in all persons to the extent possible.
44. Bedrest is ordered to
    A. _____
    B. _____
    C. _____
    D. _____
    E. _____
45. The nurse tells you the resident is on bedrest, but can use the bathroom for elimination. This type of bedrest is _____.
46. When a person has a contracture, the person is _____ deformed and disabled.
47. When a person is moved from lying or sitting to a standing position, the blood pressure may _____. This is called _____
48. Supportive devices such as bed boards are used to _____ and _____ the person in a certain position.

49. When you use a foot board the soles of the feet are _____ against it to prevent _____.

50. A trochanter roll is placed along the body to prevent the hips and legs from _____.

51. Hand rolls or grips prevent _____ of the thumb, fingers, and wrists.

52. A device used to keep the wrist, thumb, and fingers in normal position is a _____.

53. Bed cradles are used because the weight of top linens can cause _____ and _____.

54. A trapeze bar allows the person to lift the _____ off the bed. It also allows the person to _____ and _____ in bed.

55. When a person does exercises with some help they are doing _____ range-of-motion exercises.

56. When range-of-motion exercises are done what should be reported or recorded?
    A. _____
    B. _____
    C. _____
    D. _____
    E. _____

57. When performing range-of-motion, each movement should be repeated _____ times or the _____.

58. List the safety measures to follow when performing range-of-motion.
    A. _____
    B. _____
    C. _____
    D. _____
    E. _____
    F. _____
    G. _____
    H. _____
    I. _____

59. When you help a person to walk, you should walk to the _____ and _____ the person. Provide support with the _____ or have _____ and the other _____.

60. Many people prefer a walker because it gives more support than a _____.

Use Focus on PRIDE in the Textbook to complete questions 61–63.

61. You can promote activity, exercise, and well-being when you
    A. _____
    B. _____
    C. _____
    D. _____
    E. _____

62. OBRA requires _____ programs for nursing center residents. These programs are important for _____.

63. Activities in nursing centers must meet the interests and needs of each resident. These needs are
    A. _____
    B. _____
    C. _____

Labeling

64. ROM exercises for the _Shoulder_ joint are shown in these drawings.

Name the movements shown in each drawing.
    A. _Flexion, extension, hyperextension_
    B. _Abduction & adduction_
    C. _External and internal rotation_

65. ROM exercises for the _____ are shown in these drawings.

Name the movements shown in each drawing.
    A. _Flexion, extension, hyperextension_
    B. _Ulnar & radial_

66. ROM exercises for the _Hip_ are shown in these drawings.

Name the movements shown in each drawing.

A. _Flexion_

B. _abduction & adduction_

C. _External rotation_

D. _Internal rotation_

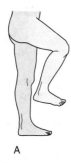 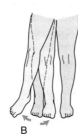 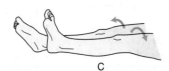 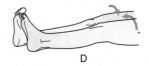

A   B   C   D

Crossword

Fill in the following crossword by answering the clues with the words from this list:

Abduction	Flexion	Rotation	External rotation	Pronation
Adduction	Hyperextension	Internal rotation	Plantar flexion	Supination
Extension	Dorsiflexion			

Across
5. Turning the joint upward
7. Turning the joint inward
10. Straightening a body part
11. Bending the toes and foot up at the ankle
12. Turning the joint downward

Down
1. Bending a body part
2. Bending the foot down at the ankle
3. Turning the joint outward
4. Excessive straightening of a body part
6. Turning the joint
8. Moving a body part away from the midline of the body
9. Moving a body part toward the midline of the body

Optional Learning Exercises

67. What kind of range-of-motion would be used with each of these residents?

    A. The resident needs complete care for bathing, grooming, and feeding.

    _____

    B. The resident takes part in many activities in the center. She walks to most activities independently.

    _____

    C. The resident has weakness on his left side. He is able to feed himself, but needs help with bathing and dressing. _____

68. As you plan to help a person out of bed, you are concerned about orthostatic hypotension. In order to make sure the person is able to stand and get up safely, you plan to take the blood pressure, pulse, and respirations several times. When would you take the blood pressure?

    A. _____

    B. _____

    C. _____

    D. _____

    E. _____

69. When doing range-of-motion exercises, you should ask the person if he or she

    A. _____

    B. _____

    C. _____

70. When you ambulate a person, what observations are reported and recorded?

    A. _____

    B. _____

    C. _____

    D. _____

    E. _____

71. When using a cane, the person walks as follows:

    A. Step A: _____

    _____

    B. Step B: _____

    _____

    C. Step C: _____

    _____

72. Why does the nurse assess the skin under braces every shift? _____

    _____

Independent Learning Activities

Role-play with a classmate and take turns acting as the nursing assistant and a person with left-sided weakness. Perform range-of-motion exercises on the person. Answer these questions about how you felt after this activity.

- What did the nursing assistant explain to you before performing the exercises?
- How were you positioned for exercising? What did the nursing assistant ask about your comfort and personal wishes in the position used?
- How was your privacy maintained? Was there anything that made you feel exposed or embarrassed?
- How were your joints supported during the exercises? Did you feel any discomfort or pain during the exercises?
- What exercises were you encouraged to carry out independently? With some assistance?
- Which exercises were done first? Were the exercises carried out in an organized pattern? How did you know what exercise would be done next?
- After this activity, what will you do differently when giving range-of-motion exercises to a person?

With a classmate, role-play assisting a weak, older person to ambulate. Take turns acting as the person and the nursing assistant. Answer these questions about how you felt and what you learned.

- What did the nursing assistant tell you before preparing to walk with you? What choices were offered about the time you were to ambulate, what clothing to wear, and where you were going to walk?
- What safety devices were used? What did the nursing assistant tell you about the devices or equipment used?
- What assessments were made before you sat up? When you dangled? After walking?
- How did the nursing assistant make you feel secure during ambulation? How did the nursing assistant hold you?
- What did you learn from this activity that will help you when you ambulate a person?

28 Comfort, Rest, and Sleep

Fill in the Blank: Key Terms

Acute pain
Chronic pain
Circadian rhythm
Comfort

Discomfort
Distraction
Enuresis
Guided imagery

Insomnia
NREM sleep
Pain
Persistent pain

Phantom pain
Radiating pain
Relaxation

REM sleep
Rest
Sleep

1. Another name for discomfort is
   Pain.

2. _Acute pain_ is pain that is felt suddenly from injury, disease, trauma, or surgery.

3. _Distraction_ is a way to change a person's center of attention.

4. A state of unconsciousness, reduced voluntary muscle activity, and lowered metabolism is
   Sleep.

5. Pain lasting longer than 6 months is
   Chronic Pain. It is constant or occurs off and on.

6. _Relaxation_ is to be free from mental or physical stress.

7. _Comfort_ is a state of well-being. The person has no physical or emotional pain and is calm and at peace.

8. To be calm, at ease, and relaxed is to _rest_. The person is free of anxiety and stress.

9. Creating and focusing on an image is
   Guided imagery.

10. The stage of sleep when there is rapid eye movement is
    REM sleep.

11. _Insomnia_ is a chronic condition in which the person cannot sleep or stay asleep all night.

12. The day-night cycle or body rhythm is also called
    Circadian _Rythm_. This daily rhythm is based on a 24-hour cycle.

13. _Radiating pain_ is pain felt at the site of tissue damage and in nearby areas.

14. To ache, hurt, or be sore is _discomfort_. It is also called pain.

15. _NREM sleep_ is the phase of deep sleep when there is no rapid eye movement.

16. Pain felt in a body part that is no longer there is
    Phantom Pain.

17. Urinary incontinence in bed at night is
    enuresis.

18. Another name for chronic pain is
    Persistent pain.

Circle the Best Answer

19. Rest and sleep are needed to
    A. Restore well-being and energy
    B. Decrease function and quality of life
    C. Increase muscle strength
    D. Relieve pain

20. OBRA and CMS requirements related to comfort, rest, and sleep include
    A. Only 2 people in a room
    B. Bright lighting in all areas
    C. Room temperature between 65° F and 71° F
    D. Adequate ventilation and room humidity

21. When a person complains of pain or discomfort
    A. The person has pain or discomfort
    B. It must be carefully measured to see if the person really has pain
    C. You can easily measure to find out how much pain is present
    D. You can tell if the person really has pain by the way he or she acts

22. When a person complains of pain that is nearby an area of tissue damage, this is _____ pain.
    A. Acute
    B. Chronic
    C. Radiating
    D. Phantom

23. If pain is ignored or denied it may be because the person thinks pain is a sign of weakness. Which factor that affects pain would this be?
    A. Attention
    B. Past experience
    C. Value or meaning of pain
    D. Support from others

24. A person from Mexico may react to pain by
    A. Showing a strong emotional response
    B. Appearing very stoic
    C. Accepting pain quietly
    D. Viewing it as the will of God

25. When a person has anxiety, the person
    A. Will usually feel increased pain
    B. Will usually feel less pain
    C. May deny having pain
    D. May be stoic and show no reaction to pain

26. When you ask a person, "Where is the pain?" you are asking the person to
    A. Describe the pain
    B. Explain the intensity of the pain
    C. Tell you the onset and duration of the pain
    D. Tell you the location of the pain

27. A child may deal with pain by
    A. Restricting play or school activities
    B. Describing pain to an adult
    C. Asking for pain medications
    D. Concentrating on reading, watching TV, or playing quietly

28. Older persons may ignore new pain because they
    A. Cannot verbally communicate pain
    B. May think it is related to a known health problem
    C. Have increased anxiety
    D. Are used to being in pain

29. When a person tells you he has pain when coughing or deep breathing, this is
    A. A factor causing pain
    B. A measurement of the onset of pain
    C. Words used to describe the pain
    D. The location of the pain

30. A distraction measure to promote comfort and relieve pain may be
    A. Asking the person to focus on an image
    B. Learning to breathe deeply and slowly
    C. Listening to music or playing games
    D. Contracting and relaxing muscle groups

31. If the nurse has given a person pain medication, it is best if you
    A. Give the person a bath
    B. Walk the person according to the care plan
    C. Wait 30 minutes before giving care
    D. Give care before the medication makes the person sleepy

32. You may help to promote comfort and relieve pain by doing all of these *except*
    A. Allow family members and friends at the bedside as requested by the person
    B. Keep the room brightly lit and play loud music
    C. Provide blankets for warmth and to prevent chilling
    D. Use touch to provide comfort

33. You can help to promote rest by doing all of these *except*
    A. Meeting physical needs such as thirst, hunger, and elimination needs
    B. Making sure the person feels safe
    C. Allowing the person to practice rituals or routines before resting
    D. Giving care at a time most convenient to you

34. When caring for an ill or injured person, you know the person may need more rest. You can help the person to get rest by making sure you
    A. Provide plenty of exercise to prevent weakness
    B. Provide rest periods during or after a procedure
    C. Give complete hygiene and grooming measures quickly
    D. Spend time talking with the person to distract him or her

35. Which of these does *not* occur during sleep?
    A. The person is unaware of the environment.
    B. Metabolism is reduced during sleep.
    C. Vital signs (blood pressure, temperature, pulse, respirations) increase.
    D. There are no voluntary arm or leg movements.

36. Some people function better in the morning because of
    A. The circadian rhythm
    B. Getting enough sleep
    C. Interference with the body rhythm
    D. Changes in the work schedule

37. During REM sleep, the person
    A. Is hard to arouse
    B. Has a gradual fall in vital signs
    C. Is easily aroused
    D. Has tension in voluntary muscles

38. Which stage of sleep is usually not repeated during the cycles of sleep?
    A. REM   C. Stage 2: NREM
    B. Stage 1: NREM   D. Stage 3: NREM

39. Which age group requires the least amount of sleep?
    A. Toddlers   C. Adolescents
    B. Young adults   D. Older adults

40. Which of these factors increases the need for sleep?
    A. Illness
    B. Weight loss
    C. Emotional problems
    D. Drugs and other substances

41. When a person takes sleeping pills, sleep may not restore the person mentally because
    A. Caffeine prevents sleep
    B. Some have difficulty falling asleep
    C. The length of REM sleep is reduced
    D. It upsets the usual sleep routines

42. Exercise should be avoided for 2 hours before sleep because
    A. It requires energy
    B. People usually feel good after exercise
    C. It causes the release of substances in the bloodstream that stimulate the body
    D. The person tires after exercise

43. Persons who are ill, in pain, or receiving hospital care are at risk for
    A. Sleep deprivation
    B. Sleepwalking
    C. Insomnia
    D. Increased sleep times

44. If a person has decreased reasoning; red, puffy eyes; and coordination problems, report this to the nurse because the person
    A. Is having a reaction to sleeping medications
    B. Has signs and symptoms of sleep disorders
    C. Needs more exercise before bedtime
    D. May need an increase in sleeping pills

45. Which of these measures would *not* help to promote sleep?
    A. Provide blankets or socks for those who tend to be cold.
    B. Have the person void or make sure incontinent persons are clean and dry.
    C. Follow bedtime rituals.
    D. Offer the person a cup of coffee or tea at bedtime.

Fill in the Blank

46. Write out the abbreviations.

   A. CMS _____

   B. F _____

   C. NREM _____

   D. OBRA _____

   E. REM _____

47. OBRA and CMS have requirements about the person's room. List the requirements that relate to each of these

   A. Suspended curtain _____

   B. Linens _____

   C. Bed _____

   D. Room temperature _____

   E. Persons in room _____

48. Name the type of pain described.

   A. A person with an amputated leg may still sense leg pain. _____

   B. There is tissue damage. The pain decreases with healing. _____

   C. Pain from a heart attack is often felt in the left chest, left jaw, left shoulder, and left arm.

   _____

   D. The pain remains long after healing. Common causes are arthritis and cancer.

   _____

49. What is the reason persons from the Phillipines may appear stoic in reaction to pain?

   _____

50. Older persons may ignore or deny new pain because

   A. _____

   B. _____

51. Changes _____

   may signal pain in persons with demention.

52. When gathering information about a person in pain, you can use a scale of 1 to 10. Which end of the scale is the most severe pain? _____

53. What happens to vital signs when the person has acute pain? _____

54. When the person uses words to describe pain such as aching, knifelike, or sore, what do you report to the nurse? _____

55. What body responses that you can see or measure (objective signs) may mean the person has pain?

   A. _____

   B. _____

   C. _____

   D. _____

56. What changes in these behaviors may be symptoms of pain?

   A. Speech _____

   B. Affected body part _____

   C. Body position _____

57. List nursing measures to promote comfort and relieve pain related to these clues.

   A. Position of the person _____

   B. Linens _____

   C. Blankets _____

   D. Pain medications _____

   E. Family members _____

58. If a person is receiving strong pain medication or sedatives, what safety measures are important?

   A. _____

   B. _____

   C. _____

   D. _____

59. When you explain the procedure before performing it, you may help a person to rest better because you met the need for _____.

60. A clean, neat, and uncluttered room can promote rest by meeting _____ needs.

61. The mind and body rest, the body saves energy, and body functions slow during

   _____

62. Mental restoration occurs during a phase of sleep called _____.

63. The deepest stage of sleep occurs during

   _____

64. If work hours change it can affect the normal _____ cycle or _____ rhythm.

65. Alcohol tends to cause drowsiness and sleep, but it interferes with _____.

66. Insomnia may be caused by

   A. Fear of _____

   B. Afraid of not _____

   C. Fear of not being able _____

   D. Physical and emotional _____

67. When a person has dementia and wanders at night the best approach for some persons is to allow

   _____

Use Focus on PRIDE in the Textbook to complete questions 68–71.

68. When you are caring for persons who have pain, what is your responsibility?

   A. Report _____ and _____

   B. Report what the person _____ and what

   _____

69. It is important to report signs and symptoms of pain, because the nurse uses this information to

_____ .

70. Take pride in providing care that focuses on the

person as a _____ .

71. You can affect the person's well-being by meeting these needs.

    A. _____

    B. _____

    C. _____

Optional Learning Exercises

72. You are caring for 2 residents who both have arthritis. Mr. Forman tells you this is the first time he has had any health problems. Mrs. Wegman tells you she has had several surgeries and has had 3 children. Which of these 2 persons is likely to be more anxious about the pain and to be unable to

handle the pain well? _____ Why?

_____

_____

73. Mr. Forman tells you his pain seems much worse at night. What could be the reason for this reaction?

_____

_____

74. You are caring for Mrs. Reynolds. She tells you she misses her children who have moved to another state. Today, Mrs. Reynolds is complaining of pain in her abdomen. In spite of providing nursing comfort measures, she still rates her pain at a 7. What is a possible reason Mrs. Reynolds is not getting relief of

her pain? _____

_____

75. When a person is ill, how do these affect sleep?

    A. Treatments and therapies

    _____

    B. Care devices such as traction or a cast

    _____

    C. Emotions that affect sleep include

    _____

76. Certain foods affect sleep. Tell how these foods affect sleep and list foods that contain the substances.

    A. Caffeine _____ sleep. It is found in

    _____

    _____ .

    B. Tryptophan _____ sleep. It is found

    in _____

    _____ .

Independent Learning Activities

Form a group with several classmates and share your personal experiences with pain. Discuss these questions to understand the different ways you respond to pain and treat the pain.

- What experiences have you had with pain? Accidents? Illnesses? Childbirth? Surgery?
- What type of pain have you had? Acute? Chronic? Other types?
- How would you rate your pain on a scale of 1 to 10? How long did it last?
- How did your family and friends respond to your pain? How much support did you receive from them? How did the support (or lack of it) affect the pain?
- What measures were used to treat the pain? What was the most effective? The least effective?
- What did you learn from this discussion with others about their pain? How will this help you as you care for others with pain?

Form a group with several classmates to talk about differences in sleep habits. Answer these questions to understand differences in personal practices concerning rest and sleep.

- How many hours do you sleep each day? How many hours of sleep do you think you *should* get each day?
- If you did not have to follow a schedule (work, school, etc.), when would you go to bed and wake up?
- What rituals do you perform before going to bed? How is your sleep affected if you cannot perform these rituals?
- What factors interfere with your sleep? What do you do to avoid these factors?
- When do you feel most alert? Morning? Afternoon? Night?
- How do you feel when you wake up? Alert? Pleasant? Grouchy? Tired?
- How often do you take naps? What time of day do you like to nap? How do you feel when you wake from a nap?
- How will this discussion help you to understand differences in sleep patterns when you are caring for others? How will it affect how you help the persons you care for to get the rest and sleep they need?

29 Admissions, Transfers, and Discharges

Fill in the Blank: Key Terms

Admission   Discharge   Transfer

1. _Transfer_ _____ is moving a person from one room or nursing unit to another.

2. The official entry of a person into a nursing agency is _Admission_ _____ .

3. _Discharge_ _____ occurs with the official departure of a person from a nursing agency.

Circle the Best Answer

4. Admission to a hospital or nursing center
   A. Causes anxiety and fear
   B. Is a time when being kind, courteous, and respectful to the person is important
   C. Causes the person to be separated from family and friends
   D. All of the above

5. Usually, _____ is a happy time.
   A. Admission   C. Transfer
   B. Discharge   D. Home care

6. The admissions process starts with the
   A. Doctor
   B. Nurse on the nursing unit
   C. Admitting office
   D. Activities director

7. When a person with dementia is admitted to a nursing center, the person
   A. Is usually depressed
   B. May have an increase in confusion
   C. May have a decrease in confusion
   D. Usually feels safer in the new setting

8. Persons being admitted are
   A. Always admitted by the RN
   B. Usually admitted by the nursing assistant
   C. May be admitted by the nursing assistant if the person has no discomfort or distress
   D. Never admitted by the nursing assistant

9. If a person being admitted is arriving by stretcher, you should
   A. Raise the bed to its highest level
   B. Leave the bed closed
   C. Raise the head of the bed to Fowler's position
   D. Lower the bed to its lowest level

10. During admission you can help the person feel more comfortable by
    A. Offering the person and the family beverages to drink
    B. Introduce the person to other residents
    C. Assist the person to hang pictures or display photos
    D. All of the above

11. When weighing a resident, have the person
    A. Wear socks and shoes and bathrobe
    B. Remove regular clothes and wear a gown or pajamas
    C. Wear regular street clothes
    D. Remove clothing after weighing and then weigh the clothes

12. A chair scale is used when a person
    A. Cannot transfer from a wheelchair
    B. Cannot stand
    C. Can stand and walk independently
    D. Is in the supine position

13. When a person cannot stand on the scale to have the height measured
    A. Ask the person or the family the height of the person
    B. Have the person sit in a chair and use a tape measure from head to toe to measure the person
    C. Position the person in supine position if the position is allowed and measure with a tape measure
    D. Estimate the height of the person by observing him or her

14. When a person is being transferred, who is told about the transfer?
    A. The doctor
    B. The social worker
    C. The family and business office
    D. The person's roommate

15. When you are transferring a person you should do all of these *except*
    A. Identify the person by checking the ID bracelet with the transfer slip
    B. Explain the reasons for the transfer
    C. Collect the person's personal belongings and bedside equipment
    D. Report to the receiving nurse

16. If a person wishes to leave the center without the doctor's permission, you should
    A. Tell the person this is not allowed
    B. Prevent the person from leaving
    C. Tell the nurse at once
    D. Try to convince the person to stay

17. When you are assisting a person who is being discharged, you should
    A. Check all drawers and closet
    B. Check off the clothing list and personal belongings list
    C. Help the person dress as needed
    D. All of the above

Fill in the Blank

18. Write out the abbreviations.

   A. CMS _____

   B. ID _____

   C. lb _____

   D. OBRA _____

19. OBRA and CMS have standards for transfers and discharges. List the ways these standards affect the person's rights.

   A. Reasons for _____ are

   part of the person's _____.

   B. The _____ and

   _____ are told of transfer or

   discharge plans.

   C. A procedure is followed if the person

   _____.

   D. An _____ often

   works with the person and family to assure that

   _____.

20. When you are delegated to assist with admissions, transfers, or discharges, what information do you need from the nurse?

   A. _____

   B. _____

   C. _____

   D. _____

   E. _____

   F. _____

   G. _____

   H. _____

   I. _____

   J. _____

21. When a person is being admitted, what information is obtained for the admission record?

   A. _____

   B. _____

   C. _____

   D. _____

   E. _____

22. During admission, what is the person given

   to allow the staff to identify the person?

   _____ and

   _____.

23. The person may also have a _____

   ID taken.

24. When you are asked to admit a person, what can you do to make a good first impression?

   A. _____

   B. _____

   C. _____

   D. _____

   E. _____

25. Why is it important to have a person void before

   being weighed? _____

26. What is done to the balance scale before having the person step on?

   A. _____

   B. _____

   C. _____

   _____

27. When measuring a person in the supine position, the

   ruler is placed _____.

28. When you transfer or discharge a person, tell the nurse when the person is ready, so that the nurse can

   A. _____

   B. _____

   C. _____

   D. _____

29. When you assist with a discharge, you should report and record

   A. _____

   B. _____

   C. _____

   D. _____

   E. _____

   F. _____

Use Focus on PRIDE in the Textbook to complete questions 30–31.

30. When you admit, transfer, or discharge a person it is your responsibility to help the person adjust by

   A. _____

   B. _____

   C. _____

   D. _____

   _____

   E. _____

   _____

31. If a person tells you he or she does *not* want certain

   people to visit, you should tell _____. The

   staff must _____ the person's wishes.

Optional Learning Exercises

Answer the questions about the following person and situation. Rosa Romirez, 65, had a stroke (CVA) last week and is being admitted to a rehabilitation unit in the nursing care center where you work.

32. Since you know Mrs. R. is arriving by wheelchair, you

    leave the bed _____ and _____

    the bed to its _____.

33. The nurse instructs you to collect the needed equipment to admit a new person. You collect

    A. _____

    B. _____

    C. _____

    D. _____

    E. _____

    F. _____

    G. _____

    H. _____

    I. _____

    J. _____

34. When Mrs. R. arrives with her husband it may help them feel more comfortable if you offer them

    _____.

35. You greet Mrs. Romirez by name and ask her if a

    certain _____.

36. Mrs. R. has some weakness on her left side and cannot stand alone, but can safely transfer from the wheelchair to chairs or the bed. The nurse tells you to

    weigh Mrs. R. with the _____ scale.

    When you arrive at work one day, you are told Mrs. Romirez is being transferred to another nursing unit, and you are asked to assist. Answer these questions about transferring her.

37. When you transport Mrs. R. in a wheelchair, she is

    covered with a _____.

38. What items are taken with Mrs. R. to the new unit?

    _____

39. What information is recorded and reported about the transfer?

    A. _____

    B. _____

    C. _____

    D. _____

    E. _____

    F. _____

    G. _____

Several weeks later, you are sent to the nursing unit where Mrs. R. is living and find she is going home. Answer these questions about her discharge.

40. Mrs. R. tells you she and her family have been taught

    about her _____, _____,

    and _____.

41. Good communication skills should be used when assisting with the discharge. When Mrs. R. and her

    family leave, you should _____.

Independent Learning Activities

Have a discussion with 3 or 4 classmates to share experiences you have had with admissions to care centers. You may have had personal experience, or you may have observed a friend or family member being admitted. If you have not had this experience, perhaps you can relate the feelings you have had when visiting a doctor's office. Use these questions during the discussion.

- Who was the first person you met when you arrived to be admitted? How were you greeted? Did you feel welcome?
- How did you arrive at your room? Were you escorted or did you have to find your way?
- How long did you wait in the room before a staff member came to admit you? How did this affect your feelings about the place?
- How were you addressed? First name? Last name? Did anyone ask you what you preferred?
- What information were you given to make you feel more comfortable? What printed information was provided?
- Overall, how did the admission procedure affect your feelings about the facility? Negative? Positive?
- How will your personal experience and the experiences of others in this group affect your approach to new persons in a care facility?

Fill in the Blank: Key Terms

Dorsal recumbent position
Genupectoral position
Horizontal recumbent position

Knee-chest position
Laryngeal mirror
Lithotomy position

Nasal speculum
Ophthalmoscope
Otoscope

Percussion hammer
Tuning fork
Vaginal speculum

1. An instrument vibrated to test hearing is a

_____.

2. In the _____ the woman lies on her back with her hips at the edge of the exam table, her knees are flexed, her hips are externally rotated, and her feet are in stirrups.

3. The supine position with the legs together is called the

_____.

4. An _____ is a lighted instrument used to examine the external ear and the eardrum (tympanic membrane).

5. A _____ is an instrument used to open the vagina so it and the cervix can be examined.

6. When a person kneels and rests the body on the knees and chest, and the head is turned to one side, the arms are above the head or flexed at the elbows, the back is straight, and the body is flexed about 90 degrees at the hip, the person is in the

_____.

7. A _____ is an instrument used to tap body parts to test reflexes.

8. An instrument used to examine the mouth, teeth, and throat is called a _____.

9. An instrument used to examine the inside of the nose is a _____.

10. The dorsal recumbent position is also called the

_____.

11. An _____ is a lighted instrument used to examine the internal structures of the eye.

12. Another name for knee-chest position is

_____.

Circle the Best Answer

13. In nursing centers, residents have a physical examination
    A. Only when the person is admitted
    B. Once a month
    C. At least once a year
    D. Only when the person is ill

14. If a person is having a physical examination, you may be asked to do all of these *except*
    A. Measure vital signs, height, and weight
    B. Hand equipment and supplies to the examiner
    C. Explain why the examination is being done and what to expect
    D. Position and drape the person

15. When the doctor is examining the person's mouth, teeth, and throat, you may be asked to hand him or her the
    A. Ophthalmoscope
    B. Percussion hammer
    C. Tuning fork
    D. Laryngeal mirror

16. Which of these would provide for privacy for a person having a physical examination?
    A. Having the person urinate before the examination begins
    B. Telling the person who will do the exam and when it will be done
    C. Screening the person and closing the room door
    D. Allowing a family member to decide who will be in the examination during the exam

17. When a child is examined, all of the following are true *except*
    A. All clothing is removed
    B. Parents are allowed to be present
    C. Underpants are worn by toddlers, preschool children, school-age children
    D. Protect the child from chilling

18. It is important to have a person empty the bladder before an examination because
    A. An empty bladder allows the examiner to feel the abdominal organs
    B. A full bladder can change the normal position and shape of organs
    C. A full bladder can cause discomfort when the abdominal organs are felt
    D. All of the above

19. Which of these steps would *not* promote safety and comfort during an exam?
    A. The procedure is not explained to the person.
    B. Have an extra bath blanket nearby
    C. Prevent drafts to protect the person from chilling
    D. Do not leave the person unattended

20. After you have taken the person to the exam room and placed the person in position, you should
    A. Put the signal light on for the examiner
    B. Leave the room
    C. Go to the examiner to report the person is ready
    D. Open the door, so the examiner knows you are ready
21. When the abdomen, chest, and breasts are to be examined, you will place the person in the
    A. Lithotomy position
    B. Sims position
    C. Dorsal recumbent (horizontal recumbent) position
    D. Knee-chest position
22. If a person is asked to stand on the floor during an exam, you should
    A. Assist the person to put on shoes or slippers
    B. Place paper or paper towels on the floor
    C. Place a sheet on the floor
    D. Wipe the floor carefully with an antiseptic cleaner before the person stands on it

Fill in the Blank

23. List the equipment you need to collect when the ears are being examined.
    A. _____
    B. _____
24. What equipment is needed to examine the eyes?
    A. _____
    B. _____
25. When the nose, mouth, and throat are being examined, you should collect
    A. _____
    B. _____
    C. _____
    D. _____
26. What are concerns the person may have when a physical examination is done?
    A. _____
    B. _____
    C. _____
27. When the examiner is a man and the person being examined is female, who else should be in the examination room? _____
    Why? _____
    _____
28. What should you do to the exam room after the examination is completed? _____
    _____

Use Focus on PRIDE in the Textbook to complete questions 29–31.

29. Fears about the exam affect the person's well-being. Common fears are
    A. _____
    B. _____

C. _____
D. _____
30. You violate the Health Insurance Portability and Accountability Act of 1996 (HIPAA) when you
    _____
    _____.
31. Failure to follow HIPAA can result in
    _____.

Labeling
Look at the instruments and answer questions 32-36.
32. Name the instruments

A. _____
B. _____
C. _____
D. _____
E. _____
F. _____
G. _____

33. Which instrument is used to examine the nose?

   _____

34. When the eye is examined, the examiner uses the

   _____

35. If a person has a sore throat, the examiner will look at the throat with the _____.

36. The reflexes are examined by using the

   _____

Use these figures to answer questions 37–40

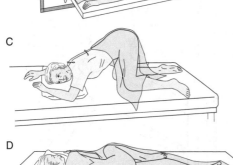

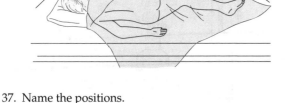

37. Name the positions.

   A. _____
   B. _____
   C. _____
   D. _____

38. Which positions may be used when a rectal examination is done?

   A. _____
   B. _____

39. When the abdomen, chest, and breasts are examined, the person is placed in _____.

40. The _____ is used for a vaginal exam.

Optional Learning Exercises

41. When you are delegated the job of preparing a person for an exam, why do you need the following information?

   A. What time is the examination? _____
   B. What are 2 reasons it would helpful to know which examinations will be done? _____

   _____

   C. What equipment will you need if you are assigned to take vital signs? _____

42. You are a female nursing assistant assisting a male examiner with an examination of a female resident. The nurse tells you to stay in the exam room during the entire procedure. Why is this important to the examiner and to the woman? _____

   _____

Independent Learning Activities

You probably have had a physical examination at some time. Perhaps you needed one to be a student in this class. Answer these questions about your experience when you had the physical done to you.

- Who explained what to expect during the exam? What were you told about any discomfort?
- What steps were taken to give you privacy? While you changed clothes? During the exam?
- Who was present during the exam? Were you given a choice of having another person in the room with you and the examiner? How did you feel about having (or not having) another person in the room?
- How did you know what was being done? How much information were you given about procedures? Positions? Tests?
- What positions were used during the exam? Which positions shown in this chapter were used? How comfortable did you feel? How did the examiner and assistant help to make you more comfortable with the positions?
- What questions did you have during the exam? Who was able to answer these? How well were they answered to make you understand what was being done?
- How comfortable did you feel about the exam? What could have been done to make you more comfortable physically and psychologically?
- How did this experience help you to understand the feelings of persons you may assist during an exam?

31 Collecting and Testing Specimens

Fill in the Blank: Key Terms

Acetone	Glycosuria	Hematuria	Ketone	Melena
Glucosuria	Hematoma	Hemoptysis	Ketone body	Sputum

1. Bloody sputum is _hemoptysis_.

2. Ketone or acetone is also called _Ketone body_.

3. A black, tarry stool is _melena_.

4. _Glycosuria_ is glucosuria or sugar in the urine.

5. _Sputum_ is mucus from the respiratory system that is expectorated through the mouth.

6. _ketone_ is a substance that appears in urine from the rapid breakdown of fat for energy.

7. Another name for ketone or ketone body is _acetone_.

8. Sugar in the urine is called glycosuria or _glucosuria_.

9. _Hematuria_ is blood in the urine.

10. A swelling that contains blood is a _hematoma_.

Circle the Best Answer

11. Specimens are collected and tested for all of these reasons *except*
    A. To measure the specimen
    B. To prevent diseases
    C. To detect diseases
    D. To treat diseases

12. When you are collecting a specimen, which of these is *incorrect*?
    A. Use a clean container for each specimen
    B. Gloves are not needed
    C. Do not touch the inside of the container or lid
    D. Place the specimen container in a BIOHAZARD plastic bag

13. When collecting a urine specimen from some people, including children, the specimen may be placed in a paper bag to
    A. Prevent embarrassing the person
    B. Protect the specimen from light
    C. Follow Standard Precautions
    D. To keep the specimen sterile

14. A random urine specimen is collected
    A. First thing in the morning
    B. After meals
    C. At any time
    D. At bedtime

15. When a person is collecting a random urine specimen, remind the person to put the toilet tissue in
    A. The wastebasket or toilet
    B. In the specimen container
    C. In the specimen pan
    D. Any of the above

16. When obtaining a midstream specimen, the perineal area is cleaned to
    A. Remove all microbes from the area
    B. Reduce the number of microbes in the urethral area
    C. Follow Standard Precautions and Bloodborne Pathogen Standards
    D. Reduce infection during the specimen collection

17. When collecting a midstream specimen, which of these is correct?
    A. Collect the entire amount of urine voided.
    B. Collect about 4 oz (120 mL) of urine.
    C. Have the person start to void, and then stop. A sterile specimen container is positioned to catch urine as the person begins to void again.
    D. Collect several specimens and mix them together.

18. When collecting a 24-hour urine specimen, the urine is kept
    A. Chilled on ice or refrigerated during the entire time
    B. At room temperature
    C. In a sterile container at the nurses station
    D. In a drainage collection bag at the bedside

19. A 24-hour urine specimen collection is started
    A. At the beginning of a shift
    B. After a meal
    C. At night
    D. After the person voids and that urine is discarded
20. At the end of 24-hour specimen collection
    A. The person voids and that urine is saved
    B. Write down any missed or spilled urine
    C. Record the amount of urine collected
    D. The person voids and that urine is discarded
21. When a urine specimen is needed from infants or very young children, it is obtained by
    A. Inserting a straight catheter
    B. Using a collection bag applied over the urethra
    C. Having the parent hold the child on a potty chair until the child voids
    D. Applying a diaper and then squeezing the urine out of the diaper
22. A child may be able to void for a specimen if you give the child fluids
    A. 5–10 minutes before the test
    B. 30 minutes before the test
    C. One hour before the test
    D. While you are obtaining the specimen
23. When you test urine with a reagent strip, it is important that you
    A. Follow the manufacturer's instructions
    B. Use a sterile urine specimen
    C. Wear sterile gloves
    D. Make sure the urine is cold
24. When you are assigned to strain a person's urine, you
    A. Have the person void directly into the strainer
    B. Send all urine to the lab
    C. Have the person void into the voiding device and then pour the urine through the strainer
    D. Discard the strainer if it contains any stones
25. If a warm stool specimen is required, it is
    A. Placed it in an insulated container
    B. Stored on the nursing unit until the end of the shift
    C. Tested at once on the nursing unit
    D. Taken at once to the laboratory or the storage area
26. When collecting a stool specimen, ask the person to
    A. Void and have a bowel movement in a bedpan
    B. Use only a bedpan or commode to collect the specimen
    C. Urinate into the toilet and collect the stool in the specimen pan
    D. Place the toilet tissue in the bedpan, commode, or specimen pan with the stool
27. When collecting the stool specimen
    A. Pour it into the specimen container
    B. Use your gloved hand to obtain a specimen to place in the container
    C. Use a tongue blade to take about 2 tablespoons of stool from the middle of the formed stool
    D. Use a tongue blade to place the entire stool specimen in the container

28. When you test a stool specimen for blood
    A. It must be sent to the laboratory
    B. The specimen must be sterile
    C. You will need to test the entire stool specimen
    D. Use a tongue blade to obtain a small of amount of stool
29. A sputum specimen is more easily collected
    A. Upon awakening   C. At bedtime
    B. After eating   D. After activity
30. Before obtaining a sputum specimen, ask the person to
    A. Rinse the mouth with clear water
    B. Brush the teeth and use mouthwash
    C. Cough and discard the first sputum expectorated
    D. Sit in an upright position to loosen secretions
31. Postural drainage is used when collecting a sputum specimen to
    A. Collect sterile specimens
    B. Make the sputum specimen more liquid
    C. Stimulate coughing
    D. Help secretions drain by gravity
32. If a sputum specimen is needed from an infant or small child, you may assist the nurse by
    A. Positioning the child for postural drainage
    B. Holding the child's head and arms still
    C. Positioning the sputum specimen cup near the child's mouth
    D. Explaining the procedure to the child
33. If you are delegated to do blood glucose testing, the most common site for testing is
    A. The earlobe   C. The forearm
    B. A fingertip   D. The abdomen
34. It is important to do glucose testing at correct times because
    A. The nurse uses the results to make decisions about the diet and drug dosages for the person
    B. It must be done before meals
    C. It must be done after meals
    D. It must be done at a time when the person is not sleeping

Fill in the Blank

35. Write out the abbreviations.
    A. BM _Bowel Movement_
    B. ID _Identification_
    C. I&O _Intake and output_
    D. mL _milliliter_
    E. oz _Ounce_
36. When collecting urine specimens, what observations are reported and recorded?
    A. _Problems obtaining_
    B. _Color clarity odor_

C. _Blood_

D. _Particles_

E. _Complaints_

F. _Time_

37. How much urine is collected for a random urine specimen? _120 mL_

38. When collecting a midstream urine specimen, the person may not be able to stop voiding. If so, you will pass _The specimen container_.

39. When you are obtaining a midstream specimen from a female, spread the labia with your thumb and index finger with your _gloved_ hand.

40. When cleaning the female perineum for a midstream specimen, clean from _Clean to dirty_

41. When cleaning the male perineum for a midstream specimen, clean the penis starting

_____

42. When you make labels for a 24-hour urine collection container, what information is marked?

_____

_____

43. Urine pH measures if the urine is _____

or _____.

44. When you use reagent strips, you read the strip by comparing it to the _____

_____.

45. When you strain urine, you are looking for stones that can develop in the _____.

46. The strainer or gauze are placed in the specimen container if any _____ appear.

47. Stool specimens are studied and checked for

A. _____

B. _____

C. _____

D. _____

E. _____

48. After collecting a stool specimen, place the container in a _____

_____

49. When you are delegated to collect a stool specimen, what observations are reported and recorded?

A. _____

B. _____

C. _____

D. _____

E. _____

F. _____

50. When stools are black and tarry, there is bleeding in the _____.

51. Blood in the stool that is hidden is called

_____.

52. Mouthwash is *not* used before a sputum specimen is collected because it _____.

53. When you are delegated to collect a sputum specimen, report and record

A. _____

B. _____

C. _____

D. _____

E. _____

F. _____

G. _____

H. _____

I. _____

54. When you are assisting a person to collect a sputum specimen, ask the person to take 2 or 3

_____ and

_____ the sputum.

55. When you make a skin puncture for a blood glucose test, avoid sites that are _____,

_____, _____,

_____ or _____.

These sites are avoided because

_____.

56. Why do you avoid the center, fleshy part of the fingertip when you make a skin puncture? _____

_____.

57. When you test for blood glucose, what should you report and record?

A. _____

B. _____

C. _____

D. _____

E. _____

F. _____

G. _____

H. _____

Use Focus on PRIDE in the Textbook to complete questions 58–61.

58. When collecting a specimen, you are responsible to correctly _____ the person.

59. What information may you need to place on the specimen container?

   A. _____

   B. _____

   C. _____

60. When collecting specimens, you respect the person's right to privacy when you

   A. _____

   B. _____

   C. _____
      _____

   D. _____
      _____

   E. _____
      _____

61. If you did not collect a specimen correctly, why is it important to report this to the nurse?

   _____

Crossword

Fill in the following crossword by answering the clues with the words from this list:

Calculi	Expectorated	Midstream	Postural	Specimens
Dysuria	Labia	Occult	Random	Suctioning

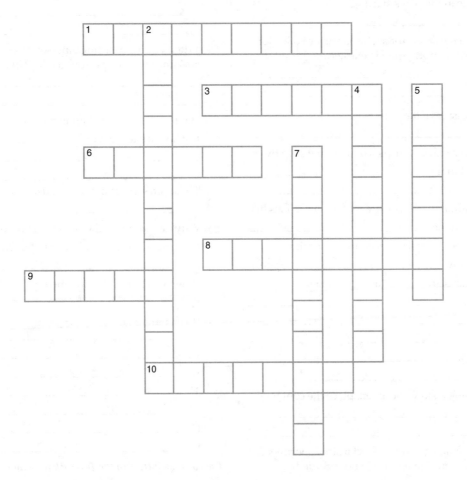

Across
1. Samples
3. Urine specimen that can be collected at any time
6. Hidden, as in blood in stool
8. Position with head lower than body used to cause fluid to flow downward
9. Folds of tissue on each side of the vagina
10. Pain when urinating

Down
2. Expelled, as in sputum through the mouth
4. Urine specimen that is collected after the person starts to void
5. Stones that develop in kidneys, ureters, or bladder
7. Removal of sputum from the trachea with a machine

Optional Learning Exercises

62. If you are collecting a midstream specimen, what should you do if it is hard for the person to stop the stream of urine? _____

_____

63. You are caring for a person who is having a 24-hour urine specimen test. He tells you he forgot to save a specimen an hour ago. What should you do and why?

_____

64. What is normal pH for urine?

_____ What can cause changes in the normal pH? _____

65. When the body cannot use sugar for energy, it uses fat. When this happens _____ appear in the urine.

66. Why is privacy important when collecting a sputum specimen? _____

_____

Independent Learning Activities

Answer these questions about collecting specimens.

- What specimens may be collected by nursing assistants in your state?
- What special training is given to make sure nursing assistants know how to collect specimens?
- Ask permission to look at specimen containers used in your clinical site.
  - Are any directions included with the containers?
- Where is information about collecting specimen kept at the clinical site?

32 The Person Having Surgery

Fill in the Blank: Key Terms

Anesthesia   Emergency surgery   Postoperative   Sedation
Elective surgery   General anesthesia   Preoperative   Thrombus
Embolus   Local anesthesia   Regional anesthesia   Urgent surgery

1. The loss of consciousness and all feeling or sensation is _general anesthesia_

2. _Elective surgency_ is surgery done by choice to improve the person's life or well-being.

3. A blood clot is called a _thrombus_.

4. _Anesthesia_ is the loss of feeling or sensation produced by a drug.

5. An _embolus_ is a blood clot that travels through the vascular system until it lodges in a blood vessel.

6. _Pre-operative_ is before surgery.

7. _Urgent surgery_ is surgery needed for the person's health. It is done soon to prevent further damage or disease.

8. _Post-operative_ is after surgery.

9. The loss of feeling or sensation in a large area of the body is _regional anesthesia_

10. Surgery done immediately to save life or function is _emergency surgery_.

11. _Local anesthesia_ is the loss of feeling or sensation in a small area.

12. A state of quiet, calmness, or sleep produced by a drug is _sedation_

Circle the Best Answer

13. Surgery is done to
    A. Remove a diseased body part
    B. Make a diagnosis
    C. Restore or improve function
    D. All of the above

14. A surgery that is done to prevent further damage or disease is
    A. Emergency surgery   C. Urgent surgery
    B. Elective surgery   D. General surgery

15. When an accident occurs, the person often requires
    A. Elective surgery   C. General anesthesia
    B. Emergency surgery   D. Urgent surgery

16. When a person tells you about fears and concerns before surgery, you should
    A. Explain that the surgeon is very skilled
    B. Tell the person not to worry
    C. Listen to the person; use verbal and nonverbal communication
    D. Change the subject and talk about something else

17. When a patient asks you about test results or the diagnosis
    A. Answer the questions honestly
    B. Tell the person you will get the nurse
    C. Tell the person that information is not available
    D. Explain that you do not know but will find out

18. Which of these is *not* part of your role when caring for a surgical patient?
    A. Explain the care you will give
    B. Perform procedures and tasks with skill and ease
    C. Tell the person about your own experience with the same surgery
    D. Report a request to see a member of the clergy to the nurse

19. The nurse will tell the patient that deep breathing and coughing exercises will be done after surgery
    A. Once a shift
    B. Every 1 or 2 hours when the person is awake
    C. Every 4 hours
    D. Every 2 hours for the first 48 hours after surgery

20. How is a child prepared for surgery?
    A. The parents are responsible for explaining the surgery to the child.
    B. A doll may be used to show the site of the surgery.
    C. Children are not told about the surgery because it may frighten them.
    D. A child does not need an explanation because the idea of surgery is too difficult for the child to understand.

21. If blood loss is expected during surgery, what test is done preoperatively?
    A. Type and crossmatch
    B. Complete blood count
    C. Urinalysis
    D. Electrocardiogram

22. A person is NPO 6 to 8 hours before surgery to reduce
    A. Breathing problems after surgery
    B. Pain postoperatively
    C. Diarrhea
    D. Vomiting and aspiration during and after surgery
23. Cleansing enemas may be ordered before surgery to
    A. Clear the bowel of feces
    B. Prevent incontinence after surgery
    C. Prevent diarrhea after surgery
    D. Prevent pain
24. The person being prepared for surgery needs to void
    A. Right before leaving the room
    B. The morning of surgery
    C. Before the nurse gives the preoperative drugs
    D. Before an enema is given
25. Makeup, nail polish, and fake nails are removed before surgery because
    A. This reduces wound infection
    B. It reduces the number of microbes on the body
    C. The skin, lips, and nail beds are observed for color during and after surgery
    D. It makes the person more comfortable after surgery
26. When preparing a child for surgery, it is important to report
    A. A dry mouth
    B. Any loose teeth
    C. Any missing teeth
    D. That you removed hair clips from the hair
27. If a person is allowed to wear a wedding ring during surgery, you should
    A. Record this information on the chart
    B. Secure it in place with gauze and tape
    C. Make sure it fits well and will not come off
    D. Put a clean glove on the person's hand
28. If you are assigned to do a skin prep with a razor preoperatively, you should be careful
    A. Not to cut, scratch, or nick the skin
    B. To shave against the direction of hair growth
    C. To shave the entire body
    D. Not to shave too closely to the skin
29. The surgery consent
    A. Is signed by the person and sometimes the nearest relative
    B. Is signed by the person's attorney
    C. May be obtained by nursing assistant
    D. Is not needed for emergency surgery
30. Preoperative medications are given
    A. To prevent pain
    B. Before the person is transported to the OR
    C. Immediately before surgery
    D. In the operating room
31. When you are delegated to assist with the preoperative checklist, it must be completed before
    A. The nurse gives the preoperative drugs
    B. The patient falls asleep after receiving the preoperative drugs
    C. The patient leaves the unit for surgery
    D. The night before the surgery

32. When a child is transported to the operating room, the

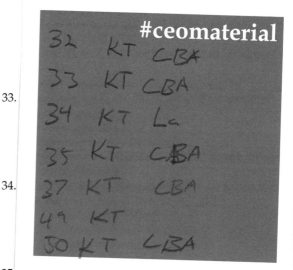

33.

34.

35. You may be assigned to take ___ after surgery. They are usually measured
    A. Once a shift
    B. Every 15 minutes until the person is stable
    C. Every 2 hours
    D. Every 5 minutes for the first hour
36. Postoperatively, the person is positioned to
    A. Prevent aspiration
    B. Allow for easy and comfortable breathing
    C. Prevent stress on the incision
    D. All of the above
37. Coughing and deep breathing exercises are done after surgery to
    A. Make the person more comfortable
    B. Prevent complications such as pneumonia and atelectasis
    C. Decrease pain and discomfort
    D. Prevent nausea and vomiting
38. Leg exercises are important to prevent
    A. Pneumonia and atelectasis
    B. Thrombus and embolus (blood clots) from forming
    C. Pain at the surgical site
    D. Low blood pressure
39. Leg exercises are done
    A. At least every 1 to 2 hours while the person is awake
    B. Once a shift
    C. When the person is able to do them independently
    D. After the person begins to ambulate
40. Elastic stockings help to
    A. Prevent swelling in the legs
    B. Prevent orthostatic hypotension
    C. Promote venous blood return to the heart and prevent blood clots
    D. Increase blood pressure

41. When applying elastic stockings, you should have the person
    A. Lie in a supine position
    B. Sit in a chair
    C. In a Fowler's position
    D. First walk around the room for few minutes
42. When applying elastic bandages
    A. Start at the proximal part of the extremity
    B. Completely cover the fingers or toes
    C. Apply the bandages very loosely
    D. Expose the fingers and toes if possible
43. When you assist a person to walk after surgery, you first measure
    A. The person's temperature
    B. The blood pressure and pulse
    C. The distance from the bed to the door
    D. The person's weight
44. If a person is NPO after surgery, important personal hygiene is
    A. Frequent oral hygiene
    B. Giving ice chips frequently
    C. Offering sips of cool water
    D. Giving a complete bed bath
45. It is important to report the time and amount of the first voiding after surgery, because the person must void
    A. Within 2 hours after surgery
    B. During the first 24 hours after surgery
    C. Within 8 hours after surgery
    D. At least 1000 mL within the first 4 hours after surgery
46. You can help the person be comfortable postoperatively by
    A. Offering frequent oral care
    B. Changing the gown whenever it is wet or soiled
    C. Telling the nurse promptly when the person complains of pain
    D. All of the above

Fill in the Blank

47. Write out the abbreviation.
    A. AE _____
    B. CBC _____
    C. ECG _____
    D. EKG _____
    E. ID _____
    F. I&O _____
    G. IV _____
    H. NG _____
    I. NPO _____
    J. OR _____
    K. PACU _____
    L. SCD _____
    M. TED _____
48. If a person has outpatient, one-day, or ambulatory surgery, the person is admitted in the morning and
    _____.

49. Before surgery, special personal care is done. Describe the care given and the reasons it is important.
    A. Baths _____
    _____.
    B. Removing makeup, nail polish, and fake nails
    _____
    _____
    C. Hair care _____
    _____
    D. Oral hygiene _____
    _____
50. Some people do not like being seen without their dentures. How can you promote dignity and self-esteem when dentures must be removed before surgery? _____
51. When you are delegated a skin prep, what is reported and recorded?
    A. _____
    B. _____
    C. _____
    D. _____
52. What vital signs are recorded on the preoperative checklist? _____
    _____
53. After the preoperative drugs are given, the person is *not* allowed _____.
54. When a person returns to the room after surgery how often are vital signs usually measured?
    A. _____
    B. _____
    C. _____
    D. _____
55. What post-operative observations of the vital signs should be reported to the nurse?
    A. Temperature _____
    B. Pulse
       1) _____
       2) _____
       3) _____
       4) _____
    C. Respirations
       1) _____
       2) _____
       3) _____
       4) _____
       5) _____
       6) _____
       7) _____
       8) _____
    D. Blood pressure _____

56. You may be able to turn a person who has had surgery by yourself when the person's condition

    _____.

57. Why are older persons at risk for respiratory complications?

    A. _____

    B. _____

    C. _____

58. Leg exercises are done at least every

    _____.

    These exercises are done _____ times.

59. Leg exercises are

    A. _____

    B. _____

    C. _____

    D. _____

60. When you apply elastic stockings, you avoid twists

    because they can _____. Creases

    and wrinkles can cause _____.

61. When you apply elastic bandages, what observations are reported and recorded?

    A. _____

    B. _____

    C. _____

    D. _____

    E. _____

    F. _____

    G. _____

    H. _____

62. Early ambulation prevents

    A. _____

    B. _____

    C. _____

    D. _____

    E. _____

Use Focus on PRIDE in the Textbook to complete questions 63–65.

63. How can you ease a person's fears and concerns when he or she has surgery?

    A. _____

    B. _____

    C. _____

    D. _____

64. What questions can you answer when caring for a

    person having surgery? _____

65. When you are delegated to take post-operative vital signs, what should you report at once to the nurse?

    A. _____

    B. _____

    C. _____

Labeling

66. Color in the area on the figure that needs a skin prep for the surgery listed

    A. Breast surgery

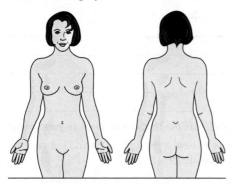

    B. Cervical spine surgery

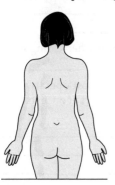

C. Knee surgery

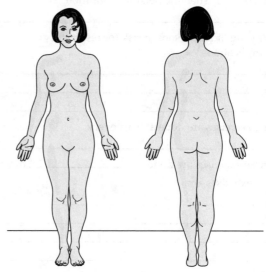

D. Abdominal and leg surgery

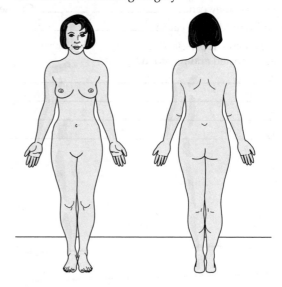

67. A preoperative checklist is completed before a person
    is sent to surgery. Mark the steps that a nursing
    assistant can do and report to the nurse.

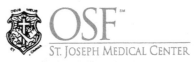

OSF
ST. JOSEPH MEDICAL CENTER

2200 E. Washington Street, Bloomington, Illinois 61701
Phone (309) 662-3311

PRE-OPERATIVE CHECKLIST

DATE OF SURGERY: _____

CHART PREPARATION	ADEQUATE INITIAL HERE	NOT ADEQUATE INITIAL HERE AND EXPLAIN
1. HISTORY AND PHYSICAL ON CHART HT. _____ WT. _____		
2. SURGICAL CONSENT ON CHART, SIGNED		
3. CONSENT FOR ADM BLOOD/BLOOD PROD.		
4. PREGNANCY TEST OBTAINED WHEN INDICATED		
5. URINALYSIS REPORT ON CHART		
6. BLOOD WORK TYPE _____		
7. TYPE AND CROSSMATCH		
8. CHEST X-RAY REPORT ON CHART		
9. EKG REPORT ON CHART READ _____		
10. KNOWN ALLERGIES AND SENSITIVITIES NOTED ON CHART		
11. KNOWN EXPOSURE AND/OR ALLERGY TO **LATEX** NOTED ON CHART		

PATIENT PREPARATION	ADEQUATE INITIAL HERE	NOT ADEQUATE INITIAL HERE AND EXPLAIN
12. FAMILY NOTIFIED OF SURGERY NAME _____ DATE/TIME _____		
13. PATIENT IDENTIFICATION ON WRIST		
14. ALL PROSTHESIS REMOVED (INCLUDING DENTURES, WIGS, HAIRPINS, CONTACT LENSES, COSMETICS, NAIL POLISH, ARTIFICIAL EYES, LIMBS, ETC.)		
15. ALL JEWELRY REMOVED		
16. CLOTHING REMOVED EXCEPT HOSPITAL GOWN WITH TIES		
17. SURGICAL PREP DONE		
18. TIME OF LAST MEAL OR FLUIDS _____ TIME		
19. PRE-OP TPR AND BP: T_____ P_____ R_____ BP_____		
20. VOIDED TIME _____ OR FOLEY		
21. PRE-OP IV AND/OR ANTIBIOTIC: TIME:		

	DRUG	DOSAGE	ROUTE		
PREOPERATIVE MEDICATION GIVEN,	_____	_____	_____	TIME _____ GIVEN BY _____

☐ SIDE RAILS UP

READY FOR O.R.   DATE _____ TIME _____   SIGNATURE _____

PATIENT IDENTIFIED BY TRANSPORTER AND STAFF NURSE   TIME _____

FLOOR NURSE SIGNATURE _____   OR TRANSPORTER SIGNATURE _____   OR NURSE SIGNATURE _____

IDENTIFICATION OF INITIALS			
INITIALS	SIGNATURE	INITIALS	SIGNATURE

Optional Learning Exercises

Mr. Shafer is an 82-year-old man admitted for knee replacement surgery. Answer questions 68–71 about Mr. Shafer and his preoperative care.

68. This surgery is done by choice and is an

_____ surgery.

69. When you are in the room, you listen quietly while Mr. Shafer talks about his fears and concerns. By sitting quietly and showing concern for his feelings, you can assist in Mr. Shafer's

_____ care.

70. The nurse comes to Mr. Shafer's room. What kind of preoperative teaching will be given to him?

A. _____

B. _____

C. _____

D. _____

E. _____

F. _____

G. _____

H. _____

I. _____

J. _____

K. _____

71. The nurse tells you she will give Mr. Shafer his preoperative drugs in 10 minutes. What should you do? _____

_____

Mrs. Johnson is a 70-year-old woman who is scheduled for abdominal surgery. Answer questions 72–76 about her care.

72. The nurse tells you she is busy and asks you to have Mrs. Johnson sign the operative permit. What should you do? _____

_____

73. Mrs. Johnson returns to her room 2 hours after the surgery is completed. You know she is returned to her room when

A. _____

B. _____

C. _____

74. How is the room prepared for Mrs. Johnson's return?

A. _____

B. _____

C. _____

75. When Mrs. Johnson returns to her room, she has sequential compression devices (SCD) on her legs. What is the purpose of SCD?

_____

_____

76. You are caring for Mrs. Johnson 3 days after her surgery. She tells you she has not had a bowel movement since before surgery. You know that one reason for constipation can be drugs given for

_____.

Independent Learning Activities

Answer these questions about a person's experience with surgery. If you have had surgery, use your own experience. If you have not had surgery, ask a family member or friend who has had surgery to answer the questions.

- What type of surgery did you have—elective, urgent, or emergency?
- What information were you given before surgery? Who gave you the information? If you did not understand the information, how well were your questions answered?
- What preparations were needed before surgery—skin prep, enemas, etc.? Who explained the procedures needed? How did you feel about having these done?
- What fears did you have about the surgery? How did you express these feelings to others? How did the person respond to your concerns?
- How much pain did you have after surgery? How was it treated? Did you get relief from the medications and care?

33 Wound Care

Fill in the Blank: Key Terms

Abrasion
Arterial ulcer
Chronic wound
Circulatory ulcer
Clean-contaminated
   wound
Clean wound
Closed wound
Contaminated
   wound
Contusion
Dehiscence

Diabetic foot ulcer
Dirty wound
Edema
Embolus
Evisceration
Excoriation
Full-thickness
   wound
Gangrene
Hematoma
Hemorrhage
Incision

Infected wound
Intentional wound
Laceration
Open wound
Partial-thickness wound
Penetrating wound
Phlebitis
Puncture wound
Purulent drainage
Sanguineous drainage
Serosanguineous
   drainage

Serous drainage
Shock
Skin tear
Stasis ulcer
Trauma
Ulcer
Unintentional
   wound
Vascular ulcer
Venous ulcer
Wound

1. A __skin tear__ is a break or rip in the skin that separates the epidermis from underlying tissues.

2. An open wound with clean, straight edges, usually intentional from a sharp instrument is an __incision__.

3. A shallow or deep crater-like sore of the skin or mucous membrane is an __ulcer__.

4. When tissues are injured but the skin is *not* broken it is a __closed wound__.

5. __Purulent drainage__ is thick green, yellow, or brown drainage.

6. When the dermis and epidermis of the skin are broken, it is called a _____.

7. A __wound__ is a break in the skin or mucous membrane.

8. A wound that is not infected and microbes have not entered the wound is a __clean wound__.

9. An __abrasion__ is a partial-thickness wound caused by the scraping away or rubbing of the skin.

10. A __diabetic foot ulcer__ is an open wound on the foot caused by complications from diabetes.

11. Thin, watery drainage that is blood-tinged is called __serosanguineous drainage__.

12. An __infected wound__ is a wound containing large amounts of bacteria and that shows signs of infection; dirty wound.

13. An open sore on the lower legs or feet caused by decreased blood flow through arteries or veins is a __stasis ulcer__.

14. A swelling that contains blood is a __hematoma__.

15. __Phlebitis__ is an inflammation of a vein.

16. A wound with a high risk of infection is a __contaminated wound__.

17. A condition in which there is death of tissue is __gangrene__.

18. A __laceration__ is an open wound with torn tissues and jagged edges.

19. A wound resulting from trauma is an __unintentional wound__.

20. An __arterial ulcer__ is an open wound on the lower legs and feet caused by poor arterial blood flow.

21. Clear, watery fluid is __serous drainage__.

22. The excessive loss of blood in a short time is __hemorrhage__.

23. An infected wound is a __dirty wound__.

24. A wound that occurs from surgical entry of the urinary, reproductive, respiratory, gastrointestinal system is a __clean-contaminated wound__.

25. A __chronic wound__ is a wound that does *not* heal easily.

26. An open sore on the lower legs or feet caused by poor blood flow through the veins is a __venous ulcer__; stasis ulcer.

27. An open wound made by a sharp object is a ___incision___ _____. The entry of the skin and underlying tissues may be intentional or unintentional.

28. A wound created for therapy is an ___intentional wound___.

29. A ___penetrating wound___ is an open wound that breaks the skin and enters a body area, organ, or cavity.

30. ___dehiscence___ is the separation of wound layers.

31. A circulatory ulcer is also called a ___vascular ulcer___.

32. Swelling that is caused by fluid collecting in tissues is ___edema___.

33. A ___full-thickness wound___ occurs when the dermis, epidermis, and subcutaneous tissue are penetrated. Muscle and bone may be involved.

34. An accident or violent act that injures the skin, mucous membranes, bones, and internal organs is called _____.

35. The separation of the wound along with the protrusion of abdominal organs is ___evisceration___.

36. A ___stasis ulcer___ is another name for a venous ulcer.

37. Bloody drainage is called ___sanguineous drainage___.

38. A closed wound caused by a blow to the body is a ___contusion___.

39. An ___open wound___ occurs when the skin or mucous membrane is broken.

40. ___Shock___ results when tissues do *not* get enough oxygen.

41. A blood clot that travels through the vascular system until it lodges in a vessel is an _____.

42. ___Excoriation___ is the loss of epidermis caused by scratching or when skin rubs against skin, clothing, or other materials.

Circle the Best Answer

43. When you inspect a resident's elbow, you find some of the skin is rubbed away. You would report this to the nurse as an
    A. Laceration
    B. Abrasion
    C. Contusion
    D. Incision

44. When you look at a resident's arm that caught on the wheelchair, the tissue is torn with jagged edges. You know this is a
    A. Puncture wound
    B. Abrasion
    C. Penetrating wound
    D. Laceration

45. Which of these would *not* place a person at risk for skin tears?
    A. The person is obese
    B. The person requires total help in moving
    C. The person has poor nutrition
    D. The person has altered mental awareness

46. Applying lotion will help to prevent skin breakdown or skin tears because it may prevent
    A. Loss of fatty layer under the skin
    B. General thinning of the skin
    C. Dryness of the skin by keeping the skin moisturized
    D. Moisture in areas of the body where perspiration occurs

47. Ulcers of the feet and legs are caused by
    A. Poorly fitted shoes
    B. Decreased blood flow through arteries or veins
    C. Increased activity
    D. Increased fluid intake

48. A measure to prevent circulatory ulcers is
    A. Use elastic, or rubber band type garters to hold the person's socks in place
    B. Remind the person not to sit with the legs crossed
    C. Cut the toenails to keep them short
    D. Massage the legs and feet

49. Common causes of arterial ulcers are
    A. Poor blood flow through the veins
    B. Leg or foot surgery
    C. Smoking, high blood pressure, and diabetes
    D. Surgery on bones and joints

50. It is important to check the feet of a diabetic every day because
    A. The person may not feel a cut, blister, burn, or other trauma to the foot
    B. Tissue and cells do not get needed oxygen and nutrients to heal
    C. Injuries do not heal well
    D. All of the above

51. During wound healing, what phase is happening when the wound is about 1 year old?
    A. Initial phase
    B. Inflammatory phase
    C. Maturation phase
    D. Proliferative phase

52. A surgical wound that is closed with sutures, staples, clips, special glue, or adhesive strips is an example of wound healing by
    A. Delayed intention
    B. First intention
    C. Second intention
    D. Third intention

53. A sign of internal hemorrhage is
    A. Dressings that are soaked with blood
    B. Bloody drainage
    C. An increase in the blood pressure
    D. A hematoma

54. If you observe signs of shock or hemorrhage, you should
    A. Report it to the nurse at once
    B. Reposition the person into a more comfortable position
    C. Make a note of your observations on the flow sheet
    D. Report the observations at the end of your shift

55. The nurse tells you to make sure Mrs. Reynolds supports her abdominal wound when she coughs. The nurse wants this done to protect against
    A. Secondary intention healing
    B. Infection
    C. Scarring
    D. Dehiscence
56. When you are caring for Mrs. Reynolds, you notice thin, watery drainage that is blood-tinged. When you report your observations, you would tell the nurse that the wound has _____ drainage.
    A. Purulent   C. Serous
    B. Serosanguineous   D. Sanguineous
57. Which of these methods used in wound care will prevent microbes from entering a draining wound?
    A. Wet-to-dry dressings
    B. A Hemovac suction device
    C. A Penrose drain
    D. Nonadherent gauze
58. When wet-to-damp dressings are used, they
    A. Absorb dead tissue which is removed when dressings are dry
    B. Are kept moist
    C. Allow air to reach the wound, but fluids and bacteria cannot
    D. Do not stick to the wound
59. Plastic and paper tape may be used to secure a dressing
    A. Because they allow movement of the body part
    B. When the dressing must be changed frequently
    C. If the person is allergic to adhesive tape
    D. Because they stick well to the skin
60. If you care for a person who has Montgomery ties to secure a dressing, you should
    A. Replace the cloth ties when you give care
    B. Tell the nurse if the adhesive strips are soiled
    C. Replace the adhesive strips each time you give care
    D. Retie the cloth ties when you reposition the person
61. If you are assigned to change a dressing, which of these is important information to have?
    A. What kind of medication the person receives
    B. The person's diagnosis
    C. When pain medication was given and how long until it takes effect
    D. When the dressing was last changed
62. You can make the person more comfortable when changing a dressing by doing all of the following *except*
    A. Control your nonverbal communication when looking at the wound
    B. Remove tape by pulling it toward the wound
    C. Encourage the person to look at the wound
    D. Make sure the person does not see the old dressing when it is removed

63. When you are assigned to change dressings, you should
    A. Follow Standard Precautions and Bloodborne Pathogen Standards
    B. Use sterile technique
    C. Only wear gloves to remove old dressings
    D. Use one pair of gloves throughout the dressing change
64. A binder promotes healing because it will
    A. Prevent infection
    B. Reduce drainage
    C. Reduce swelling, promote comfort, and prevent injury
    D. Stop bleeding
65. A binder should be applied
    A. With firm, even pressure over the area
    B. And secured with safety pins positioned where they are easy to reach
    C. Very loosely to prevent interfering with movement
    D. Only once a day and only removed during AM care
66. Which of these measures will *not* be helpful when a person has a wound?
    A. Tell the person the wound looks fine and he or she shouldn't be upset.
    B. Encourage the person to eat well so that the body can heal better.
    C. Remove any soiled dressings from the room as soon as possible.
    D. Allow pain medications to take effect before giving wound care.

Fill in the Blank

67. Write out the abbreviations.
    A. GI _____
    B. ID _____
    C. PPE _____
68. What are common causes of skin tears?
    A. _____
    B. _____
    C. _____
    D. _____
    E. _____
    F. _____
    G. _____
    H. _____
69. List ways to prevent skin tears in the following.
    A. Keep the person hydrated by _____
    _____.
    B. What kind of clothing would be helpful? ____
    _____
    _____

C. Nail care of the person _____

_____.

D. Lift and turn the person with a _____

_____.

E. Support the arms and legs _____

_____.

F. Pad _____

_____.

G. Keep your fingernails _____

and _____. Do not wear rings

with _____.

70. Skin tears are portals _____.

71. When the person has circulatory ulcers report any

_____.

72. If you are caring for a person with a disease that affects venous circulation. You notice her toenails are long and sharp. You should

_____ Why? _____

_____.

73. What 2 diseases are common causes of arterial ulcers?

_____

74. When a person has diabetes, what complications can occur with the following?

A. Nerves – The person does not feel

_____. Can develop

_____

B. Blood vessels – Blood flow _____.

What can occur? _____

_____

75. Explain what can happen if a person with diabetes has these foot problems.

A. Corns and calluses _____

B. Ingrown toenails _____

_____

C. Hammer toes _____

_____

D. Dry and cracked skin _____

_____

76. With primary intention healing the wound edges are held together with _____.

77. Secondary intention healing is used for _____

_____ wounds. Because healing

takes longer, the threat of _____

is great.

78. If you suspect a person has external hemorrhage, where would you check for drainage? _____

_____

79. What should you do if you find a person's wound has dehiscence or evisceration? _____

_____

80. What observations would you make about wound appearance?

A. _____

B. _____

C. _____

D. _____

E. _____

81. When you are delegated to change a dressing, what should you do if the old dressings stick to the wound?

_____

_____

82. If the person has drainage from a wound, how is it measured?

A. _____

B. _____

C. _____

83. What are the purposes of a transparent adhesive film dressing?

A. _____

B. _____

C. _____

D. _____

84. What is the difference between wet-to-damp dressings and wet-to-wet dressings? _____

_____

85. When taping a dressing in place, the tape should *not* encircle the entire body part because _____

_____.

86. When delegated to apply dressings, list what observations should be reported and recorded.

A. _____

B. _____

C. _____

D. _____

E. _____

F. _____

_____

G. _____

H. _____

I. _____

J. _____

K. _____

L. _____

M. _____

Use Focus on PRIDE in the Textbook to complete questions 87–88.

87. When you are giving care, you are responsible to protect the person's safety and well-being. What are your responsibilities regarding wound care in these situations?

    A. If you are careless during a transfer, you can cause

    a _____ .

    B. If you rush during a bath, you may not notice a

    _____ between skin folds on a bariatric person.

    C. If you do not apply shoes properly on a diabetic

    person, _____ can develop.

88. To promote comfort and interaction with family and friends for a person with a wound, you may

    A. _____

    B. _____

    C. _____

    D. _____

    E. _____

Optional Learning Exercises

You are assigned to care for Mrs. Stevens. She is 87 years old and has diabetes and high blood pressure. She walks with difficulty and spends most of her day sitting in her chair. She is somewhat overweight and tells you she had a knee replacement 5 years ago and had phlebitis after surgery. The nurse tells you to watch carefully for signs of circulatory ulcers. Answer questions 89–90.

89. What risk factors does Mrs. Stevens have that place her at risk for venous ulcers?

    A. _____

    B. _____

    C. _____

    D. _____

    E. _____

    F. _____

90. What risk factors does Mrs. Stevens have that place her at risk for arterial ulcers?

    A. _____

    B. _____

Mr. Hawkins, age 74, was in an automobile accident and has a wound on his leg that is large and open. It has become infected and he is being treated with antibiotics. When you are talking with him, he tells you he has smoked for 55 years and has poor circulation in his legs. He lives alone and generally eats takeout foods or eats cereal when he is at home. Answer questions 91–94.

91. Why is he receiving antibiotics? _____

    _____

92. What side effect of the antibiotics can cause a problem that could interfere with healing?

    _____

    _____

93. What factors would increase Mr. Hawkins risk for complications?

    A. _____

    B. _____

    C. _____

    D. _____

94. What is missing in Mr. Hawkins diet that is needed to

    help in healing the wound? _____

You are assisting the nurse with wound care. She is changing dressings for 2 different persons. Mrs. Henderson has a wound that has a large amount of drainage. Mr. Wendel has a drain in his wound that is attached to suction. Answer questions 95–99.

95. Why does the nurse weigh Mrs. Henderson's new dressings before applying them to the wound and the old dressings when they are removed?

    _____

    _____

96. How does she find out the amount of drainage from

    Mr. Wendel's wound? _____

    _____

97. What other ways can be used to measure drainage in old dressings?

    A. _____

    B. _____

    C. _____

    D. _____

    E. _____

    F. _____

98. When you are changing a nonsterile dressing, why do

    you need 2 pairs of gloves? _____

    _____

99. When a wound is infected and has poor circulation, the wound may be left open at first and then closed later. This type of wound healing is called healing

    through _____ . This

    type of healing combines _____ and

    _____ intention healing.

Independent Learning Activities

Role-play this situation with a classmate. One of you should act as the person, and one should act as the nursing assistant. Work together to answer the questions for each role.

Situation: Mr. Chavez is 45 years old and has a reddened area on his left calf. The doctor has ordered moist warm compresses to the area, and the nurse has delegated this task to you.

- As the Nursing Assistant:
  - What questions would you ask the nurse before you applied the compresses?
  - How will you check the temperature of the compress?
  - How will you keep the compresses at the correct temperature?
  - How often will you check the compresses? What will you observe when you check the area?
- As Mr. Chavez:
  - How was the treatment explained to you?
  - How were you positioned? What did the nursing assistant do to make sure you were comfortable?
  - How did the compresses feel? Was the temperature maintained? How?
  - How often was the compress checked?

34 Pressure Ulcers

Fill in the Blank: Key Terms

Avoidable pressure ulcer
Bedfast
Bony prominence
Chairfast

Colonized
Epidermal stripping
Eschar
Friction

Pressure ulcer
Shear

Slough
Unavoidable pressure ulcer

1. _Colonized_ is the presence of bacteria on the wound surface or in wound tissue; the person does *not* have signs and symptoms of an infection.

2. Dead tissue that is shed from the skin is _slough_.

3. A pressure ulcer that develops from the improper use of the nursing process is an _avoidable pressure ulcer_.

4. A _bony prominence_ is an area where the bone sticks out or projects from the flat surface of the body.

5. Thick, leathery dead tissue that may be loose or adhered to the skin is _eschar_.

6. _Shear_ occurs when layers of the skin rub against each other; when the skin remains in place and underlying tissues move and stretch and tear underlying capillaries and blood vessels, causing tissue damage.

7. _bedfast_ means confined to bed.

8. The rubbing of one surface against another is _friction_.

9. An _unavoidable pressure ulcer_ is a pressure ulcer that occurs despite efforts to prevent one through proper use of the nursing process.

10. A localized injury to the skin and/or underlying tissue, usually over a bony prominence, resulting from pressure or pressure in combination with shear is a _pressure ulcer_.

11. _Chairfast_ means confined to a chair.

12. Removing the epidermis as tape is removed from the skin is _epidermal stripping_.

Circle the Best Answer

13. A pressure ulcer occurs because
    A. The person repositions himself or herself in the bed or chair
    B. The person drinks too many fluids
    C. Skin and underlying tissue is damaged by pressure or pressure in combination with shear and/or friction
    D. The person is repositioned too frequently

14. Older and disabled persons are at great risk for pressure ulcers because of
    A. Acute illnesses
    B. Increased activity
    C. Thin and fragile skin
    D. Good nutrition

15. The first sign of a pressure ulcer in an area may be
    A. Reddened skin over a bony prominence
    B. Swelling in the area
    C. A break in the skin
    D. Exposed tissue and some drainage from the area

16. Mrs. Greene keeps sliding down in bed. The nurse tells you to raise the head of the bed no more than 30 degrees. This position will prevent tissue damage caused by
    A. Pressure over hard surfaces
    B. Shearing
    C. Poor body mechanics
    D. Poor fluid balance

17. Pressure ulcers can occur
    A. Over bony areas such as the hips
    B. Underneath the breasts
    C. Between abdominal folds
    D. All of the above

18. A stage 3 pressure ulcer would have
    A. Intact skin with redness or different skin coloring over a bony prominence
    B. Exposed subcutaneous fat and slough
    C. Full-thickness tissue loss with muscle, tendon, and bone exposure
    D. A blister or shallow ulcer

19. The most common site for a pressure ulcer is the
    A. Elbow
    B. Sacrum
    C. Thighs
    D. Ears

20. When following a repositioning schedule, the person should be repositioned
    A. According to the schedule in the person's repositioning schedule
    B. Every 2 hours
    C. Every 15 minutes
    D. As often as you have time
21. One way to prevent friction in the bed is to
    A. Use soap when cleansing the skin
    B. Rub or massage reddened areas
    C. Use pillows and blankets to prevent skin from being in contact with skin
    D. Powder sheets lightly
22. Bed cradles are used to
    A. Position the person in good body alignment
    B. Prevent pressure on the legs, feet, and toes
    C. Keep the heels off the bed
    D. Distribute body weight evenly
23. When the person is using an eggcrate-type mattress, it is covered with a special cover and
    A. Only a bottom sheet
    B. A bottom sheet and a draw sheet
    C. Waterproof materials, a lift sheet, and a bottom sheet
    D. A bottom sheet and a waterproof pad

Fill in the Blank

24. Write out the abbreviations.
    A. CMS _____
    B. TJC _____
25. Name the stage of pressure ulcer described in each of these
    A. The skin is gone, and subcutaneous fat may be exposed _____
    B. The skin is red with light skin, or red, blue, or purple with dark skin. The color does *not* return to normal when the skin is relieved of pressure.
    _____
    C. Muscle, tendon, and bone are exposed and damage. Eschar may be present
    _____
    _____
    D. The wound may involve an abrasion, blister, or shallow crater. _____
26. You can help prevent shearing by raising the head of the bed only _____. The care plan tells you
    A. _____
    B. _____
    C. _____
27. Explain how the following conditions place a person at risk for pressure ulcers.
    A. Urinary or fecal incontinence _____
    _____

B. Poor nutrition _____

C. Poor fluid balance _____
_____

D. Lowered mental awareness _____
_____

E. Circulatory problems _____
_____

F. Older age _____
_____

28. Explain how these protective devices help prevent pressure ulcers.
    A. Bed cradle prevents pressure on
    _____
    B. Heel and elbow protectors prevent
    _____
    and _____.
    C. Heel and foot elevators raise
    _____.
    D. Eggcrate-type pads distribute
    _____.
    E. Special beds distribute
    _____. There is little
    pressure on _____.

Use Focus on PRIDE in the Textbook to complete questions 29–30.

29. When you observe and report skin problems to the nurse, it can prevent _____.
30. When you speak up for your patients and residents, this is called being an _____.

Labeling

Use this figure to answer questions 31–32.

31. Name this position _____

32. Place an "X" on each of the 5 pressure points. Name the bony point for each one.

    A. _____

    B. _____

    C. _____

    D. _____

    E. _____

Use this figure to answer questions 33–34.

33. Name this position _____

34. Place an "X" on each of the 10 pressure points. Name the bony point(s) for each one.

    A. _____

    B. _____

    C. _____

    D. _____

    E. _____

    F. _____

    G. _____

    H. _____

    I. _____

    J. _____

Use this figure to answer questions 35–36.

35. Name this position _____

36. Place an "X" on each of the 10 pressure points. Name the bony point for each one.

    A. _____

    B. _____

    C. _____

    D. _____

    E. _____

    F. _____

    G. _____

    H. _____

    I. _____

    J. _____

Use this figure to answer questions 37–38.

37. Name this position _____

38. Place an "X" on each of the 6 pressure points. Name the bony point for each one.

    A. _____

    B. _____

    C. _____

    D. _____

    E. _____

    F. _____

Use this figure to answer questions 39–40.

39. Name this position _____

40. Place an "X" on each of the 5 pressure points. Name the bony point for each one.

    A. _____

    B. _____

    C. _____

    D. _____

    E. _____

Optional Learning Exercises

41. After admission to a nursing center, many pressure ulcers develop with the first

    _____ after admission.

42. How quickly can a person develop a pressure ulcer after the onset of pressure?

    _____

43. When handling, moving, and positioning a person, it is important to follow the _____

    _____ in the person's care plan.

    A. How often should a bedfast person be

       repositioned? _____

    B. How often should a chairfast person be

       repositioned? _____

    C. Why would a person be repositioned more frequently (as often as every 15 minutes)?

       _____

44. What are 2 ways pressure ulcers can occur on the ears?

    A. _____

    B. _____

45. If you are interviewed by the CMS staff about pressure ulcers, what questions may be asked?

    A. _____

    B. _____

    C. _____

    D. _____

    E. _____

Independent Learning Activities

Take turns with a classmate and carry out these exercises. They will help you understand how a person who cannot move without help feels when pressure is unrelieved. NOTE: These exercises work best if the person wears thin clothes so the discomfort is more noticeable.

- Place a pencil or similar hard object on the seat of a chair and have a classmate sit on the object for 10 minutes. Keep time, and remind the person not to move, to make it more uncomfortable. Remember, persons at risk for pressure ulcers often are unable to change position without assistance.
- Position a classmate in bed, making sure the bedclothes are wrinkled to form lumps under bony pressure points. (For example, place a wrinkle under the sacrum in the supine position, or under the hip or shoulder in the lateral position.)

Answer these questions about the exercises done.

- How long did it *seem* like when you waiting for 10 minutes to pass?
- How many times did you begin to reposition yourself without thinking about it?
- How did the pressure areas feel when you completed the 10 minutes? What color was the area?
- How will this exercise affect your care of persons who cannot move?

35 Heat and Cold Applications

Fill in the Blank: Key Terms

Compress   Cyanosis   Hyperthermia   Pack
Constrict   Dilate   Hypothermia

1. A body temperature that is much higher than the person's normal range is
   __hyperthermia__.

2. __Constrict__ means to narrow.

3. A treatment that involves wrapping a body part with a wet or dry application is a
   __pack__.

4. A __Compress__ is a soft pad applied over a body area.

5. __dilate__ means to expand or open wider.

6. __hypothermia__ occurs when the body temperature is very low.

7. A bluish color is __Cyanosis__

Circle the Best Answer

8. Before you apply heat applications it is important to know if
   A. A nurse is available to answer questions and supervise you
   B. Your state allows you to perform the procedure
   C. The procedure is in your job description
   D. All of the above

9. Heat applications can be applied
   A. Only to extremities
   B. To areas with metal implants
   C. To almost any body part
   D. To persons who have difficulty sensing heat or pain

10. When heat is applied to the skin
    A. Blood vessels in the area dilate
    B. Tissues have less oxygen
    C. Blood flow decreases
    D. Blood vessels constrict

11. When heat is applied too long, a complication that occurs is
    A. Blood vessels dilate
    B. Blood flow increases
    C. Blood vessels constrict
    D. More nutrients reach the area

12. Moist heat applications have cooler temperatures than dry heat applications because
    A. Dry heat penetrates more deeply
    B. Dry heat cannot cause burns
    C. Heat penetrates deeper with a moist application
    D. Moist heat has a slower effect than dry heat

13. When heat is applied to an area, which of these is an expected response?
    A. The skin is red and warm.
    B. The skin is pale, white, or gray.
    C. The person begins to shiver.
    D. The area is excessively red.

14. The care plan states that the person receives a heat application of 110° F. As a nursing assistant you know that you should
    A. Measure the temperature carefully before applying to the person
    B. Not apply an application that is above 106° F
    C. Ask the person if the application is too warm
    D. Apply the application and remind the person not to remove the application

15. Heat and cold applications are applied for no longer than
    A. 1 hour   C. 15 to 20 minutes
    B. 30 minutes   D. 4 hours

16. When a hot or cold application is in place, you should check the area
    A. Every 15 to 20 minutes
    B. Every 5 minutes
    C. About every 30 minutes
    D. Once an hour

17. When hot compresses are in place, you may apply an aquathermia pad over the compress
    A. To keep the compress wet
    B. To protect the area from injury
    C. To measure the temperature of the compress
    D. To maintain the correct temperature of the compress

18. A hot soak is applied
    A. By putting the body part into water
    B. By applying a soft pad to a body part
    C. And is covered with plastic wrap
    D. Only until the water temperature cools down

19. When giving a sitz bath
    A. Stay with the person if he or she is weak or unsteady
    B. Observe for signs of weakness, faintness, or fatigue
    C. Prevent the person from getting chills and burns
    D. All of the above

20. When you use an aquathermia pad
    A. The pad temperature will cool off after about 20 to 30 minutes
    B. The temperature is maintained by the flow of water through the pad
    C. It is a form of moist heat
    D. You do not need to check the person as often as with other heat applications
21. When a cold application is applied, the numbing effect helps to
    A. Reduce or relieve pain in the body part
    B. Constrict blood vessels
    C. Decrease blood flow
    D. Cool the body part
22. Which of these cold applications is moist?
    A. Ice bag   C. Ice glove
    B. Ice collar   D. Cold compress
23. You should remove the heat or cold application if
    A. The skin is red and warm with a heat application
    B. The person tells you the cold application has numbed the area and relieved some pain
    C. The skin appears pale, white, gray, or bluish in color
    D. The person is slightly chilled and asks for another blanket
24. When a person has hyperthermia, ice packs are applied to all of these areas *except*
    A. The abdomen   C. The underarms
    B. The head   D. The groin

Fill in the Blank

25. Write out the abbreviations.
    A. F _____
    B. C _____
26. What are the effects of heat applications?
    A. _____
    B. _____
    C. _____
    D. _____
    E. _____
27. When you are caring for a confused person and heat or cold is applied, how can you know if they are in pain? _____
28. What are the advantages of dry heat applications?
    A. _____
    B. _____
29. Give two examples of dry heat applications.
    _____
30. When the nurse delegates you to prepare a warm soak, what is the temperature range that is correct?
    _____
31. When you are giving a sitz bath, what observations should be reported to the nurse? _____

32. When using an aquathermia pad you should make sure the hoses do not have kinks or air bubbles to allow the water to _____
33. Name uses for cold applications.
    A. _____
    B. _____
    C. _____
    D. _____
    E. _____
34. When you prepare an ice bag, collar, or glove, remove the excess air by _____
35. When a heat or cold compress is in place, it usually needs to be changed every 5 minutes because _____
36. When a cooling blanket is being used, _____ are checked often.
37. How can you manage your time to stay in or near the person's room during a heat or cold application?
    A. _____
    B. _____
    C. _____
    D. _____
    E. _____
    F. _____

Use Focus on PRIDE in the Textbook to complete questions 38–39.

38. When applying heat or cold, you must allow time for
    A. _____
    B. _____
    C. _____
    D. _____
    E. _____
39. When applying heat and cold, harm and legal action can result if you
    A. _____
    B. _____
    C. _____
    D. _____
    E. _____
    F. _____
    G. _____

Optional Learning Exercises

Situation: The nurse instructs you to apply a cold pack to a resident who has twisted her ankle. Use the information you learned in this chapter to answer questions 40–48 about carrying out this treatment.

40. What is the purpose of the cold application for this injury? _____

41. What can you use to make a cool dry application to the ankle if no commercial packs are available?

_____

42. Why do you squeeze the application tightly after filling it with ice? _____

_____

43. How will you protect the person's skin? _____

44. How often do you check the application?

_____

45. When you check the area where the cold pack was applied, what signs and symptoms should be reported?

    A. _____
    B. _____
    C. _____
    D. _____
    E. _____
    F. _____
    G. _____

46. What should you do if any of these signs or symptoms are present? _____

47. How long should you leave the application in place?

_____

48. What happens if you leave the cold pack in place too long? _____

Independent Learning Exercises

Situation: Mr. Chavez is 45 years old and has a reddened area on his left calf. The doctor has ordered moist warm compresses to the area, and the nurse has delegated this task to you.

- Role-play this situation with a classmate. One of you should act as the person, and one should act as the nursing assistant. Work together to answer the questions for the each role.
- As the Nursing Assistant:
  - What questions would you ask the nurse before you applied the compresses?
  - What temperature range is used for this compress?
  - How did you check the temperature of the compresses?
  - How did you keep the compress at the correct temperature?
  - How often did you check the compress? What did you observe when you checked the area?
- As Mr. Chavez:
  - How was the treatment explained to you?
  - How were you positioned? How did the nursing assistant check to see if you were comfortable?
  - How did the compress feel? Was the temperature maintained? How?
  - How often was the compress checked?

36 Oxygen Needs

Fill in the Blank: Key Terms

Allergy
Apnea
Atelectasis
Biot's respirations
Bradypnea
Cheyne-Stokes respirations

Cyanosis
Dyspnea
Hemoptysis
Hyperventilation
Hypoventilation
Hypoxemia

Hypoxia
Kussmaul respirations
Orthopnea
Orthopneic position
Oxygen concentration
Pollutant

Respiratory arrest
Respiratory depression
Sputum
Tachypnea

1. _Biot's respiration_ are respirations that are rapid and deep, followed by 10 to 30 seconds of apnea.

2. Bloody sputum is called _hemoptysis_.

3. Rapid breathing where respirations are usually greater than 20 per minute is called _tachypnea_.

4. An _allergy_ is a sensitivity to a substance that causes the body to react with signs and symptoms.

5. Difficult, labored, or painful breathing is _dyspnea_.

6. Mucus from the respiratory system that is expectorated through the mouth is _sputum_.

7. Being able to breathe deeply and comfortably only while sitting is _orthopnea_.

8. Respirations that are less than 12 per minute is slow breathing or _bradypnea_.

9. A reduced amount of oxygen in the blood is _hypoxemia_.

10. _Respiratory depression_ describes slow, weak respirations that occur at a rate of fewer than 12 per minute.

11. The lack or absence of breathing is _apnea_.

12. _Kussmaul respiration_ is a pattern of respirations that is rapid and deeper than normal.

13. A harmful chemical or substance in the air or water is a _pollutant_.

14. _Cheyne-Stokes respiration_ are respirations that gradually increase in rate and depth and then become shallow and slow. Breathing may stop for 10 to 20 seconds.

15. The _orthopneic position_ is sitting up and leaning over a table to breathe.

16. When breathing stops, it is _respiratory arrest_.

17. Very deep and rapid respirations are _hyperventilation_.

18. _Oxygen concentration_ is the amount of hemoglobin containing oxygen.

19. When cells do not have enough oxygen, it is called _hypoxia_.

20. Respirations that are slow, shallow, and sometimes irregular is _hypoventilation_.

21. The collapse of a portion of the lung is _atelectasis_.

22. _Cyanosis_ is a bluish color to the skin, lips, mucous membranes, and nail beds.

Circle the Best Answer

23. Capillaries and cells must exchange O_2 and CO_2 in the
   A. Respiratory system
   B. Circulatory system
   C. Nervous system
   D. Red blood cells

24. Oxygen needs increase when
   A. The person is aging
   B. Drugs are taken
   C. The person has fever or pain
   D. The person is well-nourished

25. Respiratory depression or arrest can occur when
   A. The person exercises
   B. Allergies are present
   C. Narcotic drugs are taken in large doses
   D. The person smokes

26. Restlessness is an early sign of
   A. Hypoxia
   B. Apnea
   C. Hyperventilation
   D. Bradypnea

27. Which of these would *not* be a sign of hypoxia?
   A. Disorientation and confusion
   B. Decrease in pulse rate and respirations
   C. Apprehension and anxiety
   D. Cyanosis of the skin, mucous membranes, and nail beds

28. If a pulse oximeter is being used on a person with tremors or poor circulation, which of these sites would be best to use?
    A. A toe on a foot that is swollen
    B. A finger that has nail polish on the nail
    C. A toe with an open wound
    D. An earlobe

29. When you are delegated to place a pulse oximeter on a person, report to the nurse if
    A. The person is sleeping
    B. The pulse rate is above or below the alarm limit
    C. You remove nail polish on the nail before attaching the pulse oximeter
    D. You tape the oximeter in place

30. When a person has breathing difficulties, it is usually easier for the person to breath
    A. In the supine position
    B. Lying on one side for long periods
    C. In the semi-Fowler's or Fowler's position
    D. In the prone position

31. Deep breathing and coughing exercises
    A. Help prevent pneumonia and atelectasis
    B. Decrease pain after surgery or injury
    C. Are done once a day
    D. Cause mucus to form in the lungs

32. When assisting with coughing and deep breathing you ask the person to
    A. Inhale through the mouth
    B. Hold the breath for 30 seconds
    C. Exhale slowly through pursed lips
    D. Repeat the exercise 1 or 2 times

33. When a person uses an incentive spirometer, it allows the person to
    A. Take shallow breaths
    B. See air movement when inhaling
    C. See air movement with exhaling
    D. Exhale quickly

34. If a person is receiving oxygen, you may
    A. Set the flow rate
    B. Apply the oxygen device to the person
    C. Set up the system
    D. Turn on the oxygen

35. If you are caring for a person with oxygen therapy, you may *not*
    A. Start and maintain oxygen therapy
    B. Attach the oxygen device and connecting tube to the humidifier
    C. Tell the nurse if the rate is too high or too low
    D. Check for irritation from the device

36. If a person is receiving oxygen, it is important to
    A. Place no smoking signs in the room and on the room door
    B. Turn off electrical items before unplugging then
    C. Not use wool or synthetic fabrics in room
    D. All of the above

37. If a person receives oxygen through a nasal cannula, it is important to look for irritation
    A. On the nose, ears, and cheekbones
    B. Under the mask
    C. In the throat
    D. In the oral cavity

38. If you are delegated to set up for oxygen administration, you will do all of these *except*
    A. Collect the device with connecting tubing
    B. Attach the flowmeter to the wall outlet or tank
    C. Apply the oxygen device to the person
    D. Fill the humidifier with distilled water

39. If you are near a person receiving oxygen, which of these should you report?
    A. The humidifier is bubbling.
    B. The humidifier has enough water.
    C. The humidifier is not bubbling.
    D. The person is in a semi-Fowler's position.

Fill in the Blank

40. Write out the meaning of the abbreviations.
    A. CO_2 _Carbon dioxide_
    B. ID _identification_
    C. L/min _Liters per minute_
    D. O_2 _Oxygen_
    E. RBC _Red blood cell_
    F. SpO_2 _Saturation of peripheral oxygen_

41. As a person ages, what factors affect the person's oxygen needs?
    A. Respiratory muscles _weakens_
    B. Lung tissue _less elastic_
    C. Strength for coughing _decreases_
    D. Risk increases for developing _pneumonia_

42. Three diseases are caused by or related to smoking. They are
    A. _lung cancer_
    B. _pulmonary disease_
    C. _coronary artery disease_

43. How does alcohol increase the risk of aspiration? It depresses the _brain_, reduces the _cough reflex_, and increases _risk of aspiration_.

44. What terms can be used to describe sputum when reporting and recording?
    A. Color: _clear, white, yellow, green_
    B. Odor: _none or foul odor_
    C. Consistency: _thick, watery, frothy_
    D. Hemoptysis: _bright red, dark red, blood tinged, streaked with blood_

45. The normal range for oxygen concentration is _95% - 100%_.

46. If you are caring for a person with a pulse oximeter, what observations should be reported and recorded?
    A. _SpO_2_
    B. _pulse rate_
    C. _observations_
    D. _____

E. _____

F. _____

47. If a pulse oximeter is in place, what should be reported at once to the nurse?

A. SpO$_2$ _in alarm range_

B. Pulse rate _abnormal_

C. Signs and symptoms of _hypoxia_ and

apnea

48. If a person has difficulty breathing, he or she may prefer a position where the person is sitting

_up_ .

This position is called _orthopnea_ .

49. If a person has a productive cough, what respiratory hygiene and cough etiquette should be taught?

A. _gloves_

B. _yours_

C. _covering_

D. _____

50. If a person is using an incentive spirometer, how long is the breath held to keep the balls floating?

3 seconds

51. What observations should be reported after a person uses an incentive spirometer?

A. _observation_

B. _resident concerns_

C. _height   breaths_

D. _if person coughed tolerated_

52. When a person wears a mask to receive oxygen, what should you do when the person needs to eat?

take off

How will the person receive oxygen during the meal?

cannula prongs

53. Oxygen is humidified because it will _____

purify water .

Use Focus on PRIDE in the Textbook to complete questions 54–55.

54. When you remind the person or visitors not to smoke when NO SMOKING signs are used, you are protecting the person's right to a _clean residency_ .

55. You do *not* adjust the oxygen flow rate unless allowed by your _patient_ and _nurse_ and instructed _doctor_ .

Crossword

Fill in the following crossword by answering the clues with the words from this list:

Apnea	Bradypnea	Dyspnea	Hypoventilation	Orthopnea
Biot's	Cheyne-Stokes	Hyperventilation	Kussmaul	Tachypnea

Across

9. Respirations are rapid and deeper than normal
10. Rapid and deep respirations followed by 10 to 30 seconds of apnea; occur with nervous disorders

Down

1. Respirations gradually increase in rate and depth; common when death is near
2. Respirations are 20 or more per minute
3. Respirations are slow, shallow, and sometimes irregular
4. Very deep and rapid respirations; signal diabetic coma
5. Difficult, labored, or painful breathing
6. Breathing deeply and comfortably only when sitting
7. Lack or absence of breathing
8. Respirations are fewer than 12 per minute

Optional Learning Exercises

Situation: You are caring for Mr. R., age 84, who has chronic obstructive pulmonary disease. Answer questions 56–57.

56. What position would make it easier for Mr. R. to breathe when he is in bed? _____

_____

57. How can you increase his comfort when he sitting up? _____

_____ What is this

position called? _____

Situation: Mrs. F. is receiving oxygen through a nasal cannula at 2 L/min. Her respirations are unlabored at 16 per minute unless she is walking about or doing personal care. Then her respirations are 28 per minute and dyspneic. Answer questions 58–61.

58. Why is there no humidifier with the oxygen setup for Mrs. F.? _____

_____

59. Where should you check for signs of irritation from the cannula? _____

_____

60. You should make sure there are _____ in the tubing and that Mrs. F. does not

_____ of the tubing.

61. What are the abnormal respirations that Mrs. F. has with activity called? _____

Independent Learning Activities

Work with a classmate and carry out these exercises. They will help you to understand how it feels to a person with breathing problems.

- Have your partner count your respirations while you are at rest. Then exercise by running or jogging in place for at least 2 minutes. Now have your partner check your respirations again. How have they changed? Rate? Rhythm or pattern? Easy or labored?
- While you exercise, try first to breathe only through your nose. Then try breathing through your mouth. Which way makes you feel you are getting enough air?
- Place a drinking straw in your mouth and close your lips tightly around it. Now breathe only through the straw while at rest and during exercise. When you are at rest, how comfortable does this feel? Are you getting enough air? How is your air supply during exercise?
- Take a drinking straw and place small pieces of paper in one end so that it is fairly tight. Now try breathing through the straw at rest and exercise. What is the difference between the open and blocked straw? Imagine if every breath you take feels like it does with the blocked straw. This is how many people with breathing problems feel all the time.

37 Respiratory Support and Therapies

Fill in the Blank: Key Terms

Hemothorax   Mechanical ventilation   Pleural effusion   Suction
Intubation   Patent   Pneumothorax   Tracheostomy

1. The escape and collection of fluid in the pleural space is _pleural effusion_.

2. _hemothorax_ is blood in the pleural space.

3. A _tracheostomy_ is a surgically created opening into the trachea.

4. _Suction_ is the process of withdrawing or sucking up fluid.

5. Inserting an artificial airway is _intubation_.

6. _Pneumothorax_ is air in the pleural space.

7. _Mechanical ventilation_ is using a machine to move air into and out of the lungs.

8. _Patent_ is open or unblocked.

Circle the Best Answer

9. When caring for a person with an artificial airway, you should tell the nurse at once if
   A. The vital signs remain stable
   B. Frequent oral hygiene is done
   C. The airway comes out or is dislodged
   D. The person feels as if he or she is gagging

10. Because a person with an endotracheal tube (ET) cannot speak, it is important to
    A. Never ask questions
    B. Avoid talking to the person
    C. Always keep the signal light within reach
    D. Avoid explaining what you are going to do

11. The person with an ET can communicate by
    A. Whispering or speaking softly
    B. Using paper and pencil, magic slates, or communication boards
    C. Having a family member ask and answer questions
    D. Covering the tube opening

12. If you are caring for a person with an artificial airway, your care should always include
    A. Removing the device to clean it
    B. Comforting and reassuring the person that the airway helps breathing
    C. Suctioning to maintain the airway
    D. Making sure the person never takes a tub bath

13. The stoma or tube must be
    A. Covered when shaving
    B. Covered with plastic when outdoors
    C. Covered with a loose gauze dressing when bathing
    D. Uncovered when the person is out of doors

14. If you are assisting with tracheostomy care, you may be delegated to
    A. Use clean technique when handling the equipment
    B. Provide care every 2 to 4 hours
    C. Clean a reusable cannula with hydrogen peroxide or with normal saline or soap
    D. Remove the inner and outer cannulas to clean

15. When suctioning is done, the nurse
    A. Follows Standard Precautions and Bloodborne Pathogen Standards
    B. Make sure a suction cycle is not more than 20 to 30 seconds
    C. Waits about 5 seconds between each suction cycle
    D. Suction as many times as needed to clear the airway

16. If you are caring for a person who needs suctioning, you know that suctioning is done
    A. On a regular schedule
    B. When signs and symptoms of respiratory distress are observed
    C. When the nurse directs you to do the suctioning
    D. When the person asks for suctioning

17. When the alarm sounds on a machine used for mechanical ventilation, you should first
    A. Report to the nurse at once
    B. Reset the alarms
    C. Reassure the person that the alarm is normal
    D. Check to see if the person's tube is attached to the ventilator

18. When caring for a person with chest tubes, tell the nurse at once if bubbling in the drainage system
    A. Stops   C. All of the above
    B. Decreases   D. All of the above

19. Petrolatum gauze is kept at the bedside of a person with chest tubes to
    A. Cover the insertion site if the chest tube comes out
    B. Lubricate the site of the chest tube
    C. Cleanse the skin around the chest tube
    D. Cover the site of the chest tube insertion to prevent drainage

Fill in the Blank

20. Write out the meaning of the abbreviations
    A. CO$_2$ _____
    B. ET _____
    C. O$_2$ _____
    D. RT _____

21. When caring for a person with an artificial airway, you may be delegated to
    A. Check _____ often
    B. Observe for _____
    C. Give frequent _____
    D. Report to the nurse at once if
    _____

22. What are the three parts of a tracheostomy tube?
    A. _____
    B. _____
    C. _____

23. Which part of the tracheostomy tube is removed for cleaning and mucus removal? _____

24. Which part of the tracheostomy tube is *not* removed?
    _____

25. If a person with a tracheostomy is outdoors, what is used to cover the tracheostomy? _____
    _____

26. A suction cycle takes no more than _____ seconds. The cycle involves
    A. _____
    B. _____
    C. _____

27. A suction cycle for an infant or child is limited to
    _____ seconds.

28. Before, during, and after suctioning, what is checked and observed?
    A. _____
    B. _____
    C. _____
    D. _____

29. When you are observing a person with a tracheostomy, what should be reported to the nurse at once?
    A. _____
    B. _____
    C. _____
    D. _____
    E. _____

30. When a person has mechanical ventilation, what should you do when you enter the room? _____
    _____

    When you leave the room? _____
    _____

31. If chest tubes are in place, what should be reported to the nurse?
    A. Signs and symptoms of _____ and
    _____
    B. Complaints of _____ or
    _____

Use Focus on PRIDE in the Textbook to complete questions 32–33.

32. It is important to report signs and symptoms that a person needs suctioning because the airway must be clear for _____.

33. When a person has an ET tube, you show dignity and respect when providing care by
    A. _____
    B. _____
    C. _____
    D. _____
    E. _____

Optional Learning Exercises

34. If you are caring for a person with a tracheostomy, why is the tracheostomy covered when the person is outdoors? _____
    _____

35. What is done to protect the stoma in the following situations?
    A. Showers _____
    _____
    B. Shaving _____
    C. Shampooing _____
    _____

36. The stoma is never covered with _____,
    _____.
    Why? _____
    _____

37. What do you need to check before using an Ambu bag attached to oxygen? _____
    Why? _____
    _____

38. If a person has mechanical ventilation, where do you find a plan for communication? _____
    Why is it important for everyone to use the same signals for communication? _____
    _____

39. If a person has chest tubes, why is it important to prevent kinks in the tubing? _____
    _____

Independent Learning Activities

Try to find a person who has had a type of artificial ventilation discussed in this chapter. Ask the person these questions.

- What was the worst part of the experience?
- How did the person communicate his or her needs with others?
- What did the staff do that helped make the person comfortable?
- What would have helped to make the experience better?

38 Rehabilitation and Restorative Nursing Care

Fill in the Blank: Key Terms

Activities of daily living   Disability   Rehabilitation   Restorative nursing care
    Prosthesis   Restorative aide

1. A nursing assistant with special training in restorative nursing and rehabilitation skills is a _Restorative aide_.

2. _Activities of daily living_ are activities usually done during a normal day in a person's life.

3. An artificial replacement for a missing body part is a _prosthesis_.

4. Care that helps persons regain their health, strength, and independence is _restorative nursing care_.

5. A _disability_ is any lost, absent, or impaired physical or mental function.

6. The process of restoring the disabled person to the highest possible level of physical, psychological, social, and economic functioning is _Rehabilitation_.

Circle the Best Answer

7. The focus of rehabilitation is to
   A. Improve abilities
   B. Restore function to normal
   C. Help the person regain health and strength
   D. Prevent injury

8. Restorative nursing programs include measures that promote
   A. Self-care, elimination, and positioning
   B. Mobility, communication, and cognitive function
   C. Maintaining the highest level of function
   D. All of the above

9. If you are a restorative aide, it means you have
   A. Special training in restorative nursing and rehabilitation skills
   B. Taken required classes for restorative aides
   C. Passed a special test to show you can perform these duties
   D. The most seniority at the facility

10. When assisting with rehabilitation and restorative care, it is important to
    A. Give complete care to prevent exertion by the person
    B. Make sure you do everything for the person
    C. Encourage the person to perform ADLs to the extent possible
    D. Complete care quickly

11. Which of these would be most helpful for a person receiving rehabilitative care?
    A. Give the person pity or sympathy when tasks are difficult
    B. Remind the person not to try new skills or those that are difficult
    C. Give praise when even a little progress is made
    D. Encourage the person to perform ADLs quickly

12. Complications can be prevented by
    A. Doing all ADLs for the person
    B. Allowing the person to decide if he or she wants to move or exercise
    C. Making sure the person is in good alignment, is turned and repositioned, and has range-of-motions exercises
    D. Making sure rehabilitation is fast-paced

13. Rehabilitation begins
    A. After the person has recovered
    B. When the person first seeks health care
    C. When the person asks for help
    D. When a discharge date has been set

14. Self-help devices help to meet the goal of
    A. Recovery of all normal abilities
    B. Self-care
    C. Living alone
    D. Dependence on others

15. Rehabilitation includes ways to help the person adjust to
    A. Only physical care needs
    B. Only ambulation needs
    C. Physical, psychological, social, and economic needs
    D. Only psychological and social needs

16. The rehabilitation team meets to evaluate the person's progress
    A. Every 90 days
    B. Often, to discuss the person and make needed changes
    C. Every week
    D. Only when requested by the family or person

17. OBRA requires that nursing centers
    A. Have a full-time physical therapist
    B. Provide rehabilitation services
    C. Provide physical care only
    D. Employ full-time occupational and speech therapists

Fill in the Blank

18. Write out the abbreviations.

    A. ADL _____

    B. ROM _____

19. The goals of rehabilitation and restorative care that help residents are to

    A. _____

    B. _____

20. A person in rehabilitation needs to adjust in these areas.

    A. _____

    B. _____

    C. _____

    D. _____

21. Rehabilitation takes longer in which age group?

    _____ What are reasons for this?

    A. Changes affect _____

    B. Chronic _____

    C. Risk for _____

22. What are some self-help devices that will assist in self-feeding?

    A. _____

    B. _____

    C. _____

23. The goal for a prosthesis is for the device to _____

    _____.

24. When you are assisting with rehabilitation and restorative care, why should you practice the task that the person must perform? _____

    _____

25. When assisting with rehabilitation and restorative care, what complications can be prevented if you report early signs and symptoms?

    _____

26. What can you do to promote the person's quality of life

    A. _____

    B. _____

    C. _____

    D. _____

    E. _____

    F. _____

    G. _____

Use Focus on PRIDE in the Textbook to complete questions 27–28.

27. If a nursing assistant is being considered for promotion to a restorative aid position, what qualities are considered first?

    A. _____

    B. _____

    C. _____

28. To promote independence when a person is receiving rehabilitation and restorative care, you can:

    A. _____

    B. _____

    C. _____

    D. _____

    _____

    E. _____

Optional Learning Exercises

Situation: Mrs. Mercer is 82 years old. She is a resident in a rehabilitation unit because she had a stroke that has caused weakness on her left side. Although she is right-handed, she needs to learn to use several self-help devices as she relearns ways to carry out ADLs. She often becomes angry or depressed. Answer questions 29–34 about Mrs. Mercer and her care. <u>NOTE: Some of these questions will require information contained in other chapters as noted.</u>

29. Mrs. Mercer is having difficulty with controlling urinary and bowel elimination. What would be the goal of her care for these problems?

    _____

    _____ Her plan of care would

    include programs for _____.

30. What should you do to prepare Mrs. Mercer's food at mealtime so she can feed herself? *(Ch 24 Nutrition and Fluids)*

    _____

    _____

31. Mrs. Mercer needs help to get in and out of bed. When helping her to transfer, you remember to position the chair on her _____ side. *(Ch 17 Safely Moving and Transferring the Person)*

32. When Mrs. Mercer becomes discouraged because progress is slow, how can you help her? You can stress

    _____ and focus on

    _____.

Independent Learning Activities

Role-play the situation with a classmate. Answer the questions about how you felt when you played Mrs. Leeds, to understand how a person with a disability feels. Use your nondominant hand to attempt the activities she must do.

- *Situation: Mary Leeds is 62 and had a stroke last month. She has weakness on her dominant side and has been admitted to a rehabilitation unit to relearn activities of daily living (ADLs). She is practicing eating by using a spoon to place fluids and food in her mouth. She is also learning to button clothing. How well could you hold the spoon with your nondominant hand?*
  - What problems did you have controlling the spoon?
  - How rapidly could you eat? What type of food was easier to eat?
  - How well were you able to button your clothing? What techniques did you find that made you more successful?
  - How did this experience make you feel? How will it affect the way you interact with persons who have similar disabilities?

With your instructor's permission, borrow a wheelchair from your school to use for 1–2 hours. Have a classmate push you around in the chair in a grocery store, mall, or in your school. <u>You must stay in the chair for the entire time to experience the feelings of a person who must use a wheelchair.</u> Use a handicap-equipped bathroom during this experience.

- How comfortable was the wheelchair? Did you use any special padding or cushion in the seat?
- What difficulties were encountered moving about? Doorways? Steps? Aisles? Crowds? How did you deal with any difficulties?
- How accessible was the handicap-equipped bathroom? How much room was available for you to transfer from the wheelchair to the toilet?
- How did other people treat you? How many spoke to you? How many talked to your classmate and avoided you?
- How did this experience make you feel? How will it affect the way you interact with a person in a wheelchair?

Fill in the Blank: Key Terms

Aphasia
Blind
Braille
Broca's aphasia
Cerumen

Deafness
Expressive aphasia
Expressive-receptive
  aphasia
Global aphasia

Hearing loss
Low vision
Mixed aphasia
Motor aphasia
Receptive aphasia

Tinnitus
Vertigo
Wernicke's aphasia

1. _____ is a touch reading and writing system that uses raised dots for each letter of the alphabet.

2. Another name for receptive aphasia is

_____.

3. Another name for earwax is _____.

4. _____ is dizziness.

5. A ringing, roaring, hissing, or buzzing sound in the ears is _____.

6. The total or partial loss of the ability to use or understand language is _____.

7. _____ is not being able to hear the normal range of sounds associated with normal hearing.

8. _____ is difficulty expressing or sending out thoughts; motor aphasia, Broca's aphasia.

9. Eyesight that cannot be corrected with eyeglasses, contact lenses, medicine, or surgery is

_____.

10. _____ is also called expressive aphasia or Broca's aphasia.

11. A hearing loss in which it is impossible for the person to understand speech through hearing alone is

_____.

12. Another name for expressive aphasia or motor aphasia is _____.

13. _____ is also called expressive-receptive aphasia or mixed aphasia.

14. The absence of sight is _____.

15. Difficulty expressing or sending out thought and difficulty understanding language is

_____.

16. Another name for expressive-receptive aphasia or global aphasia is _____.

17. Difficulty understanding language is

_____. This is also called Wernicke's aphasia.

Circle the Best Answer

18. If a person has chronic otitis media, the person may develop
    A. Vertigo
    B. Permanent hearing loss
    C. Diarrhea
    D. Nausea and vomiting

19. If a young child has otitis media, you may observe
    A. The child has a problem with balance
    B. Fluid draining out of the ear
    C. The child does not respond to quiet sounds
    D. All of the above

20. How would you know when a person with dementia has otitis media?
    A. The person would tell you he or she has pain.
    B. The person would speak softly.
    C. You might notice the person tugging or pulling at one or both ears.
    D. The person would have tinnitus.

21. If you are caring for a person who has Ménière's disease, it is important to
    A. Assist with walking
    B. Assist the person to move quickly
    C. Keep the lights in the room very bright
    D. Encourage the person to be active

22. Which of these is preventable cause of hearing loss?
    A. Aging
    B. Heredity
    C. Exposure to very loud sounds and noises
    D. Birth defects

23. When you are caring for a person with a hearing loss, which of these would *not* help communication?
    A. Gain the person's attention by lightly touching the person's arm.
    B. Speak as loudly as possible.
    C. Face the person when talking to him or her.
    D. Use gestures and facial expressions to give useful clues.

24. A child with normal hearing begins to repeat sounds at
    A. Birth to 3 months
    B. 6 to 10 months
    C. 3 to 6 months
    D. 18 to 24 months

25. A person with a hearing loss may
    A. Answer questions or respond inappropriately
    B. Think others are mumbling or slurring words
    C. Shun social events to avoid embarrassment
    D. All of the above
26. When you are caring for a person with a hearing aid, report to the nurse
    A. When turning the hearing aid off at night
    B. If a new battery is inserted
    C. If the hearing aid is lost or damaged
    D. Removing the battery at night
27. If a person has expressive aphasia, he or she
    A. Would not understand simple language
    B. Would speak in complete sentences
    C. Would have difficulty hearing what was said
    D. Might speak in single words or put words in the wrong order
28. When a person cannot communicate, he or she may be
    A. Frustrated   C. Depressed
    B. Angry   D. All of the above
29. An effective measure to use when caring for a speech-impaired person is to
    A. Speak in a child-like way
    B. Ask the person questions to which you know the answer
    C. Use long, involved sentences
    D. Make sure the TV and radio are loud
30. When a person has glaucoma, he or she may have difficulty seeing objects
    A. That are far away
    B. To the right side or left side of the person
    C. Directly in front of the person
    D. That are bright colors
31. Which of these groups of persons are at risk for glaucoma?
    A. Everyone over 50 years of age
    B. Caucasian and Asians over 40 years of age
    C. Those with a family history of glaucoma
    D. Those who need corrective glasses to see clearly
32. Cataracts most commonly are caused by
    A. Aging
    B. Injury
    C. Increased pressure in the eye
    D. Surgery
33. When a person has had eye surgery for cataracts, the care includes
    A. Removing the eye shield or patch for naps and at night
    B. Having the person cover both eyes during a shower or shampoo
    C. Reminding the person not to rub or press the affected eye
    D. Placing the overbed table on the operative side
34. After cataract surgery, report to the nurse at once if
    A. The person complains of eye pain or has eye drainage
    B. Glasses need to be cleaned
    C. The person asks for equipment to clean contact lenses
    D. The person asks for help with basic needs

35. If a person has dry age-related macular degeneration (AMD)
    A. It can be treated with surgery
    B. The person will need to use eye drops for the rest of his or her life
    C. The person will eventually be blind
    D. The person will need to wear corrective glasses to see clearly
36. Which of these measures can reduce the risk of AMD?
    A. Exposing the eyes to sunlight
    B. Eating a healthy diet high in green leafy vegetables and fish
    C. Eating a diet high in red meats
    D. Decreasing the amount of exercise
37. Diabetic retinopathy is the result of
    A. High blood pressure
    B. Tiny blood vessels in the retina being damaged as a complication of diabetes
    C. A clouding of the lens
    D. Increased pressure in the eye
38. A person who is legally blind
    A. Is totally unable to see anything
    B. May sense some light but have no usable vision
    C. May have some usable vision but cannot read newsprint
    D. All of the above may be true
39. When you enter the room of a blind person, you should first
    A. Touch the person to let him or her know you are there
    B. Speak loudly to make sure the person knows you are there
    C. Make sure the lights are bright
    D. Identify yourself and give your name, title, and reason for being there
40. When a person is blind, you should not
    A. Rearrange furniture and equipment
    B. Use words such as "see," "look," or "read"
    C. Let the person move about
    D. Let the person perform self-care
41. When you assist a blind person to walk, it is best if you
    A. Walk slightly behind the person and link your arm with the person's arm
    B. Walk slightly ahead of the person and allow the person to hold onto your arm just above the elbow
    C. Grasp the person's arm firmly to guide him or her
    D. Walk very slowly to allow the person to take small steps
42. If a blind person uses a cane, you can assist by
    A. Grasping the person by the arm holding the cane
    B. Come up behind the person and grasp his or her elbow
    C. Give the person verbal cues to avoid objects in the way
    D. Ask if you can assist before trying to help

43. If a blind person uses a guide dog, it is correct to
    A. Take the person by the arm on the side opposite from the dog
    B. Avoid distracting a guide dog by petting or feeding the dog
    C. Give the dog commands to avoid danger
    D. Greet the dog and pet it
44. Eyeglasses should be cleaned with
    A. Special cleaning solution or warm water
    B. Boiling water
    C. Detergent
    D. Dry cleansing tissues
45. When cleaning an ocular prosthesis you should
    A. Wash the prosthesis with mild soap and warm water
    B. Wash the eyelid and eyelashes with warm water
    C. Rinse the eye with sterile water before the person inserts the eye
    D. All of the above

Fill in the Blank

46. Write out the abbreviations.
    A. AMD _____
    B. ASL _____
47. Otitis media often begins with _____ _____.
48. If a person has chronic otitis media, it can cause permanent _____
49. When a person has Ménière's disease, attacks can occur _____ or just _____.
50. With Ménière's disease, the person avoids turning the _____.
51. What are examples of noises that can cause hearing loss?
    A. _____
    B. _____
    C. _____
    D. _____
52. When persons are 75 years of age or older, about _____ have a hearing loss.
53. Symptoms of hearing loss include
    A. _____
    B. _____
    C. _____
    D. _____
    E. _____
    F. _____
    G. _____
    H. _____
    I. _____
    J. _____
    K. _____

54. If a woman is speaking to a hearing impaired person, why should she adjust the pitch of her voice? _____
55. Why is it important for a person with a hearing loss to see your face when you are speaking to the person? _____ _____
56. What are common causes of speech disorders?
    A. _____
    B. _____
    C. _____
57. If a person has apraxia, the brain _____ _____.
58. Measures you can use to communicate with a speech-impaired person are
    A. Listen, and give _____
    B. Repeat _____
    C. Write down _____
    D. Allow the person _____
    E. Watch _____
59. When a person has expressive aphasia, the person knows what _____ _____. Thinking is _____
60. When a person has receptive aphasia, the person may speak in _____ that have no _____.
61. Symptoms of glaucoma include
    A. Peripheral _____
    B. Blurred _____
    C. Halos _____
62. Drugs and surgery are used with glaucoma to _____ _____
63. Most cataracts are caused by _____. Other risk factors are
    A. _____
    B. _____
    C. _____
    D. _____
64. When you are caring for a person after cataract surgery, an eye shield is worn as directed, and is worn for _____.
65. When assisting a blind or visually impaired person, what can be done to provide a consistent mealtime setting?
    A. _____
    B. _____
    C. _____
    D. _____ _____
    E. _____
    F. _____

66. A person with age-related macular degeneration (AMD) would develop a blind spot _____.

67. Everyone with diabetes is at risk for _____.

68. How can a person with low vision use a computer as an adaptive device?

    A. _____

    B. _____

69. The legally blind person sees at 20 feet what a person with normal vision sees at _____.

70. When you orient a person to the room, why do you let the person move about the room?

    _____

Use Focus on PRIDE in the Textbook to complete questions 71–72.

71. When you are referring to a person who has speech, hearing, or vision problems, he or she should be referred to by _____, not by the

    _____

72. Braille signs for areas with public access are required by the _____.

Optional Learning Exercises

Mr. Herman is an 85-year-old man with a hearing loss that has developed as he has gotten older. Answer questions 73–76 about his care.

73. Two nursing assistants are caring for Mr. Herman, a male and a female. They notice that he answers questions asked by the male nursing assistant more quickly. What is the likely reason for this?

    _____

    _____

74. The nursing assistants have found that Mr. H. is alert and oriented. They are surprised when Joan, another nursing assistant, tells them he is "senile." Why would Joan make this statement? _____

    _____

75. Mr. H. says he is too tired to go to the game room for a party. He says no one likes him. What are some reasons for his actions and statements?

    A. Tired because _____

    B. No one likes him _____

    _____

76. When giving care, the nursing assistant turns off the TV and radio in Mr. H.'s room. Why is this done?

    _____

You are caring for Mrs. Sanchez, who is legally blind because of glaucoma. Answer questions 77–79 about her care.

77. When you enter the room, you notice that Mrs. Sanchez is looking at her mail with a magnifying glass. How is this possible since you thought she was blind? _____

    _____

78. When you enter the room, Mrs. S. asks you to adjust the blinds. Why? _____

79. When you are helping Mrs. S. to move about the room, you are careful to tell her where furniture is located. Why? _____

    _____

Independent Learning Activities

Cover your ears so that you cannot hear clearly. Use one of these methods or one that you devise.

- *Commercial earplugs*
- *Cotton plugs in ears*
- *Cover ears with earmuffs or similar devices*

Keep your ears covered and hearing muffled for at least one hour as you go about your daily activities. A wise student will not wear earplugs during class time! Answer the following questions about the experience.

- How did you find yourself compensating for the hearing loss? Turning up the TV or radio? Asking others to write out information? Staying away from others? Getting angry or frustrated?
- When you could not understand someone, what did you do? Ask them to repeat? Ask them to speak louder? Answer even if you were unsure of what was said? Not respond at all?
- If you answered when unsure, what was your response? Did you tend to agree or disagree with the speaker? Why?
- What methods listed in the chapter were helpful? What other methods did you use to understand what was being said? Watching the speaker? Cupping your hand around ears?
- How will this experience assist you when you care for a person with a hearing loss?

Cover your eyes with a blindfold so you cannot see. Keep the blindfold on for at least one hour as you go about your normal activities. Have someone act as a guide during this time. In addition to your normal activities, include the activities listed. Answer the questions about the experience.

- Go outside with your guide and cross a street.
- Visit a store or restaurant with your guide.
- Eat a simple snack or meal.
- Go to the toilet, wash your hands, and comb your hair.
- Have your guide take to a public area, place you in a chair or on a bench, and leave you alone for 5–10 minutes.

NOTE: You may wish to carry out this exercise using the blindfold and using this alternate method. If you wear glasses, cover the lenses with a heavy coating of petroleum jelly. This will simulate the vision experienced by a person with cataracts. Answer the questions for both experiences.

- How did you feel when you were unable to see what was going on around you? What noises or other sensory stimulants did you notice?
- When you were crossing the street, how did you feel? Safe? Frightened?

- When you were in a public area, what did you notice? How did you feel? How did others respond to you?
- How comfortable did you feel about eating when you could not see the food? How were you able to locate the food? What problems did you have?
- How did you manage in the bathroom? Were you able to find the equipment you needed? How competent did you feel about carrying out hand washing and grooming without seeing?
- What were your feelings when left alone in a public area for 5 to 10 minutes? How long did it *seem* to be before your guide returned? What concerns did you have? Safety? Fear of injury? Desertion?

- How will this experience assist you when caring for a person with a vision loss?

Have a group discussion with your classmates who have all carried out the exercises to simulate vision and hearing problems. Answer these questions.

- Which disability did you find the most difficult to tolerate? Why?
- If you had to live with one of these disabilities, which one would you choose? Why?
- What happened during these exercises that surprised you about being unable to see or hear? How does this discovery change your attitude about the disabilities?

Cancer, Immune System, and Skin Disorders

Fill in the Blank: Key Terms

Benign tumor   Malignant tumor   Stomatitis

Cancer   Metastasis   Tumor

1. A _____ is a tumor that invades and destroys nearby tissue and can spread to other body parts.

2. Inflammation of the mouth is _____.

3. A tumor that does *not* spread to other body parts is a

_____.

4. A new growth of abnormal cells that may be benign or malignant is a _____.

5. The spread of cancer to other body parts is

_____.

6. Another name for a malignant tumor is

_____.

Circle the Best Answer

7. Benign tumors
   A. Do not spread to other body parts
   B. Invade healthy tissue
   C. Are always very small
   D. Divide in an orderly and controlled way

8. When cancer occurs in children, it
   A. It is usually fatal
   B. Has a high cure rate
   C. Is treated very easily
   D. Is very rare

9. Risk factors that increase cancer include all of the following *except*
   A. Exposure to sun and tanning booths
   B. Smoking
   C. A diet high in fresh fruits and vegetables
   D. Close relatives with certain types of cancer

10. When surgery is done to treat cancer
    A. It cures the cancer
    B. It relieves the pain from advanced cancer
    C. The tumor is removed
    D. All of the above

11. When you care for a person receiving radiation therapy, you might expect the person to
    A. Have pain related to the therapy
    B. Need extra rest related to fatigue
    C. Be at risk for bleeding and infections
    D. Complain of flu-like symptoms such as chills, fever, muscle aches

12. Chemotherapy involves
    A. X-ray beams aimed at the tumor
    B. Giving drugs that prevent the production of certain hormones
    C. Therapy to help the immune system
    D. Giving drugs that kill cells

13. While caring for a person receiving chemotherapy, she tells you she is upset because her hair is falling out. You know that
    A. The hair often falls out when a person receives chemotherapy
    B. This is symptom of her disease
    C. You should report this to the nurse at once
    D. You should change the subject so she will not be so upset

14. When hormone therapy is used to treat cancer, a woman may experience
    A. Stomatitis
    B. Flu-like symptoms
    C. Weight gain, hot flashes, and fluid retention
    D. Burns and skin breakdown

15. A person with cancer may complain of constipation because of
    A. The side effects of pain relief drugs
    B. Pain
    C. A side effect from cancer treatments
    D. Fluid and nutrition intake

16. When a person has cancer and expresses anger, fear, and depression, you can help most by
    A. Telling the person not to worry or get upset
    B. Give the person privacy and time alone
    C. Being there when needed and listening to the person
    D. Change the subject to distract the person

17. Treatment for autoimmune disorders is aimed at
    A. Curing the illness
    B. Controlling the autoimmune response
    C. Removing the affected organs
    D. Preventing metastasis

18. HIV is *not* spread by
    A. Blood
    B. Semen
    C. Sneezing or coughing
    D. Breast milk

19. To protect yourself from HIV and AIDS, you should
    A. Avoid all body fluids when giving care
    B. Refuse to give care to persons diagnosed with these diseases
    C. Follow Standard Precautions and the Bloodborne Pathogen Standard when giving care
    D. Always use sterile care when giving any care
20. Shingles is caused by the same virus that causes
    A. HIV
    B. Measles
    C. Chicken pox
    D. Mumps

Fill in the Blank

21. Write out the abbreviations.
    A. AIDS _____
    B. HIV _____
    C. IV _____
22. Cancer is the _____ most common cause of death in the United States.
23. The goals of cancer treatment are
    A. _____
    B. _____
    C. _____
24. The general signs and symptoms of cancer are
    A. _____
    B. _____
    C. _____
    D. _____
    E. _____
    F. _____
    G. _____
    H. _____
    I. _____
    J. _____
25. When radiation therapy is used, _____ cells and _____ cells are both destroyed.
26. With radiation therapy, skin care measures are needed at the treatment site because _____ and _____ can occur.
27. When chemotherapy is used, it affects _____ cells and _____ cells.
28. When a person is receiving chemotherapy, what side effects might occur?
    A. _____
    B. _____
    C. _____
    D. _____

29. Biological therapy treats cancer by
    A. _____
    B. _____
30. Complementary and alternative medicine (CAM) is sometimes used with standard cancer treatment. They include:
    A. _____
    B. _____
    C. _____
    D. _____
    E. _____
    F. _____
31. When a person has an autoimmune disorder, it means the _____ system attacks the _____.
32. Autoimmune disorder treatment is aimed at
    A. _____
    B. _____
    C. _____
33. Acquired immunodeficiency syndrome (AIDS) is caused by a _____ that attacks the _____.
34. How is the human immunodeficiency virus (HIV) mainly transmitted?
    A. _____
    B. _____
    C. _____
35. When caring for a person with HIV, the main threat to health care workers is from _____.
36. Those at risk for developing shingles are
    A. _____
    B. _____
    C. _____

Use Focus on PRIDE in the Textbook to complete questions 37–38.

37. If you work on an oncology unit, staff and patients value a person who is _____, _____, _____, and _____.
38. When you work closely with oncology patients and families, you must protect the person's privacy and rights and avoid crossing _____.

Optional Learning Exercises
Situation: Mrs. Myers is a 62 year old who is having chemotherapy to treat cancer. She has not been eating well and complains of feeling very tired. When you assist her with personal care, you notice a large amount of hair on her pillow. Answer questions 39–41 about Mrs. Myers and her care.

39. Mrs. Myers may not be eating well because the

    chemotherapy _____ the

    gastrointestinal tract and causes _____,

    _____, _____, and

    _____.

40. She may also have _____,
    which is called stomatitis. You can help to relieve the
    discomfort from this side effect when

    you provide _____.

41. What is causing Mrs. Myers to lose her hair?

    _____

    This condition is called _____.

Independent Learning Activities

Interview a person who has been treated for cancer and ask the following questions.

- How was the person told about the diagnosis of cancer? What kind of reaction did the person have – was he or she frightened, angry, depressed, etc.?
- What treatment was used to treat the cancer? What side effects did the person have? Did any of the treatments affect body image? Did the treatment leave any permanent disfigurement?
- How did the cancer and the treatment affect the person's life? How able was the person to carry on normal activities such as caring for family members, or working?
- How long ago did this occur? How is the person feeling now? What long-term affects has the cancer and treatments had on the person?

If you have cared for a person with HIV/AIDS, answer these questions about the experience. If you have not, think about how you might feel in that situation.

- How did you react when you knew the person had HIV? What questions did you ask the nurse? The person?
- What special precautions did you take when you were caring for the person?
- How would you feel if you found out a person you had been caring for was diagnosed with HIV? How would this new diagnosis affect the care you give?
- When you use Standard Precautions and Bloodborne Pathogen Standards for ALL persons you care for, how does that affect your reaction to an HIV patient?

41 Nervous System and Musculo-Skeletal Disorders

Fill in the Blank: Key Terms

Amputation	Closed fracture	Gangrene	Paralysis	Simple fracture
Arthritis	Compound fracture	Hemiplegia	Paraplegia	Tetraplegia
Arthroplasty	Fracture	Open fracture	Quadriplegia	

1. An open fracture is also called a

   _____.

2. Another name for quadriplegia is

   _____.

3. The removal of all or part of an extremity is

   _____.

4. A _____ is when the
   bone is broken but the skin is intact.

5. _____ is paralysis and
   loss of sensory function in the arms, legs, and trunk. It
   can also be called tetraplegia.

6. Paralysis on one side of the body is

   _____.

7. Joint inflammation is

   _____.

8. A closed fracture can also be called

   _____.

9. A _____ is a broken
   bone.

10. An _____ occurs when
    the broken bone has come through the skin. It is also
    called a compound fracture.

11. An _____ is the surgical
    replacement of a joint.

12. Paralysis and loss of sensory function in the legs is

    _____.

13. A condition in which there is death of tissue is

    _____.

14. _____ is loss of motor
    function, loss of sensation, or both.

Circle the Best Answer

15. The leading cause of disability in the United States is
    - A. Heart disease
    - B. Cancer
    - C. Stroke
    - D. Diabetes

16. If a person has stroke-like symptoms that last a few
    minutes, it means that
    - A. The person has had a transient ischemic attack (TIA)
    - B. It is not a dangerous situation since it was temporary
    - C. The person needs to lie down at once
    - D. No further treatment is needed

17. Which of these is *not* a risk factor for stroke?
    - A. High blood pressure
    - B. Cigarette smoking
    - C. Regular physical activity
    - D. Diabetes

18. When a person has "neglect" after a stroke, it
    means that
    - A. There is paralysis on one side of the body
    - B. The person may forget about or ignore the
      weaker side
    - C. The person is incontinent
    - D. The speech is slowed or slurred

19. When a person who has had a stroke ignores the
    weaker side of the body, it is probably because the
    person has
    - A. Lost movement of that side
    - B. Lost feeling on that side
    - C. A loss of vision on that side
    - D. All of the above

20. When you are caring for a person who has had a
    stroke, the signal light
    - A. Should be removed from the room
    - B. Is placed on the weak side of the body
    - C. Is placed on the strong side of the body
    - D. Is given to a family member to use for the
      person

21. A safety concern for a person with Parkinson's disease
    would be
    - A. Changes in speech
    - B. Swallowing and chewing problems
    - C. A mask-like expression
    - D. Emotional changes

22. Multiple Sclerosis (MS) is a disease that
    - A. Is an acute illness from which the person recovers
      completely
    - B. Always follows the same course with the same
      symptoms
    - C. May have long periods without symptoms before
      a flare-up occurs
    - D. Is easily treated with medications

23. As Amyotrophic Lateral Sclerosis (ALS) progresses,
    the person is
    - A. Confused and disoriented
    - B. Able to walk with assistance even as the disease
      progresses
    - C. Incontinent of bladder and bowel functions
    - D. Unable to move the arms, legs, and body

24. If a person is in a persistent vegetative state after a head injury, he or she
    A. Is unconscious, unaware, and cannot be aroused
    B. Is unconscious and has sleep-wake cycles and periods of being alert
    C. Is unresponsive, but can be briefly aroused
    D. Is in a vegetative state for more than 1 month

25. A person who has a spinal cord injury in the lumbar region will likely have
    A. Quadriplegia   C. Hemiplegia
    B. Paraplegia   D. Tetraplegia

26. When caring for a person with paralysis, it is important to
    A. Turn and reposition the person at least every 2 hours
    B. Check bath water temperatures, heat applications, and food for proper temperature
    C. Give emotional and psychological support
    D. All of the above

27. Autonomic dysreflexia occurs in a person who has paralysis
    A. Of any kind
    B. Above the mid-thoracic level
    C. In the lumbar region
    D. That is incomplete

28. If you are caring for a person with autonomic dysreflexia, report to the nurse at once if
    A. The person has sweating above the level of the injury
    B. The blood pressure is low
    C. The person complains of pain below the level of the injury
    D. The person has sweating below the level of the injury

29. If a person is at risk for autonomic dysreflexia, it is best if only the nurse
    A. Gives basic care
    B. Makes sure the catheter is draining properly
    C. Checks for fecal impactions or gives an enema
    D. Repositions the person at least every 2 hours

30. Osteoarthritis differs from rheumatoid arthritis because osteoarthritis
    A. Is an inflammatory disease
    B. Occurs with aging
    C. The person does not feel well
    D. Occurs on both sides of the body

31. When you are caring for a person with osteoarthritis, which of these would be most helpful to the person?
    A. Allow the person to stay in bed as much as desired
    B. Keep the room cool as osteoarthritis improves with cold temperatures
    C. Help the person use good body mechanics, good posture, and get regular rest
    D. Tell the person not to exercise as the exercise will prevent healing

32. You are caring for a person who has active rheumatoid arthritis. You should do all of these *except*
    A. Make sure the person exercises more often
    B. Position the person in good alignment
    C. Encourage the person to rest more than usual
    D. Apply splints to support affected joints

33. When caring for a person who has had a total hip replacement, which of these measures should *not* be done?
    A. Have a high, firm chair for the person to use when out of bed
    B. Remove the pillow between the legs when turning the person in bed
    C. Remind the person not to cross his or her legs
    D. Make sure the person has a raised toilet seat

34. Which of these will help to strengthen bones in a person at risk for osteoporosis?
    A. Bedrest
    B. Decrease calcium intake
    C. Exercise weight-bearing joints
    D. Increase alcohol and caffeine intake

35. Which of these is *not* a sign or symptom of a fracture?
    A. Full range of motion in the affected limb
    B. Bruising and color change in the skin of the affected area
    C. Pain
    D. Swelling

36. When a closed reduction or external fixation is done, the person has
    A. A simple fracture with no bone exposed
    B. Surgery to allow the bone to be moved into alignment
    C. Devices to keep the bones in place, such as pins, screws, or wires
    D. The bone exposed so it can be moved into alignment

37. When a person has a newly applied plaster cast, it will dry in
    A. 2 to 4 hours   C. 24 to 48 hours
    B. 3 to 4 days   D. 12 to 24 hours

38. You can prevent flat spots on a cast by
    A. Positioning the cast on a hard, flat surface
    B. Supporting the entire cast with pillows
    C. Using your fingertips to lift the cast
    D. Covering the cast with a blanket

39. If a person complains of numbness in a part that is in a cast, you should
    A. Tell the person to move the limb a little to relieve the numbness
    B. Reposition the person to help the numbness
    C. Gently rub the exposed toes or fingers
    D. Tell the nurse at once

40. When giving care to a person in traction, you should
    A. Put bottom linens on the bed from the top down
    B. Remove the weights while you are giving care
    C. Turn the person from side to side to change the bed and to give care
    D. Assist the person to use the commode chair when needed

41. After surgery to repair a hip fracture, the operated leg should be
    A. Abducted at all times
    B. Adducted at all times
    C. Exercised with range-of-motion exercises every 4 hours
    D. Positioned to keep the leg in external rotation
42. When you assist a person to get up in a chair after hip surgery,
    A. Place the chair on the affected side
    B. Place the chair on the unaffected side
    C. Have a low, soft chair for the person to use
    D. Remind the person to cross the legs
43. If a person complains of pain in the amputated part,
    A. Report at once to the nurse
    B. Assume the person is confused or disoriented
    C. Reassure the person that this is a normal reaction
    D. Tell the person that this a temporary sensation that will go away shortly

Fill in the Blank

44. Write out the abbreviations.
    A. ADL _____
    B. ALS _____
    C. CVA _____
    D. JRA _____
    E. MS _____
    F. PVS _____
    G. RA _____
    H. TBI _____
    I. TIA _____
45. What are the warning signs of stroke?
    A. _____
    B. _____
    C. _____
    D. _____
    E. _____
46. What are signs and symptoms of Parkinson's disease?
    A. _____
    B. _____
    C. _____
    D. _____
    E. _____
47. Multiple sclerosis (MS) may present in many ways. For example, symptoms may last for a few _____ or a few _____
    A. When symptoms disappear, the person is in _____
    B. When symptoms flare up, the person is in a _____

48. What effect does amyotrophic lateral sclerosis have on
    A. Mind, intelligence, memory _____
    B. Senses _____
    C. Bowel and bladder functions _____
    D. Motor nerve cells _____
49. When traumatic brain injury occurs
    A. Brain tissue is _____
    B. Bleeding can be in the _Brain_ _____ or _nearby tissue_ _____
    C. Spinal cord injuries are _likely_ _____
50. _____ are the major cause of head trauma in newborns.
51. When caring for a person with paralysis, you must check the person often if he or she is unable to use _____
52. Range-of-motion exercises are important when caring for a person with paralysis because they will maintain _____ and prevent _____
53. If the nurse delegates you to raise the head of the bed 45 degrees or more for a person with a spinal cord injury, the person may have signs or symptoms of _____.
54. If you are caring for a person with osteoarthritis, exercise is important because it
    A. Decreases _____
    B. Increases _____
    C. Improves _____
    D. It also helps with _____ and promotes _____
55. Rest and joint care are also used to treat osteoarthritis. Explain how these treatments help.
    A. Regular rest _____
    B. Canes and walkers _____
    C. Splints _____
56. Which type of arthritis generally develops between the ages of 20 to 50? _____
57. What are the treatment goals for rheumatoid arthritis?
    A. _____
    B. _____
    C. _____
    D. _____
58. When caring for a person who has had a hip replacement, what measures are used to protect the hip?
    A. _____
    B. _____
    C. _____
    D. _____
    E. _____
    F. _____

59. List how these risk factors affect developing osteoporosis
    A. Women risk increases _____
    B. Family _____
    C. Weight _____

60. Calcium is lost from bone if it does not _____. What happens to the bone when calcium is lost? _____ _____

61. What joints are exercised to help prevent osteoporosis? _____
    What types of exercise are used on these joints? _____

62. When a person has a cast on a fracture, what do these symptoms mean?
    A. Pain _____
    B. Odor _____
    C. Numbness _____
    D. Cool skin _____
    E. Hot skin _____

63. When caring for a person in traction, what would you do in these situations?
    A. Rope is frayed _____
    B. ROM exercises are performed on _____
    C. Usual position allowed _____
    D. Redness, drainage, and odor noted at pin site _____
    E. Person complains of numbness _____

64. How should the fractured hip be supported in these situations?
    A. Prevent external rotation _____
    B. Keep leg abducted _____

65. When turning and positioning a person after hip surgery, usually the person is *not* positioned on _____.

66. If the person has an internal fixation device, the operative leg is not elevated when sitting in a chair because _____.

67. _____ is a common cause of vascular changes that can lead to an amputation.

68. Phantom pain after an amputation may occur for a _____ or for _____.

Use Focus on PRIDE in the Textbook to complete question 69.

69. To promote independence when a person has disorders discussed in this chapter, it is important to
    A. _____
    B. _____
    C. _____
    D. _____

Optional Learning Exercises
You are caring for Mrs. Huber, who has had a stroke. Questions 70–74 relate to Mrs. Huber and her care. Explain the reason(s) the care plan gives each of the following instructions.

70. Position Mrs. Huber in a side-lying position _____

71. Approach Mrs. Huber from the unaffected side _____

72. Mrs. Huber is given a dysphagia diet _____

73. Elastic stockings are applied as part of her care _____

74. Range-of-motion exercises are given _____

You are caring for 2 persons who have arthritis. Read the information about each of them and answer questions 75–77 about these 2 persons.
- *Mr. Miller is 78 years old. He worked in construction for many years where he did heavy physical work. He complains about pain in his hips and right knee. His fingers are deformed by the arthritis and interfere with good range of motion.*
- *Mrs. Haxton is 40 years old. She has swelling, warmth, and tenderness in her wrists, several finger joints on both hands, and both knees. She tells you that she has had arthritis for about 10 years and it "comes and goes." At present, Mrs. Haxton has a temperature of 100.2° F, and she states she is tired and does not feel well.*

75. Which type of arthritis does Mr. Miller have? _____ Joint stiffness occurs with _____ and _____.

76. Mrs. Haxton has _____ arthritis. She complains of not feeling well because the arthritis affects _____ as well as the joints.

77. It is cold and raining today. Which of these persons is more likely to be affected by the weather? _____

Independent Learning Activities

Many people have had a fracture at some time. If you have had a broken bone, answer these questions about the experience.

- When did you know the bone was broken? Immediately? Several hours or days later? How did you find out?
- What signs and symptoms did you have? Describe these signs and symptoms.
- What treatment was done? Cast? Surgery? Pins, plates, screws, traction? Describe the treatment and how you felt about it.
- How did the fracture affect your day-to-day life? Work? School? Leisure activities?
- What changes were needed for you to carry out ADL? How much help did you need from others? How did the need for help make you feel?
- How was your mobility affected? Walking? Getting out of bed or out of a chair? Driving?
- What discomfort did you have during healing process? With the cast or surgical site?
- What permanent or long-range problems happened? Periodic pain? Limited mobility?

Try this experiment to have a "fractured leg." It will help you to understand how a fracture interferes with normal activities. Make an immobilizer for your leg. Use one of the methods suggested, or devise one of your own.

- *Find 4 pieces of sturdy cardboard that are long enough to reach from the ankle to mid-thigh. Place them on the front, back, and sides of the leg and secure with elastic bandages or cloth strips. You should not be able to bend the knee.*

- *Use several layers of newspaper or magazines and wrap them around the leg from the ankle to above the knee. Secure with elastic bandages or cloth strips. You should not be able to bend the knee.*

After the "cast" is in place, leave it on for 1 to 2 hours and go about your normal routine. Answer these questions about the experience.

- How much did the cast interfere with your routine?
- How did the cast affect ADL? Driving? Walking?
- What other problems did you have with the cast?
- How did you feel when you were in the cast? Awkward? Embarrassed?
- How do think this short experience may help you when you care for a person with a cast?

Try this experiment to understand how osteoporosis affects bone.

Fold a piece of standard 8½ × 11 paper in half the long way 3 times. (It will now be about 1 inch by 11 inches). Try to tear it in half along the fold and along the 1-inch edge.

- What happens?

Unfold the paper once (it will be 2 inches by 11 inches) and cut pieces out along all of the edges. This step will make the paper porous much like the bone becomes with osteoporosis. Refold the paper to the 1-inch by 11-inch size and try to tear it again.

- What happens now?

42 Cardiovascular and Respiratory Disorders

Fill in the Blank: Key Terms

Congenital   High blood pressure   Lymphedema   Sleep apnea
Dysrhythmia   Hypertension   Pre-hypertension

1. An abnormal heart rhythm is
   _____dysrhythmic_____.

2. Pauses in breathing that occur during sleep is
   _____sleep apnea_____.

3. When the systolic pressure is 140 mm Hg or higher, or the diastolic pressure is 90 mm Hg or higher, it is
   _____hypertension_____.

4. _____Congenital_____ means to be born with a condition.

5. A buildup of lymph in the tissues causing edema is
   _____lymphedema_____.

6. _____Pre-hypertension_____ is when the systolic pressure is between 120 and 139 mm Hg or the diastolic pressure is between 80 and 89 mm Hg.

7. Another name for hypertension is
   _____high blood pressure_____.

Circle the Best Answer

8. The leading cause of death in the United States is
   A. Cardiovascular and respiratory system disorders
   B. Cancer
   C. Strokes
   D. Accidents

9. Hypertension (high blood pressure) would be a reading of
   A. 120/70   C. 140/90
   B. 100/60   D. 130/60

10. A risk factor for hypertension that cannot change is
    A. Stress   C. Age
    B. Being overweight   D. Lack of exercise

11. The most common cause of coronary artery disease is
    A. Lack of exercise   C. Family history
    B. Atherosclerosis   D. Stress

12. Cardiac Rehab includes all of these *except*
    A. Exercise training
    B. Learning about his or her heart condition
    C. Strict bedrest
    D. Learning how to deal with fears about the future

13. When a person has angina pectoris, the chest pain occurs when
    A. Oxygen does not reach the lungs
    B. The heart needs more oxygen
    C. The blood pressure is too high
    D. Heart muscle dies

14. If a person has angina pain, it will usually be relieved by
    A. Resting for 3 to 15 minutes
    B. Taking narcotic drugs
    C. Using oxygen therapy
    D. Getting up and walking for exercise

15. If a person takes a nitroglycerin tablet for angina, you should
    A. Give them a large glass of water to swallow the pill
    B. Take the pills back to the nurse's station
    C. Make sure the person tells the nurse a pill was taken
    D. Encourage the person to walk around the room

16. When a myocardial infarction occurs, it means that
    A. Part of the heart muscle dies
    B. The heart muscle is not receiving enough oxygen
    C. Pain can be relieved by rest
    D. Blood backs up into the lungs

17. If a person complains of pain or numbness in the back, neck, jaw, or stomach, you should tell the nurse at once because the person
    A. Is having an angina attack
    B. May be having a stroke
    C. May be having a myocardial infarction
    D. Has symptoms of COPD

18. When heart failure occurs, the person may have
    A. Fluid in the lungs
    B. Swelling in the feet and ankles
    C. Confusion, dizziness, and fainting
    D. All of the above

19. An older person with heart failure is at risk for
    A. Contractures
    B. Skin breakdown
    C. Fractures
    D. Urinary tract infections

20. When a person has a pacemaker
    A. He or she can never take a tub bath or go swimming
    B. He or she may feel dizzy or lightheaded and have fluttering in the chest
    C. The function and battery life of the pacemaker must be checked regularly
    D. It is removed after the heart becomes stronger

21. The most important risk factor for chronic obstructive pulmonary disease (COPD) is
    A. Family history
    B. Respiratory infections
    C. Cigarette smoking
    D. Exercise

22. When a person has COPD, it interferes with
    A. Oxygen (O_2) and carbon dioxide (CO_2) exchange in the lungs
    B. Airflow in the lungs
    C. Elasticity in the airways and alveoli
    D. All of the above

23. If a person has chronic bronchitis, a common symptom is
    A. Wheezing and tightening in the chest
    B. Shortness of breath on exertion
    C. A smoker's cough in the morning
    D. A high temperature for several days

24. Asthma is often triggered by
    A. Smoking and second-hand smoke
    B. Air pollutants and irritants
    C. Cold air
    D. All of the above

25. If an older person has influenza, they may have
    A. A body temperature below normal
    B. An increased appetite
    C. A feeling of more energy than usual
    D. No symptoms of illness

26. Which of these symptoms is more likely to be from a cold rather than the flu?
    A. Sinus congestion
    B. High fever (100° F to 102° F)
    C. Fatigue for 2 to 3 weeks
    D. Bronchitis or pneumonia

27. The flu vaccine would be recommended for all of these persons *except*
    A. A man with diabetes and chronic heart disease
    B. A woman with an immune system disease
    C. A healthy 30 year old
    D. A 75-year-old man in good health

28. When a person has pneumonia, fluid intake is increased to
    A. Decrease the amount of bacteria in the lungs
    B. Dilute medication given to treat the disease
    C. Thin secretions
    D. Decrease inflammation of the breathing passages

29. Breathing is easier for a person with pneumonia when the person is positioned in
    A. Semi-Fowler's position   C. Supine position
    B. Side-lying position   D. A soft chair

30. When you care for a person with tuberculosis, you should
    A. Wash your hands if you have contact with sputum
    B. Flush tissues down the toilet, place in a BIOHAZARD bag, or place in a paper bag and burn
    C. Remind the person to cover the mouth and nose with tissues when coughing and sneezing
    D. All of the above

31. When a person has lymphedema, it is important that you
    A. Never use an affected arm to take a blood pressure
    B. Keep the affected arm or leg elevated at all times
    C. Keep the person on strict bedrest
    D. Strict fluid intake

Fill in the Blank

32. Write out the abbreviations.
    A. CAD _____
    B. CDC _____
    C. CO_2 _____
    D. COPD _____
    E. MI _____
    F. mm Hg _____
    G. O_2 _____
    H. TB _____
    I. WBC _____

33. What risk factors that increase blood pressure cannot be changed?
    A. _____
    B. _____
    C. _____
    D. _____

34. The most common cause of coronary artery disease (CAD) is _____. When this occurs, _____ collects on the _____.

35. When a person has CAD, what life-style changes are needed?
    A. _____
    B. _____
    C. _____
    D. _____

36. What activities or other factors can cause angina?
    A. _____
    B. _____
    C. _____
    D. _____
    E. _____
    F. _____

37. Where are nitroglycerin tablets kept?

    _____

38. Signs and symptoms of a myocardial infarction may be chest pain that is
    A. _____
    B. _____
    C. _____
    D. _____

39. The goals of cardiac rehabilitation after a myocardial infarction are

A. _____

B. _____

C. _____

40. When left-sided heart failure occurs, blood backs up into _____. What effect does this have on these areas of the body?

A. Brain _____

B. Kidneys _____

C. Skin _____

D. Blood pressure _____

41. When the person has right-sided heart failure, the signs and symptoms listed above occur. In addition, what happens to these areas?

A. Feet and ankles _____

B. Liver _____

C. Abdomen _____

42. Older persons with heart failure are at risk for skin breakdown because of

A. _____

B. _____

C. _____

43. How can you help to prevent skin breakdown in older persons with heart failure?

_____

44. Dysrhythmias are caused by changes in the heart's

_____

45. What changes occur in the lungs when a person has chronic obstructive pulmonary disease (COPD)?

A. _____

B. _____

C. _____

D. _____

46. If a person has bronchitis or emphysema, the person must stop _____.

47. Signs and symptoms of sleep apnea are

A. _____

B. _____

C. _____

D. _____

E. _____

F. _____

G. _____

48. A common complication of influenza is

_____

49. If an older person has pneumonia, typical signs and symptoms may be masked by

_____ and other

_____.

50. What signs and symptoms may be present if a person has active tuberculosis (TB)?

A. _____

B. _____

C. _____

D. _____

E. _____

F. _____

G. _____

H. _____

51. Why does TB sometimes become active as a person ages? _____

52. The goals of treating lymphedema are

A. _____

B. _____

C. _____

D. _____

E. _____

53. Lymphoma is cancer involving cells in the

_____.

Use Focus on PRIDE in the Textbook to complete questions 54–56.

54. When a person makes unhealthy choices, such as smoking, the health team

A. Teaches the person the

_____ and

encourages _____

B. Cannot force _____

C. Must be sure the person understands

_____

55. Color-coded wristbands communicate

_____ or

_____

56. If a color-coded bracelet says "limb alert" or "forbidden extremity," it means that an arm must *not* be used for

A. _____

B. _____

C. _____

Matching

Match the symptom listed with disorders of coronary artery disease.

A. Angina
B. Myocardial infarction
C. Heart failure

57. _____A_____ Chest pain occurs with exertion
58. _____B_____ Blood flow to the heart is suddenly blocked
59. _____C_____ Blood backs up into the venous system
60. _____C_____ Fluid in the lungs
61. _____B_____ Rest and nitroglycerin often relieves the symptoms
62. _____A_____ Pain is described as crushing, stabbing, or squeezing

Match the form of chronic obstructive pulmonary disease (COPD) with the related symptom.

A. Chronic bronchitis
B. Emphysema
C. Asthma

63. _____B_____ Person develops a barrel chest
64. _____A_____ Mucus and inflamed breathing passages obstruct airflow
65. _____B_____ Alveoli become less elastic
66. _____C_____ Air passages narrow
67. _____A_____ First symptom is often a smoker's cough in morning
68. _____B_____ Normal O_2 and CO_2 exchange cannot occur in affected alveoli
69. _____C_____ Allergies and air pollutants are common causes

Optional Learning Exercises

70. A parent with a congenital heart defect is at risk of having a child with one. What are other risk factors that may cause a congenital heart defect?

A. _____

B. _____

C. _____

D. _____

E. _____

71. Why is hypertension called "the silent killer?"

_____

_____

72. Older persons may not have typical symptoms of flu. Older persons may have these symptoms that signal flu:

A. _____

B. _____

C. _____

D. _____

E. _____

Independent Learning Activities

If possible, visit a cardiac rehabilitation center. Observe and ask the staff:

- What exercises are included for a person recovering from an MI? Cardiac surgery?
- How is the person monitored while exercising?
- How long does the person need to continue the program?
- How often does the person come to the rehab center? How much time is spent each time?

Get permission from the staff to ask questions of one the persons exercising.

- What condition do you have that needed this program?
- When did your rehab begin after your diagnosis?
- How long will you need to continue the rehab program?
- What benefits do you feel you are getting from the program?
- What exercise will you continue after the rehab program is completed?
- What other life-style changes have you made?

Try this experiment: Use a straw to drink water. Now, put small pieces of paper towel into the end of the straw and try to drink.

- What happens?

Add more paper and try to drink again.

- How does this experiment relate to coronary artery disease?

43 Digestive and Endocrine Disorders

Fill in the Blank: Key Terms

Emesis   Hyperglycemia   Jaundice
Heartburn   Hypoglycemia   Vomitus

1. High sugar in the blood is
   _hyperglycemia_____.

2. __Vomitus_____ is when food and
   fluids are expelled from the stomach through the
   mouth.

3. Low sugar in the blood is
   _hypoglycemia_____.

4. Another word for vomitus is
   __emesis_____.

5. __Jaundice_____ is yellowish color of
   the skin or whites of the eyes.

6. A burning sensation in the chest and sometimes the
   throat is __heartburn_____.

Circle the Best Answer

7. A risk factor for gastroesophageal reflux disease
   (GERD) is
   A. Eating small, frequent meals
   B. Alcohol use
   C. Maintaining normal weight
   D. Respiratory illnesses

8. If you are caring for a person with GERD, the person
   may be
   A. Given small meals
   B. Instructed not to lie down for 3 hours after eating
   C. Wearing loose belts and loose-fitting clothes
   D. All of the above

9. Aspirated vomitus
   A. Can lead to shock
   B. Can obstruct an airway
   C. Contains undigested food
   D. Has a bitter taste

10. If vomitus looks like coffee grounds, you should
    report at once to the nurse because
    A. It signals bleeding
    B. The person may need a diet change
    C. This indicates an infection
    D. The person may need pain medication

11. Diverticular disease may occur because of
    A. A high fiber diet
    B. Regular bowel movements
    C. Aging
    D. Infections

12. Gallstones are
    A. Needed for digestion of fats
    B. Formed in the small intestine
    C. Sometimes the reason bile flow is trapped
    D. Easily passed through the kidneys

13. A symptom of gallstones is
    A. Pain radiating down one or both arms
    B. Diarrhea
    C. Constipation
    D. Pain in the back between the shoulder blades

14. When hepatitis is contracted by eating or drinking
    food or water contaminated by feces, it is
    A. Hepatitis A   C. Hepatitis C
    B. Hepatitis B   D. Hepatitis D

15. A person with cirrhosis will need good skin care
    because of
    A. Muscle aches
    B. Itching
    C. Nausea and vomiting
    D. Diarrhea or constipation

16. An obese 50-year-old woman with hypertension is
    diagnosed with diabetes. She most likely has
    A. Type 1   C. Gestational
    B. Type 2   D. None of the above

17. A diabetic complains of thirst and frequent urination.
    You notice the person has a flushed face and rapid,
    deep, and labored respirations. You know these are
    signs and symptoms of
    A. Hyperglycemia   C. Diabetic coma
    B. Hypoglycemia   D. An infection

Fill in the Blank

18. Write out the meaning of the abbreviations.
    A. GERD _____
    B. HBV _____
    C. I&O _____
    D. IV _____

19. What life-style changes may be needed for a person
    with GERD?
    A. _____
    B. _____
    C. _____
    D. _____
    E. _____

20. What measures will help the person who is vomiting?
    A. Turn _____
    B. Place _____
    C. Move_____
    D. Provide _____
    E. Eliminate _____

21. Risk factors related to diverticular disease are
    A. Age _____
    B. Diet _____
    C. Bowel function _____

22. If a person with gallstones has jaundice, the skin and whites of the eyes will appear

    _____.

23. A gallbladder attack often follows a

    _____

24. List the characteristics of the types of hepatitis.
    A. Hepatitis A is spread by the

       _____ route.

    B. Hepatitis B is present in the

       _____ of infected persons.

    C. Hepatitis C can be transmitted even when the

       person has _____.

    D. Hepatitis D occurs only in people with

       _____.

    E. Hepatitis E is not common in

       _____.

25. Signs and symptoms of cirrhosis that may occur are
    A. _____
    B. _____
    C. _____
    D. _____
    E. _____
    F. _____
    G. _____

26. A person with _____ diabetes will be treated with healthy eating, exercise, and sometimes oral drugs.

27. A person with _____ diabetes will be treated with daily insulin therapy, as well as healthy diet and exercise.

Use Focus on PRIDE in the Textbook to complete questions 28–29.

28. When you are caring for a person with diabetes, it is important to report if the person is

    _____, _____,

    and _____.

29. When a person has health problems related to life-style choices, it is important that you
    A. Do not judge _____
    B. Always treat the person _____

Matching
Match the type of hepatitis with the correct statement.
    A. Hepatitis A
    B. Hepatitis B
    C. Hepatitis C
    D. Hepatitis D

30. __D__ This hepatitis occurs in person infected with hepatitis B
31. __A__ Caused by poor sanitation, crowded living conditions
32. __B__ Caused by HBV
33. __A__ Ingested when eating contaminated food or water
34. __C__ Person may have virus but no symptoms
35. __D__ Serious liver damage shows up years later

Match the symptom with either hypoglycemia or hyperglycemia.
    A. Hypoglycemia
    B. Hyperglycemia

36. __A__ Trembling, shakiness
37. __B__ Sweet breath odor
38. __A__ Tingling around the mouth
39. __A__ Cold, clammy skin
40. __B__ Rapid, deep, and labored respirations
41. __B__ Leg cramps
42. __B__ Flushed face
43. __A__ Frequent urination

Optional Learning Exercises
You are caring for several persons with diabetes. Answer questions 44–52 about these persons.
    Mr. Jones, a 75-year-old African-American man
    Ms. Miller, a 45-year-old white, overweight woman
    Mrs. Thorpe, a 32-year-old pregnant woman
    Ms. Hernandez, a 60-year-old Hispanic woman with hypertension
    Emily F., 12-year-old girl who has lost 15 pounds recently without dieting

44. Three of these persons are most likely to have Type 2 diabetes. They are
    A. _____
    B. _____
    C. _____

45. The 32-year-old probably has

_____ diabetes. She is at

risk to develop _____

later in life.

46. The 12 year old probably has

_____ diabetes.

47. Which type of diabetes develops rapidly?

_____

48. Ms. Hernandez has an open wound on her ankle. Why is this wound a concern?

_____

_____

49. Emily F. is scheduled for a visit to the dentist. What will the dentist look for when her mouth is examined?

_____ Why?

_____

50. Why is Ms. Miller instructed to decrease her food

intake? _____

51. Mr. Jones tells you he feels shaky, dizzy, and has a headache when he misses a meal. He probably is

experiencing _____.

52. Why does Emily F. take a snack with her when she

goes to school? _____

_____

Independent Learning Activities

Talk with a person who has gastroesophageal reflux disease (GERD) and ask these questions.
- What symptoms does the person have related to GERD?
- What risk factors does the person have that may have caused the GERD?
- What life-style changes has the person made since the diagnosis?

Talk with a person who has had gallstones and ask these questions.
- What risk factors does the person have related to gallstone formation?
- What signs and symptoms did the person have that helped the doctor diagnose gallstones?
- What treatment did the person have to relieve the symptoms?
- After treatment, what signs or symptoms have changed?

Talk with a person with diabetes and ask these questions.
- What type of diabetes does the person have – type 1 or type 2?
- How old was the person when diabetes was diagnosed?
- What life-style changes have been made to treat the diabetes?
- What complications of diabetes have occurred?

Ask your instructor to help you arrange to attend a diabetic education class if these are available at your agency. Answer these questions.
- What are the ages of the members of the class? Were other family members included in the class?
- What information is given to the class about diet?
- What exercise programs are recommended to the class?
- What information is given about medications used to treat diabetes?

44 Urinary and Reproductive Disorders

Fill in the Blank: Key Terms

Dialysis   Dysuria   Oliguria   Urinary diversion
Diuresis   Hematuria   Pyuria   Urostomy

1. Scant urine is _Oliguria_.
2. Difficult or painful urination is _dysuria_.
3. A _urostomy_ is a surgically created opening between the ureter and the abdomen.
4. _diuresis_ is the process of passing urine; large amounts of urine are produced – 1000 to 5000 mL a day.
5. A new pathway for urine to exit the body is a _urinary diversion_.
6. Blood in the urine is _hematuria_.
7. _Pyuria_ is pus in the urine.
8. The process of removing waste products from the blood is _dialysis_.

Circle the Best Answer

9. Women have a higher risk of urinary tract infections because of
   A. Hormone levels in the body
   B. The short female urethra
   C. Bacteria
   D. Prostrate gland secretions
10. If a person has cystitis, the care plan will include
    A. Restricting fluid intake
    B. Assisting the person to ambulate frequently
    C. Straining the urine
    D. Encouraging the person to drink 2000 mL of fluid a day
11. If a man has prostate enlargement, he will probably
    A. Be incontinent of urine
    B. Have frequent voiding at night
    C. Have increased urine output
    D. Have renal failure
12. After surgery to correct benign prostatic hyperplasia (BPH), the care plan may include
    A. A balanced diet to prevent constipation
    B. Increased activity with an exercise plan
    C. Restricted fluid intake
    D. Care of the surgical incision

13. When caring for a person with a urinary diversion, the pouch is changed
    A. Every shift
    B. Every 3 to 4 hours
    C. When the person showers or takes a tub bath
    D. Every 5 to 7 days or if it leaks
14. If you are caring for a person with kidney stones, your care will include
    A. Restricting fluids
    B. Keeping the person on strict bedrest
    C. Straining all urine
    D. Maintaining a strict diet
15. When you care for a person with acute renal failure, the care plan will include
    A. Increasing fluid intake to 2000–3000 mL per day
    B. Measuring and recording urine output every hour
    C. Making sure the person does not drink any fluids
    D. Measuring weight weekly
16. Chronic renal failure
    A. Occurs suddenly
    B. Generally improves and kidney function returns to normal within 1 year
    C. Occurs when nephrons of the kidney are destroyed over many years
    D. Has very little effect on the person's overall health
17. If a person has chronic renal failure, which of these would be included in the care plan?
    A. A diet high in protein, potassium, and sodium
    B. Plenty of exercise
    C. Measures to prevent itching
    D. Frequent bathing with soap
18. A woman who complains about frothy, thick, foul smelling vaginal discharge most likely has
    A. Gonorrhea
    B. Genital warts
    C. Syphilis
    D. Trichomoniasis

Fill in the Blank

19. Write out the meaning of the abbreviations.

    A. AIDS _____

    B. BPH _____

    C. HIV _____

    D. mL _____

    E. STD _____

    F. UTI _____

20. Why are older persons at high risk for urinary tract infections?

    A. _____

    B. _____

    C. _____

    D. _____

21. After a transurethral resection of the prostate (TURP), the person's care plan may include

    A. _____

    B. _____

    C. _____

    D. _____

    E. _____

22. What are the risk factors for developing kidney stones?

    A. _____

    B. _____

    C. _____

    D. What is the most common race, sex, and age of person at risk?

    _____

23. A person with kidney stones needs to drink 2000 to 3000 mL of fluid a day to help

    _____

24. When acute renal failure occurs, there are 2 phases. Name and explain each phase.

    A. At first, _____ occurs. Urine output is _____. This phase lasts _____.

    B. Then, _____ occurs. Urine output is _____. This phase lasts _____.

25. When caring for a person with acute renal failure, report to the nurse at once if the person has

    _____

26. Signs and symptoms of chronic renal failure appear when _____ is lost.

27. You may need to assist a person in chronic renal failure with nutritional needs. List what the care plan is likely to included for the following:

    A. Diet _____

    B. Fluids _____

28. Sexually transmitted diseases are transmitted by

    _____

29. Using _____ helps prevents the spread of STDs.

30. When caring for a person with an STD, you should follow _____ and _____.

Use Focus on PRIDE in the Textbook to complete questions 31–32.

31. You can help to prevent UTIs when giving care to females by always cleaning the perineal area from

    _____

32. When a person has an STD, you protect the person's right and give respect when you do *not* _____ about the person with coworkers.

Matching

Match the sexually transmitted disease with the correct statement.

  A. Herpes
  B. Genital warts
  C. Gonorrhea
  D. Chlamydia
  E. Syphilis
  F. Trichomoniasis

33. _____ Surgical removal if ointment is not effective

34. _____ Sores may have a watery discharge

35. _____ No symptoms in men, only in women

36. _____ May have vaginal bleeding

37. _____ Urinary urgency and frequency is present

38. _____ Treated with anti-viral drugs

39. _____ Painless sores appear on genitals 10–90 days after exposure

40. _____ May not show symptoms

Optional Learning Exercises

You give home care to Mrs. Eunice Weber twice a week. She is 92 years old and lives alone. She has severe osteoporosis and uses a walker to move about in her home. She receives Meals on Wheels and spends most of the day sitting on the sofa. She has periods of incontinence or dribbling because of poor bladder control. When you arrive to care for her today, she tells you she is not feeling well. She tells you it burns when she urinates and when she needs to urinate, the urge comes on suddenly and she often does not get to the toilet in time. Answer questions 41–47 about Mrs. Weber.

41. You should tell the _____, because these symptoms may mean Mrs. Weber has

    _____

42. When the feeling to urinate comes on suddenly, it is called _____

43. How does Mrs. Weber's immobility affect the following:

   A. Fluid intake _____

   _____ .

   B. Perineal care _____

   _____ .

44. Why is she at high risk for urinary tract infections

   because she is a woman? _____

45. The doctor will probably order _____ to treat the condition.

46. The care plan will probably include, "Encourage

   fluids to _____ per day."

Two weeks later you notice that Mrs. Weber has chills. When you take her temperature, it is 102° F. She tells you she has been vomiting since yesterday. You observe her urine and see that is very cloudy.

47. You report these symptoms to the nurse, because it

   can indicate Mrs. Weber now has _____ .
   This means the infection has moved from the

   _____ to the _____ .

Independent Learning Activities

Talk with someone who has had urinary tract infections (UTIs). If you have had a UTI, answer these questions about your own experience.

- What signs and symptoms were present?
- How many UTIs have occurred?
- What risk factors may have placed the person (or you) at risk to develop UTIs?
- What treatment was used to treat the UTI?
- What life-style changes were recommended to prevent a recurrence of the UTI?

Talk with someone who has had renal calculi and ask these questions.

- What signs and symptoms were present?
- How was the problem treated?
- What dietary changes have been prescribed to prevent future attacks?

45 Mental Health Problems

Fill in the Blank: Key Terms

- Affect
- Anxiety
- Compulsion
- Conscious
- Defense
  mechanism
- Delusion

- Delusion of
  grandeur
- Delusion of
  persecution
- Emotional illness
- Flashback
- Hallucination

- Mental
- Mental disorder
- Mental health
- Mental illness
- Obsession
- Panic
- Paranoia

- Personality
- Phobia
- Psychiatric
  disorder
- Psychosis
- Stress
- Stressor

- Subconscious
- Suicide
- Suicide contagion
- Unconscious
- Withdrawal
  syndrome

1. When a person has an exaggerated belief about one's own importance, wealth, power, or talents, it is called ___delusion of grandeur___.

2. A disturbance in the ability to cope with or adjust to stress; behavior and function are impaired; mental illness, emotional illness, or psychiatric disorder is also a ___mental disorder___

3. A ___stressor___ is any event or factor that causes stress.

4. ___Affect___ is feelings and emotions.

5. ___Mental___ is relating to the mind. It is something that exists in the mind or is performed by the mind.

6. A recurrent, unwanted thought or idea is an ___obsession___

7. The response or change in the body caused by any emotional, physical, social, or economic factor is ___stress___

8. ___Anxiety___ is a vague, uneasy feeling that occurs in response to stress.

9. Emotional ___illness___ is another name for a mental disorder.

10. A ___phobia___ is an intense fear.

11. Awareness of the environment and experiences is ___conscious___. The person knows what is happening and can control thoughts and behaviors.

12. A false belief is a ___delusion___

13. Mental ___illness___ is another name for a mental disorder.

14. Experiences and feelings that cannot be recalled are ___unconscious___

15. A state of severe mental impairment is ___psychosis___.

16. A ___hallucination___ is seeing, hearing, or feeling something that is not real.

17. ___Paranoia___ is a disorder of the mind. The person has false beliefs and suspicion about a person or situation.

18. The repeating of an act over and over is ___compulsion___.

19. ___Mental health___ is when the person copes with and adjusts to everyday stresses in ways accepted by society.

20. The set of attitudes, values, behaviors, and traits of a person is ___personality___.

21. The ___subconscious___ is memory, past experiences, and thoughts of which the person is not aware. They are easily recalled.

22. ___Delusion of persecution___ is a false belief that one is being mistreated, abused, or harassed.

23. An intense and sudden feeling of fear, anxiety, terror, or dread is ___panic___.

24. ___Psychiatric disorder___ is another name for emotional illness, mental disorder, or mental illness

25. A ___defense mechanism___ is an unconscious reaction that blocks unpleasant or threatening feelings.

26. ___Suicide contagion___ occurs with exposure to suicide or suicidal behaviors within one's family, peer group, or media reports of suicide.

27. Reliving the trauma in thoughts during the day and in nightmares at night is ___flashback___.

28. The person's physical and mental response after stopping or severely reducing the use of a substance that was used regularly. ___withdrawal syndrome___

29. To kill oneself is called ___suicide___

Circle the Best Answer

30. The causes of mental health disorders include
   A. Physical illness
   B. Growth and development tasks
   C. Not being able to cope or adjust to stress
   D. Personality development

31. The part of the personality that deals with reality is the
   A. Ego   C. Id
   B. Subconscious   D. Superego

32. Which of these statements about anxiety is *not* true?
   A. Anxiety often occurs when needs are not met.
   B. All anxiety is normal.
   C. Increases in pulse, respirations, and blood pressure may be due to anxiety.
   D. The anxiety level depends on the stressor.

33. An unhealthy coping mechanism would be
   A. Talking about the problem
   B. Playing music
   C. Smoking
   D. Exercising

34. A student fails a test and blames a friend for not helping with studying. This is an example of a defense mechanism called
   A. Conversion   C. Repression
   B. Projection   D. Displacement

35. Panic is
   A. The highest level of anxiety
   B. A disorder that occurs gradually
   C. A psychosis
   D. A condition that continues for many months or years

36. When a person washes his hands over and over, it may be a sign of
   A. Schizophrenia
   B. Hallucinations
   C. A phobia
   D. Obsessive-compulsive disorder

37. A person who was abused as a child may have difficulty feeling close to people or trusting people. The person may have
   A. Paranoia
   B. Panic disorder
   C. Post-traumatic stress disorder
   D. Conversion

38. A person you are caring for tells you he is the President of the United States. He has a delusion of grandeur, which is a part of
   A. Obsessive-compulsive disorder
   B. Phobias
   C. Bipolar disorders
   D. Schizophrenia

39. A person with bipolar disorder may
   A. Be more depressed than manic
   B. Be more manic than depressed
   C. Alternate between depression and mania
   D. Have any of the above

40. A safety risk of depression is that the person
   A. May be very sad
   B. Has thoughts of suicide and death
   C. Has depressed body functions
   D. Cannot concentrate

41. Depression may be overlooked in older persons because
   A. It does not occur often in older persons
   B. Depression is very mild in the elderly
   C. The person may be diagnosed with a cognitive disorder
   D. Physical problems are more important

42. A person with an antisocial personality may
   A. Be suspicious and distrust others
   B. Have emotional highs and lows
   C. See, hear, or feel something that is not real
   D. Blame others for actions and behaviors

43. All abused drugs
   A. Depress the nervous system
   B. Stimulate the nervous system
   C. Affect the mind and thinking
   D. Are illegal substances

44. When alcohol is ingested, it will
   A. Make the person more alert
   B. Slow down brain activity
   C. Have little effect on the organs of the body
   D. Do permanent damage to organs even in small amounts

45. Older persons have more risks when drinking alcohol because they have
   A. Slower reaction times
   B. Hearing and vision problems
   C. A lower tolerance for alcohol
   D. All of the above

46. When a person uses drugs or alcohol over a period of time, a sign of addiction is
   A. The person uses the substance once or twice a month
   B. More and more of the substance is needed to get the same "high"
   C. Using the substance occasionally in a social setting
   D. Being on time for job and meeting family obligations

47. Abused drugs are
   A. Drugs prescribed by a doctor
   B. Illegal street drugs
   C. Legal drugs obtained from a friend
   D. All of the above

48. When a young woman eats large amounts of food and then purges the body, she has
   A. Anorexia nervosa   C. Anxiety
   B. Depression   D. Bulimia nervosa

49. If a person mentions suicide
   A. It means they will not act on carrying it out
   B. The person has anxiety
   C. Take the person seriously
   D. It means the person has psychosis

Fill in the Blank

50. Write out the meaning of the abbreviations.

    A. BPD _____

    B. CDC _____

    C. GI _____

    D. OCD _____

    E. PTSD _____

51. What are causes of mental health disorders?

    A. _____

    B. _____

    C. _____

    D. _____

    E. _____

    F. _____

52. Name the defense mechanism being used in these situations.

    A. A girl fails a test. She blames the other girl for not helping her study.

    _____

    B. A man does not like his boss. He buys the boss an expensive Christmas present.

    _____

    C. A girl complains of a stomachache, so she will not have to read aloud.

    _____

    D. A child is angry with his teacher. He hits his brother. _____

    E. A woman misses work frequently and is often late. She gets a bad evaluation. She says that the boss does not like her.

    _____

53. What is the phobia in each example?

    A. _____ Being afraid of strangers

    B. _____ Fear of pain or seeing others in pain

    C. _____ Being trapped in an enclosed area

    D. _____ Fear of darkness

54. During a _____, the person may lose touch with reality and believe the trauma is happening all over again. This occurs when the person has _____.

55. Below are examples of problems that occur with schizophrenia. Name each one.

    A. A man believes his neighbor is poisoning his water. _____

    B. A woman says that voices told her to set fire to her apartment. _____

    C. A man believes that others can hear his thoughts on the radio. _____

    D. A woman tells you she owns 3 BMW cars and is the president of McDonald's.

    _____

Use Focus on PRIDE in the Textbook to complete questions 56–58.

56. You treat the person with mental health disorders with dignity and respect when you

    A. do not _____ or _____ the person

    B. do not _____ the others about the person

57. When caring for a person with mental illness, the team must react quickly to

    _____

58. When caring for a person with a mental illness, you can take pride in working as a team when you

    A. _____ when the person calls for help

    B. _____ as the nurse directs

Optional Learning Exercises

59. An infant wants to be fed immediately. At this stage of development, the part of the personality that is making the infant want to satisfied almost right away is the _____.

60. A teenager is with friends who are drinking alcohol and he does not join them. What parts of the personality may be affecting his behavior?

    _____

61. Mr. Johnson is very worried about his surgery tomorrow. You notice that he is talking very fast and is sweating. You give him directions to collect a urine specimen. Five minutes later, he turns on his call light to ask you to repeat the directions. He tells you he is using the toilet "all the time" because he has diarrhea and frequent urination. The nurse tells you all of these things are signs and symptoms of

    _____

62. You are assigned to care for Mrs. Grand, a new resident. She is getting ready to go to the dining room. You assist her to get dressed, and she tells you she wants to wash her hands before going to the dining room. She goes to the bathroom and washes her hands for several minutes. As she leaves the room, she stops to turn off the light. Then she tells you she must wash her hands again. She repeats washing her hands and turning the lights on and off 4 or 5 times. You report this to the nurse who tells you Mrs. Grand has

    _____

Independent Learning Activities

Try this experiment with a group of classmates. Make up labels with various roles for "staff members" and "mentally ill" persons. A list is provided, but you may add or subtract according to the size of your group. Make sure that the group includes a mixture of people with mental health problems and staff or visitors such as:

- Doctor
- Nurse
- Visitor
- Nursing Assistant
- Recreational Therapist
- Dietician

- A person with bipolar disorder
- A person with delusions of grandeur
- A person with obsessive compulsive disorder
- A person with schizophrenia with paranoia
- A person with hallucinations
- A person with anorexia nervosa

Attach a label to each person so that he or she cannot read it. (It may be placed on the back or the forehead.) Have everyone move about the group and talk to each other based on how the person thinks he or she should approach the person with a certain "label." Continue the experiment for about 15 minutes, and then use the questions to guide a group discussion.

- How did you feel talking to a person with a mental health disorder?
- How were the people with a mental health disorder approached? How quickly were the "mentally ill" able to sense that this was their label? What cues did they receive from others?
- How quickly did "staff members" recognize the label they had? What cues did they receive from others?
- In what ways did the approach of others cause people to respond in a way expected? Did the people with mental health problems show signs of the illness based on the reaction of others?
- What did the group learn about approaching a person with a mental health problem?

Consider this situation and answer the questions concerning how you would feel about caring for a person with a mental health problem.

SITUATION: Marion Cross, 65, is a patient in an acute care hospital with a diagnosis of pneumonia. The nurse tells you Mrs. Cross has a history of schizophrenia. You are assigned to provide AM care for Mrs. Cross.

- How would you approach Mrs. Cross when you enter her room? How would your knowledge about her mental health problem affect your initial contact with her?
- What would you do if Mrs. Cross told you she sees an elephant in the room? What would you say to her?
- How would you react if Mrs. Cross told you that she owns Disney World and goes there free anytime she wants? How would you respond?
- How would you provide good oral hygiene if Mrs. Cross refuses to cooperate because she is sure the staff is trying to poison her? What could you try that might be helpful?
- What would you do if Mrs. Cross curls up in a tight ball and refuses to talk or cooperate during AM care? What could you do to maintain her hygiene?
- How would you feel about caring for a person with abnormal behavior? Why?

46 Confusion and Dementia

Fill in the Blank: Key Terms

Cognitive function   Delusion   Elopement   Paranoia   Sundowning
Delirium   Dementia   Hallucination   Pseudodementia

1. _Elopement_ occurs when a person leaves the agency without staff knowledge.
2. A false belief is a _delusion_.
3. Seeing, hearing, smelling, or feeling something that is not real is _hallucination_.
4. Increased signs, symptoms, and behavior of AD during hours of darkness is _Sundowning_.
5. _Delirium_ is a state of temporary but acute mental confusion that comes on suddenly.
6. The loss of cognitive function and social function that interferes with routine personal, social, and occupational activities is _dementia_.
7. _Pseudodementia_ is false dementia.
8. _Cognitive function_ involves memory, thinking, reasoning, ability to understand, judgment, and behavior.
9. _Paranoa_ is a disorder of the mind; the person has false beliefs and suspicion about a person or situation.

Circle the Best Answer

10. Confusion caused by aging
    A. Occurs suddenly
    B. Is due to reduced blood flow to the brain
    C. Can be cured
    D. Is usually temporary
11. Acute confusion
    A. Is usually temporary
    B. Is the result of aging
    C. Cannot be cured
    D. Is the result of physical changes
12. When a person is confused, it is helpful if you
    A. Repeat the date and time as often as necessary
    B. Change the routine each day to stimulate the person
    C. Keep the drapes pulled during the day
    D. Give complex answers to questions

13. Vision and hearing decrease with confusion, so you should
    A. Speak in a loud voice
    B. Write out directions to the person
    C. Face the person and speak clearly
    D. Keep the lighting dim in the room
14. Dementia can be treated if it is caused by
    A. AIDS
    B. Depression
    C. Permanent changes in the brain
    D. Alzheimer's disease
15. Dementia
    A. Is the same as changes in the brain that occur with aging
    B. Causes the person to have problems with common tasks
    C. Is always temporary and can be cured
    D. Affects most older people
16. The most common type of permanent dementia in older persons is
    A. Alzheimer's disease   C. Depression
    B. Dementia   D. Delirium
17. If a person has an infection, it may cause
    A. Alzheimer's disease   C. Delirium
    B. Pseudodementia   D. Depression
18. Depression is often overlooked in older persons because
    A. Signs and symptoms are similar to aging and some drug side effects
    B. Depression is rare in older persons
    C. It is a temporary condition that passes without treatment
    D. It is always the result of a physical problem
19. The classic sign of Alzheimer's Disease (AD) is
    A. Mood and personality changes
    B. Gradual loss of short-term memory
    C. Acute confusion and delirium
    D. Wandering and sundowning

20. In mild AD, the person may
    A. Walk slowly with a shuffling gait
    B. Be totally incontinent
    C. Have problems making new memories
    D. Become agitated and may be violent
21. As AD progresses to moderate AD, the person
    A. Has difficulty performing everyday tasks
    B. Needs assistance with activities of daily living
    C. Is disoriented to time and place
    D. Has seizures
22. In severe AD, the person may
    A. Forget recent events
    B. Lose impulse control and use foul language or have poor table manners
    C. Be less interested in things or be less outgoing
    D. Cry out when touched or transferred
23. At what stage as described by the Alzheimer's Association, would a person forget names, but recognize faces?
    A. Moderate cognitive decline
    B. Severe cognitive decline
    C. Very severe decline
    D. Mild cognitive decline
24. When a person with AD wanders, the major risk is
    A. The person's comfort
    B. Life-threatening accidents can occur
    C. Inconvenience of the family or facility
    D. Making sure the person gets enough rest and sleep
25. When a person with AD has symptoms of sundowning, it may be due to
    A. Being tired or hungry
    B. Having poor judgment
    C. Impaired vision or hearing
    D. The person looking for something or someone
26. Too much stimuli from being asked too many questions all at once can overwhelm a person and cause
    A. Delusions
    B. Catastrophic reactions
    C. Hallucinations
    D. Sundowning
27. A caregiver may cause agitation and restlessness by
    A. Calling the person by name
    B. Selecting tasks and activities specific to the person's cognitive abilities and interests
    C. Encouraging activity early in the day
    D. Rushing the person to complete care quickly
28. When a person with AD screams, it may be because the person
    A. Has hearing and vision problems
    B. Is trying to communicate
    C. Has too much stimulation in the environment
    D. All of the above
29. When the person with AD has abnormal sexual behaviors, it may be due to
    A. Disorientation to person, time, and place
    B. Poor hygiene
    C. Infection, pain, or discomfort in the urinary or reproductive systems
    D. All of the above
30. If a person with AD displays sexual behaviors, the nurse may tell you to
    A. Tell the person this behavior is not acceptable
    B. Make sure the person has good hygiene to prevent itching
    C. Avoid caring for the person
    D. Ignore the behavior because the disease causes it
31. What should you do when a person repeats the same motions or repeats the same words over and over?
    A. Remind the person to stop the repeating.
    B. Report this to the nurse immediately.
    C. Take the person for a walk, or distract the person with music or picture books.
    D. Isolate the person in his or her room until the repeating behavior stops.
32. A person with AD is encouraged to take part in therapies and activities that
    A. Increase the level of confusion
    B. Help the person to feel useful, worthwhile, and active
    C. Will prevent aggressive behaviors
    D. Improve physical problems such as incontinence and contractures
33. How do AD special care units differ from other areas of a care facility?
    A. Complete care is provided.
    B. Entrances and exits may be locked.
    C. Meals are served in the person's room.
    D. No activities are provided.
34. A person with AD can no longer stay in a secured unit when
    A. The condition improves
    B. The family requests a move to another unit
    C. The person cannot sit or walk
    D. Aggressive behaviors disrupt the unit
35. A family who cares for a person with dementia at home
    A. May feel anger and resentment towards the person
    B. May feel guilty
    C. Needs assistance from others to cope with the person
    D. All of the above

Fill in the Blank

36. Write out the meaning of the abbreviations.
    A. AD _____
    B. ADL _____
    C. NIA _____
    D. OBRA _____
37. Cognitive functioning involves
    A. _____
    B. _____
    C. _____
    D. _____
    E. _____
    F. _____

38. What senses decrease with changes in the nervous system from aging?

    A. _____

    B. _____

    C. _____

    D. _____

    E. _____

39. Some early warning signs of dementia affect these areas. Explain or give an example for each one.

    A. Recent memory _____

    B. Common tasks _____

    C. Language _____

    D. Judgment _____

40. What substances can cause treatable dementia?

    A. _____

    B. _____

41. Pseudodementia can occur with _____

    and _____.

42. With delirium, the onset is _____.

    It often lasts for about _____.

    It may take _____ for normal mental function to return.

43. Alzheimer's disease (AD) damages brain cells that control these functions.

    A. _____

    B. _____

    C. _____

    D. _____

    E. _____

    F. _____

    G. _____

    H. _____

44. Certain behaviors are common with AD. Name the behavior for each of these examples.

    A. The person becomes more anxious, confused, or restless during the night.

    _____

    B. The person sits in a chair and folds the same napkin over and over.

    _____

    C. The person begins to scream and cry when a visitor asks many questions.

    _____

    D. The person walks away from home and cannot find the way back home.

    _____

    E. The person begins to pace when he needs to eliminate or when he is hungry.

    _____

F. The person tells you he sees his dog sitting in the room, but you do not see anything.

G. The person hits and pinches the staff when a shower is given. _____

H. The person tries to hug and kiss other residents of the facility. _____

_____

Use Focus on PRIDE in the Textbook to complete questions 45–47.

45. You demonstrate personal and professional responsibility when you report changes

    _____.

46. You show that you respect the rights of a person when you keep personal items _____.

    It is important to protect the person's belongings from

    _____ or

    _____.

47. You help to maintain independence for a person with AD by maintaining the person's _____ when giving ADLs.

Optional Learning Exercises

You are caring for Mr. Harris, a 78-year-old who is confused. You know there are ways to help a person to be more oriented. Answer questions 48–50 about ways to help a confused person.

48. How can you help to orient Mr. Harris every time you are in contact with him?

    _____

49. What are ways you can help to orient Mr. Harris to time?

    A. _____

    B. _____

    _____

50. What are ways you can maintain the day-night cycle?

    A. _____

    B. _____

    C. _____

You are caring for Mrs. Matthews, an 82-year-old resident. The nurse tells you she lived with her daughter for the last 2 years, but the family is now concerned for her safety. She left the home when the temperature was 35° F and was found 2 miles away, wearing a light sweater. On another occasion, she turned on the gas stove and could not remember how to turn it off. Sometimes, she did not recognize her daughter and resisted getting a bath or changing clothes. Since admission to the care facility, she repeatedly tells everyone she must leave to go to her birthday party. She brushes her arms and legs and tells you "bugs" are crawling on her. Answer questions 51–53 about Mrs. Matthews and her care.

51. What is the most important reason that Mrs. Matthews is living in a special care unit in the nursing facility? _____

    _____

52. Mrs. Matthews is diagnosed with

    _____ stage AD. What
    activities would indicate she is in this stage?

    A. _____

    B. _____

    C. _____

    D. _____

    E. _____

53. The nurse may encourage Mrs. Matthew's daughter

    to join a _____ group.
    How can this be helpful to the daughter?

    A. _____

    B. _____

    C. _____

Independent Learning Activities

Consider the situation and answer the questions about how you would feel.

SITUATION: Imagine you are in a strange country where people talk to you, but you do not understand what they are saying. They use strange tools to eat and you cannot figure out how to use them. They try to feed you food you do not recognize. Sometimes, these people seem friendly and caring, but at other times, they become angry because you are not doing what they ask you to do. You become frightened when they try to remove your clothes and take you in a room to shower you. You become frightened and upset because you do not know what will happen next. At times, other strangers come to your room and bring gifts. They talk kindly to you, but you do not know them. They seem upset when you do not respond to their gifts and gestures. The doors and windows in this country are all locked and you cannot find a way out so that you can go home.

- How does this situation relate to the information in this chapter?

- How would you react if you were the person in this situation? Why?
- What methods might you use to try to communicate with the person in this situation?
- Why would the person want to go home? What does "home" mean to him or her?
- How will this exercise help you when you care for a person who is confused?

Consider the situation and answer the questions about how you would care for a person who has dementia.

SITUATION: You are assigned to care for Ronald Myers, 85 years old, who has Alzheimer's disease. He often wanders from room to room and tries to open the outside doors. He frequently becomes agitated and restless, especially in the evening. Most of the time, Mr. Myers is unable to feed himself and is often incontinent. He keeps repeating, "Help me, help me," all day.

- How do you feel about caring for a person like this? Frightened? Angry? Impatient? How do you deal with your feelings so that you can give care to the person?
- At what stage of Alzheimer's disease is Mr. Myers? What signs and symptoms support your answer?
- Why would it be ineffective to remind Mr. Myers of the date and time during your shift? Why is this a good technique with some confused persons and not with others?
- Why does Mr. Myers become more agitated toward evening? What is this called?
- What methods could you use to make sure Mr. Myers receives the care needed to maintain good personal hygiene? How could you get him to cooperate or participate in his care?
- What parts of Mr. Myers behavior would be most difficult for you to tolerate? What would you do if you found yourself becoming irritated and angry with Mr. Myers?
- What information in this chapter has helped you to understand persons like Mr. Myers better? How will this information help you to give better care to these persons and to maintain their quality of life?

47 Developmental Disabilities

Fill in the Blank: Key Terms

Birth defect

Developmental disability

Diplegia

Disability

Inherited

Intellectual disability

Spastic

1. _____ involves severe limits in intellectual function and adaptive behavior occurring before age 18.

2. An abnormality present at birth that can involve body structure or function is a _____.

3. When similar body parts are affected on both sides of the body, it is called _____.

4. The uncontrolled contraction of skeletal muscles is _____

5. That which is passed down from parents to children is _____

6. A disability that occurs before 22 years of age is _____

7. Any lost, absent, or impaired physical or mental function is a _____.

Circle the Best Answer

8. A developmental disability (DD)
   A. Occurs before, during, or after birth
   B. Is usually temporary
   C. Limits function in 3 or more life skills
   D. Is present before the age of 12

9. Developmentally disabled adults
   A. Need lifelong assistance, support, and special services
   B. Usually can live independently after they become adults
   C. Always need to be in long-term care in special centers
   D. Generally outgrow the problems as they mature

10. A person is considered to have intellectual disabilities if
    A. The IQ score is below 70
    B. The condition is present before 18 years of age
    C. The person is limited in the skills needed to live, work, and play
    D. All of the above

11. The Arc of the United States is a national organization
    A. Related to Alzheimer's disease
    B. That focuses on people with intellectual and related developmental disabilities
    C. That provides care for people with physical disability
    D. For persons with cerebral palsy

12. Down syndrome (DS) is caused by
    A. An extra 21st chromosome
    B. Head injury during birth
    C. Diseases of the mother during pregnancy
    D. Lack of oxygen to the brain

13. A person with Down syndrome is at risk for
    A. Cerebral palsy   C. Leukemia
    B. Diplegia   D. Poor nutrition

14. Fragile X syndrome occurs because
    A. Of a birth injury
    B. Of an extra 21st chromosome
    C. Of a change in a gene that makes a protein needed for brain development
    D. The mother had rubella (German measles) during pregnancy

15. Cerebral palsy is a group of disorders involving
    A. Intellectual disabilities
    B. Muscle weakness or poor muscle control
    C. Abnormal genes from one or both parents
    D. An increased risk of developing leukemia

16. When a person has spastic cerebral palsy, the symptoms include
    A. Constant slow weaving or writhing motions
    B. Uncontrolled contractions of skeletal muscles
    C. Using little or no eye contact
    D. A strong attachment to a single item, idea, activity, or person

17. A person with autism may
    A. Not like being held or cuddled
    B. Have bladder and bowel control problems
    C. Have generalized seizures
    D. Have diplegia or hemiplegia

18. The person with autism
    A. Needs to develop social and work skills
    B. Will outgrow the condition
    C. Will always live in group homes or residential care centers
    D. Will have severe physical problems

19. Spina bifida occurs
    A. At birth, because of injury during delivery
    B. Because of traumatic injury in childhood
    C. During the first month of pregnancy
    D. As a result of child abuse

20. Which of these types of spina bifida cause the person to have leg paralysis and lack of bowel and bladder control?
    A. Spina bifida cystica
    B. Myelomeningocele
    C. Spina bifida occulta
    D. Meningocele
21. A shunt placed in the brain of a child with hydrocephalus will
    A. Increase pressure on the brain
    B. Drain fluid from the brain to a body cavity
    C. Cause intellectual disabilities or neurological damage
    D. Cure the hydrocephalus

Fill in the Blank

22. Write out the abbreviations.
    A. ADA _____
    B. CP _____
    C. DD _____
    D. DS _____
    E. FXS _____
    F. IQ _____
    G. OBRA _____
    H. SB _____
23. A developmental disability is present when function is limited in 3 or more of these life skills:
    A. _____
    B. _____
    C. _____
    D. _____
    E. _____
    F. _____
    G. _____
24. What genetic conditions can cause intellectual disabilities?
    A. _____
    B. _____
    C. _____
    D. _____
    E. _____
25. Intellectual disabilities may be caused after birth by childhood diseases, such as
    A. _____
    B. _____
    C. _____
    D. _____
    E. _____
    F. _____
26. According to the Arc of the United States, intellectual disabilities involve the condition being present before _____

27. The Arc beliefs about sexuality include the rights to
    A. _____
    B. _____
    C. _____
    D. _____
    E. _____
    F. _____
    G. _____
    H. _____
    I. _____
    J. _____
    K. _____
28. If a child has Down syndrome (DS), what features are present in these areas?
    A. Head _____
    B. Eyes _____
    C. Tongue _____
    D. Nose _____
    E. Hands and fingers _____
29. Persons with Down syndrome need therapy in these areas.
    A. _____
    B. _____
    C. _____
    D. _____
30. The usual cause of cerebral palsy is a lack of _____.
31. Which type of cerebral palsy is described in each example?
    A. Arm and leg on one side are paralyzed. _____
    B. Muscles contract or shorten. They are stiff and cannot relax. _____
    C. Both arms and both legs are paralyzed. _____
    D. The person has constant, slow, weaving, or writhing motions. _____
    E. Both arms or both legs are paralyzed. _____
32. The goal for a person with cerebral palsy is to be _____.
33. A person with autism has
    A. _____
    B. _____
    C. _____
34. Spina bifida is a defect of the _____.

35. Children with spina bifida may have difficulty learning because of problems with

   A. _____

   B. _____

   C. _____

   D. _____

36. Which type of spina bifida would cause the problems in each of the examples given?

   A. The person has leg paralysis and a lack of bowel and bladder control. _____

   B. The person may have no symptoms.

   _____

   C. Nerve damage usually does not occur and surgery corrects the defect. _____

37. If a hydrocephalus is not treated, pressure increases in the head and causes _____ and _____.

Use Focus on PRIDE in the Textbook to complete questions 38–40.

38. Persons with developmental disabilities have a right to enjoy and maintain a good quality of life. Such a life involves

   A. _____

   B. _____

   C. _____

39. The goal for children with developmental disabilities is independence _____

40. Signs of abuse of a developmentally disabled person may be

   A. _____

   B. _____

   C. _____

   D. _____

   E. _____

Optional Learning Exercises

Mr. Murphy is one of the residents you care for. He has Down syndrome. Answer questions 41–43 that relate to this person.

41. Mr. Murphy is 40 years old. What disease is a risk for an adult with Down syndrome?

   _____

42. Mr. Murphy is encouraged to eat a well-balanced diet and to attend regular exercise classes. Including these in the care plan will help to prevent the problems of

   _____ and _____.

43. What 2 therapies may help Mr. Murphy to communicate more clearly?

   _____ and _____.

You care for Mary Reynolds, who has cerebral palsy. Answer questions 44–45 about Ms. Reynolds.

44. It is difficult to feed Ms. Reynolds because she drools, grimaces, and moves her head constantly. You know that she does this because she has a type of cerebral palsy called _____.

45. Because Ms. Reynolds remains in bed or a special chair all the time, she is at special risk for _____ because of immobility. She needs to be repositioned at least every _____.

Independent Learning Activities

Many communities have services available to families with children and adults who are developmentally disabled. Some communities have sheltered workshops, day care, sheltered living centers, or physical and occupational therapy programs available. If your community has these services, ask permission to visit them and observe the persons being served there. Answer these questions when you observe in the agency.

- What age groups are served in this program?
- What activities are available to the group?
- What training is required for the people who work there?
- How do the persons in the program act? Happy? Bored? Withdrawn? Other reactions?
- What other services are available to these individuals in the agency? In the community?
- Where do the persons in this program live? With family? Group homes? Other?

Do you know a family who has a developmentally disabled family member? Ask the family if they will answer these questions about living with this person.

- How old is the developmentally disabled person? Where does the person live?
- What abilities does the person have? What disabilities interfere with the activities of daily living for the person?
- What therapies are being done to help the person reach his or her highest level of function?
- What community programs have been helpful for the person?
- How does this person's disability affect the family? Physical? Emotional? Financial? Day-to-day activities?

48 Sexuality

Fill in the Blank: Key Terms

Bisexual   Heterosexual   Impotence   Sexuality   Transsexual
Erectile dysfunction   Homosexual   Sex   Transgender   Transvestite

1. _____ is a broad term to describe people who express their sexuality or gender in other than the expected way.

2. Another name for impotence is

_____.

3. _____ is the physical, psychological, social, cultural, and spiritual factors that affect a person's feelings and attitudes about his or her sex.

4. A _____ is a person who dresses and behaves like the other sex for emotional and sexual relief.

5. A person attracted to both sexes is _____.

6. A _____ is a person who believes that he or she is really a member of the other sex.

7. A _____ is a person who is attracted to members of the same sex.

8. The physical activities involving the reproductive organs is _____.

9. A person who is attracted to members of the other sex is _____.

10. The inability of the male to have an erection is erectile dysfunction or

_____.

Circle the Best Answer

11. Sexuality
    A. Involves the whole person
    B. Is the physical activities involving reproductive organs
    C. Is unimportant in old age
    D. Is done for pleasure or to have children

12. A women who is attracted to men is
    A. Homosexual   C. Lesbian
    B. Heterosexual   D. Bisexual

13. Transvestites are often
    A. Homosexual
    B. Transsexual
    C. Married and heterosexual
    D. Bisexual

14. Diabetes, spinal cord injuries, and multiple sclerosis may cause
    A. Impotence   C. Sexual aggression
    B. Menopause   D. Heterosexuality

15. Which of these are *not* true about sexuality and older persons?
    A. An orgasm is less forceful than in younger persons
    B. Arousal takes longer.
    C. Older persons lose sexual needs and desires.
    D. Love, affection, and intimacy are needed throughout life.

16. When older adult couples live in a nursing center, OBRA requires that they
    A. Are allowed to share the same room
    B. Are placed in separate rooms
    C. Are not encouraged to be intimate
    D. Cannot share a bed

17. When a person in a nursing center is sexually aggressive, it may be the result of
    A. Confusion
    B. Using a way to gain your attention
    C. Genital soreness or itching
    D. All of the above

18. If a person touches you in the wrong way, you should
    A. Ignore it and realize the person is not responsible
    B. Tell the person you do not like him or her
    C. Tell the person that those behaviors make you uncomfortable
    D. Refuse to give care to the person

Fill in the Blank

19. ED is an abbreviation for _____.

20. Sexuality develops when the baby's _____.

21. Children know their own sex at age _____.

22. Bisexuals often _____ and have

_____.

23. Sexual function may be affected by chronic illnesses such as
    A. _____
    B. _____
    C. _____
    D. _____

24. What reproductive surgeries may affect sexuality?

A. Men _____

B. Women _____

25. Some older people do not have intercourse. They may express their sexual needs or desires

by _____ .

26. When you are assisting persons, what grooming practices will promote sexuality for residents?

A. Men _____

B. Women _____

_____

27. What can you do to allow privacy for a person and a partner?

A. Close _____

B. Let the person and partner know _____

C. Tell other _____

D. Knock _____

28. Masturbation is a normal _____ .

29. What health-related problems may cause a person to touch his or her genitals?

A. _____ or _____

system disorders

B. Poor _____

C. Being _____ or _____ from urine and feces

Use Focus on PRIDE in the Textbook to complete questions 30–33.

30. When you are caring for a person, it is important to get consent before touching _____, _____,

or _____ .

31. If you touch these areas without consent, you may be accused of _____ .

32. Sexuality includes _____, _____,

_____, _____, and _____ factors.

33. When giving care, you can promote sexuality when you

A. _____

_____

B. _____

_____

C. _____

_____

D. _____

_____

Optional Learning Exercises

Mr. and Mrs. Davis are 78-year-old residents in a nursing center, where they share a room. They need assistance with ADLs, but are mentally alert. They are an affectionate couple and care deeply for each other. Answer this question about meeting their sexuality needs.

34. Mr. Davis has diabetes and high blood pressure. What effect can these disorders have on sexuality?

_____

_____

Independent Learning Activities

Consider this situation about a sexually aggressive person, and answer the questions about how you would respond.

SITUATION: John James is 72 and has paraplegia because of an accident several years ago. His caregivers report that recently he has begun to make sexually suggestive remarks. While you are giving his morning care, he touches you several times in private areas and makes frequent sexually suggestive remarks. The other nursing assistants tell you they just ignore him or joke around with him about the actions.

- What would you say to Mr. James when he touched you in private areas?
- How would you respond to his suggestive remarks?
- What would you say to your colleagues who suggest you ignore or joke with Mr. James?
- Has this type of situation ever occurred to you? How did you handle it then? What would you do differently after studying this chapter?

Consider this situation about caring for a person who is gay. Answer the questions about how you would respond.

SITUATION: Bobbie Freeman is 45 and has had gallbladder surgery. While assisting her to ambulate, she begins to talk about her friend, Judy. She tells you that they have been lovers for 15 years.

- What would you say to a person who tells you she is gay?
- What effect would this information have on the care you provide for the person?
- Has this type of situation ever occurred when you were caring for a person? How did you respond? How would you respond after studying this chapter?

49 Caring for Mothers and Newborns

Fill in the Blank: Key Terms

Breast-feeding   Episiotomy   Meconium   Postpartum
Circumcision   Lochia   Nursing   Umbilical cord

1. An _episiotomy_ is an incision into the perineum.
2. Breast-feeding is also called _nursing_.
3. After childbirth is called _postpartum_.
4. _Circumcision_ is the surgical removal of foreskin from the penis.
5. The vaginal discharge that occurs after childbirth is _lochia_.
6. The structure that carries blood, oxygen, and nutrients from the mother to the fetus is the _umbilical cord_.
7. A dark green to black, tarry bowel movement is _meconium_.
8. Feeding a baby milk from the mother's breast is _breast-feeding_.

Circle the Best Answer

9. You lift a newborn by
   - A. The arms
   - B. Using only one hand
   - C. Supporting the head and upper back
   - D. Using two hands – one to support the head and back, the other to support the legs
10. Babies cry when they
    - A. Are hungry
    - B. Are uncomfortable, wet, frightened, or tired
    - C. Want attention
    - D. All of the above
11. Babies should not be placed on an adult's or child's bed because
    - A. The beds will not provide enough support
    - B. The baby can get trapped between the bed and the wall or between the bed and another object
    - C. Babies must sleep on their backs
    - D. The beds are too firm for comfort
12. When a crib is checked for safety, which of these is *not* correct?
    - A. There should be less than a 2-finger width between the edge of the mattress and crib side
    - B. Corner posts are no higher than ¹⁄₁₆ inch (1.5 mm)
    - C. Slats are spaced no more than 4 inches apart
    - D. There are no cutouts in the headboard or footboard to allow head entrapment

13. Toys or squeeze toys can safely have
    - A. Ball-shaped ends or squeakers
    - B. A ribbon, strings, or cords attached
    - C. Small parts that can be detached for the baby to chew on
    - D. Handles that are too large to lodge in the baby's throat
14. Which of these should be reported to the nurse at once?
    - A. The baby has a rectal temperature of 99.6° F.
    - B. The baby has a soft, unformed stool after being breast-fed.
    - C. The baby turns his or her head to one side or puts a hand to one ear.
    - D. The baby cries when the diaper is wet, or when he or she is hungry.
15. A breast-fed newborn baby generally nurses
    - A. Every 2 to 3 hours
    - B. Every 8 to 12 hours
    - C. About once an hour for very short periods of time
    - D. On a very strict schedule
16. When a mother is breast-feeding, she should avoid
    - A. Drinking whole milk
    - B. Certain foods that cause the baby to have cramping or diarrhea
    - C. Foods that are high in calories or calcium
    - D. Moderate intake of foods with caffeine
17. When the mother is breast-feeding, she should
    - A. Position the baby by using a pillow to prop the baby
    - B. Begin by stroking the baby's cheek with her nipple
    - C. Nurse only from one breast at each feeding
    - D. Lay the baby on his or her stomach after feeding
18. When preparing bottles for feeding babies, you should
    - A. Prepare, then refrigerate bottles that can be used within 24 hours
    - B. Sterilize the bottles by boiling them for 20 minutes
    - C. Rinse bottles and nipples that have been used only in cool water
    - D. Not use any soap when cleaning the equipment as it can cause serious stomach and intestinal irritation

19. When preparing to give a bottle to a baby
    A. It may be used from the refrigerator without heating
    B. Warm the bottle in warm running tap water
    C. Set the bottle out of the refrigerator and allow it to warm
    D. Heat the bottle in a microwave oven
20. When diapering a baby, report to the nurse if
    A. The stool is soft and unformed
    B. The stool is hard and formed or watery
    C. If the diaper is wet 6 to 8 times a day
    D. If the baby has 3 stools in one day
21. The umbilical cord stump falls off
    A. At birth
    B. Within 2 to 3 days after birth
    C. About 2 weeks after birth
    D. About one month after birth
22. Circumcision care includes
    A. Washing the area with mild soap and water or commercial wipes
    B. Cleaning the area with a sterile solution
    C. Applying a snug dressing to the area
    D. Cleaning the area once a day
23. Sponge baths are given
    A. To protect the dry skin of an infant
    B. Until the cord site and circumcision heal
    C. Because it is unsafe to give a baby a tub bath
    D. Until the baby is able to support the head without assistance
24. When giving a bath to a baby, the water should be
    A. Room temperature   C. 100° to 105° F
    B. 75° to 80° F   D. 110° to 115° F
25. An important safety measure when giving a bath to a baby is
    A. Apply lotion when the bath is finished
    B. Clean the ears and nostrils with cotton swabs
    C. Use a mild soap when bathing the baby
    D. Always keep one hand on the baby if you must look away
26. When a baby is breast-fed, the baby is weighed
    A. Once a day
    B. Before and after each breast-feeding
    C. After every diaper change
    D. Once a week
27. When a mother breast-feeds, she
    A. Can expect a menstrual period within 2 to 4 weeks
    B. Cannot get pregnant as long as she continues to breast-feed
    C. Needs to use birth control measures to prevent pregnancy
    D. Will have difficulty losing weight gained during the pregnancy
28. You are caring for a mother who had a baby 4 weeks ago. She tells you she is concerned because she has whitish vaginal drainage. You know that this is
    A. Abnormal and should be reported to the nurse at once
    B. Unusual, because her discharge should be pinkish brown in color
    C. Normal at this time after having a baby
    D. An indication that she has an infection

29. A mother may have emotional swings after having a baby, which are caused by
    A. Hormone changes   C. Lack of sleep
    B. Life-style changes   D. All of the above

Fill in the Blank

30. C-section is an abbreviation for _____.
31. When you hold and cuddle infants, it helps them learn to feel _____ and

    _____
32. You should not place pillows, quilts, or soft toys in the crib, because they may

    cause _____.
33. Babies are not placed on their stomachs for sleep, because this position can _____
34. A toy chest should have no latch so the child cannot

    be _____.
35. What signs or symptoms related to each of these may indicate the baby is ill?
    A. Skin color _____
    B. Respirations _____
    C. Eyes _____
    D. Stools _____
36. When a mother is breast-feeding, if the baby finished the last feeding at the right breast, the baby

    starts the next feeding at the _____ breast.
37. The baby is burped at least twice when breast-feeding. Burping is done
    A. _____
    B. _____
38. When planning meals or grocery shopping for a mother who is breast-feeding, what should you know about her diet?
    A. Calories _____
    B. Milk, yogurt, and cheese group _____

    _____
    C. Calcium _____
    D. What foods should be avoided? _____
       _____ Why? _____

    _____
    E. What foods are used in moderation? _____
       _____ Why? _____

    _____
    F. She should not drink _____
39. Why is it important to thoroughly rinse baby bottles, caps, and nipples to remove all

    soap? _____

    _____

40. You can prevent having air in the neck of the bottle or in the nipple by _____.

41. When you are burping a baby, you should support the _____ for the first _____ months.

42. If you are using cloth diapers, rinse the soiled diaper in _____.

43. When changing a baby's diaper, what observations should be reported and recorded?
    A. _____
    B. _____
    C. _____
    D. _____

44. When diapering a newborn, what should you do if the baby has an unhealed circumcision or a cord stump still attached?
    A. Circumcision _____
    B. Cord stump _____

45. The base of the cord stump is washed with _____ and _____. The stump heals faster if allowed to _____.

46. When caring for the umbilical cord, you should report to the nurse the following:
    A. _____
    B. _____
    C. _____

47. Petrolatum gauze dressing or jelly is applied to an unhealed circumcision to
    A. _____
    B. _____

48. To protect an infant during a bath, what safety measures are followed?
    A. Room temperature _____
    B. Bath water temperature _____
    C. Never _____
    D. Always _____
    E. Hold _____

49. What steps are used to wash a baby's head?
    A. _____
    B. _____
    C. _____
    D. _____
    E. _____

50. In order to protect a baby from falling when you weigh him or her, always keep _____.

51. Describe the vaginal discharge that occurs after childbirth.
    A. Lochia rubra _____ It is seen during the _____.
    B. Lochia serosa _____ It lasts about _____.
    C. Lochia alba _____ It continues for _____.

52. What signs and symptoms of postpartum complications should be reported to the nurse at once?
    A. _____
    B. _____
    C. _____
    D. _____
    E. _____
    F. _____
    G. _____
    H. _____
    I. _____
    J. _____
    K. _____

Use Focus on PRIDE in the Textbook to complete questions 53–55.

53. When you return a newborn to the mother, it is your professional responsibility to follow the agency policy for _____.

54. Parents will learn to be independent and gain confidence by performing _____.

55. Newborns wear a security bracelet that will signal the agency when he or she is carried _____.

Optional Learning Exercises
You are caring for Marilyn Hansen and her newborn son, Samuel, at home. Answer questions 56–63 about their care.

56. Ms. Hansen asks you if the playpen she was given is safe. What safety guidelines are important for a playpen?
    A. _____
    B. _____
    C. _____
    D. _____
    E. _____
    F. _____
    G. _____

57. Ms. Hansen is breast-feeding. When she strokes the baby's cheek with her nipple, what does the baby do? _____

    This is called the _____.

58. Ms. Hansen is having difficulty in removing Samuel from her breast. You tell her to break the suction, she can _____.

59. You notice that the nipples are dry and cracking. What can Ms. Hansen do to prevent this from happening?

    A. _____

    B. _____

    C. _____

    D. _____

60. When you are changing Samuel's diaper, clean the genital area from _____.

61. The cord stump is still in place. Ms. Hansen asks you when it will fall off. You tell her it dries up and falls off in _____.

62. Samuel has been circumcised and Ms. Hansen is concerned because the penis looks red, swollen, and sore. You know that this is _____.
    However, you should observe the circumcision for signs of

    A. _____ and _____

    B. There should be no _____

63. Ms. Hansen asks whether she should bathe Samuel in the morning or in the evening. You tell her an evening bath might help Samuel sleep longer because a bath is _____.

Independent Learning Activities

Many communities offer baby care classes, parenting classes, and breast-feeding classes. Find out what is available in your community and ask permission to attend one or more of these classes. Answer these questions about what you learned.

- Where were the classes offered? How many classes were offered for each topic?
- What new information did you get from attending the classes? How did studying this chapter help you when you went to the classes?

Talk with a friend or family member who has recently had a baby. Ask the following questions.

- How did the mother learn about caring for herself and a newborn? Classes? Family members? Friends?
- How did she feel when she brought the new baby home? What help did she have from her family or friends? How did she cope when she felt tired or overwhelmed?
- How did she care for the umbilical cord? How long did the cord stump stay attached? What problems did she have with cord care? What signs and symptoms did she know were signs of a problem?
- If the baby was a boy, was he circumcised? What care did she give to the circumcision? What problems did she have with the circumcision?
- How did she feed the baby – breast or bottle? What were the reasons she chose the method used? If breast-feeding, how long did she continue to breast-feed? What were the advantages of the method chosen? What were the disadvantages?

50 Assisted Living

Fill in the Blank: Key Terms

Assisted living   Medication reminder   Service plan

1. A _medication reminder_ is reminding the person to take drugs, observing them being taken as prescribed, and charting that they were taken.

2. A written plan that lists the services needed by the person and who provides them is a _service plan_.

3. _Assisted living_ provides a housing option for older persons who need help with activities of daily living yet wish to remain independent as long as possible.

Circle the Best Answer

4. Which of these persons would *not* be living in an ALR?
   A. A person who needs medication management or help taking drugs
   B. Someone who needs help with shopping, banking, and money management
   C. A person who needs complete help with ADLs
   D. Someone who is lonely and wants to live with people.

5. When a person lives in an ALR, one requirement is
   A. At least 2 rooms and a bath
   B. Both a bathtub and a shower
   C. A door that locks and the person keeps the key
   D. A double or queen-sized bed

6. Environmental requirements in an ALR include
   A. Common bathrooms have toilet paper, soap, and cloth towels or a dryer
   B. Pets or animals must be kept in kennels
   C. Hot water temperatures are between 110° F and 130° F
   D. Garbage is stored in covered containers lined with plastic bags that are removed at least once day

7. Which of these is *not* included in the Assisted Living Resident's Rights?
   A. May participate in religious, social, community, and other activities
   B. May communicate privately and freely with any person
   C. Has a doctor or pharmacist assigned by the facility
   D. Is given information on how residents and others can file complaints

8. A staff member in an ALR would be expected to have training in all of these areas *except*
   A. Assisting with drugs
   B. Early signs of illness and the need for health care
   C. Food preparation, service, and storage
   D. Measuring and giving medications

9. Which of these is often a requirement of a resident in an ALR?
   A. The person must be able to leave the building in an emergency.
   B. The person requires skilled nursing services.
   C. The person has complex nursing problems.
   D. The person must not be paralyzed or be chronically ill.

10. Which of these is a service offered in an ALR?
   A. Daily housekeeping
   B. A garage for cars owned by residents
   C. A 24-hour emergency communication system
   D. A bank in the facility

11. Meals in an ALR
   A. Are always served in the person's room
   B. Include the noon meal only
   C. May provide a nutritious snack in the evening
   D. Cannot meet special dietary needs

12. When you assist with housekeeping, you will be expected to
   A. Clean the tub or shower after each use
   B. Put out clean towels and washcloths every week
   C. Use a disinfectant or water and detergent to clean bathroom surfaces once a week
   D. Dust furniture every day

13. A measure you should follow when handling, preparing, or storing foods is
   A. Use leftover food within 4 or 5 days
   B. Wash all pots and pans in a dishwasher
   C. Date and refrigerate containers of leftovers and refrigerate as soon as possible
   D. Clean kitchen appliances, counters, tables and other surfaces once a day

14. When practicing food safety, which of these is *incorrect*?
   A. Use a garbage disposer for food and liquid garbage.
   B. Place leftover food in a refrigerator as soon as possible.
   C. Use leftover food within one week.
   D. Place washed eating and cooking items in a drainer to dry.

15. When assisting with laundry, a guideline to follow is
    A. Sort items according to the amount of soil on the items
    B. Wear gloves when handling soiled laundry
    C. Use hot water to wash all items
    D. Use the highest setting on the dryer to sanitize the items

16. When you assist a person with medication, it may involve
    A. Opening containers for a person who cannot do so
    B. Measuring the medications for the person
    C. Explaining to a person the action of the medication
    D. Preparing a pill organizer for the person each week

17. If a drug error occurs, you should
    A. Tell the person not to do it again
    B. Make sure the person takes the correct medication at the next scheduled time
    C. Report the error to the nurse
    D. Take all medications away from the person immediately

18. An attendant is needed in an ALR 24 hours a day to
    A. Give care to those who need it
    B. Make sure medications are dispensed when ordered
    C. To assist those who need assistance if an emergency occurs
    D. To provide activities for the residents

19. A resident can be transferred, discharged, or evicted from the ALR if
    A. The ALR closes
    B. The person is a threat to the health and safety of self or others
    C. The person fails to pay for services as agreed upon
    D. All of the above

20. Which of these is *not* a right of a resident in assisted living?
    A. The right to expect medical records to be confidential
    B. The right to have overnight guests whenever the resident wishes
    C. The right to leave the facility and return without unreasonable restriction
    D. The right to be free from unjustified room transfers or discharges from the facility

Fill in the Blank

21. Write out the meaning of the abbreviations.
    A. AD _____
    B. ADL _____
    C. ALR _____

22. When working in an assisted living setting, you should follow _____ when contact with blood, body fluids, secretions, excretions, or potentially contaminated items is likely.

23. Most persons living in ALRs need help with one or more ADLs, such as
    A. _____
    B. _____
    C. _____
    D. _____
    E. _____
    F. _____

24. A bathroom in an ALR must provide privacy and
    A. _____
    B. _____
    C. _____
    D. _____
    E. _____

25. The ALR cannot employ a person with a _____.

26. The service plan is a written plan listing
    A. _____
    B. _____
    C. _____

27. The service plan also relates to
    A. _____
    B. _____
    C. _____
    D. _____
    E. _____
    F. _____
    G. _____

28. What 24-hour services are usually provided by the ALR?
    A. _____
    B. _____
    C. _____

29. The time between the evening meal and breakfast usually is no more than _____. It can be longer if _____.

30. When you wash eating and cooking items by hand, what is the order in which they are washed?
    _____

31. If you are assisting the person with taking medications, you should know the 6 rights of drug administration. They are
    A. _____
    B. _____
    C. _____
    D. _____
    E. _____
    F. _____

32. If a person is taking his or her drugs and tells you that a pill looks different, what should you do?

33. If a person needs a medication reminder it means reminding _____,
observing _____, and charting _____.

34. If you are assisting in drug administration, you should report any drug error to the RN. Errors would include:
    A. _____
    B. _____
    C. _____
    D. _____
    E. _____
    F. _____
    G. _____
    H. _____
    I. _____

Use Focus on PRIDE in the Textbook to complete questions 35–37.

35. Take pride in protecting the person's rights when you work in an ALR. These include
    A. Quality _____
    B. Self- _____
    C. _____
    D. Protection against _____
    E. Access to _____
    F. _____

36. In order to make the room in an ALR feel home-like, residents are allowed to _____.

37. It is important to know your state's laws when you assist with drugs, because if you act beyond those limits, you can lose _____ and your ability to work _____.

Optional Learning Exercises
You are working in an assisting living facility. What would you do in these situations?

38. You are providing housekeeping assistance to Mrs. Miller who lives alone. The stove is on and a pan has burning food in it. Mrs. Miller tells you she did not put the pan on the stove. What should you do?

    What is a likely reason for her behavior?

39. A resident in the facility has lived there for 2 years and has needed little assistance. He recently had a stroke and now needs care for all of his ADLs. Why is he being moved to a nursing facility? _____

40. Mrs. Jenkins tells you she is expecting an important phone call and wants to eat her lunch in her room. What should you do? _____

41. Mr. Shante asks you to get his medicines ready for him to take. What assistance are you allowed to give when the nurse has trained you?
    A. _____
    B. _____
    C. _____
    D. _____
    E. _____
    F. _____
    G. _____
    H. _____

42. When you are assisting Mrs. Clyde with her medicines, you notice two of the labels have an expired date. What should you do? _____

43. Mrs. Johnson asks you when the next meeting of the quilting group will be held. She also asks what days the community crafts fair is planned. Where would you direct her to find this information? _____

Independent Learning Activities
Find out if your community has any assisted living facilities. They may be part of another facility or may be an independent facility. Visit the facility to answer these questions.
- What services are offered in the facility? Who provides the services? Nursing assistants? Other assistants? What training is required?
- What kinds of living quarters are provided? What belongings can the person bring from home?
- What activities are scheduled? How are residents given information about these activities?
- How do the residents act? Happy? Withdrawn? Sad? How do the staff members act?

Find out what laws in your state apply to assisted living facilities. Answer these questions about the laws.
- What type of license is required for an assisted living facility? Do the laws apply to independent facilities as well as those attached to other facilities?
- What laws apply to staff training for these facilities? Does the state require workers to be nursing assistants with special training?
- What does the state law say about assisting with medications? What non-licensed persons can assist with medications? What training is required?

51 Basic Emergency Care

Fill in the Blank: Key Terms

Anaphylaxis   Convulsion   First aid   Respiratory arrest   Shock
Cardiac arrest   Fainting   Hemorrhage   Seizure   Sudden cardiac arrest

1. Another term for sudden cardiac arrest is
   _____.

2. In _____, breathing stops but the heart action continues for several minutes.

3. The sudden loss of consciousness from an inadequate blood supply to the brain is _____.

4. When the heart and breathing stops suddenly and without warning it is _____ or cardiac arrest.

5. _____ results when there is *not* enough blood supply to organs and tissues.

6. Emergency care given to an ill or injured person before medical help arrives is _____.

7. Violent and sudden contractions or tremors of muscle groups is a convulsion or _____.

8. _____ is the excessive loss of blood in a short period of time.

9. A life-threatening sensitivity to an antigen is
   _____.

10. Another term for a seizure is _____.

Circle the Best Answer

11. When an emergency occurs in nursing centers, the nurse determines when to
    A. Call the doctor for orders
    B. Activate the EMS system
    C. Call the supervisor
    D. Assist the person to bed

12. If you find a person lying on the floor, you should
    A. Keep the person lying down
    B. Help the person back to bed
    C. Elevate the head
    D. Help the person to a chair

13. If the nurse instructs you to activate the EMS system, you should do all of these *except*
    A. Tell the operator your location
    B. Explain to the operator what has happened
    C. Describe aid that is being given
    D. Hang up as soon as you have finished giving the information

14. It is important to restore breathing and circulation quickly because
    A. The lungs will be damaged
    B. The person will lose consciousness
    C. Permanent brain and other organ damage occurs
    D. Hemorrhage will occur

15. Which of these is *not* a major sign of sudden cardiac arrest (SCA)?
    A. Complaints of chest pain   C. No breathing
    B. No pulse   D. No response

16. The purpose of chest compressions is to
    A. Deflate the lungs
    B. Increase oxygen in the blood
    C. Force blood through the circulatory system
    D. Help the heart work more effectively

17. In order for chest compressions to be effective, the person must be
    A. In prone position
    B. On a soft surface
    C. Supine on a hard, flat surface
    D. In a semi-Fowler's position

18. When preparing to give chest compressions locate the hands
    A. On the sternum between the nipples
    B. On the lower half of the sternum
    C. Side by side over the sternum
    D. Slightly below the end of the sternum

19. When giving chest compressions to an adult, depress the sternum
    A. About 1 to 1½ inches   C. At least 2 inches
    B. No more than 1 inch   D. About 3 inches

20. The purpose of the head-tilt/chin-lift maneuver is to
    A. Make the person more comfortable
    B. Open the airway
    C. Practice Standard Precautions
    D. Stimulate the heart to beat

21. When a person is given breaths, you should
    A. Allow the person's chin to relax against the neck
    B. Place your mouth loosely over the person's mouth
    C. Give a breath for about 1 second each. You should see the chest rise with each breath
    D. Apply pressure on the chin to close the mouth

22. Barrier device breathing is used
    A. Whenever possible to avoid contact with body fluids
    B. In order to make a better seal for breathing
    C. When you cannot ventilate through the person's mouth
    D. Only when other methods will not work
23. Mouth-to-nose breathing is used when
    A. You cannot breathe through the person's mouth
    B. You want to avoid contact with body fluids
    C. When giving rescue breaths to a child
    D. When chest compressions are not needed
24. If an automated external defibrillator (AED) is available
    A. Use it only after other methods have been unsuccessful
    B. It can only be used by a RN or doctor
    C. Attach and use the AED as soon as it is available
    D. Use it once the person is responsive
25. When an automated external defibrillator (AED) is used, it
    A. Stops the heart
    B. Slows the heartbeat down
    C. Stops ventricular fibrillation and restores a regular heartbeat
    D. Starts the heartbeat
26. CPR is done when the person
    A. Does not respond when you shout, "Are you OK?"
    B. Is not breathing
    C. Is unconscious
    D. Does not respond, is not breathing, and has no pulse
27. Before starting chest compressions
    A. Make sure the person is breathing
    B. Check for a carotid pulse for 5–10 seconds
    C. Wait 30 seconds to see if the person regains consciousness
    D. Turn the person to the side
28. When one rescuer CPR is started, you first give
    A. 30 chest compressions
    B. 2 breaths
    C. 5 breaths
    D. 15 chest compressions
29. If the person is not breathing or not breathing adequately, give 2 breaths that
    A. Last about 1 second each
    B. Last about 5 seconds each
    C. Last 5 to 10 seconds each
    D. Last 15 seconds each
30. When performing one rescuer CPR, chest compressions are at a rate of
    A. 15 compressions per minute
    B. 100 compressions per minute
    C. 60 compressions per minute
    D. 12 compressions per minute
31. When performing one rescuer CPR, continue cycle of compressions and breathing
    A. For 5 minutes
    B. For 30 minutes
    C. Until an AED arrives
    D. For 4 cycles of 15 compressions and 2 breaths

32. The recovery position is used
    A. Because it helps keep the airway open
    B. Because it prevents aspiration
    C. When the person is breathing and has a pulse but is not responding
    D. All of the above
33. When giving CPR to children or infants, chest compressions
    A. Move the sternum 1½ to 2 inches
    B. Are done with enough pressure to press down ⅓ the depth of the chest
    C. Are not done
    D. The sternum is compressed ½ to 1 inch
34. When giving breaths to an infant, you should
    A. Tip the head back as far as possible to open the airway
    B. Pinch the nose closed and breath through the mouth
    C. Cover the infant's mouth and nose with your mouth
    D. Always use a mouth barrier
35. Which of these is a sign of internal hemorrhage?
    A. Steady flow of blood from a wound
    B. Pain, shock, vomiting blood, or coughing up blood
    C. Bleeding that occurs in spurts
    D. Dried blood at the site of an injury
36. To control external bleeding, you should do all of these *except*
    A. Remove any objects that have pierced or stabbed the person
    B. Place a sterile dressing directly over the wound
    C. Apply pressure with your hand directly over the bleeding site
    D. Bind the wound when bleeding stops
37. If a person tells you she feels faint
    A. Have the person lie down in a supine position
    B. Let the person walk around to increase circulation
    C. Have the person sit or lie down before fainting occurs
    D. If the person is lying down, raise the head with pillows
38. If a person is in shock, it is helpful if you
    A. Have the person sit in a chair
    B. Keep the person cool by removing some of the clothing
    C. Stay calm. This helps the person feels more secure
    D. Give the person something to drink or eat
39. Anaphylactic shock occurs because of
    A. Hemorrhage
    B. An allergy to foods, insects, chemicals, or drugs
    C. Sudden cardiac arrest
    D. Seizures
40. If the person has signs of a stroke, position the person in
    A. A chair   C. The recovery position
    B. Semi-Fowler's position   D. A supine position
41. If a person has a seizure, you should
    A. Place an object between the teeth
    B. Distract the person to stop the seizure
    C. Position the person in bed
    D. Move furniture, equipment, and sharp objects away from the person

42. If you are assisting a person with burns,
    A. Remove burned clothing
    B. Cover the burn wounds with a sterile or clean, cool, moist covering
    C. Give the person plenty of fluids
    D. Apply oils or ointments to the burns

Fill in the Blank

43. Write out the abbreviations.
    A. AED _____
    B. AHA _____
    C. BLS _____
    D. CPR _____
    E. EMS _____
    F. RRT _____
    G. SCA _____
    H. VF _____
    I. V-fib _____

44. If you activate the EMS system, what information should you give to the operator?
    A. _____
    B. _____
    C. _____
    D. _____
    E. _____
    F. _____

45. Chain of Survival actions are
    A. _____
    B. _____
    C. _____
    D. _____
    E. _____

46. The three major signs of sudden cardiac arrest (SCA) are
    A. _____
    B. _____
    C. _____

47. Rescue breaths are given when there is a _____ but no _____. To give rescue breaths
    A. _____
    B. _____
    C. _____
    D. _____
    E. _____

48. To find the carotid pulse, place _____.
    Slide your fingers down _____.

49. When doing chest compressions, the AHA recommends that you
    A. _____
    B. _____
    C. _____
    D. _____

50. When performing the head-tilt/chin-lift maneuver, explain how you tilt the head and lift the chin.
    A. Place the palm _____
    B. Tilt _____
    C. Place the fingers _____
    D. Lift _____

51. When you perform mouth-to-mouth breathing, it is likely you will have contact with _____
    _____.

52. A bag valve mask is a _____ device. It is squeezed to give _____ during rescue breathing. It can be connected to an _____.

53. Mouth-to-nose breathing is used when
    A. _____
    B. _____
    C. _____
    D. _____
    E. _____

54. A cycle of _____ compressions is followed by _____ rescue breaths.

55. When defibrillation is used, the AHA recommends that rescuers
    A. Attach and use _____
    B. Minimize _____
    _____
    C. Give _____
    _____
    D. Check _____

56. The AHA pediatric Chain of Survival involves these steps.
    A. _____
    B. _____
    C. _____
    D. _____
    E. _____

57. For children, CPR rules for the following are
    A. Start CPR if the child's heart rate is _____
    B. Give chest compressions with enough pressure to _____.
    C. Give only enough air to _____

58. When giving CPR to an infant when you are alone, you should
    A. Check for a pulse, using the _____ artery. This artery is found _____.
    B. Start CPR if the infant's pulse rate is _____
    C. Locate the hand position for compression by _____
    D. Place 2 _____ on the _____

59. If direct pressure does not stop hemorrhage, apply pressure over the artery _____

60. Common causes of fainting are
    A. _____
    B. _____
    C. _____
    D. _____

61. Signs and symptoms of shock include
    A. _____
    B. _____
    C. _____
    D. _____
    E. _____
    F. _____
    G. _____

62. Anaphylaxis is an emergency because the reaction occurs within _____

63. Penicillin causes _____ shock in many people.

64. Describe the 2 phases of a generalized tonic-clonic seizure.
    A. Tonic phase _____
    _____
    _____
    B. Clonic phase _____
    _____
    _____

65. The following relate to the emergency care of a person having a seizure.
    A. How do you protect the person's head? _____
    _____
    B. How is the person positioned? _____
    _____

C. Why is furniture moved? _____
_____

D. What two times are noted? _____
_____

66. Partial-thickness burns involve the _____.

67. Full-thickness burns involve _____.

68. A _____ burn is very painful because _____.

Use Focus on PRIDE in the Textbook to complete questions 69–71.

69. You demonstrate professional responsibility when you take a _____ course that you can use to save a life.

70. If a person has an emergency in a public place, you protect the person's right to privacy when you do what you can to_____.

71. When an emergency happens, it is good ethics when you keep the person's _____.

Optional Learning Exercises

You are visiting a neighbor and she is washing dishes. As she washes a glass, it shatters and she sustains a deep cut on her wrist. Answer questions 72–76 about how you would respond.

72. Your neighbor is crying and walking around the room. What is the best thing you can do to help her?
    _____
    _____

73. Clean rubber gloves are laying on the counter. How can they be useful to you? _____
    _____

74. What materials in the home could be used to place over the wound? _____
    _____

75. Your neighbor is restless, and has a rapid and weak pulse. You notice her skin is cold, moist, and pale. These signs indicate she may be in _____.

76. Her wound is still bleeding, and she loses consciousness. What should you do before you continue to give first aid? _____

Independent Learning Activities

You have learned some basic emergency care in this chapter. Find out where in your community a more advanced first aid course is available. Answer these questions about the course.
- What agency or agencies offer a course in first aid?
- How long does the course last? How much does it cost?
- Who may take the course? The public? Medical personnel? Others, such as police and firefighters?

- What subjects are covered in the course?
- Would taking this course help you on your job? In your family? In your community?

Most health care facilities require employees to take a course in basic CPR. You may be required to take CPR as part of this course. Answer these questions about CPR training in your community.

- What agency or agencies offer CPR courses?

- How long does the course take? How much does it cost?
- Who can take the courses? The public? Medical personnel? Are different classes offered to the medical personnel? If so, what is the difference?
- How often does the person need to be re-certified? How does the re-certification course differ from the beginning class?

52 End-of-Life Care

Fill in the Blank: Key Terms

Advance directive   End-of-life care   Post-mortem care   Rigor mortis
Autopsy   Palliative care   Reincarnation   Terminal illness

1. The support and care given during the time surrounding death is _____.
2. The stiffness or rigidity of skeletal muscles that occurs after death is _____.
3. An _____ is a document stating a person's wishes about health care when that person cannot make his or her own decisions.
4. Care of the body after death is _____.
5. An illness or injury for which there is no reasonable expectation of recovery is a _____.
6. _____ is the belief that the spirit or soul is reborn in another human body or in another form of life.
7. The examination of the body after death is an _____.
8. _____ is care that involves relieving or reducing the intensity of uncomfortable symptoms without producing a cure.

Circle the Best Answer

9. When a person has a terminal illness
   A. The doctor is able to accurately predict when the person will die
   B. Modern medicine can cure the disease
   C. He or she often lives longer than expected because of a strong will to live
   D. He or she will die when expected
10. When palliative care is done
    A. The person has an acute illness that can be cured
    B. The focus is on relief of symptoms
    C. Life-saving measures will be taken to prolong life
    D. The person always remains at home
11. Hospice care
    A. Is only available when the person remains at home
    B. Is used when the person is receiving rehabilitation therapy after an illness
    C. Stresses pain relief and comfort
    D. Is given until the person recovers from the illness
12. Practices and attitudes among people from India include
    A. Placing small pillows under the body's neck, feet, and wrists
    B. White clothing is worn for mourning
    C. A time and place for prayer are essential for the family and the person
    D. Having an aversion to death

13. Children between ages 2 and 6 years may see death as
    A. Final
    B. Punishment for being bad
    C. Suffering and pain
    D. A reunion with those who have died
14. Older persons see death as
    A. A temporary state
    B. Freedom from pain, suffering, and disability
    C. Something that happens to other people
    D. Something that affects plans, hopes, dreams, and ambitions
15. In which stage of dying does the person make promises and make "just one more" requests?
    A. Acceptance   C. Depression
    B. Anger   D. Bargaining
16. If a dying person begins to talk about worries and concerns, you should
    A. Call a spiritual leader
    B. Tell the nurse
    C. Listen quietly and use touch
    D. Change the subject to more pleasant topics
17. When a person is dying and weakens, care is given
    A. Only if the person requests it
    B. To meet basic needs
    C. Often, to keep the person active
    D. Only while the person is conscious
18. Because vision fails as death approaches, you should
    A. Explain what you are doing to the person when you are in the room
    B. Have the room very brightly lit
    C. Turn out all the lights
    D. Keep the eyes covered at all times
19. Hearing is one of the last functions lost, so it is important to
    A. Speak in a normal voice
    B. Offer words of comfort
    C. Provide reassurance and explanations about care
    D. All of the above
20. As death nears, oral hygiene is
    A. Given routinely
    B. More frequently given when taking oral fluids is difficult.
    C. Given very infrequently to avoid disturbing the person
    D. Never given because the person cannot swallow

21. Which of these does *not* occur as death nears?
    A. Body temperature rises.
    B. The skin is cool, pale, and mottled.
    C. Perspiration decreases.
    D. Circulation fails.
22. Because of breathing difficulties, the dying person is generally more comfortable in
    A. The supine position
    B. A side-lying position
    C. A prone position
    D. A semi-Fowler's position
23. When a person is dying, you can help the family by
    A. Allowing the family to stay as long as they wish
    B. Staying away from the room and delay giving care
    C. Telling the family that they need to leave so you can give care
    D. Telling the family that the person dying is not in pain
24. If a person has a living will, it may instruct doctors
    A. Not to start measures that will save the person's life
    B. To start CPR whenever necessary
    C. Not to start measures that prolong dying
    D. Never to activate the EMS system for a person
25. If the doctor writes a "Do Not Resuscitate" (DNR) order, it means that
    A. The person will not be resuscitated
    B. The person will be resuscitated if it is an emergency
    C. The doctor will decide whether or not to resuscitate
    D. The RN may decide that in a particular situation, resuscitation is needed
26. A sign that death is near would be
    A. Deep, rapid respirations
    B. The body temperature increases
    C. Muscles tense and contract in spasms
    D. Peristalsis increases
27. When the family wishes to see the body after death, it should be
    A. Positioned in normal alignment
    B. Positioned to appear comfortable and natural
    C. Soiled areas are bathed and cleaned.
    D. All of the above
28. When you are assisting with post-mortem care, you should
    A. Place the body in good alignment in side-lying position without pillows
    B. Tape all jewelry in place
    C. Gently pull eyelids over the eyes
    D. Dress the person in their regular clothing
29. An ID tag is attached to the big toe or
    A. Wrist   C. Upper arm
    B. Ankle   D. Upper leg
30. The Dying Person's Bill of Rights includes all of these *except*
    A. The right to privacy before and after death
    B. The right to be free from abuse, mistreatment, and neglect
    C. The right to participate in resident and family groups
    D. The right to personal choice

Fill in the Blank

31. Write out the abbreviations.
    A. DNR _____
    B. ID _____
    C. OBRA _____
32. It is important to examine your own feelings about death, because they will affect _____.
33. When you understand the dying process, you can approach the dying person with _____
    _____.
34. Hospice care focuses on these needs of the dying person and families.
    A. _____
    B. _____
    C. _____
    D. _____
35. Religious beliefs strengthen when dying, and they often provide _____
    _____.
36. Adults fear death because they fear
    A. _____ and _____
    B. Dying _____
    C. Invasion _____
    D. _____
    E. Separation from _____
37. Name the 5 stages of dying.
    A. _____
    B. _____
    C. _____
    D. _____
    E. _____
38. The goals of comfort needs are
    A. _____
    B. _____
39. When caring for a dying person, do not ask questions that need long answers because _____
    _____
    _____.
40. Because crusting and irritation of the nostrils can occur, you should _____
    _____.
41. What kinds of elimination problems can occur in the dying person?
    A. _____ and _____ incontinence
    B. _____
    C. _____ retention

42. The Patient Self-Determination Act and OBRA give 2 rights that affect the rights of a dying person. They are

    A. _____

    B. _____

43. A living will instructs doctors

    A. _____

    B. _____

44. When a person cannot make health care decisions, the authority to do so is given to the person with

    _____

45. What are the signs that death is near?

    A. _____

    B. _____

    C. _____

    D. _____

    E. _____

    F. _____

46. The signs of death include no _____. The _____ pupils are _____ and _____.

47. When assisting with post-mortem care, you need this information from the nurse.

    A. _____

    B. _____

    C. _____

    D. _____

    E. _____

48. The Dying Patient's Bill of Last Rights are the Right to

    A. _____

    B. _____

    C. _____

    D. _____

    E. _____

    F. _____

    G. _____

    H. _____

    I. _____

Use Focus on PRIDE in the Textbook to complete questions 49–51.

49. You are giving quality care to a dying person when you

    A. _____

    B. _____

    C. _____

    D. _____

50. According to OBRA, the right to confidentiality before and after death means that _____

    _____.

51. When a dying person refuses treatment, the health team must respect these choices because of the person's right to _____.

Optional Learning Exercises

You are assigned to care for Mrs. Adams, who is dying. Answer the questions regarding this situation.

52. You find Mrs. Adams crying in her room. When you ask her what is wrong, she tells you no one gave her fresh water this morning and she has not had her bath yet. She tells you just to go away. What stage of dying is she displaying? _____

53. Later in the day, Mrs. Adams tells you she can't wait until she is better to go home and plant her garden. She states that she knows the tests done last week were wrong and she will recover quickly from her illness. Now what stage is she displaying? _____. Why is she displaying 2 different stages so rapidly? _____

    _____

54. A minister comes to visit Mrs. Adams while you are giving care. What should you do? _____

55. You are working one night and find Mrs. Adams awake during the night. She asks you to sit with her. She begins to talk about her fears, worries, and anxieties. What are 2 things you can do to convey caring to her? _____

56. As Mrs. Adams becomes weaker, a family member is always at her bedside. When they ask to assist with her care, you know that this is acceptable because

    _____

57. Mrs. Adams dies while you are working, and the nurse asks you to assist with post-mortem care. As you clean soiled areas, you assist the nurse to turn the body and air is expelled. This occurs because

    _____

    _____

    _____.

58. You wear gloves during post-mortem care to protect you from _____.

Independent Learning Activities

It is important to explore your own beliefs about death and dying before you care for persons who are dying. Answer these questions to understand your own feelings.

- Have you attended a funeral or visited a funeral home? How did you feel?
- Has anyone close to you died? How did you assist with any of the funeral arrangements? What kinds of preparation did the family do?
- What cultural or religious practices in your family affect death and funeral arrangements? How do you think these practices will affect you when you care for those who are dying?

- Have you ever been present when someone died? In your personal life? As a student? At your job? How did you respond? What were you asked to do in this situation?
- What is your personal belief about a living will? How will you respond if a person or family refuses a feeding tube or a ventilator? How will you respond if they ask to have these measures discontinued and the person dies?
- What is your personal belief about a "Do Not Resuscitate" order? How would you feel if a person you are caring for has this order? How will you respond when the person dies and no effort is made to help the person?

Procedure Checklists

Relieving Choking—Adult or Child (Over 1 Year of Age)

Name: _____   Date: _____

Procedure	S	U	Comments

Procedure

1. Asked the person if he or she was choking.
   Helped if he or she nodded "yes" and could not talk.   _____ _____ _____
2. Called or had someone call for help.
   a. *In a public area:*
      (1) Had someone activate the EMS system by calling 911.   _____ _____ _____
      (2) Sent someone to get an automated external defibrillator (AED).   _____ _____ _____
   b. *In an agency:*
      (1) Had someone call the rapid response team (RRT).   _____ _____ _____
      (2) Sent someone to get the AED.   _____ _____ _____
3. *If person was standing or sitting,* gave abdominal thrusts:
   a. Stood or kneeled behind the person.   _____ _____ _____
   b. Wrapped your arms around the person's waist.   _____ _____ _____
   c. Made a fist with one hand.   _____ _____ _____
   d. Placed thumb side of fist against the abdomen.
      The fist was in the middle above the navel and well below the end of the sternum (breastbone).   _____ _____ _____
   e. Grasped the fist with other hand.   _____ _____ _____
   f. Pressed fist into the person's abdomen with a quick, upward thrust.   _____ _____ _____
   g. Repeated thrusts until the object was expelled or the person became unresponsive.   _____ _____ _____
4. *If the person was lying down but responsive,* gave abdominal thrusts:
   a. Straddled the person's thighs.   _____ _____ _____
   b. Placed the heel of one hand against the abdomen.
      It was in the middle slightly above the navel and well below the end of the sternum (breastbone).   _____ _____ _____
   c. Placed your second hand on top of your first hand.   _____ _____ _____
   d. Pressed both hands into the abdomen with a quick, upward thrust.   _____ _____ _____
   e. Repeated thrusts until the object was expelled or the person was unresponsive.   _____ _____ _____
5. *If the object was dislodged,* encouraged the person to go to the hospital. Injuries could have occurred from abdominal thrusts.   _____ _____ _____
6. *If the person became unresponsive:*
   Lowered the person to the floor or ground. Positioned the person supine (laid flat on the back). Made sure EMS or the RRT was called. If alone, provided 5 cycles (2 minutes) of CPR first. Then called EMS or RRT.   _____ _____ _____

Date of Satisfactory Completion _____   Instructor's Initials _____

Procedure—cont'd	**S**	**U**	**Comments**
7. Started CPR.			
a. Did not check for pulse. Began compressions. Gave 30 compressions.	_____	_____	_____
b. Used head tilt-chin lift method to open airway. Opened the person's mouth. Mouth was wide open. Looked for an object. Removed the object if you saw it and could remove it easily. Used your fingers.	_____	_____	_____
c. Gave 2 breaths.	_____	_____	_____
d. Continued cycles of 30 compressions and 2 breaths. Looked for an object every time you opened the airway for rescue breaths.	_____	_____	_____
8. *If you relieved choking in an unresponsive person:*			
a. Checked for a response, breathing, and a pulse.	_____	_____	_____
(1) *If no response, normal breathing, or pulse*–continued CPR. Attached an AED.	_____	_____	_____
(2) *If no response and no normal breathing but there is a pulse*–gave rescue breaths. For an adult, gave 1 breath every 5 to 6 seconds (10 to 12 breaths per minute). For a child, gave 1 breath every 3 to 5 seconds (12 to 20 breaths per minute). Checked for pulse every 2 minutes. If no pulse, began CPR.	_____	_____	_____
(3) *If the person had normal breathing and a pulse*–placed the person in the recovery position if there was no response. Continued to check the person until help arrived. Encouraged the person to go to the hospital if the person responded.	_____	_____	_____

Date of Satisfactory Completion _____   Instructor's Initials _____

Relieving Choking—In The Infant (Less Than 1 Year of Age)

Name: _____   Date: _____

Procedure	S	U	Comments
1. Had someone call for help:			
a. *In a public area,* had someone call the EMS system by calling 911. Sent someone to get AED.	___	___	_____
b. *In an agency,* had someone call the RRT and get a defribrillator (AED).	___	___	_____
2. Knelt next to the infant. Or sat with the infant in your lap.	___	___	_____
3. Exposed the infant's chest and back. Performed this step if it was done easily.	___	___	_____
4. Held the infant face down over your forearm. (Supported your arm on your thigh or lap.) The infant's head was lower than the trunk. Supported the head and jaw with your hand.	___	___	_____
5. Gave up to 5 forceful back slaps (back blows). Used the heel of your hand. Gave the back slaps between the shoulder blades. (Stopped the back slaps if the object was expelled.)	___	___	_____
6. Turned the infant as a unit:			
a. Continued to support the infant's face, jaw, head, neck, and chest with one hand.	___	___	_____
b. Supported the back and the back of the infant's head with your other hand. Your palm supported the back of the head.	___	___	_____
c. Turned the infant as a unit. The infant was in a back-lying position on your forearm. Your forearm rested on your thigh. The infant's head was lower than the trunk.	___	___	_____
7. Gave up to 5 chest thrusts. The chest thrusts were quick and downward.			
a. Located hand position as for chest compressions. The location was just below the nipple line.	___	___	_____
b. Gave chest thrusts at a rate of about 1 every second.	___	___	_____
c. Stopped chest thrusts if the object was expelled.	___	___	_____
8. Continued giving 5 back slaps followed by 5 chest thrusts until:			
a. The object was expelled.	___	___	_____
b. The infant became unresponsive.	___	___	_____
9. Did the following if the infant became unresponsive:			
a. Sent someone to activate EMS system or RRT if not already done. If alone, did so after 2 minutes of CPR.	___	___	_____
b. Placed infant on a firm, flat surface.	___	___	_____
c. Started CPR. Began with compressions. Gave 30 compressions.	___	___	_____
d. Opened the airway. Used head tilt-chin method. Opened the infant's mouth. Looked for object. Removed the object if you saw it and could remove it easily. Used your fingers.	___	___	_____
e. Give 2 breaths.	___	___	_____
f. Continued cycles of 30 compressions and 2 breaths. Looked for object each time you opened the airway.	___	___	_____
g. Continued CPR until help arrived or until choking is relieved.	___	___	_____

Date of Satisfactory Completion _____   Instructor's Initials _____

Using a Fire Extinguisher

Name: _____   Date: _____

Procedure	S	U	Comments
1. Pulled the fire alarm.	____	____	_____
2. Got the nearest fire extinguisher.	____	____	_____
3. Carried it upright.	____	____	_____
4. Took it to the fire.	____	____	_____
5. Followed the word *PASS:*			
a. *P* – for pulled the safety pin. This unlocked the handle.	____	____	_____
b. *A* – for aimed low. Directed the hose or nozzle at the base of the fire. Did not try to spray the tops of the flames.	____	____	_____
c. *S* – for squeezed the lever. Squeezed or push down on the lever, handle, or button to start the stream. Released the lever, handle, or button to stop the stream.	____	____	_____
d. *S* – for swept back and forth. Swept the stream back and forth (side to side) at the base of the fire.	____	____	_____

Date of Satisfactory Completion _____   Instructor's Initials _____

Applying a Transfer/Gait Belt

Name: _____   Date: _____

Quality of Life	S	U	Comments

Remembered to:
- Knock before entering the person's room
- Address the person by name
- Introduce yourself by name and title
- Explain the procedure to the person before beginning and during the procedure
- Protect the person's rights during the procedure
- Handle the person gently during the procedure

Procedure

1. Reviewed *Promoting Safety and Comfort: Transfer/Gait Belts.*
2. Practiced hand hygiene.
3. Identified the person. Checked the indentification (ID) bracelet against the assignment sheet. Called the person by name.
4. Provided for privacy.
5. Assisted the person to a sitting position.
6. Applied the belt:
   a. Wrapped the belt around the person's waist. Applied the belt over clothing. Did not apply it over bare skin.
   b. Inserted the belt's metal tip into the buckle. Passed the belt through the side with the teeth first.
   c. Brought the belt tip across the front of the buckle. Inserted the tip through the buckle's smooth side.
7. Tightened the belt so it was snug. It should not have caused discomfort or impaired breathing. You were able to slide your open, flat hand under the belt. Asked the person about his or her comfort.
8. Made sure that a woman's breasts were not caught under the belt.
9. Placed the buckle off center in the front or off center in the back for the person's comfort. The buckle was not over the spine.
10. Tucked any excess strap into the belt.

Date of Satisfactory Completion _____   Instructor's Initials _____

Helping the Falling Person

Name: _____   Date: _____

Procedure	S	U	Comments
1. Stood behind the person with your feet apart. Kept your back straight.	_____	_____	_____
2. Brought the person close to your body as fast as possible. Used the transfer/gait belt. Or wrapped your arms around the person's waist. If necessary, you held the person under the arms.	_____	_____	_____
3. Moved your leg so the person's buttocks rested on it. Moved the leg near the person.	_____	_____	_____
4. Lowered the person to the floor. The person slid down your leg to the floor. You were bent at your hips and knees as you lowered the person.	_____	_____	_____
5. Called a nurse to check the person. Stayed with the person.	_____	_____	_____
6. Helped the nurse return the person to bed. Asked other staff to help if needed.	_____	_____	_____

Post-Procedure

	S	U	Comments
7. Provided for comfort.	_____	_____	_____
8. Placed the signal light within reach.	_____	_____	_____
9. Raised or lowered the bed rails. Followed the care plan.	_____	_____	_____
10. Completed a safety check of the room.	_____	_____	_____
11. Practiced hand hygiene.	_____	_____	_____
12. Reported and recorded the following:			
• How the fall occurred	_____	_____	_____
• How far the person walked.	_____	_____	_____
• How activity was tolerated before the fall.	_____	_____	_____
• Complaints before the fall.	_____	_____	_____
• How much help the person needed while walking.	_____	_____	_____
13. Completed an incident report.	_____	_____	_____

Date of Satisfactory Completion _____   Instructor's Initials _____

Applying Restraints

Name: _____   Date: _____

Quality of Life	S	U	Comments

Remembered to:
- Knock before entering the person's room
- Address the person by name
- Introduce yourself by name and title
- Explain the procedure to the person before beginning and during the procedure
- Protect the person's rights during the procedure
- Handle the person gently during the procedure

Pre-Procedure

1. Followed *Delegation Guidelines: Applying Restraints.* Reviewed *Promoting Safety and Comfort: Applying Restraints.*
2. Collected the following as instructed by the nurse:
   a. Correct type and size of restraints
   b. Padding for skin and bony areas
   c. Bed rail pads or gap protectors (if needed)
3. Practiced hand hygiene.
4. Identified the person. Checked the ID bracelet against the assignment sheet. Called the person by name.
5. Provided for privacy.

Procedure

6. Made sure the person was comfortable and in good alignment.
7. Put the bed rail pads or gap protectors (if needed) on the bed if the person was in bed. Followed the manufacturer's instructions.
8. Padded bony areas. Followed the nurse's instructions and the care plan.
9. Read the manufacturer's instructions. Noted the front and back of the restraint.
10. *For wrist restraints:*
    a. Applied the restraint following the manufacturer's instructions. Placed the soft part or foam part toward the skin.
    b. Secured the restraint so it was snug but not tight. Made sure you could slide 1 finger under the restraint. Followed the manufacturer's instructions. Adjusted the straps if the restraint was too loose or too tight. Checked for snugness again.
    c. Secured the straps to the movable part of the bed frame out of the person's reach. Used the buckle or quick-release tie.
    d. Repeated steps for the other wrist.
       (1) Applied the restraint following the manufacturer's instructions. Placed the soft or foam part toward the skin.
       (2) Secured the restraint so it is snug but not tight. Made sure you could slide 1 finger under the restraint. Followed the manufacturer's instructions. Adjusted the straps if the restraint was too loose or too tight. Checked for snugness again.
       (3) Secured the straps to the movable part of the bed frame out of the person's reach. Used the buckle or a quick-release tie.

Date of Satisfactory Completion _____   Instructor's Initials _____

Procedure—cont'd	**S**	**U**	**Comments**

11. *For mitt restraints:*
   a. Made sure the person's hands were clean and dry.
   b. Inserted the person's hand into the restraint with the palm down. Followed the manufacturer's instructions.
   c. Secured the restraint to the bed if directed by the nurse. Secured the straps to the movable part of the bed frame. Used the buckle or a quick-release tie.
   d. Made sure the restraint was snug. Slid 1 finger between the restraint and the wrist. Followed the manufacturer's instructions. Adjusted the straps if the restraint was too loose or too tight. Checked for snugness again.
   e. Repeated steps for the other hand.
      (1) Inserted the person's hand into the restraint with the palm down. Followed the manufacturer's instructions.
      (2) Secured the restraint to the bed if directed to do so by the nurse. Secured the straps to the movable part of the bed frame. Used the buckle or a quick-release tie.
      (3) Made sure the restraint was snug. Slid 1 finger between the restraint and the wrist. Followed the manufacturer's instructions. Adjusted the straps if the restraint was too loose or too tight. Checked for snugness again.
12. *For a belt restraint:*
   a. Assisted the person to a sitting position.
   b. Applied the restraint following the manufacturer's instructions.
   c. Removed wrinkles or creases from the front and back of the restraint.
   d. Brought the ties through the slots in the belt.
   e. Positioned the straps at a 45-degree angle between the wheelchair seat and sides. Or helped the person lie down if he or she was in bed.
   f. Made sure the person was comfortable and in alignment.
   g. Secured the straps to the movable part of the bed frame out of the person's reach or to the chair or wheelchair. Used the buckle or quick-release tie. The buckle or tie was out of the person's reach. For a wheelchair, criss-crossed and secured the straps.
   h. Made sure the belt was snug. Slid an open hand between the restraint and the person. Adjusted the restraint if it was too loose or too tight. Checked for snugness again.
13. *For a vest restraint:*
   a. Assisted the person to a sitting position. If the person was in a wheelchair:
      (1) Position the person as far back in the wheelchair as possible.
      (2) Made sure the buttocks were against the chairback.
   b. Applied the restraint and followed the manufacturer's instructions. The "V" part of the vest crossed in front.
   c. Brought the straps through the slots.
   d. Positioned the straps at a 45-degree angle between the wheelchair seat and sides. (Omitted this step if the person was in bed.)
   e. Made sure the vest was free of wrinkles in the front and back.
   f. Helped the person to lie down if he or she was in bed.
   g. Made sure the person was comfortable and in good alignment.
   h. Secured the straps to the movable part of the bed frame at waist level. Used the buckle or quick-release tie. The buckle or tie was out of the person's reach. For a wheelchair, criss-crossed and secured the straps.

Date of Satisfactory Completion _____   Instructor's Initials _____

Procedure—cont'd	S	U	Comments

14. *For a jacket restraint:*

a. Assisted the person to a sitting position. Or if the person was in a wheelchair:

    (1) Positioned the person as far back in the wheelchair as possible.

    (2) Made sure the buttocks were against the chair back

b. Applied the restraint and followed the manufacturer's instructions. Remembered the jacket opening goes in the back.

c. Closed the back with the zipper, ties, or hook and loop closures.

d. Made sure the side seams are under the arms. Removed any wrinkles in the front and back.

e. Positioned the straps at a 45-degree angle between the wheelchair seat and sides. Or helped the person lie down if in bed.

f. Made sure the person was comfortable and in good alignment.

g. Secured the straps to the chair or to the movable part of the bed frame at waist level. Used the buckle or a quick-release tie. The buckle or tie was out of the person's reach. For a wheelchair, criss-crossed and secured the straps.

h. Made sure the jacket was snug. Slid an open hand between the restraint and the person. Adjusted the restraint if it was too tight. Checked for snugness again.

Post-Procedure

15. Positioned the person as the nurse directs.

16. Provided for comfort.

17. Placed the signal light within the person's reach.

18. Raised or lowered bed rails. Followed the care plan and the manufacturer's instructions for the restraint.

19. Unscreened the person.

20. Completed a safety check of the room.

21. Practiced hand hygiene.

22. Checked the person and the restraint at least every 15 minutes. Reported and recorded your observations:

a. For wrist and mitt restraints: checked the pulse, color, and temperature of the restrained parts.

b. For vest, jacket, and belt restraints: checked the person's breathing. *Called for the nurse at once if the person was not breathing or was having problems breathing.* Made sure the restraint was properly positioned in the front and back.

23. Did the following at least every 2 hours for at least 10 minutes:

a. Removed or released the restraint.

b. Measured vital signs.

c. Re-positioned the person.

d. Met food, fluid, hygiene, and elimination needs.

e. Gave skin care.

f. Performed range-of-motion exercises or helped the person walk. Followed the care plan.

g. Provided for physical and emotional comfort.

h. Re-applied the restraints.

24. Completed a safety check of the room.

25. Practiced hand hygiene.

26. Reported and recorded your observations and the care given.

Date of Satisfactory Completion _____   Instructor's Initials _____

Hand Washing (NNAAP®)

Name: _____   Date: _____

Procedure	S	U	Comments
1. Reviewed *Promoting Safety and Comfort: Hand Hygiene.*	_____	_____	_____
2. Made sure you had soap, paper towels, an orange stick or nail file, and a wastebasket. Collected missing items.	_____	_____	_____
3. Pushed your watch up your arm 4 to 5 inches. If your uniform sleeves were long, pushed them up too.	_____	_____	_____
4. Stood away from the sink so your clothes did not touch the sink. Stood so the soap and faucet were easy to reach. Did not touch the inside of the sink at any time.	_____	_____	_____
5. Turned on and adjusted the water until it felt warm.	_____	_____	_____
6. Wet your wrists and hands. Kept your hands lower than your elbows. Was sure to wet the area 3 to 4 inches above your wrists.	_____	_____	_____
7. Applied about 1 teaspoon of soap to your hands.	_____	_____	_____
8. Rubbed your palms together and interlaced your fingers to work up a good lather. Lathered your wrists, hands, and fingers. Kept your hands lower than your elbows. This step lasted at least 15 to 20 seconds.	_____	_____	_____
9. Washed each hand and wrist thoroughly. Cleaned the back of your fingers and between your fingers.	_____	_____	_____
10. Cleaned under the fingernails. Rubbed your fingertips against your palms.	_____	_____	_____
11. Cleaned under fingernails with a nail file or orange stick. This step was done for the first hand washing of the day and when hands were highly soiled.	_____	_____	_____
12. Rinsed your wrists, hands, and fingers well. Water flowed from your wrists to your fingertips.	_____	_____	_____
13. Repeated, if needed:			
a. Applied about 1 teaspoon of soap to your hands.	_____	_____	_____
b. Rubbed your palms together and interlaced your fingers to work up a good lather. This step lasted at least 15 to 20 seconds.	_____	_____	_____
c. Washed each hand and wrist thoroughly. Cleaned the back of your fingers and between your fingers.	_____	_____	_____
d. Cleaned under the fingernails. Rubbed your fingertips against your palms.	_____	_____	_____
e. Cleaned under the fingernails with a nail file or orange stick. This step was done for the first hand washing of the day and when your hands were highly soiled.	_____	_____	_____
f. Rinsed your wrists and hands well. Water flowed from your wrists to your fingertips.	_____	_____	_____
14. Dried your wrists and hands well with clean, dry paper towels. Patted dry. Started at fingertips.	_____	_____	_____
15. Discarded the paper towels into the wastebasket.	_____	_____	_____
16. Turned off faucets with clean, dry paper towels. This prevented you from contaminating your hands. Used a clean paper towel for each faucet or used knee or foot controls to turn off the faucet.	_____	_____	_____
17. Discarded the paper towels into the wastebasket.	_____	_____	_____

Date of Satisfactory Completion _____   Instructor's Initials _____

Using an Alcohol-Based Hand Rub

Name: _____   Date: _____

Procedure

	S	U	Comments
1. Reviewed *Promoting Safety and Comfort: Hand Hygiene*.	___	___	_____
2. Applied a palmful of an alcohol-based rub into a cupped hand.	___	___	_____
3. Rubbed palms together.	___	___	_____
4. Rubbed the palm of one hand over the back of the other. Did the same for the other hand.	___	___	_____
5. Rubbed your palms together with your fingers interlaced.	___	___	_____
6. Interlocked your fingers. Rubbed your fingers back and forth.	___	___	_____
7. Rubbed the thumb of one hand in the palm of the other hand. Used a circular motion. Did the same for the fingers on the other hand.	___	___	_____
8. Rubbed the fingers of one hand into the palm of the other hand. Used a circular motion. Did the same for the fingers of the other hand.	___	___	_____
9. Continued rubbing your hands until they were dry.	___	___	_____

Date of Satisfactory Completion _____   Instructor's Initials _____

Removing Gloves (NNAAP®)

Name: _____   Date: _____

Procedure	S	U	Comments
1. Reviewed *Promoting Safety and Comfort: Gloves.*	___	___	_____
2. Made sure that glove only touched glove.	___	___	_____
3. Grasped a glove at the palm. Grasped it on the outside.	___	___	_____
4. Pulled the glove down over your hand so it was inside out.	___	___	_____
5. Held the removed glove with your other gloved hand.	___	___	_____
6. Reached inside the other glove. Used the first two fingers of the ungloved hand.	___	___	_____
7. Pulled the glove down (inside out) over your hand and the other glove.	___	___	_____
8. Discarded the gloves. Followed agency policy.	___	___	_____
9. Practiced hand hygiene.	___	___	_____

Date of Satisfactory Completion _____   Instructor's Initials _____

Donning and Removing a Gown (NNAAP®)

Name: _____   Date: _____

Procedure	S	U	Comments
1. Removed your watch and all jewelry.			
2. Rolled up uniform sleeves.			
3. Practiced hand hygiene.			
4. Held a clean gown out in front of you. Allowed it to unfold. Did not shake the gown.			
5. Put your hands and arms through the sleeves.			
6. Made sure the gown covered you from your neck to your knees. It covered your arms to the end of your wrists.			
7. Tied the strings at the back of the neck.			
8. Overlapped the back of the gown. Made sure it covered your uniform. The gown was snug, not loose.			
9. Tied the waist strings. Tied them at the back or the side. Did not tie them in front.			
10. Put on other PPE.			
a. Mask or respirator (if needed).			
b. Goggles or face shield (if needed).			
c. Gloves. Made sure gloves covered gown cuff.			
11. Provided care.			
12. Removed and discarded the gloves.			
13. Removed and discarded the goggles or face shield if worn.			
14. Removed the gown. Did not touch outside of gown.			
a. Untied the neck and waist strings.			
b. Pulled the gown down from each shoulder toward the same hand.			
c. Turned the gown inside out as it was removed. Held it at the inside shoulder seams and brought your hands together.			
15. Held and rolled up the gown away from you. Kept it inside out. Did not let the gown touch the floor.			
16. Discarded the gown.			
17. Removed and discarded the mask if worn.			
18. Practiced hand hygiene.			

Date of Satisfactory Completion _____   Instructor's Initials _____

VIDEO Donning and Removing a Mask

Name: _____   Date: _____

Procedure	S	U	Comments
1. Practiced hand hygiene.	____	____	_____
2. Put on a gown if required.	____	____	_____
3. Picked up a mask by its upper ties. Did not touch the part that covered your face.	____	____	_____
4. Placed the mask over your nose and mouth.	____	____	_____
5. Placed the upper strings above your ears. Tied them at the back in the middle of your head.	____	____	_____
6. Tied the lower strings at the back of your neck. The lower part of the mask was under your chin.	____	____	_____
7. Pinched the metal band around your nose. The top of the mask was snug over your nose. If you wore eyeglasses, the mask was snug under the bottom of the eyeglasses.	____	____	_____
8. Made sure the mask was snug over your face and under your chin.	____	____	_____
9. Put on goggles or a face shield if needed and not part of the mask.	____	____	_____
10. Put on gloves.	____	____	_____
11. Provided care. Avoided coughing, sneezing, and unnecessary talking.	____	____	_____
12. Changed the mask if it became wet or contaminated.	____	____	_____
13. Removed and discarded the gloves. Removed the goggles or face shield and gown if worn.	____	____	_____
14. Removed the mask.			
a. Untied the lower strings of the mask.	____	____	_____
b. Untied the top strings.	____	____	_____
c. Held the top strings. Removed the mask.	____	____	_____
15. Discarded the mask.	____	____	_____
16. Practiced hand hygiene.	____	____	_____

Date of Satisfactory Completion _____   Instructor's Initials _____

Double-Bagging

Name: _____   Date: _____

Procedure	S	U	Comments
1. Asked a co-worker to help you.			
2. Placed soiled linen, re-usable items, disposable supplies, and trash in the right containers. Containers were lined with leak-proof *BIOHAZARD* bags.			
3. Sealed the bags securely.			
4. Asked your co-worker to make a wide cuff on the clean bag. It was held wide open. The cuff protected the hands from contamination.			
5. Placed the contaminated bag into the clean bag. Did not touch the outside of the clean bag.			
6. Asked co-worker to seal bag. Had the bag labeled according to agency policy.			
7. Repeated steps for other contaminated bags:			
a. Asked your co-worker to make a wide cuff on the clean bag. It was held wide open. The cuff protected the hands from contamination.			
b. Placed the contaminated bag into the clean bag. Did not touch the outside of the bag.			
c. Asked co-worker to seal bag. Had the bag labeled according to agency policy.			
8. Asked co-worker to take or send the bags to appropriate department for disposal, disinfection, or sterilization.			

Date of Satisfactory Completion _____   Instructor's Initials _____

Sterile Gloving

Name: _____   Date: _____

Procedure	S	U	Comments
1. Followed *Delegation Guidelines: Assisting With Sterile Procedures.* Reviewed *Promoting Safety and Comfort:*			
a. *Assisting With Sterile Procedures*	___	___	_____
b. *Sterile Gloving*	___	___	_____
2. Practiced hand hygiene.	___	___	_____
3. Inspected the package of sterile gloves for sterility.			
a. Checked the expiration date.	___	___	_____
b. Saw if the package was dry.	___	___	_____
c. Checked for tears, holes, punctures, and watermarks.	___	___	_____
4. Arranged a work surface.			
a. Made sure you had enough room.	___	___	_____
b. Arranged the work surface at waist level and within your vision.	___	___	_____
c. Cleaned and dried the work surface.	___	___	_____
d. Did not reach over or turn your back on the work surface.	___	___	_____
5. Opened the package. Grasped the flaps. Gently peeled them back.	___	___	_____
6. Removed the inner package. Placed it on the work surface.	___	___	_____
7. Read the manufacturer's instructions on the inner package. It may be labeled with *left, right, up,* and *down.*	___	___	_____
8. Arranged the inner package for left, right, up, and down. The left glove was on your left. The right glove was on your right. The cuffs were near you with the fingers pointing away from you.	___	___	_____
9. Grasped the folded edges of the inner package. Used the thumb and index finger of each hand.	___	___	_____
10. Folded back the inner package to expose the gloves. Did not touch or otherwise contaminate the inside of the package or the gloves. The inside of the inner package is a sterile field.	___	___	_____
11. Noted that each glove had a cuff about 2 to 3 inches wide. The cuffs and insides of the gloves are *not considered sterile.*	___	___	_____
12. Put on the right glove, if you were right handed. Put on the left glove if you were left handed.			
a. Picked up the glove with your other hand. Used your thumb, index, and middle fingers.	___	___	_____
b. Touched only the cuff and inside of the glove.	___	___	_____
c. Turned the hand to be gloved palm side up.	___	___	_____
d. Lifted the cuff up. Slid your fingers and hand into the glove.	___	___	_____
e. Pulled the glove up over your hand. If some fingers got stuck, left them that way until the other glove was on. *Did not use your ungloved hand to straighten the glove. Did not let the outside of the glove touch any non-sterile surface.*	___	___	_____
f. Left the cuff turned down.	___	___	_____
13. Put on the other glove. Used your gloved hand.			
a. Reached under the cuff of the second glove. Used the four fingers of your gloved hand. Kept your gloved thumb close to your gloved palm.	___	___	_____
b. Pulled on the second glove. Your gloved hand did not touch the cuff or any surface. Held the thumb of your first gloved hand away from the gloved palm.	___	___	_____
14. Adjusted each glove with the other hand. The gloves were smooth and comfortable.	___	___	_____
15. Slid your fingers under the cuffs to pull them up.	___	___	_____
16. Touched only sterile items.	___	___	_____
17. Removed and discarded the gloves.	___	___	_____
18. Practiced hand hygiene.	___	___	_____

Date of Satisfactory Completion _____   Instructor's Initials _____

Raising the Person's Head and Shoulders

Name: _____   Date: _____

Quality of Life	S	U	Comments
Remembered to:			
• Knock before entering the person's room	___	___	_____
• Address the person by name	___	___	_____
• Introduce yourself by name and title	___	___	_____
• Explain the procedure to the person before beginning and during the procedure	___	___	_____
• Protect the person's rights during the procedure	___	___	_____
• Handle the person gently during the procedure	___	___	_____

Pre-Procedure

1. Followed *Delegation Guidelines:*
   a. *Preventing Work-Related Injuries* ___ ___ _____
   b. *Moving Persons in Bed* ___ ___ _____
   Reviewed *Promoting Safety and Comfort:*
   a. *Safe Resident Handling, Moving, and Transfers* ___ ___ _____
   b. *Preventing Work-Related Injuries* ___ ___ _____
2. Asked a co-worker to assist if needed help. ___ ___ _____
3. Practiced hand hygiene. ___ ___ _____
4. Identified the person. Checked the ID bracelet against the assignment sheet. Called the person by name. ___ ___ _____
5. Provided for privacy. ___ ___ _____
6. Locked the bed wheels. ___ ___ _____
7. Raised the bed for good body mechanics. Bed rails were up if used. ___ ___ _____

Procedure

8. Had your co-worker stand on the other side of the bed. Lowered the bed rail if up. ___ ___ _____
9. Asked the person to put the near arm under your near arm and behind your shoulder. His or her hand rested on top of your shoulder. If you stood on the right side, the person's right hand rested on your shoulder. The person did the same with your co-worker. The person's left hand rested on your co-worker's left shoulder. ___ ___ _____
10. Put your arm nearest to the person under his or her arm. Your hand was on the person's shoulder. Your co-worker did the same. ___ ___ _____
11. Put your free arm under the person's neck and shoulders. Your co-worker did the same. Supported the neck. ___ ___ _____
12. Helped the person rise to a sitting or semi-sitting position on the "count of 3." ___ ___ _____
13. Used the arm and hand that supported the person's neck and shoulders to give care. Your co-worker supported the person. ___ ___ _____
14. Helped the person lie down. Provided support with your locked arm. Supported the person's neck and shoulders with your other arm. Your co-worker did the same. ___ ___ _____

Post-Procedure

15. Provided for comfort. ___ ___ _____
16. Placed the signal light within reach. ___ ___ _____
17. Lowered the bed to its lowest position. ___ ___ _____
18. Raised or lowered bed rails. Followed the care plan. ___ ___ _____
19. Unscreened the person. ___ ___ _____
20. Completed a safety check of the room. ___ ___ _____
21. Practiced hand hygiene. ___ ___ _____
22. Reported and recorded your observations. ___ ___ _____

Date of Satisfactory Completion _____   Instructor's Initials _____

Moving the Person Up in Bed

Name: _____   Date: _____

	S	U	Comments

Quality of Life

Remembered to:
- Knock before entering the person's room
- Address the person by name
- Introduce yourself by name and title
- Explain the procedure to the person before beginning and during the procedure
- Protect the person's rights during the procedure
- Handle the person gently during the procedure

Pre-Procedure

1. Followed *Delegation Guidelines:*
   a. *Preventing Work-Related Injuries*
   b. *Moving Persons in Bed*
   Reviewed *Promoting Safety and Comfort:*
   a. *Safely Handling, Moving, and Transferring Persons*
   b. *Preventing Work-Related Injuries*
   c. *Moving the Person Up in Bed*
2. Asked a co-worker to help.
3. Practiced hand hygiene.
4. Identified the person. Checked the ID bracelet against the assignment sheet. Called the person by name.
5. Provided for privacy.
6. Locked the bed wheels.
7. Raised the bed for good body mechanics. Bed rails were up if used.

Procedure

8. Lowered the head of the bed to a level appropriate for the person. It was as flat as possible.
9. Stood on one side of the bed. Your co-worker stood on the other side.
10. Lowered the bed rails if up.
11. Removed pillows as directed by the nurse. Placed a pillow upright against the headboard if the person could be without it.
12. Stood with a wide base of support. Pointed the foot near the head of the bed toward the head of the bed. Faced the head of the bed.
13. Bent your hips and knees. Kept your back straight.
14. Placed one arm under the person's shoulders and one arm under the thighs. Your co-worker did the same.
    Grasped each other's forearms.
15. Asked the person to grasp the trapeze.
16. Had the person flex both knees.
17. Explained that:
    a. You will count "1, 2, 3."
    b. The move will be on "3."
    c. On "3," the person pushes against the bed with their feet if able. And the person pulls up with the trapeze.
18. Moved the person to the head of the bed on the count of "3." Shifted your weight from your rear leg to your front leg. Your co-worker did the same.

Date of Satisfactory Completion _____   Instructor's Initials _____

Procedure—cont'd	S	U	Comments
19. Repeated steps 12 through 18 if necessary.			
a. Stood with a wide base of support. Pointed the foot near the head of the bed toward the head of the bed. Faced the head of the bed.	_____	_____	_____
b. Bent your hips and knees. Kept your back straight.	_____	_____	_____
c. Placed one arm under the person's shoulder and one arm under the thighs. Your co-worker did the same. Grasped each other's forearms.	_____	_____	_____
d. Asked the person to grasp the trapeze.	_____	_____	_____
e. Had the person flex both knees.	_____	_____	_____
f. Explained the following:			
• You will count "1, 2, 3."	_____	_____	_____
• The move will be on "3."	_____	_____	_____
• On "3," the person pushes against the bed with the feet if able. And the person pulls up with the trapeze.	_____	_____	_____
g. Moved the person to the head of the bed on the count of "3." Shifted your weight from your rear leg to your front leg. Your co-worker did the same.	_____	_____	_____

Post-Procedure

	S	U	Comments
20. Placed the pillow under the person's head and shoulders. Straightened linens.	_____	_____	_____
21. Positioned the person in good alignment. Raised the head of the bed to a level appropriate for the person.	_____	_____	_____
22. Provided for comfort.	_____	_____	_____
23. Placed the signal light within reach.	_____	_____	_____
24. Lowered the bed to its lowest position.	_____	_____	_____
25. Raised or lowered bed rails. Followed the care plan.	_____	_____	_____
26. Unscreened the person.	_____	_____	_____
27. Completed a safety check of the room.	_____	_____	_____
28. Practiced hand hygiene.	_____	_____	_____
29. Reported and recorded your observations.	_____	_____	_____

Date of Satisfactory Completion _____   Instructor's Initials _____

Moving the Person Up in Bed With an Assist Device

Name: _____   Date: _____

Quality of Life	S	U	Comments
Remembered to:			
• Knock before entering the person's room	____	____	_____
• Address the person by name	____	____	_____
• Introduce yourself by name and title	____	____	_____
• Explain the procedure to the person before beginning and during the procedure	____	____	_____
• Protect the person's rights during the procedure	____	____	_____
• Handle the person gently during the procedure	____	____	_____

Pre-Procedure

	S	U	Comments
1. Followed *Delegation Guidelines:*			
a. *Preventing Work-Related Injuries*	____	____	_____
b. *Moving Persons in Bed*	____	____	_____
Reviewed *Promoting Safety and Comfort:*			
a. *Safely Handling, Moving, and Transferring Persons*	____	____	_____
b. *Preventing Work-Related Injuries*	____	____	_____
c. *Moving the Person Up in Bed*	____	____	_____
d. *Moving the Person Up in Bed With an Assist Device*	____	____	_____
2. Asked a co-worker to help.	____	____	_____
3. Practiced hand hygiene.	____	____	_____
4. Identified the person. Checked the ID bracelet against the assignment sheet. Called the person by name.	____	____	_____
5. Provided for privacy.	____	____	_____
6. Locked the bed wheels.	____	____	_____
7. Raised the bed for good body mechanics. Bed rails were up if used.	____	____	_____

Procedure

	S	U	Comments
8. Lowered the head of the bed to a level appropriate for the person. It was as flat as possible.	____	____	_____
9. Stood on one side of the bed. Your co-worker stood on the other side.	____	____	_____
10. Lowered the bed rails if up.	____	____	_____
11. Removed pillows as directed by the nurse. Placed a pillow upright against the headboard if the person could be without it.	____	____	_____
12. Stood with a wide base of support. Pointed the foot near the head of the bed toward the head of the bed. Faced that direction.	____	____	_____
13. Rolled the sides of the assist device up close to the person. (NOTE: Omitted this step if the device had handles.)	____	____	_____
14. Grasped the rolled-up assist device firmly near the person's shoulders and hips. Or grasped it by the handles. Supported the head.	____	____	_____
15. Bent your hips and knees.	____	____	_____
16. Moved the person up in bed on the count of "3." Shifted your weight from your rear leg to your front leg.	____	____	_____

Date of Satisfactory Completion _____   Instructor's Initials _____

	S	U	Comments

Procedure—cont'd

17. Repeated steps 12 through 16 if necessary.
    a. Stood with a wide base of support. Pointed the foot near
       the head of the bed toward the head of the bed.
       Faced that direction.   ____ ____ _____
    b. Rolled the sides of the assist device up close to the person.
       (NOTE: Omitted this step if the device had handles.)   ____ ____ _____
    c. Grasped the rolled-up assist device firmly near
       the person's shoulders and hips. Or grasped it by
       the handles. Supported the head.   ____ ____ _____
    d. Bent your hips and knees.   ____ ____ _____
    e. Moved the person up in bed on the count of "3." Shifted
       your weight from your rear leg to your front leg.   ____ ____ _____
18. Unrolled the assist device. (NOTE: Omitted this step if
    the device had handles.)   ____ ____ _____

Post-Procedure

19. Put the pillow under the person's head and shoulders.   ____ ____ _____
20. Positioned the person in good alignment. Raised the head of
    the bed to a level appropriate for the person.   ____ ____ _____
21. Provided for comfort.   ____ ____ _____
22. Placed the signal light within reach.   ____ ____ _____
23. Lowered the bed to its lowest position.   ____ ____ _____
24. Raised or lowered bed rails. Followed the care plan.   ____ ____ _____
25. Unscreened the person.   ____ ____ _____
26. Completed a safety check of the room.   ____ ____ _____
27. Practiced hand hygiene.   ____ ____ _____
28. Reported and recorded your observations.   ____ ____ _____

Date of Satisfactory Completion _____   Instructor's Initials _____

Moving the Person to the Side of the Bed

Name: _____   Date: _____

Quality of Life	S	U	Comments

Remembered to:

- Knock before entering the person's room
- Address the person by name
- Introduce yourself by name and title
- Explain the procedure to the person before beginning and during the procedure
- Protect the person's rights during the procedure
- Handle the person gently during the procedure

Pre-Procedure

1. Followed *Delegation Guidelines:*
   a. *Preventing Work-Related Injuries*
   b. *Moving Persons in Bed*
   Reviewed *Promoting Safety and Comfort:*
   a. *Safely Handling, Moving, and Transferring Persons*
   b. *Preventing Work-Related Injuries*
   c. *Moving the Person to the Side of the Bed*
2. Asked 1 or 2 co-workers to help if using an assist device.
3. Practiced hand hygiene.
4. Identified the person. Checked the ID bracelet against the assignment sheet. Called the person by name.
5. Provided for privacy.
6. Locked the bed wheels.
7. Raised the bed for good body mechanics. Bed rails were up if used.

Procedure

8. Lowered the head of the bed to a level appropriate for the person. It was as flat as possible.
9. Stood on the side of the bed to which you moved the person.
10. Lowered the bed rails if bed rails were used. (Both bed rails were lowered for step 15.)
11. Removed pillows as directed by the nurse.
12. Stood with your feet about 12 inches apart. One foot was in front of the other. Flexed your knees.
13. Crossed the person's arms over the person's chest.
14. *Method 1: Moving the person in segments:*
    a. Placed your arm under the person's neck and shoulders. Grasped the far shoulder.
    b. Placed your other arm under the mid-back.
    c. Moved the upper part of the person's body toward you. Rocked backward and shifted your weight to your rear leg.
    d. Placed one arm under the person's waist and one under the thighs.
    e. Rocked backward to move the lower part of the person toward you.
    f. Repeated the procedure for the legs and feet. Your arms should have been under the person's thighs and calves.

Date of Satisfactory Completion _____   Instructor's Initials _____

Procedure—cont'd	**S**	**U**	**Comments**
15. *Method 2: Moving the person with a drawsheet:*			
a. Rolled up the drawsheet close to the person.	———	———	———————
b. Grasped the rolled-up drawsheet near the person's shoulders and hips. Your co-worker did the same. Supported the person's head.	———	———	———————
c. Rocked backward and on the count of "3" moved the person toward you. Your co-worker rocked backward slightly and then forward toward you with arms kept straight.	———	———	———————
d. Unrolled the drawsheet. Removed any wrinkles.	———	———	———————

Post-Procedure

	S	**U**	**Comments**
16. Positioned the person in good alignment.	———	———	———————
17. Provided for comfort.	———	———	———————
18. Placed the signal light within reach.	———	———	———————
19. Lowered the bed to its lowest position.	———	———	———————
20. Raised or lowered bed rails. Followed the care plan.	———	———	———————
21. Unscreened the person.	———	———	———————
22. Completed a safety check of the room.	———	———	———————
23. Practiced hand hygiene.	———	———	———————
24. Reported and recorded your observations.	———	———	———————

Date of Satisfactory Completion ————————————   Instructor's Initials ————————————

Turning and Re-Positioning the Person (NNAAP®)

Name: _____   Date: _____

Quality of Life	S	U	Comments
Remembered to:			
• Knock before entering the person's room	___	___	_____
• Address the person by name	___	___	_____
• Introduce yourself by name and title	___	___	_____
• Explain the procedure to the person before beginning and during the procedure	___	___	_____
• Protect the person's rights during the procedure	___	___	_____
• Handle the person gently during the procedure	___	___	_____

Pre-Procedure

1. Followed *Delegation Guidelines:*
   a. *Preventing Work-Related Injuries*   ___ ___ _____
   b. *Moving Persons in Bed*   ___ ___ _____
   c. *Turning Persons*   ___ ___ _____
   Reviewed *Promoting Safety and Comfort:*
   a. *Safely Handling, Moving, and Transferring Persons*   ___ ___ _____
   b. *Preventing Work-Related Injuries*   ___ ___ _____
   c. *Moving the Person to the Side of the Bed*   ___ ___ _____
   d. *Turning Persons*   ___ ___ _____
2. Practiced hand hygiene.   ___ ___ _____
3. Identified the person. Checked the ID bracelet against the assignment sheet. Called the person by name.   ___ ___ _____
4. Provided for privacy.   ___ ___ _____
5. Locked the bed wheels.   ___ ___ _____
6. Raised the bed for good body mechanics. Bed rails were up if used.   ___ ___ _____

Procedure

7. Lowered the head of the bed to a level appropriate for the person. It was as flat as possible.   ___ ___ _____
8. Stood on the side of the bed opposite to where you turned the person.   ___ ___ _____
9. Lowered the near bed rail.   ___ ___ _____
10. Moved the person to the side near you.   ___ ___ _____
11. Crossed the person's arms over the person's chest. Crossed the leg near you over the far leg.   ___ ___ _____
12. *Turned the person away from you:*
    a. Stood with a wide base of support. Flexed the knees.   ___ ___ _____
    b. Placed one hand on the person's shoulder. Placed the other on the hip near you.   ___ ___ _____
    c. Rolled the person gently away from you toward the raised bed rail. Shifted your weight from your rear leg to your front leg.   ___ ___ _____
13. *Turned the person toward you:*
    a. Raised the bed rail.   ___ ___ _____
    b. Went to the other side of the bed. Lowered the bed rail.   ___ ___ _____
    c. Stood with a wide base of support. Flexed your knees.   ___ ___ _____
    d. Placed one hand on the person's far shoulder. Placed the other on the far hip.   ___ ___ _____
    e. Rolled the person toward you gently.   ___ ___ _____

Date of Satisfactory Completion _____   Instructor's Initials _____

Procedure—cont'd	S	U	Comments

Procedure—cont'd

14. Positioned the person. Followed the nurse's directions, the care plan, and these common measures:
    a. Placed a pillow under the head and neck. ___ ___ _____
    b. Adjusted the shoulder. The person did not lie on an arm. ___ ___ _____
    c. Placed a pillow under the upper hand and arm. ___ ___ _____
    d. Positioned a pillow against the back. ___ ___ _____
    e. Flexed the upper knee. Positioned the upper leg in front of the lower leg. ___ ___ _____
    f. Supported the upper leg and thigh on pillows. Made sure the ankle was supported. ___ ___ _____

Post-Procedure

15. Provided for comfort. ___ ___ _____
16. Placed the signal light within reach. ___ ___ _____
17. Lowered the bed to its lowest position. ___ ___ _____
18. Raised or lowered bed rails. Followed the care plan. ___ ___ _____
19. Unscreened the person. ___ ___ _____
20. Completed a safety check of the room. ___ ___ _____
21. Practiced hand hygiene. ___ ___ _____
22. Reported and recorded your observations. ___ ___ _____

Date of Satisfactory Completion _____   Instructor's Initials _____

Logrolling the Person

Name: _____   Date: _____

Quality of Life	S	U	Comments
Remembered to:			
• Knock before entering the person's room	_____	_____	_____
• Address the person by name	_____	_____	_____
• Introduce yourself by name and title	_____	_____	_____
• Explain the procedure to the person before beginning and during the procedure	_____	_____	_____
• Protect the person's rights during the procedure	_____	_____	_____
• Handle the person gently during the procedure	_____	_____	_____

Pre-Procedure

1. Followed *Delegation Guidelines:*
   a. *Preventing Work-Related Injuries*   _____ _____ _____
   b. *Moving Persons in Bed*   _____ _____ _____
   c. *Turning Persons*   _____ _____ _____
   Reviewed *Promoting Safety and Comfort:*
   a. *Safely Handling, Moving, and Transferring Persons*   _____ _____ _____
   b. *Preventing Work-Related Injuries*   _____ _____ _____
   c. *Turning Persons*   _____ _____ _____
   d. *Logrolling*   _____ _____ _____
2. Asked a co-worker to help you.   _____ _____ _____
3. Practiced hand hygiene.   _____ _____ _____
4. Identified the person. Checked the ID bracelet against the assignment sheet. Called the person by name.   _____ _____ _____
5. Provided for privacy.   _____ _____ _____
6. Locked the bed wheels.   _____ _____ _____
7. Raised the bed for good body mechanics. Bed rails were up if used.   _____ _____ _____

Procedure

8. Made sure the bed was flat.   _____ _____ _____
9. Stood on the side opposite to which you turned the person. Your co-worker stood on the other side.   _____ _____ _____
10. Lowered the bed rails if used.   _____ _____ _____
11. Moved the person as a unit to the side of the bed near you. Used the assist device. (If person had spinal cord injury, assisted the nurse as directed.)   _____ _____ _____
12. Placed the person's arms across the chest. Placed a pillow between the knees.   _____ _____ _____
13. Raised the bed rail if used.   _____ _____ _____
14. Went to the other side.   _____ _____ _____
15. Stood near the shoulders and chest. Your co-worker stood near the hips and thighs.   _____ _____ _____
16. Stood with a broad base of support. One foot was in front of the other.   _____ _____ _____
17. Asked the person to hold his or her body rigid.   _____ _____ _____
18. Rolled the person toward you. Or used the assist device. Turned the person as a unit.   _____ _____ _____
19. Positioned the person in good alignment. Used pillows as directed by the nurse and the care plan. Followed these common measures (unless the spinal cord was involved):
    a. One pillow against the back for support   _____ _____ _____
    b. One pillow under the head and neck if allowed   _____ _____ _____
    c. One pillow or a folded bath blanket between the legs   _____ _____ _____
    d. A small pillow under the upper arm and hand   _____ _____ _____

Date of Satisfactory Completion _____   Instructor's Initials _____

Post-Procedure

20. Provided for comfort.
21. Placed the signal light within reach.
22. Lowered the bed to its lowest position.
23. Raised or lowered bed rails. Followed the care plan.
24. Unscreened the person.
25. Completed a safety check of the room.
26. Practiced hand hygiene.
27. Reported and recorded your observations.

Date of Satisfactory Completion _____ Instructor's Initials _____

Sitting on the Side of the Bed (Dangling)

Name: _____   Date: _____

Quality of Life	S	U	Comments

Remember to:
- Knock before entering the person's room
- Address the person by name
- Introduce yourself by name and title
- Explain the procedure to the person before beginning and during the procedure
- Protect the person's rights during the procedure
- Handle the person gently during the procedure

Pre-Procedure

1. Followed *Delegation Guidelines:*
   a. *Preventing Work-Related Injuries*
   b. *Dangling*
   Reviewed *Promoting Safety and Comfort:*
   a. *Safely Handling, Moving, and Transferring Persons*
   b. *Preventing Work-Related Injuries*
   c. *Dangling*
2. Asked a co-worker to assist you as needed.
3. Practiced hand hygiene.
4. Identified the person. Checked the ID bracelet against the assignment sheet. Called the person by name.
5. Provided for privacy.
6. Decided what side of the bed to use.
7. Moved furniture to provide moving space.
8. Locked the bed wheels.
9. Raised the bed for good body mechanics. Bed rails were up if used.

Procedure

10. Lowered the bed rail if up.
11. Positioned the person in a side-lying position facing you. The person laid on the strong side.
12. Raised the head of the bed to a sitting position.
13. Stood near the person's hips. Faced the foot of the bed.
14. Stood with your feet apart. The foot near the head of the bed was in front of the other foot.
15. Slid one arm under the person's neck and shoulders. Grasped the far shoulder. Placed your other hand over the thighs near the knees.
16. Pivoted toward the foot of the bed while moving the person's legs and feet over the side of the bed. As the legs went over the edge of the mattress, the trunk was upright.
17. Asked the person to hold onto the edge of the mattress. This supported the person in the sitting position. If possible, raised a half-length bed rail for the person to grasp. Raised the bed rail on the person's strong side. Had your co-worker support the person at all times.
18. Did not leave the person alone. Provided support at all times.
19. Checked the person's condition:
    a. Asked how the person felt. Asked if the person felt dizzy or light-headed.
    b. Checked pulse and respiration.
    c. Checked for difficulty breathing.
    d. Noted if the skin was pale or bluish in color *(cyanosis).*

Date of Satisfactory Completion _____   Instructor's Initials _____

Procedure—cont'd	S	U	Comments
20. Reversed the procedure to return the person to bed. (Or prepared to transfer the person to a chair or wheelchair. Lowered the bed to its lowest position so the person's feet were flat on the floor. Supported the person at all times.)	____	____	_____
21. Lowered the head of the bed after the person returned to bed. Helped him or her move to the center of the bed.	____	____	_____
22. Positioned the person in good alignment.	____	____	_____

Post-Procedure

	S	U	Comments
23. Provided for comfort.	____	____	_____
24. Placed the signal light within reach.	____	____	_____
25. Lowered the bed to its lowest position.	____	____	_____
26. Raised or lowered bed rails. Followed the care plan.	____	____	_____
27. Returned furniture to its proper place.	____	____	_____
28. Unscreened the person.	____	____	_____
29. Completed a safety check of the room.	____	____	_____
30. Practiced hand hygiene.	____	____	_____
31. Reported and recorded your observations.	____	____	_____

Date of Satisfactory Completion _____ Instructor's Initials _____

Transferring the Person to a Chair or Wheelchair (NNAAP®)

Name: _____   Date: _____

Quality of Life	S	U	Comments
Remembered to:			
• Knock before entering the person's room	_____	_____	_____
• Address the person by name	_____	_____	_____
• Introduce yourself by name and title	_____	_____	_____
• Explain the procedure to the person before beginning and during the procedure	_____	_____	_____
• Protect the person's rights during the procedure	_____	_____	_____
• Handle the person gently during the procedure	_____	_____	_____

Pre-Procedure

1. Followed *Delegation Guidelines:*
   a. *Preventing Work-Related Injuries*
   b. *Transferring Persons*
   Reviewed *Promoting Safety and Comfort:*
   a. *Transfer/Gait Belts*
   b. *Safely Handling, Moving, and Transferring Persons*
   c. *Preventing Work-Related Injuries*
   d. *Transferring Persons*
   e. *Bed to Chair or Wheelchair Transfers*
2. Collected:
   a. Wheelchair or arm chair
   b. Bath blanket
   c. Lap blanket
   d. Robe and non-skid footwear
   e. Paper or sheet
   f. Transfer belt (if needed)
   g. Seat cushion (if needed)
3. Practiced hand hygiene.
4. Identified the person. Checked the ID bracelet against the assignment sheet. Called the person by name.
5. Provided for privacy.
6. Decided what side of the bed to use. Moved furniture for a safe transfer.

Procedure

7. Raised the wheelchair footplates. Removed or swung front rigging out of the way if possible. Positioned the chair or wheelchair near the bed on the person's strong side.
   a. If at the head of the bed, it faced the foot of the bed.
   b. If at the foot of the bed, it faced the head of the bed.
   c. The armrest almost touched the bed.
8. Placed a folded bath blanket or cushion on the seat (if needed).
9. Locked the wheelchair wheels. Raised the footplates. Removed or swung the front rigging out of the way.
10. Lowered the bed to its lowest position. Locked the bed wheels.
11. Fan-folded top linens to the foot of the bed.
12. Placed the paper or sheet under the person's feet. (This protected the person's linens from the footwear.) Put footwear on the person.
13. Helped the person sit on the side of bed. His or her feet touched the floor.
14. Helped the person put on a robe.
15. Applied the transfer belt if needed. It was applied at the waist over clothing.

Date of Satisfactory Completion _____   Instructor's Initials _____

Procedure—cont'd	**S**	**U**	**Comments**

16. *Method 1: Using a transfer belt:*
    a. Stood in front of the person.
    b. Had the person hold onto the mattress.
    c. Made sure the person's feet were flat on the floor.
    d. Had the person lean forward.
    e. Grasped the transfer belt at each side. Grasped the handles or grasped the belt from underneath.
    f. Prevented the person from sliding or falling by doing one of the following:
       (1) Braced your knees against the person's knees. Blocked his or her feet with your feet.
       (2) Used the knee and foot of one leg to block the person's weak leg or foot. Placed your other foot slightly behind your own for balance.
       (3) Straddled your legs around the person's weak leg.
    g. Explained the following:
       (1) You will count "1, 2, 3."
       (2) The move will be on "3."
       (3) On "3," the person pushes down on the mattress and stands.
    h. Asked the person to push down on the mattress and to stand on the count of "3." Pulled the person to a standing position as you straightened your knees.
17. *Method 2: No transfer belt:* (NOTE: Use this method only if directed by the nurse and the care plan.)
    a. Followed steps 16, a-c:
       (1) Stood in front of the person.
       (2) Had the person hold onto the mattress.
       (3) Made sure the person's feet were flat on the floor.
    b. Placed your hands under the person's arms. Your hands were around the person's shoulder blades.
    c. Had the person lean forward.
    d. Prevented the person from sliding or falling by doing one of the following:
       (1) Braced your knees against the person's knees. Blocked his or her feet with your feet.
       (2) Used the knee and foot of one leg to block the person's weak leg or foot. Placed your other foot slightly behind you for balance.
       (3) Straddled your legs around the person's weak leg.
    e. Explained the "count of 3."
       (1) You will count "1, 2, 3."
       (2) The move will be on "3."
       (3) On "3," the person pushes down on the mattress and stands.
    f. Asked the person to push down on the mattress and to stand on the count of "3." Pulled the person up into a standing position as you straightened your knees.
18. Supported the person in the standing position. Held the transfer belt, or kept your hands around the person's shoulder blades. Continued to prevent the person from sliding or falling.
19. Turned the person so he or she could grasp the far arm of the chair or wheelchair. The legs touched the edge of the seat.
20. Continued to turn the person until the other armrest was grasped.
21. Lowered him or her into the chair or wheelchair as you bent your hips and knees. The person assisted by leaning forward and bending the elbows and knees.
22. Made sure the hips were to the back of the seat. Positioned person in good alignment.

Date of Satisfactory Completion _____   Instructor's Initials _____

Procedure—cont'd

	S	U	Comments
23. Attached the wheelchair front rigging. Positioned the person's feet on the wheelchair footplates.	___	___	_____
24. Covered the person's lap and legs with a lap blanket. Kept the blanket off the floor and the wheels.	___	___	_____
25. Removed the transfer belt if used.	___	___	_____
26. Positioned the chair as the person preferred. Locked the wheelchair wheels according to the care plan.	___	___	_____

Post-Procedure

	S	U	Comments
27. Provided for comfort.	___	___	_____
28. Placed the signal light within reach.	___	___	_____
29. Unscreened the person.	___	___	_____
30. Completed a safety check of the room.	___	___	_____
31. Practiced hand hygiene.	___	___	_____
32. Reported and recorded your observations.	___	___	_____

Date of Satisfactory Completion _____   Instructor's Initials _____

Transferring the Person from a Chair or Wheelchair to Bed

Name: _____   Date: _____

Procedure	S	U	Comments
Remembered to:			
• Knock before entering the person's room	___	___	_____
• Address the person by name	___	___	_____
• Introduce yourself by name and title	___	___	_____
• Explain the procedure to the person before beginning and during the procedure	___	___	_____
• Protect the person's rights during the procedure	___	___	_____
• Handle the person gently during the procedure	___	___	_____

Pre-Procedure

	S	U	Comments
1. Followed *Delegation Guidelines:*			
a. *Preventing Work-Related Injuries*	___	___	_____
b. *Transferring Persons*	___	___	_____
Reviewed *Promoting Safety and Comfort:*			
a. *Transfer/Gait Belts*	___	___	_____
b. *Safely Moving and Transferring Persons*	___	___	_____
c. *Preventing Work-Related Injuries*	___	___	_____
d. *Transferring Persons*	___	___	_____
e. *Bed to Chair or Wheelchair Transfers*	___	___	_____
2. Collected a transfer belt if needed.	___	___	_____
3. Practiced hand hygiene.	___	___	_____
4. Identified the person. Checked the ID bracelet against the assignment sheet. Called the person by name.	___	___	_____
5. Provided for privacy.	___	___	_____

Procedure

	S	U	Comments
6. Moved furniture for moving space.	___	___	_____
7. Raised the head of the bed to a sitting position. The bed is in the lowest position.	___	___	_____
8. Moved the signal light so it was on the strong side when the person was in bed.	___	___	_____
9. Positioned the chair or wheelchair so the person's strong side was next to the bed. Had a co-worker help you if necessary.	___	___	_____
10. Locked the wheelchair and the bed wheels.	___	___	_____
11. Removed and folded the lap blanket.	___	___	_____
12. Removed the person's feet from the footplates. Raised the footplates. Removed or swung the front rigging out of the way. (Person had on non-skid footwear).	___	___	_____
13. Applied the transfer belt (if needed).	___	___	_____
14. Made sure the person's feet were flat on the floor.	___	___	_____
15. Stood in front of the person.	___	___	_____
16. Asked the person to hold onto the armrest. (If directed by the nurse, placed your arms under the person's arms. Your hands were around the shoulder blades.)	___	___	_____
17. Had the person lean forward.			
18. Grasped the transfer belt on each side if used. Grasped underneath the belt.	___	___	_____
19. Prevented the person from sliding or falling by doing one of the following:			
a. Braced your knees against the person's knees. Blocked his or her feet with your feet.	___	___	_____
b. Used the knee and foot of one leg to block the person's weak leg or foot. Placed your other foot slightly behind your own for balance.	___	___	_____
c. Straddled your legs around the person's weak leg.	___	___	_____

Date of Satisfactory Completion _____   Instructor's Initials _____

Procedure—cont'd   **S**   **U**   **Comments**

20. Explained the following:
    a. You will count "1, 2, 3."
    b. The move will be on "3."
    c. On "3," the person pushes down on the mattress and stands.
21. Asked the person to push down on the armrests on the count of "3." Pulled the person to a standing position as you straightened your knees.
22. Supported the person in the standing position. Held the transfer belt, or kept hands around the person's shoulder blades. Continued to prevent the person from sliding or falling.
23. Turned the person so he or she could reach the edge of the mattress. The legs touched the mattress.
24. Continued to turn the person until he or she reached the mattress with both hands.
25. Lowered him or her into the bed as you bent your hips and knees. The person assisted by leaning forward and bending the elbows and knees.
26. Removed the transfer belt.
27. Removed the robe and footwear.
28. Helped the person lie down.

Post-Procedure
29. Provided for comfort.
30. Placed the signal light within reach and other needed items within reach.
31. Raised or lowered bed rails. Followed the care plan.
32. Arranged furniture to meet the person's needs.
33. Unscreened the person.
34. Completed a safety check of the room.
35. Practiced hand hygiene.
36. Reported and recorded your observations.

Date of Satisfactory Completion _____   Instructor's Initials _____

Transferring the Person Using a Mechanical Lift

Name: _____   Date: _____

Quality of Life	S	U	Comments
Remembered to:			
• Knock before entering the person's room	___	___	_____
• Address the person by name	___	___	_____
• Introduce yourself by name and title	___	___	_____
• Explain the procedure to the person before beginning and during the procedure	___	___	_____
• Protect the person's rights during the procedure	___	___	_____
• Handle the person gently during the procedure	___	___	_____

Pre-Procedure

	S	U	Comments
1. Followed *Delegation Guidelines:*			
a. *Preventing Work-Related Injuries*	___	___	_____
b. *Transferring Persons*	___	___	_____
c. *Using Mechanical Lifts*	___	___	_____
Reviewed *Promoting Safety and Comfort:*			
a. *Safely Moving and Transferring Persons*	___	___	_____
b. *Preventing Work-Related Injuries*	___	___	_____
c. *Transferring Persons*	___	___	_____
d. *Using Mechanical Lifts*	___	___	_____
2. Asked a co-worker to help you.	___	___	_____
3. Collected:			
a. Mechanical lift and sling	___	___	_____
b. Arm chair or wheelchair	___	___	_____
c. Footwear	___	___	_____
d. Bath blanket or cushion	___	___	_____
e. Lap blanket	___	___	_____
4. Practiced hand hygiene.	___	___	_____
5. Identified the person. Checked the ID bracelet against the assignment sheet. Called the person by name.	___	___	_____
6. Provided for privacy.	___	___	_____

Procedure

	S	U	Comments
7. Raised the bed for body mechanics. Bed rails were up if used.	___	___	_____
8. Lowered the head of the bed to a level appropriate for the person. It was as flat as possible.	___	___	_____
9. Stood on one side of the bed. Your co-worker stood on the other side.	___	___	_____
10. Lowered the bed rails if up. Locked the bed wheels.	___	___	_____
11. Centered the sling under the person. To position the sling, turned the person from side to side as if making an occupied bed. Positioned the sling according to the manufacturer's instructions.	___	___	_____
12. Positioned the person in semi-Fowler's position.	___	___	_____
13. Placed the chair at the head of the bed. It was even with the head-board and about 1 foot away from the bed. Placed a folded bath blanket or cushion in the chair.	___	___	_____
14. Lowered the bed to its lowest position.	___	___	_____
15. Raised the lift so you could position it over the person.	___	___	_____
16. Positioned the lift over the person.	___	___	_____
17. Locked the lift wheels in position.	___	___	_____
18. Attached the sling to the swivel bar.	___	___	_____
19. Raised the head of the bed to a sitting position.	___	___	_____
20. Crossed the person's arms over the chest.	___	___	_____

Date of Satisfactory Completion _____   Instructor's Initials _____

Procedure—cont'd	S	U	Comments
21. Raised the lift high enough until the person and the sling were free of the bed.	_____	_____	_____
22. Had your co-worker support the person's legs as you moved the lift and the person away from the bed.	_____	_____	_____
23. Positioned the lift so the person's back was toward the chair.	_____	_____	_____
24. Positioned the chair so you could lower the person into it.	_____	_____	_____
25. Lowered the person into the chair. Guided the person into the chair.	_____	_____	_____
26. Lowered the spreader bar to unhook the sling. Removed the sling from under the person unless otherwise indicated.	_____	_____	_____
27. Put footwear on the person. Positioned the person's feet on the wheelchair footplates.	_____	_____	_____
28. Covered the person's lap and legs with a lap blanket. Kept it off the floor and wheels.	_____	_____	_____
29. Positioned the chair as the person preferred. Locked the wheelchair wheels according to the care plan.	_____	_____	_____

Post-Procedure

	S	U	Comments
30. Provided for comfort.	_____	_____	_____
31. Placed the signal light within reach and other needed items within reach.	_____	_____	_____
32. Unscreened the person.	_____	_____	_____
33. Completed a safety check of the room.	_____	_____	_____
34. Practiced hand hygiene.	_____	_____	_____
35. Reported and recorded your observations.	_____	_____	_____
36. Reversed the procedure to return the person to bed.	_____	_____	_____

Date of Satisfactory Completion _____   Instructor's Initials _____

Transferring the Person to and From the Toilet

Name: _____   Date: _____

Quality of Life	S	U	Comments

Remembered to:
- Knock before entering the person's room
- Address the person by name
- Introduce yourself by name and title
- Explain the procedure to the person before beginning and during the procedure
- Protect the person's rights during the procedure
- Handle the person gently during the procedure

Pre-Procedure

1. Followed *Delegation Guidelines:*
   a. *Preventing Work-Related Injuries*
   b. *Transferring Persons*
   Reviewed *Promoting Safety and Comfort:*
   a. *Transfer/Gait Belts*
   b. *Safely Moving and Transferring Persons*
   c. *Preventing Work-Related Injuries*
   d. *Transferring Persons*
   e. *Bed to Chair or Wheelchair Transfers*
   f. *Transferring the Person to and from a Toilet*
2. Practiced hand hygiene.

Procedure

3. Had the person wear non-skid footwear.
4. Positioned the wheelchair next to the toilet if there was enough room. If not, positioned the chair at a right angle (90 degrees) to the toilet. Best if the person's strong side was near the toilet.
5. Locked the wheelchair wheels.
6. Raised the footplates. Removed or swung the front rigging out of the way.
7. Applied the transfer belt.
8. Helped the person unfasten clothing.
9. Used the transfer belt to help the person stand and to turn to the toilet. The person used the grab bars to turn to the toilet.
10. Supported the person with the transfer belt while he or she lowered clothing. Or had the person hold onto the grab bars for support. Lowered the person's pants and undergarments.
11. Used the transfer belt to lower the person onto the toilet seat. Made sure he or she was properly positioned on the toilet.
12. Removed the transfer belt.
13. Told the person you will stay nearby. Reminded the person to use the signal light or call for you when help is needed. Stayed with the person if required by the care plan.
14. Closed the bathroom door to provide privacy.
15. Stayed near the bathroom. Completed other tasks in the person's room. Checked on the person every 5 minutes.
16. Knocked on the bathroom door when the person called for you.
17. Helped with wiping, perineal care, flushing, and hand washing as needed. Wore gloves and practiced hand hygiene after removing the gloves.
18. Applied the transfer belt.
19. Used the transfer belt to help the person stand.
20. Helped the person raise and secure clothing.
21. Used the transfer belt to transfer the person to the wheelchair.

Date of Satisfactory Completion _____   Instructor's Initials _____

Procedure—cont'd	S	U	Comments
22. Made sure the person's buttocks were to the back of the seat. Positioned the person in good alignment.	___	___	_____
23. Positioned the person's feet on the footplates.	___	___	_____
24. Removed the transfer belt.	___	___	_____
25. Covered the person's lap and legs with a lap blanket. Kept the blanket off the floor and wheels.	___	___	_____
26. Positioned the chair as the person preferred. Locked the wheelchair wheels according to the care plan.	___	___	_____

Post-Procedure

	S	U	Comments
27. Provided for comfort.	___	___	_____
28. Placed the signal light and other needed items within the person's reach.	___	___	_____
29. Unscreened the person.	___	___	_____
30. Completed a safety check of the room.	___	___	_____
31. Practiced hand hygiene.	___	___	_____
32. Reported and recorded your observations.	___	___	_____

Date of Satisfactory Completion _____   Instructor's Initials _____

Moving the Person to a Stretcher

Name: _____   Date: _____

Procedure	S	U	Comments

Procedure
Remembered to:
- Knock before entering the person's room
- Address the person by name
- Introduce yourself by name and title
- Explain the procedure to the person before beginning and during the procedure
- Protect the person's rights during the procedure
- Handle the person gently during the procedure

Pre-Procedure
1. Followed *Delegation Guidelines:*
   a. *Preventing Work-Related Injuries*
   b. *Transferring Persons*
   Reviewed *Promoting Safety and Comfort:*
   a. *Safely Moving and Transferring Persons*
   b. *Preventing Work-Related Injuries*
   c. *Transferring Persons*
   d. *Moving the Person to a Stretcher*
2. Asked 1 or 2 staff members to help.
3. Collected:
   a. Stretcher covered with a sheet or bath blanket
   b. Bath blanket
   c. Pillow(s) if needed
   d. Slide sheet, lateral transfer device with sliding board, drawsheet, or other assist device
4. Practiced hand hygiene.
5. Identified the person. Checked the ID bracelet against the assignment sheet. Called the person by name.
6. Provided for privacy.
7. Raised the bed and stretcher for body mechanics.

Procedure
8. Positioned yourself and co-worker.
   a. One or two workers stood on the side of the bed where the stretcher was.
   b. One worker stood on the other side of the bed.
9. Lowered the head of the bed. It was as flat as possible.
10. Lowered the bed rails if used.
11. Covered the person with a bath blanket. Fan-folded top linens to the foot of the bed.
12. Positioned the assist device. Or loosened the drawsheet on each side.
13. Used the assist device to move the person to the side of the bed where the stretcher was.
14. Protected the person from falling. Held the far arm and leg.
15. Had your co-workers position the stretcher next to the bed. They stood behind the stretcher.
16. Locked the bed and stretcher wheels.
17. Grasped the assist device.
18. Transferred the person to the stretcher on the count of "3." Centered the person on the stretcher.
19. Placed a pillow or pillows under the person's head and shoulders if allowed. Raised the head of the stretcher if allowed.
20. Covered the person. Provided for comfort.
21. Fastened the safety straps. Raised the side rails.
22. Unlocked the stretcher wheels. Transported the person.

Date of Satisfactory Completion _____   Instructor's Initials _____

Post-Procedure

23. Practiced hand hygiene.   _____ _____ _____
24. Reported and recorded:
    a. The time of the transport   _____ _____ _____
    b. Where the person was transported to   _____ _____ _____
    c. Who went with him of her   _____ _____ _____
    d. How the transfer was tolerated   _____ _____ _____
25. Reversed the procedure to return the person to bed.   _____ _____ _____

Date of Satisfactory Completion _____   Instructor's Initials _____

Making a Closed Bed

Name: _____   Date: _____

Quality of Life	S	U	Comments

Remembered to:
- Knock before entering the person's room
- Address the person by name
- Introduce yourself by name and title
- Explain the procedure to the person before beginning and during the procedure
- Protect the person's rights during the procedure
- Handle the person gently during the procedure

Pre-Procedure

1. Followed *Delegation Guidelines: Making Beds.*
   Reviewed *Promoting Safety and Comfort: Making Beds.*
2. Practiced hand hygiene.
3. Collected clean linen:
   a. Mattress pad (if needed)
   b. Bottom sheet (flat or fitted)
   c. Plastic drawsheet or waterproof pad (if needed)
   d. Cotton drawsheet (if needed)
   e. Top sheet
   f. Blanket
   g. Bedspread
   h. Pillowcase for each pillow
   i. Bath towel(s)
   j. Hand towel
   k. Washcloth
   l. Gown or pajamas
   m. Bath blanket
   n. Gloves
   o. Laundry bag
   p. Paper towels (if needed as barrier for clean linens)
4. Placed linen on a clean surface. Used the paper towels as a barrier between the clean surface and clean linen, if required by agency policy.
5. Raised the bed for body mechanics. Bed rails were down.

Procedure

6. Put on gloves.
7. Removed linen. Rolled each piece away from you. Placed each piece in a laundry bag. (NOTE: Discarded incontinence products or disposable bed protectors in the trash. Did not put them in the laundry bag.)
8. Cleaned the bed frame and mattress if this was part of your job.
9. Removed and discarded gloves. Practiced hand hygiene.
10. Moved the mattress to the head of the bed.
11. Put the mattress pad on the mattress. It was even with the top of the mattress.
12. Placed the bottom sheet on the mattress pad. Unfolded it length-wise. Placed the center crease in the middle of the bed. If used a flat sheet:
    a. Positioned the lower edge even with the bottom of the mattress.
    b. Placed the large hem at the top and the small hem at the bottom.
    c. Faced hem-stitching downward, away from the person.
13. Opened the sheet. Fan-folded it to the other side of the bed.

Date of Satisfactory Completion _____   Instructor's Initials _____

Procedure—cont'd   S   U   **Comments**

14. Tucked the corners of a fitted sheet over the mattress, at the top
    and then the foot of the bed. For flat sheet, tucked the top of the
    sheet under the mattress. The sheet was tight and smooth.   _____ _____ _____

15. Made a mitered corner if using a flat sheet.   _____ _____ _____

16. Placed the waterproof drawsheet on the bed. It was in the middle
    of the mattress. Or put the waterproof pad on the bed.   _____ _____ _____

17. Opened the waterproof drawsheet. Fan-folded it to the other
    side of the bed.   _____ _____ _____

18. Placed a cotton drawsheet over the waterproof drawsheet.
    It covered the entire waterproof drawsheet.   _____ _____ _____

19. Opened the cotton drawsheet. Fan-folded it to the other
    side of the bed.   _____ _____ _____

20. Tucked both drawsheets under the mattress. Or tucked
    each in separately.   _____ _____ _____

21. Went to the other side of the bed.   _____ _____ _____

22. Mitered the top corner of the flat bottom sheet.   _____ _____ _____

23. Pulled the bottom sheet tight so there were no wrinkles.
    Tucked in the sheet.   _____ _____ _____

24. Pulled the drawsheets tight so there were no wrinkles.
    Tucked both in together or separately.   _____ _____ _____

25. Went to the other side of the bed.   _____ _____ _____

26. Put the top sheet on the bed. Placed the center crease in
    the middle.
    a. Unfolded it length-wise.   _____ _____ _____
    b. Placed the large hem even with the top of the mattress.   _____ _____ _____
    c. Opened the sheet. Fan-folded it to the other side.   _____ _____ _____
    d. Faced hem-stitching outward, away from the person.   _____ _____ _____
    e. Did not tuck the bottom in yet.   _____ _____ _____
    f. Never tucked top linens in on the sides.   _____ _____ _____

27. Placed the blanket on the bed:
    a. Unfolded it so the center crease was in the middle.   _____ _____ _____
    b. Put the upper hem about 6 to 8 inches from the top
       of the mattress.   _____ _____ _____
    c. Opened the blanket. Fan-folded it to the other side.   _____ _____ _____
    d. Turned the top sheet down over the blanket. Hem-stitching
       was down, away from the person. (NOTE: If cuff was not made.)   _____ _____ _____

28. Placed the bedspread on the bed:
    a. Unfolded it so the center crease was in the middle.   _____ _____ _____
    b. Placed the upper hem even with the top of the mattress.   _____ _____ _____
    c. Opened and fan-folded the spread to the other side.   _____ _____ _____
    d. Made sure the spread facing the door was even.
       It covered all top linens.   _____ _____ _____

29. Tucked in top linens together at the foot of the bed.
    They were smooth and tight. Made a mitered corner.   _____ _____ _____

30. Went to the other side.   _____ _____ _____

31. Straightened all top linens. Worked from the head of the
    bed to the foot.   _____ _____ _____

32. Tucked in top linens together at the foot of the bed.
    Made a mitered corner.   _____ _____ _____

33. Turned the top hem of the spread under the blanket to make
    a cuff.   _____ _____ _____

34. Turned the top sheet down over the spread. Hem-stitching
    was down. (NOTE: Steps 33 & 34 not done in some centers.)
    The spread covered the pillow and it was tucked under the pillow. _____ _____ _____

35. Put the pillowcase on the pillow. Folded extra material under
    the pillow at the seam end of the pillowcase.   _____ _____ _____

36. Placed the pillow on the bed. The open end of the pillowcase
    was away from the door. The seam was toward the head
    of the bed.   _____ _____ _____

Date of Satisfactory Completion _____ Instructor's Initials _____

Post-Procedure

37. Provided for comfort. (NOTE: Omitted this step if the bed was prepared for a new person.)   ——— ——— ——————————

38. Attached the signal light to the bed. Or placed it within the person's reach.   ——— ——— ——————————

39. Lowered bed to its lowest position. Locked the bed wheels.   ——— ——— ——————————

40. Put the towels, washcloth, gown or pajamas, and bath blanket in the bedside stand.   ——— ——— ——————————

41. Completed a safety check of the room.   ——— ——— ——————————

42. Followed agency policy for dirty linen.   ——— ——— ——————————

43. Practiced hand hygiene.   ——— ——— ——————————

Date of Satisfactory Completion _____   Instructor's Initials _____

Making an Open Bed

Name: _____   Date: _____

Quality of Life	S	U	Comments
Remembered to:			
• Knock before entering the person's room	_____	_____	_____
• Address the person by name	_____	_____	_____
• Introduce yourself by name and title	_____	_____	_____
• Explain the procedure to the person before beginning and during the procedure	_____	_____	_____
• Protect the person's rights during the procedure	_____	_____	_____
• Handle the person gently during the procedure	_____	_____	_____

Procedure

	S	U	Comments
1. Followed *Delegation Guidelines: Making Beds.* Reviewed *Promoting Safety and Comfort: Making Beds.*	_____	_____	_____
2. Practiced hand hygiene.	_____	_____	_____
3. Collected linen for a closed bed.	_____	_____	_____
4. Made a closed bed:	_____	_____	_____
• placed linen on a clean surface.	_____	_____	_____
• raised the bed for body mechanics.	_____	_____	_____
• put on gloves.	_____	_____	_____
• removed linen. Rolled each piece away from you. Placed each piece in a laundry bag. (NOTE: Discarded incontinence products or disposable bed protectors in the trash. Did not put them in the laundry bag.)	_____	_____	_____
• cleaned the bed frame and mattress if this was part of your job.	_____	_____	_____
• removed and discarded gloves. Practiced hand hygiene.	_____	_____	_____
• moved the mattress to the head of the bed.	_____	_____	_____
• put the mattress pad on the mattress. It was even with the top of the mattress.	_____	_____	_____
• placed the bottom sheet on the mattress pad:			
○ unfolded it length-wise.			
○ placed the center crease in the middle of the bed.	_____	_____	_____
• positioned the lower edge even with the bottom of the mattress.	_____	_____	_____
• placed the large hem at the top and the small hem at the bottom.	_____	_____	_____
• faced hem-stitching downward, away from the person.	_____	_____	_____
• opened the sheet. Fan-folded it to the other side of the bed.	_____	_____	_____
• tucked the top of the sheet under the mattress. the sheet was tight and smooth.	_____	_____	_____
• made a mitered corner if using a flat sheet.	_____	_____	_____
• placed the plastic drawsheet on the bed. It was in the middle of the mattress. Or put the waterproof pad on the bed.	_____	_____	_____
• opened the waterproof drawsheet. Fan-folded it to the other side of the bed.	_____	_____	_____
• placed a cotton drawsheet over the waterproof drawsheet. It covered the entire waterproof drawsheet.	_____	_____	_____
• opened the cotton drawsheet. Fan-folded it to the other side of the bed.	_____	_____	_____
• tucked both drawsheets under the mattress. Or tucked each in separately.	_____	_____	_____
• went to the other side of the bed.	_____	_____	_____
• mitered the top corner of the flat bottom sheet.	_____	_____	_____
• pulled the bottom sheet tight so there were no wrinkles. Tucked in the sheet.	_____	_____	_____
• pulled the drawsheets tight so there were no wrinkles. Tucked both in together or separately.	_____	_____	_____
• went to the other side of the bed.	_____	_____	_____

Date of Satisfactory Completion _____   Instructor's Initials _____

Procedure—cont'd   S   U   Comments

- put the top sheet on the bed:
- unfolded it length-wise. ___ ___ _____
- placed the center crease in the middle. ___ ___ _____
- placed the large hem even with the top of the mattress. ___ ___ _____
- opened the sheet. Fan-folded it to the other side. ___ ___ _____
- faced hem-stitching outward, away from the person. ___ ___ _____
- did not tuck the bottom in yet. ___ ___ _____
- never tucked top linens in on the sides. ___ ___ _____
- placed the blanket on the bed:
  - unfolded it so the center crease was in the middle. ___ ___ _____
  - put the upper hem about 6 to 8 inches from the top of the mattress. ___ ___ _____
  - opened the blanket. Fan-folded it to the other side. ___ ___ _____
  - turned the top sheet down over the blanket. Hem-stitching was down, away from the person. (NOTE: Followed center procedure.) ___ ___ _____
- placed the bedspread on the bed:
  - unfolded it so the center crease was in the middle. ___ ___ _____
  - placed the upper hem even with the top of the mattress. ___ ___ _____
  - opened and fan-folded the spread to the other side. ___ ___ _____
  - made sure the spread facing the door was even. It covered all top linens. ___ ___ _____
- tucked in top linens together at the foot of the bed. They were smooth and tight. ___ ___ _____
- made a mitered corner. ___ ___ _____
- went to the other side. ___ ___ _____
- straightened all top linen. Worked from the head of the bed to the foot. ___ ___ _____
- tucked in top linens together at the foot of the bed. Made a mitered corner. ___ ___ _____
- turned the top hem of the spread under the blanket to make a cuff. ___ ___ _____
- turned the top sheet down over the spread. ___ ___ _____
- hem-stitching was down. (NOTE: Not done in some centers.) The spread covered the pillow and it was tucked under the pillow. ___ ___ _____
- put the pillowcase on the pillow. Followed agency policy. Folded extra material under the pillow at the seam end of the pillowcase. ___ ___ _____
- placed the pillow on the bed. The open end of the pillowcase was away from the door. The seam was toward the head of the bed. ___ ___ _____
5. Fan-folded top linens to the foot of the bed. ___ ___ _____

Post-Procedure

6. Attached the signal light to the bed. ___ ___ _____
7. Lowered bed to its lowest position. ___ ___ _____
8. Put the towels, washcloth, gown or pajamas, and bath blanket in the bedside stand. ___ ___ _____
9. Provided for comfort. ___ ___ _____
10. Placed the signal light within the person's reach. ___ ___ _____
11. Completed a safety check of the room. ___ ___ _____
12. Followed agency policy for dirty linen. ___ ___ _____
13. Practiced hand hygiene. ___ ___ _____

Date of Satisfactory Completion _____   Instructor's Initials _____

Making an Occupied Bed

Name: _____   Date: _____

Quality of Life	S	U	Comments

Quality of Life

Remembered to:
- Knock before entering the person's room
- Address the person by name
- Introduce yourself by name and title
- Explain the procedure to the person before beginning and during the procedure
- Protect the person's rights during the procedure
- Handle the person gently during the procedure

Pre-Procedure

1. Followed *Delegation Guidelines: Making Beds*.
   Reviewed *Promoting Safety and Comfort*:
   a. *Making Beds*
   b. *The Occupied Bed*
2. Practiced hand hygiene.
3. Collected the following:
   a. Gloves
   b. Laundry bag
   c. Clean linen
   d. Paper towels (if used for barrier for clean linen)
4. Placed linen on a clean surface. (Used paper towels between clean surface and clean linen when required by agency).
5. Identified the person. Checked the ID bracelet against the assignment sheet. Called the person by name.
6. Provided for privacy.
7. Removed the signal light.
8. Raised the bed for body mechanics. Bed rails were up if used. Bed wheels were locked.
9. Lowered the head of the bed. It was as flat as possible.

Procedure

10. Practiced hand hygiene. Put on gloves.
11. Loosened top linens at the foot of the bed.
12. Lowered the bed rail near you if up.
13. Removed the bedspread. Then removed the blanket. Placed each over the chair.
14. Covered the person with a bath blanket. Used the blanket in the bedside stand.
    a. Unfolded a bath blanket over the top sheet.
    b. Asked the person to hold onto the bath blanket. If he or she could not, tucked the top part under the person's shoulders.
    c. Grasped the top sheet under the bath blanket at the shoulders. Brought the sheet down toward the foot of the bed. Removed the sheet from under the blanket.
15. Positioned the person on the side of the bed away from you. Adjusted the pillow for comfort.
16. Loosened bottom linens from the head to the foot of the bed.
17. Fan-folded bottom linens one at a time toward the person. Started with the cotton drawsheet. If reused the mattress pad, did not fan-fold it.
18. Placed a clean mattress pad on the bed. Unfolded it length-wise. The center crease was in the middle. Fan-folded the top part toward the person. If reused the mattress pad, straightened and smoothed any wrinkles.

Date of Satisfactory Completion _____   Instructor's Initials _____

Procedure—cont'd

	S	U	Comments
19. Placed the bottom sheet on the mattress pad. Hem-stitching was away from the person. Unfolded the sheet so the crease was in the middle. The small hem was even with the bottom of the mattress. Fan-folded the top part toward the person.	___	___	_____
20. Tucked the corners of a fitted sheet over the mattress. If used a flat sheet, made a mitered corner at the head of the bed. Tucked the sheet under the mattress from the head to the foot.	___	___	_____
21. Pulled the waterproof drawsheet (if re-used) toward you over the bottom sheet. Tucked excess material under the mattress. Did the following for a clean waterproof drawsheet:			
a. Placed the waterproof drawsheet on the bed. It was in the middle of the mattress.	___	___	_____
b. Fan-folded the top part toward the person.	___	___	_____
c. Tucked in excess fabric.	___	___	_____
22. Placed the cotton drawsheet over the waterproof drawsheet. It covered the entire waterproof drawsheet. Fan-folded the top part toward the person. Tucked in excess fabric.	___	___	_____
23. Explained to the person that he or she will roll over a "bump." Assured the person that he or she would not fall.			
24. Helped the person turn to the other side. Adjusted the pillow for comfort.	___	___	_____
25. Raised the bed rail. Went to the other side, and lowered the bed rail.	___	___	_____
26. Loosened bottom linens. Removed one piece at a time. Placed each piece in the laundry bag. (NOTE: Discarded disposable bed protectors and incontinence products in the trash. Did not put them in the laundry bag.)	___	___	_____
27. Removed and discarded the gloves. Practiced hand hygiene.	___	___	_____
28. Straightened and smoothed the mattress pad.	___	___	_____
29. Pulled the clean bottom sheet toward you. Tucked the corners of a fitted sheet over the mattress. If used a flat sheet, made a mitered corner at the top. Tucked the sheet under the mattress from the head to the foot of the bed.	___	___	_____
30. Pulled the drawsheets tightly toward you. Tucked both under together or separately.	___	___	_____
31. Positioned the person supine in the center of the bed. Adjusted the pillow for comfort.	___	___	_____
32. Put the top sheet on the bed. Unfolded it length-wise. The crease was in the middle. The large hem was even with the top of the mattress. Hem-stitching was on the outside.	___	___	_____
33. Asked the person to hold onto the top sheet so you could remove the bath blanket. Or tucked the top sheet under the person's shoulders. Removed the bath blanket.	___	___	_____
34. Placed the blanket on the bed. Unfolded it so the center crease was in the middle and it covered the person. The upper hem was 6 to 8 inches from the top of the mattress.	___	___	_____
35. Placed the bedspread on the bed. Unfolded it so the center crease was in the middle and it covered the person. The top hem was even with the mattress top.	___	___	_____
36. Turned the top hem of the bedspread under the blanket to make a cuff.	___	___	_____
37. Brought the top sheet down over the spread to form a cuff.	___	___	_____
38. Went to the foot of the bed.	___	___	_____
39. Made a toe pleat. Made a 2-inch pleat across the foot of the bed. The pleat was about 6 to 8 inches from the foot of the bed.	___	___	_____
40. Lifted the mattress corner with one arm. Tucked all top linens under the mattress together. Made a mitered corner.	___	___	_____
41. Raised the bed rail. Went to the other side, and lowered the bed rail.	___	___	_____

Date of Satisfactory Completion _____   Instructor's Initials _____

Procedure—cont'd	**S**	**U**	**Comments**
42. Straightened and smoothed top linens.	_____	_____	_____
43. Tucked the top linens under the bottom of the mattress. Made a mitered corner.	_____	_____	_____
44. Changed the pillowcase(s).	_____	_____	_____

Post-Procedure

45. Provided for comfort.	_____	_____	_____
46. Placed the signal light within reach.	_____	_____	_____
47. Lowered bed to its lowest position. Locked the bed wheels.	_____	_____	_____
48. Raised or lowered bed rails. Followed the care plan.	_____	_____	_____
49. Put the clean towels, washcloth, gown or pajamas, and bath blanket in the bedside stand.	_____	_____	_____
50. Unscreened the person.	_____	_____	_____
51. Completed a safety check of the room.	_____	_____	_____
52. Followed agency policy for dirty linen.	_____	_____	_____
53. Practiced hand hygiene.	_____	_____	_____

Date of Satisfactory Completion _____   Instructor's Initials _____

Making a Surgical Bed

Name: _____   Date: _____

Procedure	S	U	Comments
1. Followed *Delegation Guidelines: Making Beds*. Reviewed *Promoting Safety and Comfort*:	___	___	_____
a. *Making Beds*	___	___	_____
b. *Surgical Bed*	___	___	_____
2. Practiced hand hygiene.	___	___	_____
3. Collected the following:			
a. Clean linen	___	___	_____
b. Gloves	___	___	_____
c. Laundry bag	___	___	_____
d. Equipment requested by the nurse	___	___	_____
e. Papers towels (if you needed a barrier for clean linen)	___	___	_____
4. Placed linen on a clean surface. Placed the paper towels between the clean surface and clean linen if barrier was required by agency policy.	___	___	_____
5. Removed the signal light.	___	___	_____
6. Raised the bed for body mechanics.	___	___	_____
7. Removed all linens from the bed. Wore gloves. Practiced hand hygiene after removing and discarding them.	___	___	_____
8. Made a closed bed. Did not tuck top lines under the mattress.			
a. Moved the mattress to the head of the bed.	___	___	_____
b. Put the mattress pad on the mattress. It was even with the top of the mattress.	___	___	_____
c. Placed the bottom sheet on the mattress pad:			
(1) Unfolded it length-wise.	___	___	_____
(2) Placed the center crease in the middle of the bed.	___	___	_____
(3) Positioned the lower edge even with the bottom of the mattress.	___	___	_____
(4) Placed the large hem at the top and the small hem at the bottom.	___	___	_____
(5) Faced hem-stitching downward.	___	___	_____
d. Opened the sheet. Fan-folded it to the other side of the bed.	___	___	_____
e. Tucked the top of the sheet under the mattress. The sheet was tight and smooth.	___	___	_____
f. Made a mitered corner if using a flat sheet.	___	___	_____
g. Placed the waterproof drawsheet on the bed. It was in the middle of the mattress. Or put the waterproof pad on the bed.	___	___	_____
h. Opened the waterproof drawsheet. Fan-folded it to the other side of the bed.	___	___	_____
i. Placed a cotton drawsheet over the waterproof drawsheet. It covered the entire plastic drawsheet.	___	___	_____
j. Opened the cotton drawsheet. Fan-folded it to the other side of the bed.	___	___	_____
k. Tucked both drawsheets under the mattress. Or tucked each in separately.	___	___	_____
l. Went to the other side of the bed.	___	___	_____
m. Mitered the top corner of the flat bottom sheet.	___	___	_____
n. Pulled the bottom sheet tight so there were no wrinkles. Tucked in the sheet.	___	___	_____
o. Pulled the drawsheets tight so there were no wrinkles. Tucked both in together or separately.	___	___	_____
p. Went to the other side of the bed.	___	___	_____
q. Put the top sheet on the bed:			
(1) Unfolded it length-wise.	___	___	_____
(2) Placed the center crease in the middle.	___	___	_____

Date of Satisfactory Completion _____   Instructor's Initials _____

Procedure—cont'd   S   U   **Comments**

    (3) Placed the large hem even with the top of the mattress.   _____ _____ _____

    (4) Opened the sheet. Fan-folded it to the other side.   _____ _____ _____

    (5) Faced hem-stitching outward, away from the person.   _____ _____ _____

  9. Folded all top linens at the foot of the bed back onto the bed. The fold was even with the edge of the mattress.   _____ _____ _____

10. Knew on which side of the bed the stretcher would be placed. Fan-folded linen length-wise to the other side of the bed.   _____ _____ _____

11. Put the pillowcase(s) on the pillow(s).   _____ _____ _____

12. Placed the pillow(s) on a clean surface.   _____ _____ _____

13. Left the bed in its highest position.   _____ _____ _____

14. Left both bed rails down.   _____ _____ _____

15. Put the clean towels, washcloth, gown or pajamas, and bath blanket in the bedside stand.   _____ _____ _____

16. Moved furniture away from the bed. Allowed room for the stretcher and the staff.   _____ _____ _____

17. Did not attach the signal light to the bed.   _____ _____ _____

18. Completed a safety check of the room.   _____ _____ _____

19. Followed agency policy for soiled linen.   _____ _____ _____

20. Practiced hand hygiene.   _____ _____ _____

Date of Satisfactory Completion _____   Instructor's Initials _____

Assisting the Person to Brush and Floss the Teeth

Name: _____ Date: _____

Procedure	S	U	Comments
Remembered to:			
• Knock before entering the person's room	___	___	_____
• Address the person by name	___	___	_____
• Introduce yourself by name and title	___	___	_____
• Explain the procedure to the person before beginning and during the procedure	___	___	_____
• Protect the person's rights during the procedure	___	___	_____
• Handle the person gently during the procedure	___	___	_____

Pre-Procedure

	S	U	Comments
1. Followed *Delegation Guidelines: Oral Hygiene.* Reviewed *Promoting Safety and Comfort: Oral Hygiene.*	___	___	_____
2. Practiced hand hygiene.	___	___	_____
3. Collected the following:			
a. Toothbrush	___	___	_____
b. Toothpaste	___	___	_____
c. Mouthwash (or solution noted in care plan)	___	___	_____
d. Dental floss (if used)	___	___	_____
e. Water glass with cool water	___	___	_____
f. Straw	___	___	_____
g. Kidney basin	___	___	_____
h. Hand towel	___	___	_____
i. Paper towels	___	___	_____
j. Gloves	___	___	_____
4. Placed the paper towels on the overbed table. Arranged items on the top of them.	___	___	_____
5. Identified the person. Checked the ID bracelet against the assignment sheet. Called the person by name.	___	___	_____
6. Provided for privacy.	___	___	_____
7. Lowered the bed rail near you, if up.	___	___	_____

Procedure

	S	U	Comments
8. Positioned the person so he or she could brush with ease.	___	___	_____
9. Placed the towel over the person's chest. This protected garments and linens from spills.	___	___	_____
10. Adjusted the overbed table in front of the person.	___	___	_____
11. Allowed the person to perform oral hygiene. This included brushing the teeth, rinsing the mouth, flossing, and using mouthwash or other solution.	___	___	_____
12. Removed the towel when the person was done.	___	___	_____
13. Moved the overbed table to the side of the bed.	___	___	_____

Post-Procedure

	S	U	Comments
14. Provided for comfort.	___	___	_____
15. Placed the signal light within reach.	___	___	_____
16. Raised or lowered bed rails. Followed the care plan.	___	___	_____
17. Rinsed the toothbrush. Cleaned, rinsed, and dried equipment. Returned the toothbrush and equipment to their proper place. Wore gloves.	___	___	_____
18. Wiped off the overbed table with the paper towels. Discarded the paper towels.	___	___	_____
19. Unscreened the person.	___	___	_____
20. Completed a safety check of the room.	___	___	_____
21. Followed center policy for dirty linen.	___	___	_____
22. Removed and discarded the gloves. Practiced hand hygiene.	___	___	_____
23. Reported and recorded your observations.	___	___	_____

Date of Satisfactory Completion _____ Instructor's Initials _____

Brushing and Flossing the Person's Teeth (NNAAP®)

Name: _____ Date: _____

Quality of Life	S	U	Comments

Remembered to:
- Knock before entering the person's room
- Address the person by name
- Introduce yourself by name and title
- Explain the procedure to the person before beginning and during the procedure
- Protect the person's rights during the procedure
- Handle the person gently during the procedure

Pre-Procedure
1. Followed *Delegation Guidelines: Oral Hygiene.* Reviewed *Promoting Safety and Comfort: Oral Hygiene.*
2. Practiced hand hygiene.
3. Collected the following:
   a. Toothbrush with soft bristles
   b. Toothpaste
   c. Mouthwash (or solution noted in care plan)
   d. Dental floss (if used)
   e. Water cup with cool water
   f. Straw
   g. Kidney basin
   h. Hand towel
   i. Paper towels
   j. Gloves
4. Placed the paper towels on the overbed table. Arranged items on the top of them.
5. Identified the person. Checked the ID bracelet against the assignment sheet. Called the person by name.
6. Provided for privacy.
7. Raised the bed for body mechanics. Bed rails were up if used.

Procedure
8. Lowered the bed rail near you if up.
9. Assisted the person to a sitting position or to a side-lying position near you. NOTE: Some state competency tests require that the person is at 75 to 90 degree angle.
10. Placed the towel across the person's chest.
11. Adjusted the overbed table so you could reach it with ease.
12. Practiced hand hygiene. Put on gloves.
13. Held the toothbrush over the kidney basin. Poured some water over the brush.
14. Applied toothpaste to the brush.
15. Brushed the teeth gently.
16. Brushed the tongue gently.
17. Let the person rinse the mouth with water. Held the kidney basin under the person's chin. Repeated as needed.
18. Flossed the person's teeth (optional):
    a. Broke off an 18-inch piece of floss from the dispenser.
    b. Held the floss between the middle fingers of each hand.
    c. Stretched the floss with your thumb.
    d. Started at the upper back tooth on the right side. Worked around to the left side.
    e. Moved the floss gently up and down between the teeth. Moved the floss up and down against the side of the tooth. Worked from the top of the crown to the gum line.

Date of Satisfactory Completion _____ Instructor's Initials _____

Procedure—cont'd   S   U   Comments

f. Moved to a new section of floss after every second tooth.

g. Flossed the lower teeth. Used up and down motions for the upper teeth. Started on the right side. Worked around to the left side.

19. Allowed the person to use mouthwash or other solution. Held the kidney basin under the chin.

20. Wiped the person's mouth. Removed the towel.

21. Removed and discarded the gloves. Practiced hand hygiene.

Post-Procedure

22. Provided for comfort.

23. Placed the signal light within reach.

24. Lowered the bed to its lowest position.

25. Raised or lowered bed rails. Followed the care plan.

26. Rinsed the toothbrush. Cleaned, rinsed, and dried equipment. Returned the toothbrush and equipment to their proper place. Wore gloves.

27. Wiped off the overbed table with the paper towels. Discarded the paper towels.

28. Unscreened the person.

29. Completed a safety check of the room.

30. Followed agency policy for dirty linen.

31. Removed and discarded the gloves. Practiced hand hygiene.

32. Reported and recorded your observations.

Date of Satisfactory Completion _____   Instructor's Initials _____

Providing Mouth Care for the Unconscious Person

Name: _____   Date: _____

	S	**U**	**Comments**

Quality of Life

Remembered to:
- Knock before entering the person's room
- Address the person by name
- Introduce yourself by name and title
- Explain the procedure to the person before beginning and during the procedure
- Protect the person's rights during the procedure
- Handle the person gently during the procedure

Pre-Procedure

1. Followed *Delegation Guidelines: Oral Hygiene*.
   Reviewed *Promoting Safety and Comfort*:
   a. *Oral Hygiene*
   b. *Mouth Care for the Unconscious Person*
2. Practiced hand hygiene.
3. Collected the following:
   a. Cleaning agent (checked the care plan)
   b. Sponge swabs
   c. Padded tongue blade
   d. Water glass or cup with cool water
   e. Hand towel
   f. Kidney basin
   g. Lip lubricant
   h. Paper towels
   i. Gloves
4. Placed the paper towels on the overbed table. Arranged items on top of them.
5. Identified the person. Checked the ID bracelet against the assignment sheet. Called the person by name.
6. Provided for privacy.
7. Raised the bed for body mechanics. Bed rails were up if used.

Procedure

8. Lowered the bed rail near you if up.
9. Practiced hand hygiene. Put on gloves.
10. Positioned the person in a side-lying position near you. Turned his or her head to the side.
11. Placed the towel under the person's face.
12. Placed the kidney basin under the chin.
13. Separated the upper and lower teeth. Used the padded tongue blade. Was gentle. Never used force. If you had problems, asked the nurse for help.
14. Cleaned the mouth using sponge swabs moistened with the cleaning agent.
    a. Cleaned the chewing and inner surfaces of the teeth.
    b. Cleaned the gums and outer surfaces of the teeth.
    c. Swabbed the roof of the mouth, inside of the cheeks, and the lips.
    d. Swabbed the tongue.
    e. Moistened a clean swab with water. Swabbed the mouth to rinse.
    f. Placed used swabs in the kidney basin.
15. Removed the kidney basin and supplies.
16. Wiped the person's mouth. Removed the towel.
17. Applied lubricant to the lips.
18. Removed and discarded the gloves. Practiced hand hygiene.

Date of Satisfactory Completion _____   Instructor's Initials _____

Post-Procedure

19. Provided for comfort.
20. Placed the signal light within reach.
21. Lowered the bed to its lowest position.
22. Raised or lowered bed rails. Followed the care plan.
23. Cleaned, rinsed, dried, and returned equipment to its proper place. Discarded disposable items. (Wore gloves.)
24. Wiped off the overbed table with the paper towels. Discarded the paper towels.
25. Unscreened the person.
26. Completed a safety check of the room.
27. Told the person that you were leaving the room. Told him or her when you will return.
28. Followed agency policy for dirty linen.
29. Removed and discarded the gloves. Practiced hand hygiene.
30. Reported and recorded your observations.

Date of Satisfactory Completion _____   Instructor's Initials _____

Providing Denture Care (NNAAP®)

Name: _____   Date: _____

Quality of Life	S	U	Comments

Quality of Life
Remembered to:
- Knock before entering the person's room
- Address the person by name
- Introduce yourself by name and title
- Explain the procedure to the person before beginning and during the procedure
- Protect the person's rights during the procedure
- Handle the person gently during the procedure

Pre-Procedure
1. Followed *Delegation Guidelines: Oral Hygiene.*
   Reviewed *Promoting Safety and Comfort:*
   a. *Oral Hygiene*
   b. *Denture Care*
2. Practiced hand hygiene.
3. Collected the following:
   a. Denture brush or toothbrush (for cleaning dentures)
   b. Denture cup labeled with the person's name and room and bed numbers
   c. Denture cleaning agent.
   d. Soft-bristled toothbrush or sponge swabs (for oral hygiene).
   e. Toothpaste
   f. Water cup with cool water
   g. Straw
   h. Mouthwash (or other noted solution)
   i. Kidney basin
   j. Two hand towels
   k. Gauze squares
   l. Paper towels
   m. Gloves
4. Placed the paper towels on the overbed table. Arranged items on the top of them.
5. Identified the person. Checked the ID bracelet against the assignment sheet. Called the person by name.
6. Provided for privacy.
7. Raised the bed for body mechanics.

Procedure
8. Lowered the bed rail near you if up.
9. Practiced hand hygiene. Put on gloves.
10. Placed the towel over the person's chest.
11. Asked the person to remove the dentures. Carefully placed them in the kidney basin.
12. Removed the dentures if the person could not do so. Used gauze square to get a good grip on the slippery dentures.
   a. Grasped the denture with your thumb and index finger. Moved it up and down slightly to break the seal. Gently removed the denture. Placed it in the kidney basin.
   b. Grasped and removed the lower denture with your thumb and index finger. Turned it slightly, and lifted it out of the person's mouth. Placed it in the kidney basin.
13. Followed the care plan for raising side rails.
14. Took the kidney basin, denture cup, denture brush, and denture cleaning agent to the sink.
15. Lined the bottom of the sink with a towel. Filled the sink half-way with water.

Date of Satisfactory Completion _____   Instructor's Initials _____

Procedure—cont'd   S   U   Comments

16. Rinsed each denture under warm running water. Followed agency
    policy for water temperature.   ____   ____   _____
17. Returned dentures to the kidney basin or denture cup. ____   ____   _____
18. Applied the denture cleaning agent to the brush.   ____   ____   _____
19. Brushed the dentures. Brushed the inner, outer, and chewing
    surfaces.   ____   ____   _____
20. Rinsed the dentures under running water. Used warm or cool
    water as directed by the cleaning agent manufacturer. ____   ____   _____
21. Rinsed the denture cup and lid. Placed dentures in the denture
    cup. Covered the dentures with cool water. Followed the agency
    policy for water temperature.   ____   ____   _____
22. Cleaned the kidney basin.   ____   ____   _____
23. Took the denture cup and kidney basin to the overbed table. ____   ____   _____
24. Lowered the bed rail if up.   ____   ____   _____
25. Positioned the person for oral hygiene.   ____   ____   _____
26. Cleaned the person's gums and tongue. Used toothpaste and the
    toothbrush (or sponge swab).   ____   ____   _____
27. Had the person use mouthwash (or noted solution). Held the
    kidney basin under the chin.   ____   ____   _____
28. Asked the person to insert the dentures. Inserted them if the
    person could not:
    a. Held the upper denture firmly with your thumb and index
       finger. Raised the upper lip with the other hand. Inserted the
       denture. Gently pressed on the denture with your index fingers
       to make sure it was in place.   ____   ____   _____
    b. Held the lower denture with your thumb and index finger.
       Pulled the lower lip down slightly. Inserted the denture. Gently
       pressed down on it to make sure it was in place. ____   ____   _____
29. Placed the denture cup in the top drawer of the bedside stand if
    the dentures were not worn. If not worn, the dentures are in water
    or in a denture soaking solution.   ____   ____   _____
30. Wiped the person's mouth. Removed the towel.   ____   ____   _____
31. Removed and discarded the gloves. Practiced hand hygiene. ____   ____   _____

Post-Procedure
32. Assisted with hand washing.   ____   ____   _____
33. Provided for comfort.   ____   ____   _____
34. Placed the signal light within reach.   ____   ____   _____
35. Lowered the bed to its lowest position.   ____   ____   _____
36. Raised or lowered bed rails. Followed the care plan. ____   ____   _____
37. Removed the towel from the sink. Drained the sink.   ____   ____   _____
38. Rinsed the brushes. Cleaned, rinsed, and dried equipment.
    Returned the brushes and equipment to their proper place.
    Discarded disposable items. Wore gloves.   ____   ____   _____
39. Wiped off the overbed table with the paper towels. Discarded the
    paper towels.   ____   ____   _____
40. Unscreened the person.   ____   ____   _____
41. Completed a safety check of the room.   ____   ____   _____
42. Followed agency policy for dirty linen.   ____   ____   _____
43. Removed and discarded the gloves. Practiced hand hygiene. ____   ____   _____
44. Reported and recorded your observations.   ____   ____   _____

Date of Satisfactory Completion _____   Instructor's Initials _____

Giving a Complete Bed Bath (NNAAP®)

Name: _____   Date: _____

	S	U	Comments

Quality of Life
Remembered to:
- Knock before entering the person's room
- Address the person by name
- Introduce yourself by name and title
- Explain the procedure to the person before beginning and during the procedure
- Protect the person's rights during the procedure
- Handle the person gently during the procedure

Pre-Procedure
1. Followed *Delegation Guidelines: Bathing.* Reviewed *Promoting Safety and Comfort: Bathing.*
2. Practiced hand hygiene.
3. Identified the person. Checked the ID bracelet against the assignment sheet. Called the person by name.
4. Collected clean linen for a closed bed and placed linen on a clean surface:
   a. Mattress pad (if needed)
   b. Bottom sheet
   c. Plastic drawsheet or waterproof pad (if used)
   d. Cotton drawsheet (if needed)
   e. Top sheet
   f. Blanket
   g. Bedspread
   h. Two pillowcases
   i. Gloves
   j. Laundry bag
5. Collected the following:
   a. Wash basin
   b. Soap
   c. Bath thermometer
   d. Orange stick or nail file
   e. Washcloth
   f. Two bath towels and two hand towels
   g. Bath blanket
   h. Clothing or sleepwear
   i. Lotion
   j. Powder
   k. Deodorant or antiperspirant
   l. Brush and comb
   m. Other grooming items as requested
   n. Paper towels
   o. Gloves
6. Covered the overbed table with paper towels. Arranged items on the overbed table. Adjusted the height as needed.
7. Provided for privacy.
8. Raised the bed for body mechanics. Bed rails were up if used.

Procedure
9. Removed the signal light.
10. Practiced hand hygiene. Put on gloves.
11. Removed the sleepwear. Did not expose the person. Followed agency policy for dirty sleepwear.
12. Covered the person with a bath blanket. Removed top linens.
13. Lowered the head of the bed. It was as flat as possible. The person had at least one pillow.

Date of Satisfactory Completion _____   Instructor's Initials _____

Procedure—cont'd	**S**	**U**	**Comments**
14. Filled the wash basin ⅔ (two-thirds) full with water. Followed the care plan for water temperature. Water temperature was 110° F to 115° F (43.3° C to 46.1° C) for adults. Measured water temperature. Used the bath thermometer. Or tested the water by dipping your elbow or inner wrist into the basin.	_____	_____	_____
15. Lowered the bed rail near you if up.	_____	_____	_____
16. Asked the person to check the water temperature. Adjusted the water temperature if it was too hot or too cold. Raised the bed rail before leaving the bedside. Lowered it when returned.	_____	_____	_____
17. Placed the basin on the overbed table.	_____	_____	_____
18. Placed a hand towel over the person's chest.	_____	_____	_____
19. Made a mitt with the washcloth. Used a mitt for the entire bath.	_____	_____	_____
20. Washed around the person's eyes with water. Did not use soap.			
a. Cleaned the far eye. Gently wiped from the inner to the outer aspect of the eye with a corner of the mitt.	_____	_____	_____
b. Cleaned around the eye near you. Used a clean part of the washcloth for each stroke.	_____	_____	_____
21. Asked the person if you should use soap to wash the face.	_____	_____	_____
22. Washed the face, ears, and neck. Rinsed and patted dry with the towel on the chest.	_____	_____	_____
23. Helped the person move to the side of the bed near you.	_____	_____	_____
24. Exposed the far arm. Placed a bath towel length-wise under the arm. Applied soap to the washcloth.	_____	_____	_____
25. Supported the arm with your palm under the person's elbow. His or her forearm rested on your forearm.	_____	_____	_____
26. Washed the arm, shoulder, and underarm. Used long, firm strokes. Rinsed and patted dry.	_____	_____	_____
27. Placed the basin on the towel. Put the person's hand into the water. Washed it well. Cleaned under the fingernails with an orange stick or nail file.	_____	_____	_____
28. Had the person exercise the hand and fingers.	_____	_____	_____
29. Removed the basin. Dried the hand well. Covered the arm with the bath blanket.	_____	_____	_____
30. Repeated for the near arm:			
a. Exposed the near arm. Placed a bath towel length-wise under the near arm. Applied soap to the washcloth.	_____	_____	_____
b. Supported the arm with your palm under the person's elbow. His or her forearm rested on your forearm.	_____	_____	_____
c. Washed the arm, shoulder, and underarm. Used long, firm strokes. Rinsed and patted dry.	_____	_____	_____
d. Placed the basin on the towel. Put the person's hand into the water. Washed it well. Cleaned under the fingernails with an orange stick or nail file.	_____	_____	_____
e. Had the person exercise the hand and fingers.	_____	_____	_____
f. Removed the basin. Dried the hand well. Covered the arm with the bath blanket.	_____	_____	_____
31. Placed a bath towel over the chest crosswise. Held the towel in place. Pulled the bath blanket from under the towel to the waist. Applied soap to the washcloth.	_____	_____	_____
32. Lifted the towel slightly, and washed the chest. Did not expose the person. Rinsed and patted dry, especially under the breasts.	_____	_____	_____
33. Moved the towel length-wise over the chest and abdomen. Did not expose the person. Pulled the bath blanket down to the pubic area. Applied soap to the washcloth.	_____	_____	_____
34. Lifted the towel slightly, and washed the abdomen. Rinsed and patted dry.	_____	_____	_____
35. Pulled the bath blanket up to the shoulders; covered both arms. Removed the towel.	_____	_____	_____

Date of Satisfactory Completion _____   Instructor's Initials _____

Procedure—cont'd	S	U	Comments
36. Changed soapy or cool water. Measured water temperature (110° F to 115° F, or 43.3° C to 46.1° C) for adults. Used the bath thermometer. Or tested the water by dipping your elbow or inner wrist into the basin. If bed rails were used, raised the bed rail near you before you left the bedside. Lowered it when you returned.	_____	_____	_____
37. Uncovered the far leg. Did not expose the genital area. Placed a towel length-wise under the foot and leg. Applied soap to the washcloth.	_____	_____	_____
38. Bent the knee, and supported the leg with your arm. Washed it with long, firm strokes. Rinsed and patted dry.	_____	_____	_____
39. Placed the basin on the towel near the foot.	_____	_____	_____
40. Lifted the leg slightly. Slid the basin under the foot.	_____	_____	_____
41. Placed the foot in the basin. Used an orange stick or nail file to clean under toenails if necessary. If the person could not bend the knees:			
a. Washed the foot. Carefully separated the toes. Rinsed and patted dry.	_____	_____	_____
b. Cleaned under the toenails with the orange stick or nail file if necessary.	_____	_____	_____
42. Removed the basin. Dried the leg and foot. Applied lotion to the foot if directed by the nurse and care plan. Covered the leg with the bath blanket. Removed the towel.	_____	_____	_____
43. Repeated for the near leg:			
a. Uncovered the near leg. Did not expose the genital area. Placed a towel length-wise under the foot and leg.	_____	_____	_____
b. Bent the knee and supported the leg with your arm. Washed it with long, firm strokes. Rinsed and patted dry.	_____	_____	_____
c. Placed the basin on the towel near the foot.	_____	_____	_____
d. Lifted the leg slightly. Slid the basin under the foot.	_____	_____	_____
e. Placed the foot in the basin. Used an orange stick or nail file to clean under toenails if necessary. If the person could not bend the knee:			
(1) Washed the foot. Carefully separated the toes. Rinsed and patted dry.	_____	_____	_____
(2) Cleaned under the toenails with an orange stick or nail file if necessary.	_____	_____	_____
f. Removed the basin. Dried the leg and foot. Applied lotion to the foot if directed by the nurse and care plan. Covered the leg with the bath blanket. Removed the towel.	_____	_____	_____
44. Changed the water. Measured water temperature (110° F to 115° F, or 43.3° C to 46.1° C) for adults. Used the bath thermometer. Or tested the water by dipping your elbow or inner wrist into the basin. If bed rails were used, raised the bed rail near you before you left the bedside. Lowered it when you returned.	_____	_____	_____
45. Turned the person onto the side away from you. The person was covered with the bath blanket.	_____	_____	_____
46. Uncovered the back and buttocks. Did not expose the person. Placed a towel length-wise on the bed along the back. Applied soap to the washcloth.	_____	_____	_____
47. Washed the back. Worked from the back of the neck to the lower end of the buttocks. Used long, firm, continuous strokes. Rinsed and dried well.	_____	_____	_____
48. Turned the person onto his or her back.	_____	_____	_____

Date of Satisfactory Completion _____   Instructor's Initials _____

Procedure—cont'd	S	U	Comments

Procedure—cont'd

49. Changed the water for perineal care. Measured water temperature (110° F to 115° F or 43.3° C to 46.1° C) for adults. Used the bath thermometer. Or tested the water by dipping your elbow or inner wrist into the basin. (Some state competency tests also required changing gloves and hand hygiene at this time.) Raised the bed rail near you before you left the bedside. Lowered it when you returned. _____ _____ _____

50. Provided perineal care if the person could not do so. (Practiced hand hygiene and wore gloves for perineal care.) _____ _____ _____

51. Removed and discarded the gloves. Practiced hand hygiene. _____ _____ _____

52. Gave a back massage. _____ _____ _____

53. Applied deodorant or antiperspirant. Applied lotion and powder as requested. Saw *Promoting Safety and Comfort: Bathing.* _____ _____ _____

54. Put clean garments on the person. _____ _____ _____

55. Combed and brushed the hair. _____ _____ _____

56. Made the bed. _____ _____ _____

Post-Procedure

57. Provided for comfort. _____ _____ _____

58. Placed the signal light within reach. _____ _____ _____

59. Lowered the bed to its lowest position. _____ _____ _____

60. Raised or lowered bed rails. Followed the care plan. _____ _____ _____

61. Put on clean gloves. _____ _____ _____

62. Emptied, cleaned, rinsed, and dried the wash basin. Returned it and other supplies to their proper place. _____ _____ _____

63. Wiped off the overbed table with the paper towels. Discarded the paper towels. _____ _____ _____

64. Unscreened the person. _____ _____ _____

65. Completed a safety check of the room. _____ _____ _____

66. Followed agency policy for dirty linen. _____ _____ _____

67. Removed and discarded gloves. Practiced hand hygiene. _____ _____ _____

68. Reported and recorded your observations. _____ _____ _____

Date of Satisfactory Completion _____   Instructor's Initials _____

Assisting With the Partial Bath

Name: _____   Date: _____

Quality of Life	S	U	Comments

Remembered to:
- Knock before entering the person's room
- Address the person by name
- Introduce yourself by name and title
- Explain the procedure to the person before beginning and during he procedure
- Protect the person's rights during the procedure
- Handle the person gently during the procedure

Pre-Procedure

1. Followed *Delegation Guidelines: Bathing.*
   Reviewed *Promoting Safety and Comfort: Bathing.*
2. Did the following:
   a. Practiced hand hygiene.
   b. Identified the person. Checked the ID bracelet against the assignment sheet. Called the person by name.
   d. Collected clean linen for a closed bed and placed linen on a clean surface:
   e. Collected the following:
      - Wash basin
      - Soap
      - Bath thermometer
      - Orange stick or nail file
      - Washcloth
      - Two bath towels and two hand towels
      - Bath blanket
      - Clothing or sleepwear
      - Lotion
      - Powder
      - Deodorant or antiperspirant
      - Brush and comb
      - Other grooming items as requested
      - Paper towels
      - Gloves
   f. Covered the overbed table with paper towels. Arranged items on the overbed table. Adjusted the height as needed.

Procedure

3. Made sure the bed was in the lowest position.
4. Practiced hand hygiene. Put on gloves.
5. Covered the person with a bath blanket. Removed top linens.
6. Filled the wash basin ⅔ (two-thirds) full with water. Water temperature was 110° F to 115° F (43.3° C to 46.1° C) or as directed by the nurse. Measured water temperature with the bath thermometer. Or tested bath water by dipping your elbow or inner wrist into the basin.
7. Asked the person to check the water temperature. Adjusted the water temperature if it was too hot or too cold.
8. Placed the basin on the overbed table.
9. Positioned the person in Fowler's position. Or assisted him or her to sit at the bedside.
10. Adjusted the overbed table so the person could reach the basin and supplies.
11. Helped the person undress. Provided for privacy and warmth with a bath blanket.

Date of Satisfactory Completion _____   Instructor's Initials _____

Procedure—cont'd	S	U	Comments
12. Asked the person to wash easy-to-reach body parts. Explained that you would wash the back and areas the person could not reach.	———	———	———————
13. Placed the signal light within reach. Asked him or her to signal when help was needed or bathing was complete.	———	———	———————
14. Removed and discarded the gloves. Practiced hand hygiene. Then left the room.	———	———	———————
15. Returned when the signal light was on. Knocked before entering. Practiced hand hygiene.	———	———	———————
16. Changed the bath water. Measured bath water temperature (110° F to 115° F, or 43.3° C to 46.1° C) or as directed by the nurse. Measured water temperature with the bath thermometer. Or tested bath water by dipping your elbow or inner wrist into the basin. Used the bath thermometer. Or tested the water by dipping your elbow or inner wrist into the basin.	———	———	———————
17. Raised the bed for body mechanics. The far bed rail was up if used.	———	———	———————
18. Asked what was washed. Put on gloves. Washed and dried areas the person could not reach. The face, hands, underarms, back, buttocks, and perineal area were washed for the partial bath.	———	———	———————
19. Removed and discarded the gloves. Practiced hand hygiene.	———	———	———————
20. Gave a back massage.	———	———	———————
21. Applied lotion, powder, and deodorant or antiperspirant as requested.	———	———	———————
22. Helped the person put on clean garments.	———	———	———————
23. Assisted with hair care and other grooming needs.	———	———	———————
24. Assisted the person to a chair. (Lowered the bed if the person transfers to a chair.) Or turned the person onto the side away from you.	———	———	———————
25. Made the bed. (Raised the bed for body mechanics.)	———	———	———————

Post-Procedure

	S	U	Comments
26. Provided for comfort.	———	———	———————
27. Placed the signal light within reach.	———	———	———————
28. Lowered the bed to its lowest position.	———	———	———————
29. Raised or lowered bed rails. Followed the care plan.	———	———	———————
30. Put on clean gloves.	———	———	———————
31. Emptied, cleaned, rinsed, and dried the bath basin. Returned it and other supplies to their proper place.	———	———	———————
32. Wiped off the overbed table with the paper towels. Discarded the paper towels.	———	———	———————
33. Unscreened the person.	———	———	———————
34. Completed a safety check of the room.	———	———	———————
35. Followed agency policy for dirty linen.	———	———	———————
36. Removed and discarded the gloves. Practiced hand hygiene.	———	———	———————
37. Reported and recorded your observations.	———	———	———————

Date of Satisfactory Completion ————————— Instructor's Initials —————————

Assisting With a Tub Bath or Shower

Name: _____   Date: _____

Quality of Life	S	U	Comments
Remembered to:			
• Knock before entering the person's room	___	___	_____
• Address the person by name	___	___	_____
• Introduce yourself by name and title	___	___	_____
• Explain the procedure to the person before beginning and during the procedure	___	___	_____
• Protect the person's rights during the procedure	___	___	_____
• Handle the person gently during the procedure	___	___	_____

Pre-Procedure

1. Followed *Delegation Guidelines:*
   a. *Bathing*   ___ ___ _____
   b. *Tub Baths and Showers*   ___ ___ _____
   Reviewed *Promoting Safety and Comfort:*
   a. *Bathing*   ___ ___ _____
   b. *Tub Baths and Showers*   ___ ___ _____
2. Reserved the bathtub or shower.   ___ ___ _____
3. Practiced hand hygiene.   ___ ___ _____
4. Identified the person. Checked the ID bracelet against the assignment sheet. Called the person by name.   ___ ___ _____
5. Collected the following:
   a. Washcloth and two bath towels   ___ ___ _____
   b. Soap   ___ ___ _____
   c. Bath thermometer (for a tub bath)   ___ ___ _____
   d. Clothing or sleepwear   ___ ___ _____
   e. Grooming items as requested   ___ ___ _____
   f. Robe and non-skid footwear   ___ ___ _____
   g. Rubber bath mat if needed   ___ ___ _____
   h. Disposable bath mat   ___ ___ _____
   i. Gloves   ___ ___ _____
   j. Wheelchair, shower chair, transfer bench, and so on as needed   ___ ___ _____

Procedure

6. Placed items in the tub or shower room. Used the space provided or a chair.   ___ ___ _____
7. Cleaned and disinfected the tub or shower.   ___ ___ _____
8. Placed a rubber bath mat in the tub or on the shower floor. Did not block the drain.   ___ ___ _____
9. Placed the disposable bath mat on the floor in front of the tub or shower.   ___ ___ _____
10. Placed the OCCUPIED sign on the door.   ___ ___ _____
11. Returned to the person's room. Provided for privacy. Practiced hand hygiene.   ___ ___ _____
12. Helped the person sit on the side of the bed.   ___ ___ _____
13. Helped the person put on a robe and non-skid footwear. Or the person left on clothing.   ___ ___ _____
14. Assisted or transported the person to the tub room or shower.   ___ ___ _____
15. Had the person sit on a chair if he or she walked to the tub or shower room.   ___ ___ _____
16. Provided for privacy.   ___ ___ _____
17. *For a tub bath:*
    a. Filled the tub halfway with warm water (105° F; 40.5° C). Followed the care plan for water temperature.   ___ ___ _____
    b. Measured water temperature with bath thermometer. Or checked the digital display.   ___ ___ _____
    c. Asked the person to check the water temperature. Adjusted the water temperature if it was too hot or too cold.   ___ ___ _____

Date of Satisfactory Completion _____   Instructor's Initials _____

Procedure—cont'd	S	U	Comments
18. *For a shower:*			
a. Turned on the shower.	_____	_____	_____
b. Adjusted water temperature and pressure. Checked the digital display.	_____	_____	_____
c. Asked the person to check the water temperature. Adjusted the water temperature if it was too hot or too cold.	_____	_____	_____
19. Helped the person undress and removed footwear.	_____	_____	_____
20. Helped the person into the tub or shower. Positioned the shower chair, and locked the wheels.	_____	_____	_____
21. Assisted with washing as necessary. Wore gloves.	_____	_____	_____
22. Asked the person to use the signal light when done or when help is needed. Reminded the person that a tub bath lasts no longer than 20 minutes.	_____	_____	_____
23. Placed a towel across the chair.	_____	_____	_____
24. Left the room if the person could bathe alone. If not, stayed in the room or nearby. Removed and discarded the gloves and practiced hand hygiene if you left the room.	_____	_____	_____
25. Checked the person at least every 5 minutes.	_____	_____	_____
26. Returned when he or she signaled for you. Knocked before entering. Practiced hand hygiene.	_____	_____	_____
27. Turned off the shower, or drained the tub. Covered the person while the tub drained.	_____	_____	_____
28. Helped the person out of the shower or tub and onto a chair.	_____	_____	_____
29. Helped the person dry off. Patted gently. Dried under the breasts, and between skin folds, in the perineal area, and between the toes.	_____	_____	_____
30. Assisted with lotion and other grooming items as needed.	_____	_____	_____
31. Helped the person dress and put on footwear.	_____	_____	_____
32. Helped the person return to the room. Provided for privacy.	_____	_____	_____
33. Assisted the person to a chair or into bed.	_____	_____	_____
34. Provided a back massage if the person returned to bed.	_____	_____	_____
35. Assisted with hair care and other grooming needs.	_____	_____	_____

Post-Procedure

	S	U	Comments
36. Provided for comfort.	_____	_____	_____
37. Placed the signal light within reach.	_____	_____	_____
38. Raised or lowered bed rails. Followed the care plan.	_____	_____	_____
39. Unscreened the person.	_____	_____	_____
40. Completed a safety check of the room.	_____	_____	_____
41. Cleaned and disinfected the tub or shower. Removed soiled linen. Wore gloves for this step.	_____	_____	_____
42. Discarded disposable items. Put the UNOCCUPIED sign on the door. Returned supplies to their proper place.	_____	_____	_____
43. Followed agency policy for dirty linen.	_____	_____	_____
44. Removed and discarded the gloves. Practiced hand hygiene.	_____	_____	_____
45. Reported and recorded your observations.	_____	_____	_____

Date of Satisfactory Completion _____ Instructor's Initials _____

Giving a Back Massage

Name: _____   Date: _____

Quality of Life	S	U	Comments

Remembered to:
- Knock before entering the person's room
- Address the person by name
- Introduce yourself by name and title
- Explain the procedure to the person before beginning and during the procedure
- Protect the person's rights during the procedure
- Handle the person gently during the procedure

Pre-Procedure

1. Followed *Delegation Guidelines: The Back Massage*. Reviewed *Promoting Safety and Comfort: The Back Massage*.
2. Practiced hand hygiene.
3. Identified the person. Checked the ID bracelet against the assignment sheet. Called the person by name.
4. Collected the following:
   a. Bath blanket
   b. Bath towel
   c. Lotion
5. Provided for privacy.
6. Raised the bed for body mechanics. Bed rails were up if used.

Procedure

7. Lowered the bed rail near you if up.
8. Positioned the person in the prone or side-lying position. The back was toward you.
9. Exposed the back, shoulders, upper arms, and buttocks. Covered the rest of the body with the bath blanket. Exposed the buttocks if the person gave consent.
10. Laid the towel on the bed along the back. (Did this if person was in the side-lying position.)
11. Warmed the lotion.
12. Explained that the lotion may feel cool and wet.
13. Applied lotion to the lower back area.
14. Stroked up from the buttocks to the shoulders. Then stroked down over the upper arms. Stroked up the upper arms, across the shoulders, and down the back to the buttocks. Used firm strokes. Kept your hands in contact with the person's skin. Stroked down the back to the waist and up to the shoulders, if buttocks not exposed.
15. Repeated stroking up from the buttocks to the shoulders. Then stroked down over the upper arms. Stroked up the upper arms, across the shoulders, and down the back to the buttocks. Used firm strokes. Kept your hands in contact with the person's skin. Continued this for at least 3 minutes.
16. Kneaded the back:
    a. Grasped the skin between your thumb and fingers.
    b. Kneaded half of the back. Started at the buttocks and moved up to the shoulder. Then kneaded down from the shoulder to the buttocks.
    c. Repeated on the other half of the back.
17. Applied lotion to bony areas. Used circular motions with the tips of your fingers. (Did not massage reddened bony areas.)
18. Used fast movements to stimulate. Used slow movements to relax the person.

Date of Satisfactory Completion _____   Instructor's Initials _____

Procedure—cont'd	S	U	Comments
19. Stroked with long, firm movements to end the massage. Told the person you were finishing.	———	———	—————————
20. Straightened and secured clothing or sleepwear.	———	———	—————————
21. Covered the person. Removed the towel and bath blanket.	———	———	—————————

Post-Procedure

	S	U	Comments
22. Provided for comfort.	———	———	—————————
23. Placed the signal light within reach.	———	———	—————————
24. Lowered the bed to its lowest position.	———	———	—————————
25. Raised or lowered bed rails. Followed the care plan.	———	———	—————————
26. Returned lotion to its proper place.	———	———	—————————
27. Unscreened the person.	———	———	—————————
28. Completed a safety check of the room.	———	———	—————————
29. Followed agency policy for dirty linen.	———	———	—————————
30. Practiced hand hygiene.	———	———	—————————
31. Reported and recorded your observations.	———	———	—————————

Date of Satisfactory Completion _____ Instructor's Initials _____

Giving Female Perineal Care (NNAAP®)

Name: _____   Date: _____

Quality of Life	S	U	Comments

Remembered to:
- Knock before entering the person's room
- Address the person by name
- Introduce yourself by name and title
- Explain the procedure to the person before beginning and during the procedure
- Protect the person's rights during the procedure
- Handle the person gently during the procedure

Pre-Procedure
1. Followed *Delegation Guidelines: Perineal Care.* Reviewed *Promoting Safety and Comfort: Perineal Care.*
2. Practiced hand hygiene.
3. Collected the following:
    a. Soap or other cleaning agent as directed
    b. At least 4 washcloths
    c. Bath towel
    d. Bath blanket
    e. Bath thermometer
    f. Wash basin
    g. Waterproof pad
    h. Gloves
    i. Paper towels
4. Covered the overbed table with paper towels. Arranged items on top of them.
5. Identified the person. Checked the ID bracelet against the assignment sheet. Called her by name.
6. Provided for privacy.
7. Raised the bed for body mechanics. Bed rails were up if used.

Procedure
8. Lowered the bed rail near you if up.
9. Practiced hand hygiene. Put on gloves.
10. Covered the person with a bath blanket. Moved top linens to the foot of the bed.
11. Positioned the person on her back.
12. Draped the person.
13. Raised the bed rail if used.
14. Filled the wash basin. Water temperature was 105° F to 109° F (40.5° C to 42.7° C). Followed the care plan for water temperature. Measured water temperature according to agency policy.
15. Asked the person to check the water temperature. Adjusted the water temperature if it was too hot or too cold. Raised the bed rail before you left the bedside. Lowered it when you returned.
16. Placed the basin on the overbed table.
17. Lowered the bed rail if up.
18. Helped the person flex her knees and spread her legs. Or helped her spread her legs as much as possible with the knees straight.
19. Placed a waterproof pad under her buttocks. Removed any wet or soiled incontinence products.
20. Folded the corner of the bath blanket between her legs onto her abdomen.
21. Wet the washcloths.
22. Squeezed out water from a washcloth. Made a mitted washcloth. Applied soap.

Date of Satisfactory Completion _____   Instructor's Initials _____

Procedure—cont'd	**S**	**U**	**Comments**
23. Spread the labia. Cleaned downward from front to back with one stroke.	___	___	_____
24. Repeated until area clean. Used a clean part of the washcloth for each stroke. Used more than one washcloth if needed.	___	___	_____
a. Squeezed out water from washcloth. Made a mitted washcloth. Applied soap.	___	___	_____
b. Separated the labia. Cleaned downward from front to back with one stroke.	___	___	_____
25. Rinsed the perineum with a clean washcloth. Separated the labia. Stroked downward from front to back. Repeated as necessary. Used a clean part of the washcloth for each stroke. Used more than one washcloth if needed.	___	___	_____
26. Patted the area dry with the towel. Dried from front to back.	___	___	_____
27. Folded the blanket back between her legs.	___	___	_____
28. Helped the person lower her legs and turn onto her side away from you.	___	___	_____
29. Applied soap to a mitted washcloth.	___	___	_____
30. Cleaned the rectal area. Cleaned from the vagina to the anus with one stroke.	___	___	_____
31. Repeated until the area was clean. Used a clean part of the washcloth for each stroke. Used more than one washcloth if needed.	___	___	_____
a. Applied soap to a mitted washcloth.	___	___	_____
b. Cleaned the rectal area. Cleaned from the vagina to the anus with one stroke.	___	___	_____
32. Rinsed the rectal area with a washcloth. Stroked from the vagina to the anus. Repeated as necessary. Used a clean part of the washcloth for each stroke. Used more than one washcloth if needed.	___	___	_____
33. Patted the area dry with the towel. Dried from front to back.	___	___	_____
34. Removed the waterproof pad.	___	___	_____
35. Removed and discarded the gloves. Practiced hand hygiene. Put on clean gloves.	___	___	_____
36. Provided clean and dry linens and incontinence products as needed.	___	___	_____

Post-Procedure

	S	**U**	**Comments**
37. Covered the person. Removed the bath blanket.	___	___	_____
38. Provided for comfort.	___	___	_____
39. Placed the signal light within reach.	___	___	_____
40. Lowered the bed to its lowest position.	___	___	_____
41. Raised or lowered bed rails. Followed the care plan.	___	___	_____
42. Emptied, cleaned, rinsed, and dried the wash basin.	___	___	_____
43. Returned the basin and supplies to their proper place.	___	___	_____
44. Wiped off the overbed table with the paper towels. Discarded the paper towels.	___	___	_____
45. Unscreened the person.	___	___	_____
46. Completed a safety check of the room.	___	___	_____
47. Followed agency policy for dirty linen.	___	___	_____
48. Removed and discarded the gloves. Practiced hand hygiene.	___	___	_____
49. Reported and recorded your observations.	___	___	_____

Date of Satisfactory Completion _____   Instructor's Initials _____

Giving Male Perineal Care

Name: _____   Date: _____

Quality of Life	S	U	Comments

Remembered to:
- Knock before entering the person's room
- Address the person by name
- Introduce yourself by name and title
- Explain the procedure to the person before beginning and during the procedure
- Protect the person's rights during the procedure
- Handle the person gently during the procedure

Procedure

1. Followed steps 1 through 17 in procedure: *Giving Female Perineal Care.*
   a. Followed *Delegation Guidelines: Perineal Care* Reviewed *Promoting Safety and Comfort: Perineal Care.*
   b. Practiced hand hygiene.
   c. Collected the following:
      - Soap or other cleaning agent as directed
      - At least 4 washcloths
      - Bath towel
      - Bath blanket
      - Bath thermometer
      - Wash basin
      - Waterproof pad
      - Gloves
      - Paper towels
   d. Covered the overbed table with paper towels. Arranged items on top of them.
   e. Identified the person. Checked the ID bracelet against the assignment sheet. Called him by name.
   f. Provided for privacy.
   g. Raised the bed for good body mechanics. Bed rails were up if used.
   h. Lowered the bed rail near you if up.
   i. Practiced hand hygiene. Put on gloves.
   j. Covered the person with a bath blanket. Moved top linens to the foot of the bed.
   k. Positioned the person on his back.
   l. Draped the person.
   m. Raised the bed rail if used.
   n. Filled the wash basin. Water temperature was 105° F to 109° F (40.5° C to 42.7° C). Followed the care plan for water temperature. Measured water temperature according to agency policy.
   o. Asked the person to check the water temperature. Adjusted the water temperature if it was too hot or too cold. Raised the bed rail before you left the bedside. Lowered it when you returned.
   p. Placed the basin on the overbed table.
   q. Lowered the bed rail if up.
2. Placed a waterproof pad under his buttocks. Removed any wet or soiled incontinence products.
3. Retracted the foreskin if the person was not circumcised.
4. Grasped the penis.
5. Cleaned the tip. Used a circular motion. Started at the meatus of the urethra, and worked outward. Repeated as needed. Used a clean part of the washcloth each time.
6. Rinsed the area with another washcloth.

Date of Satisfactory Completion _____   Instructor's Initials _____

Procedure—cont'd	**S**	**U**	**Comments**
7. Returned the foreskin to its natural position immediately after rinsing.	_____	_____	_____
8. Cleaned the shaft of the penis. Used firm downward strokes. Rinsed the area.	_____	_____	_____
9. Helped the person flex his knees and spread his legs. Or helped him spread his legs as much as possible with his knees straight.	_____	_____	_____
10. Cleaned the scrotum. Rinsed well. Observed for redness and irritation of the skin folds.	_____	_____	_____
11. Patted dry the penis and the scrotum. Used the towel.	_____	_____	_____
12. Folded the blanket back between his legs.	_____	_____	_____
13. Helped the person lower his legs and turn onto his side away from you.	_____	_____	_____
14. Cleaned the rectal area:			
a. Applied soap to a mitted washcloth.	_____	_____	_____
b. Cleaned from behind scrotum to the anus with one stroke.	_____	_____	_____
c. Repeated until the area was clean. Used a clean part of the washcloth for each stroke. Used more than one washcloth if needed.	_____	_____	_____
d. Rinsed and dried well.	_____	_____	_____
15. Removed the waterproof pad.	_____	_____	_____
16. Removed and discarded the gloves. Practiced hand hygiene. Put on clean gloves.	_____	_____	_____
17. Provided clean and dry linens and incontinence products.	_____	_____	_____

Post-Procedure

	S	**U**	**Comments**
18. Covered the person. Removed the bath blanket.	_____	_____	_____
19. Provided for comfort.	_____	_____	_____
20. Placed the signal light within reach.	_____	_____	_____
21. Lowered the bed to its lowest position.	_____	_____	_____
22. Raised or lowered bed rails. Followed the care plan.	_____	_____	_____
23. Emptied and cleaned the wash basin.	_____	_____	_____
24. Returned the basin and supplies to their proper place.	_____	_____	_____
25. Wiped off the overbed table with the paper towels. Discarded the paper towels.	_____	_____	_____
26. Unscreened the person.	_____	_____	_____
27. Completed a safety check of the room.	_____	_____	_____
28. Followed agency policy for dirty linen.	_____	_____	_____
29. Removed and discarded the gloves. Practiced hand hygiene.	_____	_____	_____
30. Reported and recorded your observations.	_____	_____	_____

Date of Satisfactory Completion _____ Instructor's Initials _____

Brushing and Combing the Person's Hair

Name: _____   Date: _____

	S	U	Comments

Quality of Life

Remembered to:
- Knock before entering the person's room
- Address the person by name
- Introduce yourself by name and title
- Explain the procedure to the person before beginning and during the procedure
- Protect the person's rights during the procedure
- Handle the person gently during the procedure

Pre-Procedure

1. Followed *Delegation Guidelines: Brushing and Combing Hair.* Reviewed *Promoting Safety and Comfort: Brushing and Combing Hair.*
2. Practiced hand hygiene.
3. Identified the person. Checked the ID bracelet against the assignment sheet. Called the person by name.
4. Asked the person how to style hair.
5. Collected the following:
   a. Comb and brush
   b. Bath towel
   c. Other hair items as requested
6. Arranged items on the bedside stand.
7. Provided for privacy.

Procedure

8. Lowered the bed rail if up.
9. Helped the person to the chair. The person put on a robe and non-skid footwear while up. (If the person was in bed, raised the bed for body mechanics. Bed rails were up if used. Lowered the bed rail near you. Assisted the person to a semi-Fowler's position if allowed.)
10. Placed a towel across the person's back and shoulders or across the pillow.
11. Asked the person to remove eyeglasses. Put them in the eyeglass case. Put the case inside the bedside stand.
12. *Brushed and combed hair that was not matted or tangled:*
    a. Used the comb to part the hair.
       (1) Parted hair down the middle into two sides.
       (2) Divided 1 side into two smaller sections.
    b. Brushed one of the small sections of hair. Started at the scalp, and brushed toward the hair ends. Did the same for the other small section of hair.
    c. Repeated for the other side:
       (1) Divided other side into two smaller sections.
       (2) Brushed 1 of the small sections of hair. Started at the scalp, and brushed toward the hair ends. Did the same for the other small section of hair.
13. *Brushed and combed matted and tangled hair:*
    a. Took a small section of hair near the ends.
    b. Combed or brushed through to the hair ends.
    c. Added small sections of hair as you worked up to the scalp.
    d. Combed or brushed through each longer section to the hair ends.
    e. Brushed or combed from the scalp to the hair ends.
14. Styled the hair as the person preferred.
15. Removed the towel.
16. Allowed the person to put on the eyeglasses.

Date of Satisfactory Completion _____   Instructor's Initials _____

Post-Procedure

17. Provided for comfort.
18. Placed the signal light within reach.
19. Lowered the bed to its lowest position.
20. Raised or lowered bed rails. Followed the care plan.
21. Cleaned and returned hair care items to their proper place.
22. Unscreened the person.
23. Completed a safety check of the room.
24. Followed agency policy for dirty linen.
25. Practiced hand hygiene.

Date of Satisfactory Completion _____   Instructor's Initials _____

Shampooing the Person's Hair

Name: _____   Date: _____

Quality of Life	S	U	Comments
Remembered to:			
• Knock before entering the person's room	_____	_____	_____
• Address the person by name	_____	_____	_____
• Introduce yourself by name and title	_____	_____	_____
• Explain the procedure to the person before beginning and during the procedure	_____	_____	_____
• Protect the person's rights during the procedure	_____	_____	_____
• Handle the person gently during the procedure	_____	_____	_____

Pre-Procedure

	S	U	Comments
1. Followed *Delegation Guidelines: Shampooing.* Reviewed *Promoting Safety and Comfort: Shampooing.*	_____	_____	_____
2. Practiced hand hygiene.	_____	_____	_____
3. Collected the following:			
• Two bath towels	_____	_____	_____
• Washcloth	_____	_____	_____
• Shampoo	_____	_____	_____
• Hair conditioner (if requested)	_____	_____	_____
• Bath thermometer	_____	_____	_____
• Pitcher or hand-held nozzle (if needed)	_____	_____	_____
• Shampoo tray (if needed)	_____	_____	_____
• Basin or pan (if needed)	_____	_____	_____
• Waterproof pad (if needed)	_____	_____	_____
• Gloves (if needed)	_____	_____	_____
• Comb and brush	_____	_____	_____
• Hair dryer	_____	_____	_____
4. Arranged items nearby.	_____	_____	_____
5. Identified the person. Checked the ID bracelet against the assignment sheet. Called the person by name.	_____	_____	_____
6. Provided for privacy.	_____	_____	_____
7. Raised the bed for body mechanics for a shampoo in bed. Bed rails were up if used.	_____	_____	_____
8. Practiced hand hygiene.	_____	_____	_____

Procedure

	S	U	Comments
9. Lowered the bed rail near you if up.	_____	_____	_____
10. Covered the person's chest with a bath towel.	_____	_____	_____
11. Brushed and combed hair to remove snarls and tangles.	_____	_____	_____
12. Positioned the person for the method you used. To shampoo the person in bed:			
a. Lowered the head of the bed and removed the pillow.	_____	_____	_____
b. Placed the waterproof pad and shampoo tray under the head and shoulders.	_____	_____	_____
c. Supported the head and neck with a folded towel if necessary.	_____	_____	_____
13. Raised the bed rail if used.	_____	_____	_____
14. Obtained water. Water temperature was 105° F (40.5° C). Tested water temperature according to agency policy. Also asked the person to check the water. Adjusted water temperature as needed. Raised the bed rail before you left the bedside.	_____	_____	_____
15. Lowered the bed rail near you if up.	_____	_____	_____
16. Put on gloves (if needed).	_____	_____	_____
17. Asked the person to hold a washcloth over the eyes. It did not cover the nose and mouth. (NOTE: A damp washcloth is easier to hold. It will not slip. However, some state competency tests require a dry washcloth.)	_____	_____	_____

Date of Satisfactory Completion _____   Instructor's Initials _____

Procedure—cont'd	**S**	**U**	**Comments**
18. Used the pitcher or nozzle to wet the hair.	___	___	_____
19. Applied a small amount of shampoo.	___	___	_____
20. Worked up a lather with both hands. Started at the hairline. Worked toward the back of the head.	___	___	_____
21. Massaged the scalp with your fingertips. Did not scratch the scalp with your fingernails.	___	___	_____
22. Rinsed the hair until the water ran clear.	___	___	_____
23. Repeated:			
a. Applied a small amount of shampoo.	___	___	_____
b. Worked up a lather with both hands. Started at the hairline. Worked toward the back of the head.	___	___	_____
c. Massaged the scalp with your fingertips. Did not scratch the scalp.	___	___	_____
d. Rinsed the hair until the water ran clear.	___	___	_____
24. Applied conditioner. Followed directions on the container.	___	___	_____
25. Squeezed water from the person's hair.	___	___	_____
26. Covered the hair with a bath towel.	___	___	_____
27. Removed the shampoo tray and waterproof pad.	___	___	_____
28. Dried the person's face with the towel. Used the towel on the person's chest.	___	___	_____
29. Helped the person raise the head if appropriate. For the person in bed, raised the head of the bed.	___	___	_____
30. Rubbed the hair and scalp with the towel. Used the second towel if the first one was wet.	___	___	_____
31. Combed the hair to remove snarls and tangles.	___	___	_____
32. Dried and styled hair as quickly as possible.	___	___	_____
33. Removed and discarded the gloves if used. Practiced hand hygiene.	___	___	_____

Post-Procedure	**S**	**U**	**Comments**
34. Provided for comfort.	___	___	_____
35. Placed the signal light within reach.	___	___	_____
36. Lowered the bed to its lowest position.	___	___	_____
37. Raised or lowered bed rails. Followed the care plan.	___	___	_____
38. Unscreened the person.	___	___	_____
39. Completed a safety check of the room.	___	___	_____
40. Cleaned, rinsed, dried, and returned equipment to its proper place. Remembered to clean the brush and comb. Discarded disposable items.	___	___	_____
41. Followed agency policy for dirty linen.	___	___	_____
42. Practiced hand hygiene.	___	___	_____
43. Reported and recorded your observations.	___	___	_____

Date of Satisfactory Completion _____   Instructor's Initials _____

Shaving the Person's Face With a Safety Razor

Name: _____   Date: _____

Quality of Life	S	U	Comments

Remembered to:
- Knock before entering the person's room
- Address the person by name
- Introduce yourself by name and title
- Explain the procedure to the person before beginning and during the procedure
- Protect the person's rights during the procedure
- Handle the person gently during the procedure

Pre-Procedure

1. Followed *Delegation Guidelines: Shaving.* Reviewed *Promoting Safety and Comfort: Shaving.*
2. Practiced hand hygiene.
3. Collected the following:
   - Wash basin
   - Bath towel
   - Hand towel
   - Washcloth
   - Safety razor
   - Mirror
   - Shaving cream, soap, or lotion
   - Shaving brush
   - Aftershave or lotion
   - Tissues or paper towels
   - Paper towels
   - Gloves
4. Arranged paper towels and supplies on the overbed table.
5. Identified the person. Checked the ID bracelet against the assignment sheet. Called the person by name.
6. Provided for privacy.
7. Raised the bed for body mechanics. Bed rails were up if used.

Procedure

8. Filled the wash basin with warm water.
9. Placed the basin on the overbed table.
10. Lowered the bed rail near you if up.
11. Practiced hand hygiene. Put on gloves.
12. Assisted the person to semi-Fowler's position if allowed or to the supine position.
13. Adjusted lighting to clearly see the person's face.
14. Placed the bath towel over the person's chest and shoulders.
15. Adjusted the overbed table for easy reach.
16. Tightened the razor blade to the shaver if necessary.
17. Washed the person's face. Did not dry.
18. Wet the washcloth or towel. Wrung it out.
19. Applied the washcloth or towel to the face for a few minutes.
20. Applied shaving cream with your hands. Or used a shaving brush to apply lather.
21. Held the skin taut with one hand.
22. Shaved in the direction of hair growth. Used shorter strokes around the chin and lips.
23. Rinsed the razor often. Wiped it with tissues or paper towels.
24. Applied direct pressure to any bleeding areas.
25. Washed off any remaining shaving cream or soap. Patted dry with a towel.

Date of Satisfactory Completion _____   Instructor's Initials _____

Procedure—cont'd	S	U	Comments
26. Applied aftershave or lotion if requested. (Did not apply aftershave or lotion if there were nicks or cuts.)	___	___	_____
27. Removed and discarded the towel and gloves. Practiced hand hygiene.	___	___	_____

Post-Procedure

	S	U	Comments
28. Provided for comfort.	___	___	_____
29. Placed the signal light within reach.	___	___	_____
30. Lowered the bed to its lowest position.	___	___	_____
31. Raised or lowered bed rails. Followed the care plan.	___	___	_____
32. Cleaned, rinsed, dried, and returned equipment and supplies to their proper place. Discarded a razor blade or a disposable razor into the sharps container. Discarded disposable items. Wore gloves.	___	___	_____
33. Wiped off the overbed table with paper towels. Discarded the paper towels.	___	___	_____
34. Unscreened the person.	___	___	_____
35. Completed a safety check of the room.	___	___	_____
36. Followed agency policy for dirty linen.	___	___	_____
37. Removed and discarded the gloves. Practiced hand hygiene.	___	___	_____
38. Reported nicks, cuts, irritation, or bleeding to the nurse at once. Also reported and recorded other observations.	___	___	_____

Date of Satisfactory Completion _____   Instructor's Initials _____

Giving Nail and Foot Care (NNAAP®)

Name: _____   Date: _____

	S	U	Comments

Quality of Life

Remembered to:
- Knock before entering the person's room
- Address the person by name
- Introduce yourself by name and title
- Explain the procedure to the person before beginning and during the procedure
- Protect the person's rights during the procedure
- Handle the person gently during the procedure

Pre-Procedure

1. Followed *Delegation Guidelines: Nail and Foot Care.* Reviewed *Promoting Safety and Comfort: Nail and Foot Care.*
2. Practiced hand hygiene.
3. Collected the following:
   - Wash basin or whirlpool foot bath
   - Soap
   - Bath thermometer
   - Bath towel
   - Hand towel
   - Washcloth
   - Kidney basin
   - Nail clippers
   - Orange stick
   - Emery board or nail file
   - Lotion for the hands
   - Lotion or petroleum jelly for the feet
   - Paper towels
   - Bath mat
   - Gloves
4. Arranged paper towels and supplies on the overbed table.
5. Identified the person. Checked the ID bracelet against the assignment sheet. Called the person by name.
6. Provided for privacy.
7. Assisted the person to the bedside chair. Placed the signal light within reach. Removed footwear and socks or stockings.

Procedure

8. Placed the bath mat under the feet.
9. Filled the wash basin or whirlpool foot bath ⅔ (two-thirds) full with water. The nurse told you what water temperature to use. (Measured water temperature with a bath thermometer. Or tested it by dipping your elbow or inner wrist into the basin. Followed agency policy.) Also asked the person to check the water temperature. Adjusted the water temperature as needed.
10. Placed the basin or foot bath on the bath mat.
11. Put on gloves.
12. Helped the person put his or her bare feet into the basin or foot bath. Made sure both feet were completely covered by water.
13. Adjusted the overbed table in front of the person.
14. Filled the kidney basin ⅔ (two-thirds) full with water. The nurse told you what water temperature to use. (Measured water temperature with a bath thermometer. Or tested it by dipping your elbow or inner wrist into the basin. Followed agency policy.) Also asked the person to check the water temperature. Adjusted the water temperature as needed.

Date of Satisfactory Completion _____   Instructor's Initials _____

Procedure—cont'd	S	U	Comments
15. Placed the kidney basin on the overbed table.	___	___	_____
16. Placed the person's fingers into the basin. Positioned the arms for comfort.	___	___	_____
17. Allowed the fingers to soak for 5 to 10 minutes. Allowed the feet to soak for 15 to 20 minutes. Rewarmed water as needed.	___	___	_____
18. Removed the kidney basin.	___	___	_____
19. Cleaned under the fingernails with the orange stick. Used a towel to wipe the orange stick after each nail.	___	___	_____
20. Dried the hands and between the fingers thoroughly.	___	___	_____
21. Clipped fingernails straight across with the nail clippers.	___	___	_____
22. Shaped nails with an emery board or nail file. Nails were smooth with no rough edges. Filed as needed.	___	___	_____
23. Pushed cuticles back with the orange stick or a washcloth.	___	___	_____
24. Applied lotion to the hands. Warmed the lotion before it was applied.	___	___	_____
25. Moved the overbed table to the side.	___	___	_____
26. Lifted a foot out of the water. Supported the foot and ankle with one hand. With your other hand, washed the foot and between the toes with soap and a washcloth. Returned the foot to the water to rinse. Made sure you rinsed between the toes.	___	___	_____
27. Repeated for other foot: Lifted other foot out of the water. Supported the foot and ankle with one hand. With your other hand, washed the foot and between the toes with soap and a washcloth. Returned the foot to the water to rinse. Made sure you rinsed between the toes.	___	___	_____
28. Removed the feet from the basin or foot bath. Dried thoroughly, especially between the toes. Supported the foot and ankle as needed.	___	___	_____
29. Applied lotion or petroleum jelly to the tops, soles, and heels of the feet. Did not apply between the toes. Warmed lotion or petroleum jelly before applying it. Removed excess lotion or petroleum jelly with a towel. Supported the foot and ankle as needed.	___	___	_____
30. Removed and discarded the gloves. Practiced hand hygiene.	___	___	_____
31. Helped the person put on non-skid footwear.	___	___	_____

Post-Procedure

	S	U	Comments
32. Provided for comfort.	___	___	_____
33. Placed the signal light within reach.	___	___	_____
34. Raised or lowered bed rails. Followed the care plan.	___	___	_____
35. Cleaned, rinsed, dried, and returned equipment and supplies to their proper place. Wore gloves.	___	___	_____
36. Unscreened the person.	___	___	_____
37. Completed a safety check of the room.	___	___	_____
38. Followed agency policy for dirty linen.	___	___	_____
39. Removed and discarded the gloves. Practiced hand hygiene.	___	___	_____
40. Reported and recorded your observations.	___	___	_____

Date of Satisfactory Completion _____   Instructor's Initials _____

Undressing the Person

Name: _____　　Date: _____

Quality of Life　　　　　　　　　　　　**S**　　**U**　　**Comments**

Remembered to:
- Knock before entering the person's room
- Address the person by name
- Introduce yourself by name and title
- Explain the procedure to the person before beginning and during the procedure
- Protect the person's rights during the procedure
- Handle the person gently during the procedure

Pre-Procedure
1. Followed *Delegation Guidelines: Dressing and Undressing.*
2. Practiced hand hygiene.
3. Collected a bath blanket and clothing requested by the person.
4. Identified the person. Checked the ID bracelet against the assignment sheet. Called the person by name.
5. Provided for privacy.
6. Raised the bed for body mechanics. Bed rails were up if used.
7. Lowered the bed rail on the person's weak side.
8. Positioned him or her supine.
9. Covered the person with a bath blanket. Fan-folded linens to the foot of the bed.

Procedure
10. Removed garments that opened in the back:
    a. Raised the head and shoulders. Or turned him or her onto the side away from you.
    b. Undid buttons, zippers, ties, or snaps.
    c. Brought the sides of the garment to the sides of the person. If he or she was in a side-lying position, tucked the far side under the person. Folded the near side onto the chest.
    d. Positioned the person supine.
    e. Slid the garment off the shoulder on the strong side. Removed it from the arm.
    f. Removed the garment from the weak side.
11. Removed garments that opened in the front:
    a. Undid buttons, zippers, ties, or snaps.
    b. Slid the garment off the shoulder and arm on the strong side.
    c. Assisted the person to sit up or raised the head and shoulders. Brought the garment over to the weak side.
    d. Lowered the head and shoulders. Removed the garment from the weak side.
    e. If you could not raise the head and shoulders:
        (1) Turned the person toward you. Tucked the removed part under the person.
        (2) Turned him or her onto the side away from you.
        (3) Pulled the side of the garment out from under the person. Made sure he or she was not lying on it when supine.
        (4) Returned the person to the supine position.
        (5) Removed the garment from the weak side.

Date of Satisfactory Completion _____　Instructor's Initials _____

Procedure—cont'd	**S**	**U**	**Comments**
12. Removed pullover garments:			
a. Undid any buttons, zippers, ties, or snaps.	_____	_____	_____
b. Removed the garment from the strong side.	_____	_____	_____
c. Raised the head and shoulders. Or turned the person onto the side away from you. Brought the garment up to the person's neck.	_____	_____	_____
d. Brought the garment over the person's head.	_____	_____	_____
e. Removed the garment from the weak side.	_____	_____	_____
f. Positioned him or her in the supine position.	_____	_____	_____
13. Removed pants or slacks:			
a. Removed footwear and socks.	_____	_____	_____
b. Positioned the person supine.	_____	_____	_____
c. Undid buttons, zippers, ties, snaps, or buckles.	_____	_____	_____
d. Removed the belt.	_____	_____	_____
e. Asked the person to lift the buttocks off the bed. Slid the pants down over the hips and buttocks. Had the person lower the hips and buttocks.	_____	_____	_____
f. If the person could not raise the hips off the bed:			
(1) Turned the person toward you.	_____	_____	_____
(2) Slid the pants off the hip and buttocks on the strong side.	_____	_____	_____
(3) Turned the person away from you.	_____	_____	_____
(4) Slid the pants off the hip and buttocks on the weak side.	_____	_____	_____
g. Slid the pants down the legs and over the feet.	_____	_____	_____
14. Dressed the person. Followed the procedure for *Dressing the Person*.	_____	_____	_____

Post-Procedure

	S	**U**	**Comments**
15. Provided for comfort.	_____	_____	_____
16. Placed the signal light within reach.	_____	_____	_____
17. Lowered the bed to its lowest position.	_____	_____	_____
18. Raised or lowered bed rails. Followed the care plan.	_____	_____	_____
19. Unscreened the person.	_____	_____	_____
20. Completed a safety check of the room.	_____	_____	_____
21. Followed agency policy for soiled clothing.	_____	_____	_____
22. Practiced hand hygiene.	_____	_____	_____
23. Reported and recorded your observations.	_____	_____	_____

Date of Satisfactory Completion _____   Instructor's Initials _____

Dressing the Person (NNAAP®)

Name: _____   Date: _____

Quality of Life	S	U	Comments

Remembered to:
- Knock before entering the person's room
- Address the person by name
- Introduce yourself by name and title
- Explain the procedure to the person before beginning and during the procedure
- Protect the person's rights during the procedure
- Handle the person gently during the procedure

Pre-Procedure

1. Followed *Delegation Guidelines: Dressing and Undressing*.
2. Practiced hand hygiene.
3. Asked the person what he or she would like to wear.
4. Got a bath blanket and clothing requested by the person.
5. Identified the person. Checked the ID bracelet against the assignment sheet. Called the person by name.
6. Provided for privacy.
7. Raised the bed for body mechanics. Bed rails were up if used.
8. Lowered the bed rail (if up) on the person's strong side.
9. Positioned the person supine.
10. Covered the person with a bath blanket. Fan-folded linens to the foot of the bed.
11. Undressed the person. Followed the procedure: *Undressing the Person*.

Procedure

12. Put on garments that opened in the back:
    a. Slid the garment onto the arm and shoulder of the weak side.
    b. Slid the garment onto the arm and shoulder of the strong arm.
    c. Raised the person's head and shoulders.
    d. Brought the sides to the back.
    e. If you could not raise the person's head and shoulders:
       (1) Turned the person toward you.
       (2) Brought one side of the garment to the person's back.
       (3) Turned the person away from you.
       (4) Brought the other side to the person's back.
    f. Fastened buttons, ties, snaps, zippers, or other closures.
    g. Positioned the person supine.
13. Put on garments that opened in the front:
    a. Slid the garment onto the arm and shoulder on the weak side.
    b. Raised the head and shoulders. Brought the side of the garment around to the back. Lowered the person down. Slid the garment arm onto the arm and shoulder of the strong arm.
    c. If the person could not raise the head and shoulders:
       (1) Turned the person away from you.
       (2) Tucked the garment under the person.
       (3) Turned the person toward you.
       (4) Pulled the garment out from under the person.
       (5) Turned the person back to the supine position.
       (6) Slid the garment over the arm and shoulder of the strong arm.
    d. Fastened buttons, ties, snaps, zippers, or other closures.

Date of Satisfactory Completion _____   Instructor's Initials _____

Procedure—cont'd	**S**	**U**	**Comments**
14. Put on pullover garments:			
a. Positioned the person supine.	____	____	_____
b. Slid the arm and shoulder of the garment onto the weak side.	____	____	_____
c. Raised the person's head and shoulders.	____	____	_____
d. Brought the neck of the garment over the head.	____	____	_____
e. Brought the garment down.	____	____	_____
f. Slid the arm and shoulder of the garment onto the strong side.	____	____	_____
g. If the person could not assume a semi-sitting position:			
(1) Turned the person away from you.	____	____	_____
(2) Tucked the garment under the person.	____	____	_____
(3) Turned the person toward you.	____	____	_____
(4) Pulled the garment out from under the person.	____	____	_____
(5) Positioned the person supine.	____	____	_____
(6) Slid the arm and shoulder of the garment onto the strong side.	____	____	_____
h. Fastened buttons, ties, snaps, zippers, or other closures.	____	____	_____
15. Put on pants or slacks:			
a. Slid the pants over the feet and up the legs.	____	____	_____
b. Asked the person to raise the hips and buttocks off the bed.	____	____	_____
c. Brought the pants up over the buttocks and hips.	____	____	_____
d. Asked the person to lower the hips and buttocks.	____	____	_____
e. If the person could not raise the hips and buttocks:			
(1) Turned the person onto the strong side.	____	____	_____
(2) Pulled the pants over the buttock and hip on the weak side.	____	____	_____
(3) Turned the person onto the weak side.	____	____	_____
(4) Pulled the pants over the buttock and hip on the strong side.	____	____	_____
(5) Positioned the person supine.	____	____	_____
f. Fastened buttons, ties, snaps, the zipper, belt buckle, or other closure.	____	____	_____
16. Put socks and non-skid footwear on the person. Made sure were all the way up and smooth.	____	____	_____
17. Helped the person get out of bed. If the person stayed in bed, covered the person. Removed the bath blanket.	____	____	_____

Post-Procedure

	S	**U**	**Comments**
18. Provided for comfort.	____	____	_____
19. Placed the signal light within reach.	____	____	_____
20. Lowered the bed to its lowest position.	____	____	_____
21. Raised or lowered bed rails. Followed the care plan.	____	____	_____
22. Unscreened the person.	____	____	_____
23. Completed a safety check of the room.	____	____	_____
24. Followed agency policy for soiled clothing.	____	____	_____
25. Practiced hand hygiene.	____	____	_____
26. Reported and recorded your observations.	____	____	_____

Date of Satisfactory Completion _____   Instructor's Initials _____

Changing the Gown of the Person With an IV

Name: _____   Date: _____

Quality of Life	S	U	Comments

Quality of Life

Remembered to:
- Knock before entering the person's room
- Address the person by name
- Introduce yourself by name and title
- Explain the procedure to the person before beginning and during the procedure
- Protect the person's rights during the procedure
- Handle the person gently during the procedure

Pre-Procedure
1. Followed *Delegation Guidelines: Changing Hospital Gowns.* Reviewed *Promoting Safety and Comfort: Changing Hospital Gowns.*
2. Practiced hand hygiene.
3. Got a clean gown and a bath blanket.
4. Identified the person. Checked the ID bracelet against the assignment sheet. Called the person by name.
5. Provided for privacy.
6. Raised the bed for body mechanics. Bed rails were up if used.

Procedure
7. Lowered the bed rail near you (if up).
8. Covered the person with a bath blanket. Fan-folded linens to the foot of the bed.
9. Untied the gown. Freed parts the person was lying on.
10. Removed the gown from the arm with *no IV*.
11. Gathered up the sleeve of the arm *with the IV*. Slid it over the IV site and tubing. Removed the arm and hand from the sleeve.
12. Kept the sleeve gathered. Slid your arm along the tubing to the bag.
13. Removed the bag from the pole. Slid the bag and tubing through the sleeve. Did not pull on the tubing. Kept the bag above the person.
14. Hung the IV bag on the pole.
15. Gathered the sleeve of the clean gown that went on the arm with the IV infusion.
16. Removed the bag from the pole. Slipped the sleeve over the bag at the shoulder part of the gown. Hung the bag.
17. Slid the gathered sleeve over the tubing, hand, arm, and IV site. Then slid it onto the shoulder.
18. Put the other side of the gown on the person. Fastened the gown.
19. Covered the person. Removed the bath blanket.

Post-Procedure
20. Provided for comfort.
21. Placed the signal light within reach.
22. Lowered the bed to its lowest position.
23. Raised or lowered bed rails. Followed the care plan.
24. Unscreened the person.
25. Completed a safety check of the room.
26. Followed agency policy for dirty linens.
27. Practiced hand hygiene.
28. Asked the nurse to check the flow rate.
29. Reported and recorded your observations.

Date of Satisfactory Completion _____   Instructor's Initials _____

Giving the Bedpan (NNAAP®)

Name: _____   Date: _____

	S	U	Comments

Quality of Life
Remembered to:
- Knock before entering the person's room
- Address the person by name
- Introduce yourself by name and title
- Explain the procedure to the person before beginning and during the procedure
- Protect the person's rights during the procedure
- Handle the person gently during the procedure

Pre-Procedure
1. Followed *Delegation Guidelines: Bedpans.* Reviewed *Promoting Safety and Comfort: Bedpans.*
2. Provided for privacy.
3. Practiced hand hygiene.
4. Put on gloves.
5. Collected the following:
   - Bedpan
   - Bedpan cover
   - Toilet tissue
   - Waterproof pad (if required by agency)
6. Arranged equipment on the chair or bed.

Procedure
7. Lowered the bed rail near you (if up).
8. Lowered the head of the bed. Positioned the person supine or raised the head of the bed slightly for the person's comfort.
9. Folded the top linens and gown out of the way. Kept the lower body covered.
10. Asked the person to flex the knees and raise the buttocks by pushing against the mattress with his or her feet.
11. Slid your hand under the lower back. Helped raise the buttocks. If used waterproof pad, placed it under the person's buttocks.
12. Slid the bedpan under the person.
13. If the person did not assist in getting on the bedpan:
    a. If waterproof pad used, placed it under the person's buttocks.
    b. Turned the person onto the side away from you.
    c. Placed the bedpan firmly against the buttocks.
    d. Pushed the bedpan down and toward the person.
    e. Held the bedpan securely. Turned the person onto his or her back.
    f. Made sure the bedpan was centered under the person.
14. Covered the person.
15. Raised the head of the bed so the person was in a sitting position (Fowler's position). (NOTE: Some state competency tests require that you removed gloves and washed your hands before you raised the head of the bed.)
16. Made sure the person was correctly positioned on the bedpan.
17. Raised the bed rail if used.
18. Placed the toilet tissue and signal light within reach.
    NOTE: Some state competency tests require that you ask the person to use hand wipes to clean the hands after wiping with toilet tissue.
19. Asked the person to signal when done or when help was needed.
20. Removed and discarded the gloves. Practiced hand hygiene.
21. Left the room and closed the door.
22. Returned when the person signaled. Or checked on the person every 5 minutes. Knocked before entering.
23. Practiced hand hygiene. Put on gloves.

Date of Satisfactory Completion _____   Instructor's Initials _____

Procedure—cont'd   S   U   **Comments**

24. Raised the bed for body mechanics. Lowered the bed rail
    (if used) and the head of the bed.   ___   ___   _____
25. Asked the person to raise the buttocks. Removed the bedpan.
    Or held the bedpan and turned him or her onto the side away
    from you.   ___   ___   _____
26. Cleaned the genital area if the person did not do so.
    Cleaned from front (urethra) to back (anus) with toilet tissue.
    Used fresh tissue for each wipe. Provided perineal care if needed.
    Removed and discarded the waterproof pad if used.   ___   ___   _____
27. Covered the bedpan. Took it to the bathroom. Raised the bed
    rail (if used) before leaving the bedside.   ___   ___   _____
28. Noted the color, amount, and character of the urine or feces. ___   ___   _____
29. Emptied the bedpan contents into the toilet and flushed.   ___   ___   _____
30. Rinsed the bedpan. Poured the rinse into the toilet and flushed. ___   ___   _____
31. Cleaned the bedpan with a disinfectant.   ___   ___   _____
32. Removed and discarded soiled gloves. Practiced hand hygiene
    and put on clean gloves.   ___   ___   _____
33. Returned the bedpan and clean cover to the bedside stand. ___   ___   _____
34. Helped the person with hand washing. (Wore gloves for this step.) ___   ___   _____
35. Removed and discarded the gloves. Practiced hand hygiene. ___   ___   _____

Post-Procedure
36. Provided for comfort.   ___   ___   _____
37. Placed the signal light within reach.   ___   ___   _____
38. Lowered the bed to its lowest position.   ___   ___   _____
39. Raised or lowered bed rails. Followed the care plan. ___   ___   _____
40. Unscreened the person.   ___   ___   _____
41. Completed a safety check of the room.   ___   ___   _____
42. Followed agency policy for soiled linens.   ___   ___   _____
43. Practiced hand hygiene.   ___   ___   _____
44. Reported and recorded your observations.   ___   ___   _____

Date of Satisfactory Completion _____   Instructor's Initials _____

Giving the Urinal

Name: _____   Date: _____

Quality of Life	S	U	Comments

Remembered to:
- Knock before entering the person's room
- Address the person by name
- Introduce yourself by name and title
- Explain the procedure to the person before beginning and during the procedure
- Protect the person's rights during the procedure
- Handle the person gently during the procedure

Pre-Procedure

1. Followed *Delegation Guidelines: Urinals.* Reviewed *Promoting Safety and Comfort: Urinals.*
2. Provided for privacy.
3. Determined if the man will stand, sit, or lie in bed.
4. Practiced hand hygiene.
5. Put on gloves.
6. Collected the following:
   - Urinal
   - Non-skid footwear if the person stood to void

Procedure

7. Gave him the urinal if he was in bed. Reminded him to tilt the bottom down to prevent spills.
8. If he stood:
   a. Helped him sit on the side of the bed.
   b. Put non-skid footwear on him.
   c. Helped him stand. Provided support if he was unsteady.
   d. Gave him the urinal.
9. Positioned the urinal if necessary. Placed the penis in the urinal if he could not do so.
10. Placed the signal light within reach. Asked him to signal when done or when he needed help.
11. Provided for privacy.
12. Removed and discarded the gloves. Practiced hand hygiene.
13. Left the room and closed the door.
14. Returned when he signaled. Or checked on the person every 5 minutes. Knocked before entering.
15. Practiced hand hygiene. Put on gloves.
16. Closed the cap on the urinal. Took it to the bathroom.
17. Noted the color, amount, and clarity of the urine.
18. Emptied the urinal into the toilet and flushed.
19. Rinsed the urinal with cold water. Poured rinse into the toilet and flushed.
20. Cleaned the urinal with a disinfectant.
21. Returned the urinal to its proper place.
22. Removed soiled gloves. Practiced hand hygiene and put on clean gloves.
23. Assisted with hand washing.
24. Removed and discarded the gloves. Practiced hand hygiene.

Date of Satisfactory Completion _____   Instructor's Initials _____

Post-Procedure

25. Provided for comfort.
26. Placed the signal light within reach.
27. Raised or lowered bed rails. Followed the care plan.
28. Unscreened the person.
29. Completed a safety check of the room.
30. Followed agency policy for soiled linens.
31. Practiced hand hygiene.
32. Reported and recorded your observations.

Date of Satisfactory Completion _____   Instructor's Initials _____

VIDEO **Helping the Person to the Commode**

Name: _____   Date: _____

	S	U	Comments

Quality of Life

Remembered to:
- Knock before entering the person's room
- Address the person by name
- Introduce yourself by name and title
- Explain the procedure to the person before beginning and during the procedure
- Protect the person's rights during the procedure
- Handle the person gently during the procedure

Pre-Procedure

1. Followed *Delegation Guidelines: Commodes.* Reviewed *Promoting Safety and Comfort: Commodes.*
2. Provided for privacy.
3. Practiced hand hygiene.
4. Put on gloves.
5. Collected the following:
   - Commode
   - Toilet tissue
   - Bath blanket
   - Transfer belt
   - Robe and non-skid footwear

Procedure

6. Brought the commode next to the bed. Raised the lid and removed the container cover.
7. Helped the person sit on the side of the bed. Lowered the bed rail if used.
8. Helped the person put on a robe or non-skid footwear.
9. Applied the transfer belt.
10. Assisted the person to the commode. Used the transfer belt.
11. Removed the transfer belt. Covered the person with a bath blanket for warmth.
12. Placed the toilet tissue and signal light within reach.
13. Asked the person to signal when done or when help was needed. (Stayed with the person if necessary. Was respectful. Provided as much privacy as possible.)
14. Removed and discarded the gloves. Practiced hand hygiene.
15. Left the room. Closed the door.
16. Returned when the person signaled. Or checked on the person every 5 minutes. Knocked before entering.
17. Practiced hand hygiene. Put on gloves.
18. Helped the person clean the genital area as needed. Removed and discarded the gloves. Practiced hand hygiene.
19. Applied the transfer belt. Helped the person back to bed; used the transfer belt. Removed the transfer belt, robe, and footwear. Raised the bed rail if used.
20. Put on clean gloves. Removed and covered the commode container. Cleaned the commode.
21. Took the container to the bathroom.
22. Observed urine and feces for color, amount, and character.
23. Emptied the container contents into the toilet and flushed.
24. Rinsed the container. Poured rinse into the toilet and flushed.
25. Cleaned and disinfected the container.

Date of Satisfactory Completion _____   Instructor's Initials _____

Procedure—cont'd

	S	U	Comments
26. Returned the container to the commode. Closed the lid on the commode.	___	___	_____
27. Returned other supplies to their proper place.	___	___	_____
28. Removed and discarded soiled gloves. Practiced hand hygiene and put on clean gloves.	___	___	_____
29. Assisted with hand washing.	___	___	_____
30. Removed and discarded the gloves. Practiced hand hygiene.	___	___	_____

Post-Procedure

	S	U	Comments
31. Provided for comfort.			
32. Placed the signal light within reach.	___	___	_____
33. Raised or lowered bed rails. Followed the care plan.	___	___	_____
34. Unscreened the person.	___	___	_____
35. Completed a safety check of the room.	___	___	_____
36. Followed agency policy for dirty linen.	___	___	_____
37. Practiced hand hygiene.	___	___	_____
38. Reported and recorded your observations.	___	___	_____

Date of Satisfactory Completion _____   Instructor's Initials _____

Applying Incontinence Products

Name: _____   Date: _____

Quality of Life	S	U	Comments

Remembered to:
- Knock before entering the person's room
- Address the person by name
- Introduce yourself by name and title
- Explain the procedure to the person before beginning and during the procedure
- Protect the person's rights during the procedure
- Handle the person gently during the procedure

Pre-Procedure

1. Followed *Delegation Guidelines: Applying Incontinence Products.* Reviewed *Promoting Safety and Comfort: Applying Incontinence Products.*
2. Practiced hand hygiene.
3. Collected the following:
   - Incontinence product as directed by nurse
   - Barrier cream as directed by nurse
   - Cleanser
   - Items for perineal care
   - Waterproof pad
   - Paper towels
   - Trash bag
   - Gloves
   - Non-skid footwear if the person stands
4. Covered the overbed table with paper towels. Arranged items on top of them.
5. Identified the person. Checked the ID bracelet against the assignment sheet. Called the person by name.
6. Provided for privacy.
7. Filled the wash basin. Water temperature was about 105° F (Fahrenheit) (40.5° C [Centigrade]). Measured water temperature according to agency policy. Asked the person to check the water temperature. Adjusted water temperature as needed.
8. Raised the bed for body mechanics. Bed rails were up if used. (Omitted this step if person stood.)

Procedure

9. Lowered the head of the bed. The bed was as flat as possible.
10. Lowered the bed rail near you if up.
11. Practiced hand hygiene. Put on gloves.
12. Covered the person with a bath blanket. Lowered top linens to the foot of the bed.
13. *To apply incontinence brief with the person in bed:*
    a. Placed a waterproof pad under the buttocks. Asked the person to raise the buttocks off the bed. Or turned the person from side to side.
    b. Loosened the tabs on each side of the product.
    c. Turned the person on the side away from you.
    d. Removed the product from front to back. Observed the urine as you rolled the product up.
    e. Placed the product in the trash bag. Set the bag aside.
    f. Performed perineal care.
    g. Opened the new brief. Folded it in half length-wise along the center.

Date of Satisfactory Completion _____   Instructor's Initials _____

Procedure—cont'd   **S**   **U**   **Comments**

h. Inserted the product between the legs from front to back. ___ ___ _____
i. Unfolded and spread the back panel. ___ ___ _____
j. Centered the product in the perineal area. ___ ___ _____
k. Turned the person onto his or her back. ___ ___ _____
l. Unfolded and spread the front panel. Provided a "cup" shape in the perineal area. For a man, positioned the penis downward. ___ ___ _____
m. Made sure the product was positioned high in the groin folds. This allowed the product to fit the shape of the body. ___ ___ _____
n. Secured the product.
   (1) Pulled the lower tab forward on the side near you. Attached it at a slightly upward angle. Did the same for the other side. ___ ___ _____
   (2) Pulled the upper tab forward on the side near you. Attached it in a horizontal manner. Did the same for the other side. ___ ___ _____
o. Smoothed out all wrinkles and folds. ___ ___ _____

14. *To apply a pad and undergarment with the person in bed:*
   a. Placed a waterproof pad under the buttocks. Asked the person to raise the buttocks off the bed. Or turned the person from side to side. ___ ___ _____
   b. Turned the person onto the side away from you. ___ ___ _____
   c. Pulled the undergarment down. The waistband was over the knee. ___ ___ _____
   d. Removed the pad from front to back. Observed the urine as you rolled the product up. ___ ___ _____
   e. Placed the product in the trash bag. Set the bag aside. ___ ___ _____
   f. Performed perineal care. ___ ___ _____
   g. Folded the new pad in half length-wise along the center. ___ ___ _____
   h. Inserted the pad between the legs from front to back. ___ ___ _____
   i. Unfolded and spread the back panel. ___ ___ _____
   j. Centered the pad in the perineal area. ___ ___ _____
   k. Pulled the undergarment up the back. ___ ___ _____
   l. Turned the person onto his or her back. ___ ___ _____
   m. Unfolded and spread the front panel. For a man, positioned the penis downward. ___ ___ _____
   n. Pulled the garment up in front. ___ ___ _____
   o. Checked and adjusted the pad and undergarment for a good fit. ___ ___ _____

15. *To apply pull-on underwear with the person standing:*
   a. Helped the person put on non-skid footwear. ___ ___ _____
   b. Helped the person stand. ___ ___ _____
   c. Tore the side seams to remove the used underwear. ___ ___ _____
   d. Removed the product from front to back. Observed the urine as you rolled the product up. ___ ___ _____
   e. Placed the product in the trash bag. Set the bag aside. ___ ___ _____
   f. Performed perineal care. ___ ___ _____
   g. Had the person sit on the side of the bed. ___ ___ _____
   h. Slid the underwear over the feet to past the knees. ___ ___ _____
   i. Helped the person to stand. ___ ___ _____
   j. Pulled the underwear up. ___ ___ _____
   k. Checked for a good fit. ___ ___ _____
16. Removed and discarded the gloves. Practiced hand hygiene. ___ ___ _____

Date of Satisfactory Completion _____   Instructor's Initials _____

Post-Procedure

17. Provided for comfort.
18. Placed the signal light within reach.
19. Lowered the bed to its lowest position.
20. Raised or lowered bed rails. Followed the care plan.
21. Unscreened the person.
22. Practiced hand hygiene. Put on clean gloves.
23. Estimated the amount of urine in the old product: small, moderate, large. Opened the product to observe the urine for color and blood.
24. Cleaned, rinsed, dried, and returned the wash basin and other equipment. Returned items to their proper place.
25. Removed gloves. Practiced hand hygiene.
26. Completed a safety check of the room.
27. Reported and recorded your observations.

Date of Satisfactory Completion _____   Instructor's Initials _____

Giving Catheter Care (NNAAP®)

Name: _____   Date: _____

	S	U	Comments

Quality of Life
Remembered to:
- Knock before entering the person's room
- Address the person by name
- Introduce yourself by name and title
- Explain the procedure to the person before beginning and during the procedure
- Protect the person's rights during the procedure
- Handle the person gently during the procedure

Pre-Procedure
1. Followed *Delegation Guidelines:*
   a. *Perineal Care*
   b. *Catheters*
   Reviewed *Promoting Safety and Comfort:*
   a. *Perineal Care*
   b. *Catheters*
2. Practiced hand hygiene.
3. Collected the following:
   - Items for perineal care:
   Soap or other cleaning agent as directed
   At least 4 washcloths
   Bath towel
   Bath thermometer
   Wash basin
   Waterproof pad
   Paper towels
   - Gloves
   - Bath blanket
4. Covered the overbed table with paper towels. Arranged items on top of them.
5. Identified the person. Checked the ID bracelet against the assignment sheet. Called the person by name.
6. Provided for privacy.
7. Filled the wash basin. Water temperature was about 105° F (40.5° C). Measured water temperature according to agency policy. Asked the person to check the water temperature. Adjusted water temperature as needed.
8. Raised the bed for good body mechanics. Bed rails were up if used.

Procedure
9. Lowered the bed rail near you if up.
10. Practiced hand hygiene. Put on gloves.
11. Covered the person with a bath blanket. Fan-folded top linens to the foot of the bed.
12. Draped the person for perineal care.
13. Folded back the bath blanket to expose the genital area.
14. Placed the waterproof pad under the buttocks. Asked the person to flex the knees and raise the buttocks off the bed.
15. Separated the labia (female). In an uncircumcised male, retracted the foreskin. Checked for crusts, abnormal drainage, or secretions.
16. Gave perineal care. Kept the foreskin of the uncircumcised male retracted until step 22.
17. Applied soap to clean, wet washcloth.

Date of Satisfactory Completion _____   Instructor's Initials _____

	S	U	Comments

Procedure—cont'd

18. Held the catheter at the meatus. Did so for steps 19, 20, and 21.
19. Cleaned the catheter from the meatus down the catheter at least 4 inches. Cleaned downward, away from the meatus with 1 stroke. Did not tug or pull on the catheter. Repeated as needed with a clean area of the washcloth. Used a clean area of the washcloth. Used a clean washcloth if needed.
20. Rinsed the catheter with a clean washcloth. Rinsed from the meatus down the catheter at least 4 inches. Rinsed downward, away from the meatus with 1 stroke. Did not tug or pull on the catheter. Repeated as needed with a clean area of the washcloth. Used a clean washcloth if needed.
21. Dried the catheter with towel. Dried from the meatus down the catheter at least 4 inches. Did not tug or pull on the catheter.
22. Returned the foreskin to its natural position.
23. Patted the perineal area dry. Dried from front to back.
24. Secured the catheter. Coiled and secured tubing.
25. Removed the waterproof pad.
26. Covered the person. Removed the bath blanket.
27. Removed and discarded the gloves. Practiced hand hygiene.

Post-Procedure

28. Provided for comfort.
29. Placed the signal light within reach.
30. Lowered the bed to its lowest position.
31. Raised or lowered bed rails. Followed the care plan.
32. Cleaned, rinsed, dried, and returned equipment to its proper place. Discarded disposable items. (Wore gloves for this step.)
33. Unscreened the person.
34. Completed a safety check of the room.
35. Followed agency policy for soiled linens.
36. Removed and discarded your gloves. Practiced hand hygiene.
37. Reported and recorded your observations.

Date of Satisfactory Completion _____   Instructor's Initials _____

Changing a Leg Bag to a Drainage Bag

Name: _____   Date: _____

	S	**U**	**Comments**

Quality of Life

Remembered to:
- Knock before entering the person's room
- Address the person by name
- Introduce yourself by name and title
- Explain the procedure to the person before beginning and during the procedure
- Protect the person's rights during the procedure
- Handle the person gently during the procedure

Pre-Procedure

1. Followed *Delegation Guidelines: Drainage Systems*. Reviewed *Promoting Safety and Comfort: Drainage Systems*.
2. Practiced hand hygiene.
3. Collected the following:
   - Gloves
   - Drainage bag and tubing
   - Antiseptic wipes
   - Waterproof pad
   - Sterile cap and plug
   - Catheter clamp
   - Paper towels
   - Bedpan
   - Bath blanket
4. Arranged paper towels and equipment on the overbed table.
5. Identified the person. Checked the ID bracelet against the assignment sheet. Called the person by name.
6. Provided for privacy.

Procedure

7. Had the person sit on the side of the bed.
8. Practiced hand hygiene. Put on gloves.
9. Exposed the catheter and leg bag.
10. Clamped the catheter. This prevented urine from draining from the catheter into the drainage tubing.
11. Allowed urine to drain from below the clamp into the drainage tubing. This emptied the lower end of the catheter.
12. Helped the person lie down.
13. Raised the bed rails if used. Raised the bed for body mechanics.
14. Lowered the bed rail near you if up.
15. Covered the person with a bath blanket. Fan-folded top linens to the foot of the bed. Exposed the catheter and leg bag.
16. Placed the waterproof pad under the person's leg.
17. Opened the antiseptic wipes. Placed them on paper towels.
18. Opened the package with the sterile cap and plug. Placed the package on the paper towels. Did not let anything touch the sterile cap or plug.
19. Opened the package with the drainage bag and tubing.
20. Attached the drainage bag to the bed frame.
21. Disconnected the catheter from the drainage tubing. Did not allow anything to touch the ends.
22. Inserted the sterile plug into the catheter end. Touched only the end of the plug. Did not touch the part that went inside the catheter. (If you contaminated the end of the catheter, wiped the end with an antiseptic wipe. Did so before you inserted the sterile plug.)

Date of Satisfactory Completion _____   Instructor's Initials _____

Procedure—cont'd	S	U	Comments
23. Placed the sterile cap on the end of the leg bag drainage tube. (If you contaminated the tubing end, wiped the end with an antiseptic wipe. Did so before you applied the sterile cap.)	___	___	_____
24. Removed the cap from the new drainage tubing.	___	___	_____
25. Removed the sterile plug from the catheter.	___	___	_____
26. Inserted the end of the drainage tubing into the catheter.	___	___	_____
27. Removed the clamp from the catheter.	___	___	_____
28. Looped the drainage tubing on the bed. Secured the tubing to the bottom linens.	___	___	_____
29. Removed the leg bag. Placed it in the bedpan.	___	___	_____
30. Removed and discarded the waterproof pad.	___	___	_____
31. Covered the person. Removed the bath blanket.	___	___	_____
32. Took the bedpan to the bathroom.	___	___	_____
33. Removed and discarded the gloves. Practiced hand hygiene.	___	___	_____

Post-Procedure

	S	U	Comments
34. Provided for comfort.	___	___	_____
35. Placed the signal light within reach.	___	___	_____
36. Lowered the bed to its lowest position.	___	___	_____
37. Raised or lowered bed rails. Followed the care plan.	___	___	_____
38. Unscreened the person.	___	___	_____
39. Put on clean gloves. Discarded disposable items.	___	___	_____
40. Emptied the drainage bag.	___	___	_____
41. Discarded the drainage tubing and bag following agency policy. Or cleaned the bag following agency policy.	___	___	_____
42. Cleaned and disinfected the bedpan. Placed it in a clean cover.	___	___	_____
43. Returned the bedpan and other supplies to their proper place.	___	___	_____
44. Removed and discarded the gloves. Practiced hand hygiene.	___	___	_____
45. Completed a safety check of the room.	___	___	_____
46. Followed agency policy for soiled linens.	___	___	_____
47. Practiced hand hygiene.	___	___	_____
48. Reported and recorded your observations.	___	___	_____

Date of Satisfactory Completion _____   Instructor's Initials _____

Emptying a Urinary Drainage Bag

Name: _____   Date: _____

Quality of Life	S	U	Comments

Remembered to:
- Knock before entering the person's room
- Address the person by name
- Introduce yourself by name and title
- Explain the procedure to the person before beginning and during the procedure
- Protect the person's rights during the procedure
- Handle the person gently during the procedure

Pre-Procedure
1. Followed *Delegation Guidelines: Drainage Systems.* Reviewed *Promoting Safety and Comfort: Drainage Systems.*
2. Collected the following:
   - Graduate (measuring container)
   - Gloves
   - Paper towels
   - Antiseptic wipes
3. Practiced hand hygiene.
4. Identified the person. Checked the ID bracelet against the assignment sheet. Called the person by name.
5. Provided for privacy.

Procedure
6. Put on the gloves.
7. Placed paper towel on the floor. Placed graduate on top of it.
8. Positioned the graduate under the collection bag.
9. Opened the clamp on the drain.
10. Allowed all urine to drain into the graduate. Did not let the drain touch the graduate.
11. Cleansed the end of the drain with an antiseptic wipe.
12. Closed and positioned the clamp.
13. Measured urine.
14. Removed and discarded the paper towel.
15. Emptied the contents of the graduate into the toilet and flushed.
16. Rinsed the graduate. Emptied the rinse into the toilet and flushed.
17. Cleaned and disinfected the graduate.
18. Returned the graduate to its proper place.
19. Removed and discarded the gloves. Practiced hand hygiene.
20. Recorded the time and amount of urine on the intake and output (I&O) record.

Post-Procedure
21. Provided for comfort.
22. Placed the signal light within reach.
23. Unscreened the person.
24. Completed a safety check of the room.
25. Reported and recorded the amount of urine and other observations.

Date of Satisfactory Completion _____   Instructor's Initials _____

Removing an Indwelling Catheter

Name: _____   Date: _____

Quality of Life	S	U	Comments

Remembered to:
- Knock before entering the person's room
- Address the person by name
- Introduce yourself by name and title
- Explain the procedure to the person before beginning and during the procedure
- Protect the person's rights during the procedure
- Handle the person gently during the procedure

Pre-Procedure

1. Followed *Delegation Guidelines: Removing Indwelling Catheters.* Reviewed *Promoting Safety and Comfort: Removing Indwelling Catheters.*
2. Practiced hand hygiene.
3. Collected the following:
   - Disposable towel
   - Syringe in the size as directed by the nurse
   - Disposable bag
   - Gloves
   - Bath blanket
4. Identified the person. Checked the ID bracelet against the assignment sheet. Called the person by name.
5. Provided for privacy.
6. Raised the bed for body mechanics. Bed rails were up if used.

Procedure

7. Lowered the bed rail near you if up.
8. Practiced hand hygiene. Put on the gloves.
9. Positioned and draped the person as for perineal care.
10. Covered the person with a bath blanket.
11. Removed the tape securing the catheter to the person.
12. Positioned the towel:
    a. Female—between her legs.
    b. Male—over his thighs.
13. Attached the syringe to the balloon port on the catheter.
14. Pulled back on the syringe slowly. Withdrew all water from the balloon. Called for the nurse if you could not remove all the water.
15. Pulled the catheter straight out. Removed the catheter gently. Did not remove the catheter if there was water in the balloon.
16. Discarded the catheter into the bag.
17. Dried the perineal area with the towel. Discarded the towel in the bag.
18. Removed and discarded the gloves. Practiced hand hygiene.
19. Covered the person. Removed the bath blanket.

Post-Procedure

20. Provided for comfort.
21. Placed the signal light within reach.
22. Lowered the bed to its lowest position.
23. Raised or lowered bed rails. Followed the care plan.
24. Unscreened the person.
25. Put on clean gloves. Discarded disposable items.
26. Emptied the drainage bag. Noted the amount of urine.
27. Discarded the drainage tubing and bag following agency policy.

Date of Satisfactory Completion _____   Instructor's Initials _____

Procedure—cont'd

	S	U	Comments
28. Removed and discarded the gloves. Practiced hand hygiene.	___	___	_____
29. Completed a safety check of the room.	___	___	_____
30. Practiced hand hygiene.	___	___	_____
31. Reported and recorded your observations.	___	___	_____

Date of Satisfactory Completion _____   Instructor's Initials _____

Applying a Condom Catheter

Name: _____   Date: _____

	S	U	Comments

Quality of Life

Remembered to:
- Knock before entering the person's room
- Address the person by name
- Introduce yourself by name and title
- Explain the procedure to the person before beginning and during the procedure
- Protect the person's rights during the procedure
- Handle the person gently during the procedure

Pre-Procedure

1. Followed *Delegation Guidelines*:
   a. *Perineal Care*
   b. *Condom Catheters*
   Reviewed *Promoting Safety and Comfort*:
   a. *Perineal Care*
   b. *Condom Catheters*
2. Practiced hand hygiene.
3. Collected the following:
   - Condom catheter
   - Elastic tape
   - Drainage bag or leg bag
   - Cap for the drainage bag
   - Basin of warm water
   - Soap
   - Towel and washcloth
   - Bath blanket
   - Gloves
   - Waterproof pad
   - Paper towels
4. Covered the overbed table with paper towels. Arranged item on top of them.
5. Identified the person. Checked the ID bracelet against the assignment sheet. Called the person by name.
6. Provided for privacy.
7. Filled the wash basin. Water temperature was about 105° F (40.5° C). Measured water temperature according to agency policy. Asked the person to check the water temperature. Adjusted water temperature as needed.
8. Raised the bed for body mechanics. Bed rails were up if used.

Procedure

9. Lowered the bed rail near you if up.
10. Practiced hand hygiene. Put on the gloves.
11. Covered the person with a bath blanket. Lowered top linens to the knees.
12. Asked the person to raise his buttocks off the bed. Or turned him onto his side away from you.
13. Slid the waterproof pad under his buttocks.
14. Had the person lower his buttocks. Or turned him onto his back.
15. Secured the drainage bag to the bed frame. Or had a leg bag ready. Closed the drain.
16. Exposed the genital area.

Date of Satisfactory Completion _____   Instructor's Initials _____

Procedure—cont'd	**S**	**U**	**Comments**

17. Removed the condom catheter:
    a. Removed the tape. Rolled the sheath off the penis. _____ _____ _____
    b. Disconnected the drainage tubing from the condom.
       Capped the drainage tube. _____ _____ _____
    c. Discarded the tape and condom. _____ _____ _____
18. Provided perineal care. Observed the penis for reddened areas,
    skin breakdown, and irritations. _____ _____ _____
19. Removed and discarded the gloves. Practiced hand hygiene.
    Put on clean gloves. _____ _____ _____
20. Removed the protective backing from the condom.
    This exposed the adhesive strip. _____ _____ _____
21. Held the penis firmly. Rolled the condom onto the penis.
    Left a 1-inch space between the penis and the end of the catheter. _____ _____ _____
22. Secured the condom:
    a. For a self-adhering condom: Pressed the condom to
       the penis. _____ _____ _____
    b. For a condom secured with elastic tape: Applied elastic
       tape in a spiral. Did not apply tape completely around
       the penis. _____ _____ _____
23. Made sure the penis tip did not touch the condom.
    Made sure the condom was not twisted. _____ _____ _____
24. Connected the condom to the drainage tubing. Coiled and
    secured excess tubing on the bed. Or attached a leg bag. _____ _____ _____
25. Removed the waterproof pad and gloves. Discarded them.
    Practiced hand hygiene. _____ _____ _____
26. Covered the person. Removed the bath blanket. _____ _____ _____

Post-Procedure

27. Provided for comfort. _____ _____ _____
28. Placed the signal light within reach. _____ _____ _____
29. Lowered the bed to its lowest position. _____ _____ _____
30. Raised or lowered bed rails. Followed the care plan. _____ _____ _____
31. Unscreened the person. _____ _____ _____
32. Practiced hand hygiene. Put on clean gloves. _____ _____ _____
33. Measured and recorded the amount of urine in the bag.
    Cleaned and discarded the collection bag. _____ _____ _____
34. Cleaned, rinsed, dried, and returned the wash basin and other
    equipment. Returned items to their proper place. _____ _____ _____
35. Removed and discarded the gloves. Practiced hand hygiene. _____ _____ _____
36. Completed a safety check of the room. _____ _____ _____
37. Reported and recorded your observations. _____ _____ _____

Date of Satisfactory Completion _____   Instructor's Initials _____

Checking for a Fecal Impaction

Name: _____   Date: _____

Quality of Life	S	U	Comments

Remembered to:
- Knock before entering the person's room
- Address the person by name
- Introduce yourself by name and title
- Explain the procedure to the person before beginning and during the procedure
- Protect the person's rights during the procedure
- Handle the person gently during the procedure

Pre-Procedure
1. Followed *Delegation Guidelines: Fecal Impactions.* Reviewed *Promoting Safety and Comfort: Fecal Impactions.*
2. Practiced hand hygiene.
3. Collected the following:
   - Bedpan and cover
   - Bath blanket
   - Toilet tissue
   - Gloves
   - Lubricant
   - Waterproof pad
   - Basin of warm water
   - Soap
   - Washcloth
   - Bath towel
4. Practiced hand hygiene.
5. Identified the person. Checked the ID bracelet against the assignment sheet. Called the person by name.
6. Provided for privacy.
7. Raised the bed for good body mechanics. Bed rails were up if used.

Procedure
8. Lowered the bed rail near you if up.
9. Covered the person with a bath blanket. Fan-folded top linens to the foot of the bed.
10. Positioned the person in Sims' position or in a left side-lying position.
11. Put on gloves.
12. Placed the waterproof pad under the buttocks.
13. Exposed the anal area.
14. Lubricated your gloved index finger.
15. Asked the person to take a deep breath through his or her mouth.
16. Inserted the gloved finger while the person was taking a deep breath.
17. Checked for a fecal mass.
18. Removed your finger.
19. Removed and discarded the gloves. Put on clean gloves.
20. Helped the person onto the bedpan. Raised the head of the bed, and raised the bed rail if used. Or assisted the person to the bathroom or commode. The person wore a robe and non-skid footwear while up. The bed was in the lowest position.
21. Placed the signal light and toilet tissue within reach. Reminded the person not to flush the toilet.
22. Discarded disposable items.
23. Removed and discarded the gloves. Practiced hand hygiene.
24. Left the room if the person could be left alone.

Date of Satisfactory Completion _____   Instructor's Initials _____

Procedure—cont'd

	S	U	Comments
25. Returned when the person signaled. Or checked on the person every 5 minutes. Knocked before entering.	___	___	_____
26. Practiced hand hygiene and put on gloves. Lowered the bed rail if up.	___	___	_____
27. Observed stools for amount, color, consistency, shape, and odor.	___	___	_____
28. Provided perineal care as needed.	___	___	_____
29. Removed the waterproof pad.	___	___	_____
30. Emptied, rinsed, cleaned, and disinfected equipment. Flushed the toilet after the nurse observed the bowel movement, if BM occurred.	___	___	_____
31. Returned equipment to its proper place.	___	___	_____
32. Removed and discarded the gloves. Practiced hand hygiene.	___	___	_____
33. Assisted with hand washing. Wore gloves for this step.	___	___	_____
34. Covered the person. Removed the bath blanket.	___	___	_____

Post-Procedure

	S	U	Comments
35. Provided for comfort.	___	___	_____
36. Placed the signal light within reach.	___	___	_____
37. Lowered the bed to its lowest position.	___	___	_____
38. Raised or lowered bed rails. Followed the care plan.	___	___	_____
39. Unscreened the person.	___	___	_____
40. Completed a safety check of the room.	___	___	_____
41. Followed agency policy for dirty linen and used supplies.	___	___	_____
42. Practiced hand hygiene.	___	___	_____
43. Reported and recorded your observations.	___	___	_____

Date of Satisfactory Completion _____   Instructor's Initials _____

Removing a Fecal Impaction

Name: _____ Date: _____

	S	U	Comments
Quality of Life			

Quality of Life

Remembered to:
- Knock before entering the person's room
- Address the person by name
- Introduce yourself by name and title
- Explain the procedure to the person before beginning and during the procedure
- Protect the person's rights during the procedure
- Handle the person gently during the procedure

Pre-Procedure

1. Followed steps 1–10 in procedure: *Checking for a Fecal Impaction.*
   a. Followed *Delegation Guidelines*: *Fecal Impactions.*
      Reviewed *Promoting Safety and Comfort: Fecal Impactions.*
   b. Practiced hand hygiene.
   c. Collected the following:
      - Bedpan and cover
      - Bath blanket
      - Toilet tissue
      - Gloves
      - Lubricant
      - Waterproof pad
      - Basin of warm water
      - Soap
      - Washcloth
      - Bath towel
   d. Practiced hand hygiene.
   e. Identified the person. Checked the ID bracelet against the assignment sheet. Called the person by name.
   f. Provided for privacy.
   g. Raised the bed for good body mechanics. Bed rails were up if used.
   h. Lowered the bed rail near you if up.
   i. Covered the person with a bath blanket. Fan-folded top linens to the foot of the bed.
   j. Positioned the person in Sims' position or in a left side-lying position.
2. Checked the person's pulse. Noted the rate and rhythm.
3. Practiced hand hygiene. Put on gloves.

Procedure

4. Placed the waterproof pad under the buttocks.
5. Exposed the anal area.
6. Lubricated your gloved index finger.
7. Asked the person to take a deep breath through his or her mouth.
8. Inserted your lubricated, gloved index finger.
9. Hooked your finger around a small piece of feces.
10. Removed your finger and the feces.
11. Dropped the stool into the bedpan.
12. Cleaned your finger with toilet tissue. Placed the toilet tissue in the bedpan.
13. Repeated steps 7 through 12 until you no longer felt feces:
    a. Asked the person to take a deep breath through his or her mouth.
    b. Inserted your lubricated, gloved index finger.
    c. Hooked your index finger around a small piece of feces.

Date of Satisfactory Completion _____ Instructor's Initials _____

Procedure—cont'd	S	U	Comments
d. Removed your finger and the feces.	___	___	_____
e. Dropped the stool into the bedpan.	___	___	_____
f. Cleaned your finger with toilet tissue. Placed the toilet tissue in the bedpan.	___	___	_____
14. Checked the person's pulse at intervals. Used your clean gloved hand. Noted the rate and rhythm. Stopped the procedure if the pulse rate had slowed or if the rhythm was irregular.	___	___	_____
15. Wiped the anal area with toilet tissue.	___	___	_____
16. Followed *Checking for a Fecal Impaction* steps:			
a. Removed the gloves and practiced hand hygiene. Put on clean gloves.	___	___	_____
b. Helped the person onto the bedpan. Raised the head of the bed and raised the bed rail if used. Or assisted the person to the bathroom or commode. The person wore a robe and non-skid footwear while up. The bed was in the lowest position.	___	___	_____
c. Placed the signal light and toilet tissue within reach. Reminded the person not to flush the toilet.	___	___	_____
d. Discarded disposable items.	___	___	_____
e. Removed the gloves. Practiced hand hygiene.	___	___	_____
f. Left the room if the person could be alone.	___	___	_____
g. Returned when the person signaled. Or checked on the person every 5 minutes. Knocked before entering.	___	___	_____
h. Practiced hand hygiene and put on gloves. Lowered the bed rail if up.	___	___	_____
i. Observed stools for amount, color, consistency, shape, and odor.	___	___	_____
j. Provided perineal care as needed.	___	___	_____
k. Removed the waterproof pad.	___	___	_____
l. Emptied, cleaned, and disinfected equipment. Flushed the toilet after the nurse observed the bowel movement, if BM occurred.	___	___	_____
m. Returned equipment to its proper place.	___	___	_____
n. Removed the gloves, and practiced hand hygiene.	___	___	_____
o. Assisted with hand washing. Wore gloves for this step.	___	___	_____
p. Covered the person. Removed the bath blanket.	___	___	_____

Post-Procedure

	S	U	Comments
q. Provided for comfort.	___	___	_____
r. Placed the signal light within reach.	___	___	_____
s. Lowered the bed to its lowest position.	___	___	_____
t. Raised or lowered bed rails. Followed the care plan.	___	___	_____
u. Unscreened the person.	___	___	_____
v. Completed a safety check of the room.	___	___	_____
w. Followed agency policy for dirty linen and used supplies.	___	___	_____
x. Practiced hand hygiene.	___	___	_____
y. Reported and recorded your observations.	___	___	_____

Date of Satisfactory Completion _____   Instructor's Initials _____

Giving a Cleansing Enema

Name: _____   Date: _____

Quality of Life	S	U	Comments
Remembered to:			
• Knock before entering the person's room	___	___	_____
• Address the person by name	___	___	_____
• Introduce yourself by name and title	___	___	_____
• Explain the procedure to the person before beginning and during the procedure	___	___	_____
• Protect the person's rights during the procedure	___	___	_____
• Handle the person gently during the procedure	___	___	_____

Pre-Procedure

	S	U	Comments
1. Followed *Delegation Guidelines: Enemas.* Reviewed *Promoting Safety and Comfort: Enemas.*	___	___	_____
2. Practiced hand hygiene.	___	___	_____
3. Collected the following before going to the person's room:			
• Disposable enema kit as directed by the nurse (enema bag, tube, clamp, and waterproof pad)	___	___	_____
• Bath thermometer	___	___	_____
• Waterproof pad (if not part of the enema kit)	___	___	_____
• Water-soluble lubricant	___	___	_____
• 3 to 5 ml (1 teaspoon) of castile soap or 1 to 2 teaspoons of salt	___	___	_____
• IV pole	___	___	_____
• Gloves	___	___	_____
4. Arranged items in the person's room and bathroom.	___	___	_____
5. Practiced hand hygiene.	___	___	_____
6. Identified the person. Checked the ID bracelet against the assignment sheet. Called the person by name.	___	___	_____
7. Put on gloves.	___	___	_____
8. Collected the following:			
• Commode or bedpan and cover	___	___	_____
• Toilet tissue	___	___	_____
• Bath blanket	___	___	_____
• Robe and non-skid footwear	___	___	_____
• Paper towels	___	___	_____
9. Removed and discarded the gloves. Practiced hand hygiene. Put on clean gloves.	___	___	_____
10. Provided for privacy.	___	___	_____
11. Raised the bed for good body mechanics. Bed rails were up if used.	___	___	_____

Procedure

	S	U	Comments
12. Lowered the bed rail near you if up.	___	___	_____
13. Covered the person with a bath blanket. Fan-folded top linens to the foot of the bed.	___	___	_____
14. Positioned the IV pole so the enema bag was 12 inches above the anus. Or it was at the height directed by the nurse.	___	___	_____
15. Raised the bed rail if used.	___	___	_____
16. Prepared the enema:			
a. Closed the clamp on the tube.	___	___	_____
b. Adjusted water flow until it was lukewarm.	___	___	_____
c. Filled the enema bag for the amount ordered.	___	___	_____
d. Measured water temperature with the bath thermometer. The nurse told you what temperature to use.	___	___	_____
e. Prepared the solution as directed by the nurse:	___	___	_____
(1) Tap water: added nothing			
(2) Saline enema: added salt as directed			
(3) SSE: added castile soap as directed			
f. Stirred the solution with the bath thermometer. Scooped off any suds (SSE).	___	___	_____

Date of Satisfactory Completion _____   Instructor's Initials _____

Procedure—cont'd	**S**	**U**	**Comments**
g. Sealed the bag.	___	___	_____
h. Hung the bag on the IV pole.	___	___	_____
17. Lowered the bed rail near you if up.	___	___	_____
18. Positioned the person in Sims' position or in left side-lying position.	___	___	_____
19. Placed a waterproof pad under the buttocks.	___	___	_____
20. Exposed the anal area.	___	___	_____
21. Placed the bedpan behind the person.	___	___	_____
22. Positioned the enema tube in the bedpan. Removed the cap from the tubing.	___	___	_____
23. Opened the clamp. Allowed solution to flow through the tube to remove air. Clamped the tube.	___	___	_____
24. Lubricated the tube 2 to 4 inches from the tip.	___	___	_____
25. Separated the buttocks to see the anus.	___	___	_____
26. Asked the person to take a deep breath through the mouth.	___	___	_____
27. Inserted the tube gently 2 to 4 inches into the adult's rectum. Did this when the person was exhaling. Stopped if the person complained of pain, you felt resistance, or bleeding occurred.	___	___	_____
28. Checked the amount of solution in the bag.	___	___	_____
29. Unclamped the tube. Gave the solution slowly.	___	___	_____
30. Asked the person to take slow deep breaths. This helped the person relax.	___	___	_____
31. Clamped the tube if the person needed to have a BM, had cramping, or started to expel solution. Also, clamped the tube if the person was sweating or complained of nausea or weakness. Unclamped when symptoms subsided.	___	___	_____
32. Gave the amount of solution ordered. Stopped if the person did not tolerate the procedure.	___	___	_____
33. Clamped the tube before it emptied. This prevented air from entering the bowel.	___	___	_____
34. Held toilet tissue around the tube and against the anus. Removed the tube.	___	___	_____
35. Discarded toilet tissue into the bedpan.	___	___	_____
36. Wrapped the tubing tip with paper towels. Placed it inside the enema bag.	___	___	_____
37. Assisted the person to the bathroom or commode. The person wore a robe and non-skid footwear when up. The bed was in the lowest position. Or helped the person onto the bedpan. Raised the head of the bed. Raised or lowered bed rails according to the care plan.	___	___	_____
38. Placed the signal light and toilet tissue within reach. Reminded the person not to flush the toilet.	___	___	_____
39. Discarded disposable items.	___	___	_____
40. Removed and discarded the gloves. Practiced hand hygiene.	___	___	_____
41. Left the room if the person could be left alone.	___	___	_____
42. Returned when the person signaled. Or checked on the person every 5 minutes. Knocked before entering the room or bathroom.	___	___	_____
43. Practiced hand hygiene and put on gloves. Lowered the bed rail if up.	___	___	_____
44. Observed enema results for amount, color, consistency, shape, and odor. Called the nurse to observe results.	___	___	_____
45. Provided perineal care as needed.	___	___	_____
46. Removed the waterproof pad.	___	___	_____
47. Emptied, rinsed, cleaned, and disinfected equipment. Flushed the toilet after the nurse observed the results.	___	___	_____
48. Returned equipment to its proper place.	___	___	_____
49. Removed and discarded the gloves. Practiced hand hygiene.	___	___	_____
50. Assisted with hand washing. Wore gloves for this step.	___	___	_____
51. Covered the person. Removed the bath blanket.	___	___	_____

Date of Satisfactory Completion _____   Instructor's Initials _____

Post-Procedure

52. Provided for comfort.
53. Placed the signal light within reach.
54. Lowered the bed to its lowest position.
55. Raised or lowered bed rails. Followed the care plan.
56. Unscreened the person.
57. Completed a safety check of the room.
58. Followed agency policy for dirty linen and used supplies.
59. Practiced hand hygiene.
60. Reported and recorded your observations.

Date of Satisfactory Completion _____   Instructor's Initials _____

Giving a Small-Volume Enema

Name: _____   Date: _____

Quality of Life	S	U	Comments
Remembered to:			
• Knock before entering the person's room	___	___	_____
• Address the person by name	___	___	_____
• Introduce yourself by name and title	___	___	_____
• Explain the procedure to the person before beginning and during the procedure	___	___	_____
• Protect the person's rights during the procedure	___	___	_____
• Handle the person gently during the procedure	___	___	_____

Pre-Procedure			
1. Followed *Delegation Guidelines: Enemas.* Reviewed *Promoting Safety and Comfort: Enemas.*	___	___	_____
2. Practiced hand hygiene.	___	___	_____
3. Collected the following before going to the person's room:			
• Small-volume enema	___	___	_____
• Waterproof pad	___	___	_____
• Gloves	___	___	_____
4. Arranged items in the person's room.	___	___	_____
5. Practiced hand hygiene.	___	___	_____
6. Identified the person. Checked the ID bracelet against the assignment sheet. Called the person by name.	___	___	_____
7. Put on gloves.	___	___	_____
8. Collected the following:			
• Commode or bedpan	___	___	_____
• Toilet tissue	___	___	_____
• Robe and non-skid footwear	___	___	_____
• Bath blanket	___	___	_____
9. Removed and discarded gloves. Practiced hand hygiene. Put on clean gloves.	___	___	_____
10. Provided for privacy.	___	___	_____
11. Raised the bed for body mechanics. Bed rails were up if used.	___	___	_____

Procedure			
12. Lowered the bed rail near you if up.	___	___	_____
13. Covered the person with a bath blanket. Fan-folded top linens to the foot of the bed.	___	___	_____
14. Positioned the person in Sims' position or in left side-lying position.	___	___	_____
15. Placed a waterproof pad under the buttocks.	___	___	_____
16. Exposed the anal area.	___	___	_____
17. Positioned the bedpan near the person.	___	___	_____
18. Removed the cap from the enema tip.	___	___	_____
19. Separated the buttocks to see the anus.	___	___	_____
20. Asked the person to take a deep breath through the mouth.	___	___	_____
21. Inserted the enema tip 2 inches into the rectum. Did this when the person was exhaling. Stopped if the person complained of pain, you felt resistance, or bleeding occurred.	___	___	_____
22. Squeezed and rolled the container gently. Released pressure on the container after you removed the tip from the rectum.	___	___	_____
23. Placed the container into the box, tip first. Discarded the container and box.	___	___	_____
24. Assisted the person to the bathroom or commode. The person wore a robe and non-skid footwear when up. The bed was in the lowest position. Or helped the person onto the bedpan and raised the head of the bed. Raised or lowered bed rails according to the care plan.	___	___	_____

Date of Satisfactory Completion _____   Instructor's Initials _____

Procedure—cont'd	**S**	**U**	**Comments**
25. Placed the signal light and toilet tissue within reach. Reminded the person not to flush the toilet.	____	____	_____
26. Discarded disposable items.	____	____	_____
27. Removed and discarded the gloves. Practiced hand hygiene.	____	____	_____
28. Left the room if the person could be left alone.	____	____	_____
29. Returned when the person signaled. Or checked on the person every 5 minutes. Knocked before entering the room or bathroom.	____	____	_____
30. Practiced hand hygiene. Put on gloves.	____	____	_____
31. Lowered the bed rail if up.	____	____	_____
32. Observed enema results for amount, color, consistency, shape, and odor. Called the nurse to observe results.	____	____	_____
33. Provided perineal care as needed.	____	____	_____
34. Removed the waterproof pad.	____	____	_____
35. Emptied, rinsed, cleaned, and disinfected equipment. Flushed the toilet after the nurse observed the results.	____	____	_____
36. Returned equipment to its proper place.	____	____	_____
37. Removed and discarded the gloves. Practiced hand hygiene.	____	____	_____
38. Assisted with hand washing. Wore gloves for this step.	____	____	_____
39. Covered the person. Removed the bath blanket.	____	____	_____

Post-Procedure

	S	**U**	**Comments**
40. Provided for comfort.	____	____	_____
41. Placed the signal light within reach.	____	____	_____
42. Lowered the bed to its lowest position.	____	____	_____
43. Raised or lowered bed rails. Followed the care plan.	____	____	_____
44. Unscreened the person.	____	____	_____
45. Completed a safety check of the room.	____	____	_____
46. Followed agency policy for dirty linen and used supplies.	____	____	_____
47. Practiced hand hygiene.	____	____	_____
48. Reported and recorded your observations.	____	____	_____

Date of Satisfactory Completion _____ Instructor's Initials _____

Giving an Oil-Retention Enema

Name: _____   Date: _____

Quality of Life	**S**	**U**	**Comments**

Remembered to:
- Knock before entering the person's room   _____ _____ _____
- Address the person by name   _____ _____ _____
- Introduce yourself by name and title   _____ _____ _____
- Explain the procedure to the person before beginning and during the procedure   _____ _____ _____
- Protect the person's rights during the procedure   _____ _____ _____
- Handle the person gently during the procedure   _____ _____ _____

Pre-Procedure

1. Followed *Delegation Guidelines:*
    a. *Enemas*   _____ _____ _____
    b. *Oil-Retention Enemas*   _____ _____ _____
    Reviewed *Promoting Safety and Comfort:*
    a. *Enemas*   _____ _____ _____
    b. *Oil-Retention Enemas*   _____ _____ _____
2. Practiced hand hygiene.   _____ _____ _____
3. Collected the following before going to the person's room:
    - Oil-retention enema   _____ _____ _____
    - Waterproof pad   _____ _____ _____
    - Gloves   _____ _____ _____
    - Bath blanket   _____ _____ _____
4. Arranged items in the person's room.   _____ _____ _____
5. Practiced hand hygiene.   _____ _____ _____
6. Identified the person. Checked the ID bracelet against the assignment sheet. Called the person by name.   _____ _____ _____
7. Provided for privacy.   _____ _____ _____
8. Raised the bed for good body mechanics. Bed rails were up if used.   _____ _____ _____

Procedure

9. Put on gloves.   _____ _____ _____
10. Followed these steps:
    a. Lowered the bed rail near you if up.   _____ _____ _____
    b. Covered the person with a bath blanket. Fan-folded top linens to the foot of the bed.   _____ _____ _____
    c. Positioned the person in Sims' position or in left side-lying position.   _____ _____ _____
    d. Placed a waterproof pad under the buttocks.   _____ _____ _____
    e. Exposed the anal area.   _____ _____ _____
    f. Positioned the bedpan near the person.   _____ _____ _____
    g. Removed the cap from the enema tip.   _____ _____ _____
    h. Separated the buttocks to see the anus.   _____ _____ _____
    i. Asked the person to take a deep breath through the mouth.   _____ _____ _____
    j. Inserted the enema tip 2 inches into the rectum. Did this when the person was exhaling. Stopped if the person complained of pain, you felt resistance, or bleeding occurred.   _____ _____ _____
    k. Squeezed and rolled the container gently. Released pressure on the container after you removed the tip from the rectum.   _____ _____ _____
    l. Placed the container into the box, tip first. Discarded the container and box   _____ _____ _____
11. Covered the person. Left the person in the Sims' or left side-lying position.   _____ _____ _____
12. Encouraged the person to retain the enema for the time ordered.   _____ _____ _____
13. Placed more waterproof pads on the bed if needed.   _____ _____ _____
14. Removed and discarded the gloves. Practiced hand hygiene.   _____ _____ _____

Date of Satisfactory Completion _____   Instructor's Initials _____

Post-Procedure

15. Provided for comfort.
16. Placed the signal light within reach.
17. Lowered the bed to its lowest position.
18. Raised or lowered bed rails. Followed the care plan.
19. Unscreened the person.
20. Completed a safety check of the room.
21. Followed agency policy for dirty linen and used supplies.
22. Practiced hand hygiene.
23. Reported and recorded your observations.
24. Checked the person often.

Date of Satisfactory Completion _____   Instructor's Initials _____

VIDEO **Changing an Ostomy Pouch**

Name: _____   Date: _____

Quality of Life	S	U	Comments

Remembered to:
- Knock before entering the person's room
- Address the person by name
- Introduce yourself by name and title
- Explain the procedure to the person before beginning and during the procedure
- Protect the person's rights during the procedure
- Handle the person gently during the procedure

Pre-Procedure

1. Followed *Delegation Guidelines: Ostomy Pouches.* Reviewed *Promoting Safety and Comfort: Ostomy Pouches.*
2. Practiced hand hygiene.
3. Collected the following before going to the person's room:
   - Clean pouch with skin barrier
   - Pouch clamp, clip, or wire closure
   - Clean ostomy belt (if used)
   - Gauze pads or washcloths
   - Adhesive remover wipes
   - Skin paste (optional)
   - Pouch deodorant
   - Disposable bag
   - Gloves
   - Paper towels
4. Placed the paper towels on the overbed table. Arranged supplies on top of the paper towels.
5. Practiced hand hygiene.
6. Identified the person. Checked the ID bracelet against the assignment sheet. Called the person by name.
7. Put on gloves.
8. Collected the following:
   - Bedpan with cover
   - Waterproof pad
   - Bath blanket
   - Wash basin with warm water
9. Removed and discarded gloves. Practiced hand hygiene. Put on clean gloves.
10. Provided for privacy.
11. Raised the bed for good body mechanics. Bed rails were up if used.

Procedure

12. Lowered the bed rail near you if up.
13. Covered the person with a bath blanket. Fan-folded top linens to the foot of the bed.
14. Placed a waterproof pad under the buttocks.
15. Disconnected the pouch from the belt if one was worn. Removed the belt.
16. Removed and placed the pouch and skin barrier in the bedpan. Gently pushed the skin down and lifted up on the barrier. Used adhesive remover wipes if necessary.
17. Wiped the stoma and around it with a gauze pad. This removed excess stool and mucus. Discarded the gauze pad into the disposable bag.
18. Wet the gauze or the washcloth.
19. Washed the stoma and around it with a gauze pad or washcloth. Washed gently. Did not scrub or rub the skin.
20. Patted dry with a gauze pad or towel.

Date of Satisfactory Completion _____   Instructor's Initials _____

Procedure—cont'd	S	U	Comments
21. Observed the stoma and the skin around the stoma. Reported bleeding, skin irritation, or skin breakdown.	____	____	_____
22. Removed the backing from the new pouch.	____	____	_____
23. Applied a thin layer of paste around the pouch opening. Allowed it to dry following the manufacturer's instructions.	____	____	_____
24. Pulled the skin around the stoma taut. The skin was wrinkle-free.	____	____	_____
25. Centered the pouch over the stoma. The drain was downward.	____	____	_____
26. Pressed around the pouch and skin barrier so it sealed to the skin. Applied gentle pressure with your fingers. Started at the bottom and worked up around the sides to the top.	____	____	_____
27. Maintained the pressure for 1 to 2 minutes. Followed the manufacturer's instructions.	____	____	_____
28. Tugged down on the pouch gently. Made sure the pouch was secure.	____	____	_____
29. Added deodorant to the pouch.	____	____	_____
30. Closed the pouch at the bottom. Used a clamp, clip, or wire closure.	____	____	_____
31. Attached the ostomy belt if used. The belt was not too tight. You were able to slide 2 fingers under the belt.	____	____	_____
32. Removed the waterproof pad.	____	____	_____
33. Discarded disposable supplies into a disposable bag.	____	____	_____
34. Removed and discarded the gloves. Practiced hand hygiene.	____	____	_____
35. Covered the person. Removed the bath blanket.	____	____	_____

Post-Procedure

	S	U	Comments
36. Provided for comfort.	____	____	_____
37. Placed the signal light within reach.	____	____	_____
38. Lowered the bed to its lowest position.	____	____	_____
39. Raised or lowered bed rails. Followed the care plan.	____	____	_____
40. Unscreened the person.	____	____	_____
41. Practiced hand hygiene. Put on gloves.	____	____	_____
42. Took the bedpan and disposable bag into the bathroom.	____	____	_____
43. Emptied the pouch and bedpan into the toilet. Observed the color, amount, consistency, and odor of stools. Flushed the toilet.	____	____	_____
44. Discarded the pouch into the disposable bag. Discarded the disposable bag.	____	____	_____
45. Emptied, rinsed, cleaned, and disinfected equipment. Returned equipment to its proper place.	____	____	_____
46. Removed and discarded gloves. Practiced hand hygiene.	____	____	_____
47. Completed a safety check of the room.	____	____	_____
48. Followed agency policy for dirty linens.	____	____	_____
49. Practiced hand hygiene.	____	____	_____
50. Reported and recorded your observations.	____	____	_____

Date of Satisfactory Completion _____   Instructor's Initials _____

Measuring Intake and Output (NNAAP®)

Name: _____   Date: _____

Quality of Life	S	U	Comments

Remembered to:
- Knock before entering the person's room _____ _____ _____
- Address the person by name _____ _____ _____
- Introduce yourself by name and title _____ _____ _____
- Explain the procedure to the person before beginning and during the procedure _____ _____ _____
- Protect the person's rights during the procedure _____ _____ _____
- Handle the person gently during the procedure _____ _____ _____

Pre-Procedure
1. Followed *Delegation Guidelines: Intake and Output.*
   Reviewed *Promoting Safety and Comfort: Intake and Output.* _____ _____ _____
2. Practiced hand hygiene. _____ _____ _____
3. Collected the following:
   - I&O record _____ _____ _____
   - Graduates _____ _____ _____
   - Gloves _____ _____ _____

Procedure
4. Put on gloves. _____ _____ _____
5. Measured intake:
   a. Poured liquid remaining in the container into the graduate. Avoided spills and splashes on the outside of the graduate. _____ _____ _____
   b. Measured the amount at eye level on a flat surface. Kept the container level. _____ _____ _____
   c. Checked the serving amount on the I&O record. Or checked the serving size of each container. _____ _____ _____
   d. Subtracted the remaining amount from the full serving amount. Noted the amount. _____ _____ _____
   e. Poured fluid in the graduate back into the container. _____ _____ _____
   f. Repeated steps for each liquid:
      (1) Poured liquid remaining in the container into the graduate. _____ _____ _____
      (2) Measured the amount at eye level. Kept the container level. _____ _____ _____
      (3) Checked the serving amount on the I&O record. Or checked the serving size of each container. _____ _____ _____
      (4) Subtracted the remaining amount from the full serving amount. Noted the amount. _____ _____ _____
      (5) Poured fluid in the graduate back into the container. _____ _____ _____
   g. Added the amounts from each liquid together. _____ _____ _____
   h. Recorded the time and amount on the I&O record. _____ _____ _____
6. Measured output as follows:
   a. Poured fluid into the graduate used to measure output. Avoided spills and splashes on the outside of the graduate. _____ _____ _____
   b. Measured the amount at eye level. Kept the container level. _____ _____ _____
   c. Disposed of fluid in the toilet. Avoided splashes. _____ _____ _____
7. Cleaned and rinsed the graduates. Disposed of rinse into the toilet. Returned the graduates to their proper place. _____ _____ _____
8. Cleaned and rinsed the voiding receptacle or drainage container. Disposed of the rinse into the toilet. Returned item to its proper place. _____ _____ _____
9. Removed and discarded the gloves. Practiced hand hygiene. _____ _____ _____
10. Recorded the output on the person's I&O record. _____ _____ _____

Date of Satisfactory Completion _____   Instructor's Initials _____

Post-Procedure

11. Provided for comfort.
12. Made sure the signal light was within reach.
13. Completed a safety check of the room.
14. Reported and recorded your observations.

Date of Satisfactory Completion _____ Instructor's Initials _____

Preparing the Person for a Meal

Name: _____   Date: _____

Quality of Life	S	U	Comments

Remembered to:
- Knock before entering the person's room
- Address the person by name
- Introduce yourself by name and title
- Explain the procedure to the person before beginning and during the procedure
- Protect the person's rights during the procedure
- Handle the person gently during the procedure

Pre-Procedure

1. Followed *Delegation Guidelines: Preparing for Meals.* Reviewed *Promoting Safety and Comfort: Preparing for Meals.*
2. Practiced hand hygiene.
3. Collected the following:
   - Equipment for oral hygiene
   - Bedpan and cover, urinal, commode, or specimen pan
   - Toilet tissue
   - Wash basin
   - Soap
   - Washcloth
   - Towel
   - Gloves
4. Provided for privacy.

Procedure

5. Made sure eyeglasses and hearing aids were in place.
6. Assisted with oral hygiene. Made sure dentures were in place. Wore gloves, and practiced hand hygiene after removing and discarding them.
7. Assisted with elimination. Made sure the incontinent person was clean and dry. Wore gloves, and practiced hand hygiene after removing and discarding them.
8. Assisted with hand washing. Wore gloves and practiced hand hygiene after removing and discarding them.
9. Did the following if the person was in bed:
   a. Raised the head of the bed to a comfortable position.
   b. Removed items from the overbed table. Cleaned the overbed table.
   c. Adjusted the overbed table in front of the person.
10. Did the following if the person was sitting in a chair:
    a. Positioned the person in a chair or wheelchair
    b. Removed items from the overbed table. Cleaned the table.
    c. Adjusted the overbed table in front of the person.
11. Assisted the person to the dining area, if person eats in dining area.

Post-Procedure

12. Provided for comfort.
13. Placed the signal light within reach.
14. Emptied, cleaned, and disinfected equipment. Returned equipment to its proper place. Wore gloves, and practiced hand hygiene after removing and discarding them.
15. Straightened the room. Eliminated unpleasant noise, odors, or equipment.
16. Unscreened the person.
17. Completed a safety check of the room.
18. Practiced hand hygiene.

Date of Satisfactory Completion _____   Instructor's Initials _____

Serving Meal Trays

Name: _____   Date: _____

Quality of Life	S	U	Comments

Remembered to:
- Knock before entering the person's room
- Address the person by name
- Introduce yourself by name and title
- Explain the procedure to the person before beginning and during the procedure
- Protect the person's rights during the procedure
- Handle the person gently during the procedure

Pre-Procedure

1. Followed *Delegation Guidelines: Serving Meal Trays.*
   Reviewed *Promoting Safety and Comfort: Serving Meal Trays.*
2. Practiced hand hygiene.

Procedure

3. Made sure the tray was complete. Checked items on the tray with the dietary card. Made sure adaptive equipment was included.
4. Identified the person. Checked the ID bracelet against the assignment sheet. Called the person by name.
5. Placed the tray within the person's reach. Adjusted the overbed table as needed.
6. Removed food covers. Opened cartons, cut food into bite-size pieces, buttered bread, and so on as needed. Seasoned food as the person preferred and as allowed on the care plan.
7. Placed the napkin, clothes protector, assistive devices, and eating utensils within reach.
8. Placed the signal light within reach.
9. Did the following when the person was done eating:
   a. Measured and recorded intake if ordered.
   b. Noted the amount and type of foods eaten.
   c. Checked for and removed any food in the mouth (pocketing). Wore gloves. Practiced hand hygiene after removing them.
   d. Removed the tray.
   e. Cleaned spills. Changed soiled linen and clothing.
   f. Helped the person return to bed if needed.
   g. Assisted with oral hygiene and hand washing. Wore gloves. Practiced hand hygiene after removing and discarding gloves.

Post-Procedure

10. Provided for comfort.
11. Placed the signal light within reach.
12. Raised or lowered bed rails. Followed the care plan.
13. Completed a safety check of the room.
14. Followed agency policy for soiled linen.
15. Practiced hand hygiene.
16. Reported and recorded you observations.

Date of Satisfactory Completion _____   Instructor's Initials _____

Feeding the Person (NNAAP®)

Name: _____   Date: _____

	S	U	Comments

Quality of Life
Remembered to:
- Knock before entering the person's room
- Address the person by name
- Introduce yourself by name and title
- Explain the procedure to the person before beginning and during the procedure
- Protect the person's rights during the procedure
- Handle the person gently during the procedure

Pre-Procedure
1. Followed *Delegation Guidelines: Feeding the Person.* Reviewed *Promoting Safety and Comfort: Feeding the Person.*
2. Practiced hand hygiene.
3. Positioned the person in a comfortable position for eating (usually sitting or high-Fowler's). (NOTE: Some state competency tests require that the person sit upright at least 75 to 90 degrees.)
4. Got the tray. Placed it on the overbed table or dining table where the person could see it.

Procedure
5. Identified the person. Checked the ID bracelet with the dietary card. Also called the person by name.
6. Draped a napkin across the person's chest and underneath the chin. Cleaned the person's hands with a hand wipe.
7. Told the person what foods and fluids were on the tray.
8. Prepared food for eating. Cut food into bite-size pieces. Seasoned foods as the person preferred and as was allowed on the care plan.
9. Placed a chair where you could sit comfortably. Sat facing the person.
10. Served foods in the order the person preferred. Identified foods as you served them. Alternated between solid and liquid foods. Used a spoon for safety. Allowed enough time for chewing and swallowing. Did not rush the person. Also offered water, coffee, tea, or other beverages on the tray.
11. Checked the person's mouth before offering more food or fluids. Made sure the person's mouth was empty between bites and swallows. Asked if the person was ready for the next bite or drink.
12. Used straws for liquids if person could not drink out of a glass or cup. Had one straw for each liquid. Provided short straws for weak persons.
13. Wiped the person's hands, face, and mouth as needed during the meal. Used the napkin or a hand wipe.
14. Followed the care plan if the person had dysphagia. (Some persons with dysphagia do not use straws.) Gave thickened liquids with a spoon.
15. Conversed with the person in a pleasant manner.
16. Encouraged the person to eat as much as possible.
17. Wiped the person's mouth with a napkin or a hand wipe. Discarded the napkin or a hand wipe.
18. Noted how much and which foods were eaten.
19. Measured and recorded intake if ordered.
20. Removed the tray.
21. Took the person back to his or her room (if in a dining area).
22. Assisted with oral hygiene and hand washing. Provided for privacy. Wore gloves. Practiced hand hygiene after removing and discarding the gloves.

Date of Satisfactory Completion _____   Instructor's Initials _____

Post-Procedure

23. Provided for comfort.
24. Placed the signal light within reach.
25. Raised or lowered bed rails. Followed the care plan.
26. Completed a safety check of the room.
27. Returned the food tray to the food cart.
28. Practiced hand hygiene.
29. Reported and recorded your observations.

Date of Satisfactory Completion _____   Instructor's Initials _____

Providing Drinking Water

Name: _____   Date: _____

Quality of Life	S	U	Comments
Remembered to:			
• Knock before entering the person's room	___	___	_____
• Address the person by name	___	___	_____
• Introduce yourself by name and title	___	___	_____
• Explain the procedure to the person before beginning and during the procedure	___	___	_____
• Protect the person's rights during the procedure	___	___	_____
• Handle the person gently during the procedure	___	___	_____

Pre-Procedure

	S	U	Comments
1. Followed *Delegation Guidelines: Providing Drinking Water.* Reviewed *Promoting Safety and Comfort: Providing Drinking Water.*	___	___	_____
2. Obtained a list of persons who have special fluid orders from the nurse. Or used your assignment sheet.	___	___	_____
3. Practiced hand hygiene.	___	___	_____
4. Collected the following:			
• Cart	___	___	_____
• Ice chest filled with ice	___	___	_____
• Cover for ice chest	___	___	_____
• Scoop	___	___	_____
• Water cups	___	___	_____
• Straws	___	___	_____
• Paper towels	___	___	_____
• Water pitcher for the patient and resident use	___	___	_____
• Large water pitcher filled with cold water (optional, depended on agency procedure)	___	___	_____
• Towel for the scoop	___	___	_____
5. Covered the cart with paper towels. Arranged equipment on top of the paper towels.	___	___	_____

Procedure

	S	U	Comments
6. Took the cart to the person's room door. Did not take the cart into the room.	___	___	_____
7. Checked the person's fluid orders. Used the list from the nurse.	___	___	_____
8. Identified the person. Checked the ID bracelet against the fluid order sheet or your assignment sheet. Called the person by name.	___	___	_____
9. Took the pitcher from the person's overbed table. Emptied it into the bathroom sink.			
10. Determined if a new water pitcher was needed.	___	___	_____
11. Used the scoop to fill the pitcher with ice. Did not let the scoop touch the pitcher.			
12. Placed the scoop on the towel.	___	___	_____
13. Filled the water pitcher with water. Got water from the bathroom or used the larger water pitcher on the cart.	___	___	_____
14. Placed the pitcher, cup, and straw (if used) on the overbed table. Filled the cup with water. Did not let the water pitcher touch the cup.			
15. Made sure the pitcher, cup, and straw (if used) were within the person's reach.	___	___	_____

Post-Procedure

	S	U	Comments
16. Provided for comfort.			
17. Placed the signal light within reach.	___	___	_____
18. Completed a safety check of the room.	___	___	_____
19. Practiced hand hygiene.	___	___	_____

Date of Satisfactory Completion _____   Instructor's Initials _____

Post-Procedure—cont'd   S   U   **Comments**

20. Repeated for each person:
    - Took the cart to the person's room door. Did not take the cart into the room.
    - Checked the person's fluid orders. Used the list from the nurse.
    - Identified the person. Checked the ID bracelet against the fluid order sheet or your assignment sheet. Also called the person by name.
    - Took the pitcher from the person's overbed table. Emptied it into the bathroom sink.
    - Determined if a new water pitcher was needed.
    - Used the scoop to fill the pitcher with ice. Did not let the scoop touch the rim or the inside of the pitcher.
    - Placed the scoop on the towel.
    - Filled the water pitcher with water. Got water from the bathroom or used the larger water pitcher on the cart.
    - Placed the pitcher, cup, and straw (if used) on the overbed table. Filled the cup with water. Did not let the water pitcher touch the rim or inside of the cup.
    - Made sure the pitcher, cup, and straw (if used) were within the person's reach.
    - Provided for comfort.
    - Placed the signal light within reach.
    - Completed a safety check of the room.
    - Practiced hand hygiene.

Date of Satisfactory Completion _____   Instructor's Initials _____

Taking a Temperature With an Electronic Thermometer

Name: _____   Date: _____

	S	U	Comments

Quality of Life

Remembered to:
- Knock before entering the person's room
- Address the person by name
- Introduce yourself by name and title
- Explain the procedure to the person before beginning and during the procedure
- Protect the person's rights during the procedure
- Handle the person gently during the procedure

Pre-Procedure

1. Followed *Delegation Guidelines: Taking Temperatures.* Reviewed *Promoting Safety and Comfort: Taking Temperatures.*
2. For an *oral temperature*, asked the person not to eat, drink, smoke, or chew gum for at least 15 to 20 minutes before the measurement or as required by agency policy.
3. Practiced hand hygiene.
4. Collected the following:
   - Thermometer—electronic, tympanic membrane
   - Probe (blue for an oral or ancillary temperature; red for a rectal temperature.)
   - Probe covers
   - Toilet tissue (rectal temperature)
   - Water-soluble lubricant (rectal temperature)
   - Gloves
   - Towel (axillary temperature)
5. Plugged the probe into the thermometer if used a standard electronic thermometer.
6. Practiced hand hygiene.
7. Identified the person. Checked the ID bracelet against the assignment sheet. Called the person by name.

Procedure

8. Provided for privacy. Positioned the person for an oral, rectal, axillary, or tympanic membrane temperature. The Sims' position was used for a rectal temperature.
9. Put on the gloves if contact with blood, body fluids, secretions, or excretions was likely.
10. Inserted the probe into the probe cover.
11. For an *oral temperature*:
    a. Asked the person to open the mouth and raise the tongue.
    b. Placed the covered probe at the base of the tongue and to one side.
    c. Asked the person to lower the tongue and close the mouth.
12. For a *rectal temperature*:
    a. Put some lubricant on toilet tissue.
    b. Lubricated the end of the covered probe.
    c. Exposed the anal area.
    d. Raised the upper buttock.
    e. Inserted the probe ½ inch into the rectum.
    f. Held the probe in place.
13. For *axillary temperature*:
    a. Helped the person remove an arm from the gown. Did not expose the person.
    b. Dried the axilla with a towel.

Date of Satisfactory Completion _____   Instructor's Initials _____

	S	U	Comments
Procedure—cont'd			
c. Placed the covered probe in the axilla.	___	___	___
d. Placed the person's arm over the chest.	___	___	___
e. Held the probe in place.	___	___	___
14. For a *tympanic membrane temperature:*			
a. Asked the person to turn his or her head so the ear was in front of you.	___	___	___
b. Pulled up and back on the adult's ear to straighten the ear canal.	___	___	___
c. Inserted the covered probe gently.	___	___	___
15. Started the thermometer.			
16. Held the probe in place until you heard a tone or saw a flashing or steady light.	___	___	___
17. Read the temperature on the display.	___	___	___
18. Removed the probe. Pressed the eject button to discard the cover.	___	___	___
19. Noted the person's name, temperature, and temperature site on your notepad or assignment sheet.	___	___	___
20. Returned it to the holder.	___	___	___
21. Helped the person put the gown back on (axillary temperature). For a rectal temperature:			
a. Wiped the anal area with toilet tissue to remove lubricant.	___	___	___
b. Covered the person.	___	___	___
c. Disposed of used toilet tissue.	___	___	___
d. Removed and discarded the gloves. Practiced hand hygiene.	___	___	___
Post-Procedure			
22. Provided for comfort.	___	___	___
23. Placed the signal light within reach.	___	___	___
24. Unscreened the person.	___	___	___
25. Completed a safety check of the room.	___	___	___
26. Returned the thermometer to the charging unit.	___	___	___
27. Practiced hand hygiene.	___	___	___
28. Reported and recorded the temperature. Noted the temperature site when reporting and recording. Reported any abnormal temperature at once.	___	___	___

Date of Satisfactory Completion _____   Instructor's Initials _____

Taking a Temperature With a Glass Thermometer

Name: _____   Date: _____

	S	U	Comments

Quality of Life
Remembered to:
- Knock before entering the person's room
- Address the person by name
- Introduce yourself by name and title
- Explain the procedure to the person before beginning and during the procedure
- Protect the person's rights during the procedure
- Handle the person gently during the procedure

Pre-Procedure
1. Followed *Delegation Guidelines: Taking Temperatures.* Reviewed *Promoting Safety and Comfort:*
   a. *Glass Thermometers*
   b. *Taking Temperatures*
2. For an *oral temperature,* asked the person not to eat, drink, smoke, or chew gum for at least 15 to 20 minutes before the measurement or as required by agency policy.
3. Practiced hand hygiene.
4. Collected the following:
   - Oral or rectal thermometer and holder
   - Tissues
   - Plastic covers if used
   - Gloves
   - Toilet tissue (rectal temperature)
   - Water-soluble lubricant (rectal temperature)
   - Towel (axillary temperature)
5. Practiced hand hygiene.
6. Identified the person. Checked the ID bracelet against the assignment sheet. Called the person by name.
7. Provided for privacy.

Procedure
8. Put on the gloves.
9. Rinsed the thermometer under cold running water if it soaked in disinfectant. Dried it with tissues.
10. Checked for breaks, cracks, or chips.
11. Shook down the thermometer below the lowest number. Held the thermometer by the stem.
12. Inserted it into a plastic cover if used.
13. For an *oral temperature:*
    a. Asked the person to moisten his or her lips.
    b. Placed the bulb end of the thermometer under the tongue and to one side.
    c. Asked the person to close the lips around the thermometer to hold it in place.
    d. Asked the person not to talk. Reminded the person not to bite down on the thermometer.
    e. Left it in place for 2 to 3 minutes or as required by agency policy.
14. For a *rectal temperature:*
    a. Positioned the person in Sims' position.
    b. Put a small amount of lubricant on a tissue.
    c. Lubricated the bulb end of the thermometer.
    d. Folded back top linens; exposed the anal area.
    e. Raised the upper buttock; exposed the anus.

Date of Satisfactory Completion _____   Instructor's Initials _____

Procedure—cont'd	**S**	**U**	**Comments**
f. Inserted the thermometer 1 inch into the rectum. Did not force the thermometer.	____	____	_____
g. Held the thermometer in place for 2 minutes or as required by agency policy. Did not let go of it while it was in the rectum.	____	____	_____
15. For *axillary temperature:*			
a. Helped the person remove an arm from the gown. Did not expose the person.	____	____	_____
b. Dried the axilla with a towel.	____	____	_____
c. Placed the bulb end of the thermometer in the center of the axilla.	____	____	_____
d. Asked the person to place the arm over the chest to hold the thermometer in place. Held it and the arm in place if the person did not help.	____	____	_____
e. Left the thermometer in place for 5 to 10 minutes or as required by agency policy.	____	____	_____
16. Removed the thermometer.	____	____	_____
17. Used tissues to remove plastic cover. Discarded the cover and tissues. Wiped the thermometer with a tissue if no cover was used. Wiped from the stem to the bulb end. Discarded the tissue.	____	____	_____
18. Read the thermometer.	____	____	_____
19. Noted the person's name and temperature on your notepad or assignment sheet.	____	____	_____
20. For a *rectal temperature:*			
a. Placed used toilet tissue on several thicknesses of clean toilet tissue.	____	____	_____
b. Placed the thermometer on clean toilet tissue.	____	____	_____
c. Wiped the anal area to remove excess lubricant and any feces.	____	____	_____
d. Covered the person.	____	____	_____
21. For an *axillary temperature:* Helped the person put the gown back on.	____	____	_____
22. Shook down the thermometer.	____	____	_____
23. Cleaned the thermometer according to agency policy. Returned it to the holder.	____	____	_____
24. Discarded tissues and disposed of toilet tissue.	____	____	_____
25. Removed and discarded the gloves. Practiced hand hygiene.	____	____	_____

Post-Procedure

	S	**U**	**Comments**
26. Provided for comfort.	____	____	_____
27. Placed the signal light within reach.	____	____	_____
28. Unscreened the person.	____	____	_____
29. Completed a safety check of the room.	____	____	_____
30. Practiced hand hygiene.	____	____	_____
31. Reported and recorded the temperature. Noted the temperature site when reporting and recording. Reported any abnormal temperature at once.	____	____	_____

Date of Satisfactory Completion _____   Instructor's Initials _____

Taking a Radial Pulse (NNAAP®)

Name: _____ Date: _____

Quality of Life	S	U	Comments

Remembered to:
- Knock before entering the person's room
- Address the person by name
- Introduce yourself by name and title
- Explain the procedure to the person before beginning and during the procedure
- Protect the person's rights during the procedure
- Handle the person gently during the procedure

Pre-Procedure

1. Followed *Delegation Guidelines: Taking Pulses.* Reviewed *Promoting Safety and Comfort: Taking Pulses.*
2. Practiced hand hygiene.
3. Identified the person. Checked the ID bracelet against the assignment sheet. Called the person by name.
4. Provided for privacy.

Procedure

5. Had the person sit or lie down.
6. Located the radial pulse. Used your first 2 or 3 middle fingertips.
7. Noted if the pulse was strong or weak, regular or irregular.
8. Counted the pulse for 30 seconds. Multiplied the number of beats by 2. Or counted the pulse for 1 minute if:
   a. Directed by the nurse and care plan.
   b. Required by agency policy.
   c. The pulse was irregular.
   d. Required for your state competency test.
9. Noted the person's name and pulse on your notepad or assignment sheet. Noted the strength of the pulse. Noted if it was regular or irregular.

Post-Procedure

10. Provided for comfort.
11. Placed the signal light within reach.
12. Unscreened the person.
13. Completed a safety check of the room.
14. Practiced hand hygiene.
15. Reported and recorded the pulse rate and your observations. Reported an abnormal pulse at once.

Date of Satisfactory Completion _____ Instructor's Initials _____

Taking an Apical Pulse

Name: _____   Date: _____

Quality of Life	S	U	Comments

Remembered to:
- Knock before entering the person's room
- Address the person by name
- Introduce yourself by name and title
- Explain the procedure to the person before beginning and during the procedure
- Protect the person's rights during the procedure
- Handle the person gently during the procedure

Pre-Procedure

1. Followed *Delegation Guidelines: Taking Pulses.* Reviewed *Promoting Safety and Comfort: Using a Stethoscope.*
2. Practiced hand hygiene.
3. Collected a stethoscope and antiseptic wipes.
4. Practiced hand hygiene.
5. Identified the person. Checked the ID bracelet against the assignment sheet. Called the person by name.
6. Provided for privacy.

Procedure

7. Cleaned the earpieces and diaphragm with the wipes.
8. Had the person sit or lie down.
9. Exposed the nipple area of the left chest. Exposed a woman's breasts only to the extent necessary.
10. Warmed the diaphragm in your palm.
11. Placed the earpieces in your ears.
12. Located the apical pulse. Placed the diaphragm 2 to 3 inches to the left of the breastbone and below the left nipple.
13. Counted the pulse for 1 minute. Noted if the pulse was regular or irregular.
14. Covered the person. Removed the earpieces.
15. Noted the person's name and pulse on your notepad or assignment sheet. Noted if the pulse was regular or irregular.

Post-Procedure

16. Provided for comfort.
17. Placed the signal light within reach.
18. Unscreened the person.
19. Completed a safety check of the room.
20. Cleaned the earpieces and diaphragm with the wipes.
21. Returned the stethoscope to its proper place.
22. Practiced hand hygiene.
23. Reported and recorded your observations. Reported the pulse rate with *Ap* for apical. Reported an abnormal pulse rate at once.

Date of Satisfactory Completion _____   Instructor's Initials _____

Taking an Apical-Radial Pulse

Name: _____   Date: _____

Quality of Life	S	U	Comments

Remembered to:
- Knock before entering the person's room
- Address the person by name
- Introduce yourself by name and title
- Explain the procedure to the person before beginning and during the procedure
- Protect the person's rights during the procedure
- Handle the person gently during the procedure

Pre-Procedure

1. Followed *Delegation Guidelines: Taking Pulses.*
   Reviewed *Promoting Safety and Comfort:*
   a. *Using a Stethoscope*
   b. *Taking Pulses*
2. Asked a co-worker to help you.
3. Practiced hand hygiene.
4. Collected a stethoscope and antiseptic wipes.
5. Practiced hand hygiene.
6. Identified the person. Checked the ID bracelet against the assignment sheet. Called the person by name.
7. Provided for privacy.

Procedure

8. Cleaned the earpieces and diaphragm with the wipes.
9. Had the person sit or lie down.
10. Exposed the nipple area of the left chest. Exposed a woman's breasts only to the extent necessary.
11. Warmed the diaphragm in your palm.
12. Placed the earpieces in your ears.
13. Located the apical pulse. Your helper found the radial pulse.
14. Gave the signal to begin counting.
15. Counted the pulse for 1 minute.
16. Gave the signal to stop counting.
17. Covered the person. Removed the stethoscope earpieces.
18. Noted the person's name and apical and radial pulses on your notepad or assignment sheet. Subtracted the radial pulse from the apical pulse for the pulse deficit. Noted if the pulses were regular or irregular.

Post-Procedure

19. Provided for comfort.
20. Placed the signal light within reach.
21. Unscreened the person.
22. Completed a safety check of the room.
23. Cleaned the earpieces and diaphragm with the wipes.
24. Returned the stethoscope to its proper place.
25. Practiced hand hygiene.
26. Reported and recorded your observations. (Reported an abnormal pulse at once.) Included:
    a. The apical and radial pulse rates.
    b. The pulse deficit.

Date of Satisfactory Completion _____   Instructor's Initials _____

Counting Respirations (NNAAP®)

Name: _____   Date: _____

Procedure	S	U	Comments
1. Followed *Delegation Guidelines: Respirations*.	____	____	_____
2. Kept your fingers or stethoscope over the pulse site.	____	____	_____
3. Did not tell the person you were counting respirations.	____	____	_____
4. Began counting when the chest rose. Counted each rise and fall of the chest as 1 respiration.	____	____	_____
5. Noted the following:			
a. If respirations were regular.	____	____	_____
b. If both sides of the chest rose equally.	____	____	_____
c. The depth of the respirations.	____	____	_____
d. If the person had any pain or difficulty breathing.	____	____	_____
e. An abnormal respiratory pattern.	____	____	_____
6. Counted respirations for 30 seconds. Multiplied the number by 2. Counted respirations for 1 minute if:			
a. Directed by the nurse and care plan.	____	____	_____
b. Required by agency policy.	____	____	_____
c. Respirations were abnormal or irregular.	____	____	_____
d. Required for your state competency test.	____	____	_____
7. Noted the person's name, respiratory rate, and any other observations on your notepad or assignment sheet.	____	____	_____

Post-Procedure

	S	U	Comments
8. Provided for comfort.	____	____	_____
9. Placed the signal light within reach.	____	____	_____
10. Unscreened the person.	____	____	_____
11. Completed a safety check of the room.	____	____	_____
12. Practiced hand hygiene.	____	____	_____
13. Reported and recorded the respiratory rate and your observations. Reported abnormal respirations at once.	____	____	_____

Date of Satisfactory Completion _____   Instructor's Initials _____

Measuring Blood Pressure (NNAAP®)

Name: _____   Date: _____

Quality of Life	S	U	Comments

Remembered to:
- Knock before entering the person's room
- Address the person by name
- Introduce yourself by name and title
- Explain the procedure to the person before beginning and during the procedure
- Protect the person's rights during the procedure
- Handle the person gently during the procedure

Pre-Procedure

1. Followed *Delegation Guidelines: Measuring Blood Pressure.* Reviewed *Promoting Safety and Comfort:*
   a. *Using a Stethoscope*
   b. *Equipment*
2. Practiced hand hygiene.
3. Collected the following:
   - Sphygmomanometer
   - Stethoscope
   - Antiseptic wipes
4. Practiced hand hygiene.
5. Identified the person. Checked the ID bracelet against the assignment sheet. Called the person by name.
6. Provided for privacy.

Procedure

7. Wiped the stethoscope earpieces and diaphragm with the wipes. Warmed the diaphragm in your palm.
8. Had the person sit or lie down.
9. Positioned the person's arm level with the heart. The palm was up.
10. Stood no more than 3 feet away from the manometer. The mercury type was vertical, on a flat surface, and at eye level. The aneroid type was directly in front of you.
11. Exposed the upper arm.
12. Squeezed the cuff to expel any remaining air. Closed the valve on the bulb.
13. Found the brachial artery at the inner aspect of the elbow. (The brachial artery is on the little finger side of the arm.) Used your fingertips.
14. Located the arrow on the cuff. Placed the arrow on the cuff over the brachial artery. Wrapped the cuff around the upper arm at least 1 inch above the elbow. It was even and snug.
15. Placed the stethoscope earpieces in your ears. Placed the diaphragm over the brachial artery. Did not place it under the cuff.
16. Found the radial pulse. Did this for methods 1 and 2.
17. *Method 1:*
   a. Inflated the cuff until you no longer felt the pulse. Noted that point.
   b. Inflated the cuff 30 mm Hg beyond the point where you last felt the pulse.
18. *Method 2:*
   a. Inflated the cuff until you no longer felt the pulse. Noted that point.
   b. Inflated the cuff 30 mm Hg beyond the point where you last felt the pulse.
   c. Deflated the cuff slowly. Noted the point where you felt the pulse.

Date of Satisfactory Completion _____   Instructor's Initials _____

Procedure—cont'd	S	U	Comments
d. Waited 30 seconds.	___	___	_____
e. Inflated the cuff 30 mm Hg beyond the point where you felt the pulse return.	___	___	_____
19. *Method 3:*			
a. Inflated the cuff 160 mm Hg to 180 mm Hg.	___	___	_____
b. Deflated the cuff if you heard a blood pressure sound. Re-inflated the cuff to 200 mm Hg.	___	___	_____
20. Deflated the cuff at an even rate of 2 to 4 millimeters per second. Turned the valve counterclockwise to deflate the cuff.	___	___	_____
21. Noted the point where you heard the first sound. This was the systolic reading. It was near the point where the pulse disappeared.	___	___	_____
22. Continued to deflate the cuff. Noted the point where the sound disappeared. This was the diastolic reading.	___	___	_____
23. Deflated the cuff completely. Removed it from the person's arm. Removed the stethoscope earpieces from your ears.	___	___	_____
24. Noted the person's name and blood pressure on your notepad or assignment sheet.	___	___	_____
25. Returned the cuff to the case or the wall holder.	___	___	_____

Post-Procedure

	S	U	Comments
26. Provided for comfort.	___	___	_____
27. Placed the signal light within reach.	___	___	_____
28. Unscreened the person.	___	___	_____
29. Completed a safety check of the room.	___	___	_____
30. Cleaned the earpieces and diaphragm with the wipes.	___	___	_____
31. Returned the equipment to its proper place.	___	___	_____
32. Practiced hand hygiene.	___	___	_____
33. Reported and recorded the blood pressure. Reported an abnormal blood pressure at once.	___	___	_____

Date of Satisfactory Completion _____   Instructor's Initials _____

Performing Range-of-Motion Exercises (NNAAP®)

Name: _____ Date: _____

Quality of Life	S	U	Comments

Remembered to:
- Knock before entering the person's room
- Address the person by name
- Introduce yourself by name and title
- Explain the procedure to the person before beginning and during the procedure
- Protect the person's rights during the procedure
- Handle the person gently during the procedure

Pre-Procedure

1. Followed *Delegation Guidelines: Range-of-Motion Exercises.* Reviewed *Promoting Safety and Comfort: Range-of-Motion Exercises.*
2. Practiced hand hygiene.
3. Identified the person. Checked the ID bracelet against the assignment sheet. Called the person by name.
4. Obtained a bath blanket.
5. Provided for privacy.
6. Raised the bed for body mechanics. Bed rails were up if used.

Procedure

7. Lowered the bed rail near you if up.
8. Positioned the person supine.
9. Covered the person with a bath blanket. Fan-folded top linens to the foot of the bed.
10. Exercised the neck *if allowed by the center and if the RN instructed you to do so:*
    a. Placed your hands over the person's ears to support the head. Supported the jaws with your fingers.
    b. Flexion—brought the head forward. The chin touched the chest.
    c. Extension—straightened the head.
    d. Hyperextension—brought the head backward until the chin pointed up.
    e. Rotation—turned the head from side to side.
    f. Lateral flexion—moved the head to the right and to the left.
    g. Repeated flexion, extension, hyperextension, rotation, and lateral flexion 5 times, or the number of times stated on the care plan.
11. Exercised the shoulder:
    a. Grasped the wrist with one hand. Grasped the elbow with the other hand.
    b. Flexion—raised the arm straight in front and over the head.
    c. Extension—brought the arm down to the side.
    d. Hyperextension—moved the arm behind the body. (Did this if the person was sitting in a straight-backed chair or was standing.)
    e. Abduction—moved the straight arm away from the side of the body.
    f. Adduction—moved the straight arm to the side of the body.
    g. Internal rotation—bent the elbow. Placed it at the same level as the shoulder. Moved the forearm down toward the body.
    h. External rotation—moved the forearm toward the head.
    i. Repeated flexion, extension, hyperextension, abduction, adduction, and internal and external rotation 5 times, or the number of times stated on the care plan.

Date of Satisfactory Completion _____ Instructor's Initials _____

Procedure—cont'd

	S	U	Comments
12. Exercised the elbow:			
a. Grasped the person's wrist with one hand. Grasped the elbow with your other hand.	____	____	_____
b. Flexion—bent the arm so the same-side shoulder was touched.	____	____	_____
c. Extension—straightened the arm.	____	____	_____
d. Repeated flexion and extension 5 times, or the number of times stated on the care plan.	____	____	_____
13. Exercised the forearm:			
a. Continued to support the wrist and elbow.			
b. Pronation—turned the hand so the palm was down.	____	____	_____
c. Supination—turned the hand so the palm was up.	____	____	_____
d. Repeated pronation and supination 5 times, or the number of times stated on the care plan.	____	____	_____
14. Exercised the wrist:			
a. Held the wrist with both of your hands.	____	____	_____
b. Flexion—bent the hand down.	____	____	_____
c. Extension—straightened the hand.	____	____	_____
d. Hyperextension—bent the hand back.	____	____	_____
e. Radial flexion—turned the hand toward the thumb.	____	____	_____
f. Ulnar flexion—turned the hand toward the little finger.	____	____	_____
g. Repeated flexion, extension, hyperextension, and radial and ulnar flexion 5 times, or the number of times stated on the care plan.	____	____	_____
15. Exercised the thumb:			
a. Held the person's hand with one hand. Held the thumb with your other hand.	____	____	_____
b. Abduction—moved the thumb out from the inner part of the index finger.	____	____	_____
c. Adduction—moved the thumb back next to the index finger.	____	____	_____
d. Opposition—touched each finger with the thumb.	____	____	_____
e. Flexion—bent the thumb into the hand.	____	____	_____
f. Extension—moved the thumb out to the side of the fingers.	____	____	_____
g. Repeated abduction, adduction, opposition, flexion, and extension 5 times, or the number of times stated on the care plan.	____	____	_____
16. Exercised the fingers:			
a. Abduction—spread the fingers and the thumb apart.	____	____	_____
b. Adduction—brought the fingers and thumb together.	____	____	_____
c. Extension—straightened the fingers so the fingers, hand, and arm were straight.	____	____	_____
d. Flexion—made a fist.	____	____	_____
e. Repeated abduction, adduction, flexion, and extension 5 times, or the number of times stated on the care plan.	____	____	_____
17. Exercised the hip:			
a. Supported the leg. Placed one hand under the knee. Placed your other hand under the ankle.	____	____	_____
b. Flexion—raised the leg.	____	____	_____
c. Extension—straightened the leg.	____	____	_____
d. Abduction—moved the leg away from the body.	____	____	_____
e. Adduction—moved the leg toward the other leg.	____	____	_____
f. Internal rotation—turned the leg inward.	____	____	_____
g. External rotation—turned the leg outward.	____	____	_____
h. Repeated flexion, extension, abduction, adduction, and internal and external rotation 5 times, or the number of times stated on the care plan.	____	____	_____

Date of Satisfactory Completion _____   Instructor's Initials _____

Procedure—cont'd   **S**   **U**   **Comments**

18. Exercised the knee:
    a. Supported the knee. Placed one hand under the knee.
       Placed your other hand under the ankle.   _____ _____ _____
    b. Flexion—bent the leg.   _____ _____ _____
    c. Extension—straightened the leg.   _____ _____ _____
    d. Repeated flexion and extension of the knee 5 times, or
       the number of times stated on the care plan.   _____ _____ _____
19. Exercised the ankle:
    a. Supported the foot and ankle. Placed one hand under
       the foot. Placed your other hand under the ankle.   _____ _____ _____
    b. Dorsiflexion—pulled the foot forward. Pushed down on
       the heel at the same time.   _____ _____ _____
    c. Plantar flexion—turned the foot down. Or pointed the toes. _____ _____ _____
    d. Repeated dorsiflexion and plantar flexion 5 times, or
       the number of times stated on the care plan.   _____ _____ _____
20. Exercised the foot:
    a. Continued to support the foot and ankle.   _____ _____ _____
    b. Pronation—turned the outside of the foot up and
       the inside down.   _____ _____ _____
    c. Supination—turned the inside of the foot up and
       outside down.   _____ _____ _____
    d. Repeated pronation and supination 5 times, or
       the number of times stated on the care plan.   _____ _____ _____
21. Exercised the toes:
    a. Flexion—curled the toes.   _____ _____ _____
    b. Extension—straightened the toes.   _____ _____ _____
    c. Abduction—spread the toes apart.   _____ _____ _____
    d. Adduction—pulled the toes together.   _____ _____ _____
    e. Repeated flexion, extension, abduction, and adduction
       5 times, or the number of times stated on the care plan. _____ _____ _____
22. Covered the leg. Raised the bed rail if used.   _____ _____ _____
23. Went to the other side. Lowered the bed rail near you if up. _____ _____ _____
24. Repeated exercises:
    a. Exercised the shoulder:
       (1) Grasped the wrist with one hand. Grasped
           the elbow with the other hand.   _____ _____ _____
       (2) Flexion—raised the arm straight in front and over the head. _____ _____ _____
       (3) Extension—brought the arm down to the side.   _____ _____ _____
       (4) Hyperextension—moved the arm behind the body.
           (Did this if the person was sitting in a straight-backed
           chair or was standing.)   _____ _____ _____
       (5) Abduction—moved the straight arm away from
           the side of the body.   _____ _____ _____
       (6) Adduction—moved the straight arm to the side of the body. _____ _____ _____
       (7) Internal rotation—bent the elbow. Placed it at
           the same level as the shoulder. Moved the forearm
           down toward the body.   _____ _____ _____
       (8) External rotation—moved the forearm toward the head. _____ _____ _____
       (9) Repeated flexion, extension, hyperextension,
           abduction, adduction, and internal and external rotation
           5 times, or the number of times stated on the care plan. _____ _____ _____
    b. Exercised the elbow:
       (1) Grasped the person's wrist with one hand.
           Grasped the elbow with your other hand.   _____ _____ _____
       (2) Flexion—bent the arm so the same-side shoulder
           was touched.   _____ _____ _____
       (3) Extension—straightened the arm.   _____ _____ _____
       (4) Repeated flexion and extension 5 times, or
           the number of times stated on the care plan.   _____ _____ _____

Date of Satisfactory Completion _____   Instructor's Initials _____

Procedure—cont'd	S	U	Comments

c. Exercised the forearm:
  (1) Pronation—turned the hand so the palm was down.
  (2) Supination—turned the hand so the palm was up.
  (3) Repeated pronation and supination 5 times, or
      the number of times stated on the care plan.

d. Exercised the wrist:
  (1) Held the wrist with both of your hands.
  (2) Flexion—bent the hand down.
  (3) Extension—straightened the hand.
  (4) Hyperextension—bent the hand back.
  (5) Radial flexion—turned the hand toward the thumb.
  (6) Ulnar flexion—turned the hand toward the little finger.
  (7) Repeated flexion, extension, hyperextension, and
      radial and ulnar flexion 5 times, or the number
      of times stated on the care plan.

e. Exercised the thumb:
  (1) Held the person's hand with one hand. Held
      the thumb with your other hand.
  (2) Abduction—moved the thumb out from the
      inner part of the index finger.
  (3) Adduction—moved the thumb back next to the index finger.
  (4) Opposition—touched each finger with the thumb.
  (5) Flexion—bent the thumb into the hand.
  (6) Extension—moved the thumb out to the side of the fingers.
  (7) Repeated abduction, adduction, opposition, flexion,
      and extension 5 times, or the number of times stated
      on the care plan.

f. Exercised the fingers:
  (1) Abduction—spread the fingers and the thumb apart.
  (2) Adduction—brought the fingers and thumb together.
  (3) Extension—straightened the fingers so the fingers,
      hand, and arm were straight.
  (4) Flexion—made a fist.
  (5) Repeated abduction, adduction, flexion, and extension
      5 times, or the number of times stated on the care plan.

g. Exercised the hip:
  (1) Supported the leg. Placed one hand under the knee.
      Placed your other hand under the ankle.
  (2) Flexion—raised the leg.
  (3) Extension—straightened the leg.
  (4) Abduction—moved the leg away from the body.
  (5) Adduction—moved the leg toward the other leg.
  (6) Internal rotation—turned the leg inward.
  (7) External rotation—turned the leg outward.
  (8) Repeated flexion, extension, abduction, adduction,
      and internal and external rotation 5 times, or the
      number of times stated on the care plan.

h. Exercised the knee:
  (1) Supported the knee. Placed one hand under the knee.
      Placed your other hand under the ankle.
  (2) Flexion—bent the leg.
  (3) Extension—straightened the leg.
  (4) Repeated flexion and extension of the knee 5 times, or
      the number of times stated on the care plan.

Date of Satisfactory Completion _____   Instructor's Initials _____

Procedure—cont'd	S	U	Comments
i. Exercised the ankle:			
(1) Supported the foot and ankle. Placed one hand under the foot. Placed your other hand under the ankle.	___	___	_____
(2) Dorsiflexion—pulled the foot forward. Pushed down on the heel at the same time.	___	___	_____
(3) Plantar flexion—turned the foot down. Or pointed the toes.	___	___	_____
(4) Repeated dorsiflexion and plantar flexion 5 times, or the number of times stated on the care plan.	___	___	_____
j. Exercised the foot:			
(1) Continued to support the foot and ankle.	___	___	_____
(2) Pronation—turned the outside of the foot up and the inside down.	___	___	_____
(3) Supination—turned the inside of the foot up and outside down.	___	___	_____
(4) Repeated pronation and supination 5 times, or the number of times stated on the care plan.	___	___	_____
k. Exercised the toes:			
(1) Flexion—curled the toes.	___	___	_____
(2) Extension—straightened the toes.	___	___	_____
(3) Abduction—spread the toes apart.	___	___	_____
(4) Adduction—pulled the toes together.	___	___	_____
(5) Repeated flexion, extension, abduction, and adduction 5 times, or the number of times stated on the care plan.	___	___	_____

Post-Procedure

	S	U	Comments
25. Provided for comfort.	___	___	_____
26. Removed the bath blanket.	___	___	_____
27. Placed the signal light within reach.	___	___	_____
28. Lowered the bed to its lowest position.	___	___	_____
29. Raised or lowered bed rails. Followed the care plan.	___	___	_____
30. Folded and returned the bath blanket its proper place.	___	___	_____
31. Unscreened the person.	___	___	_____
32. Completed a safety check of the room.	___	___	_____
33. Practiced hand hygiene.	___	___	_____
34. Reported and recorded your observations.	___	___	_____

Date of Satisfactory Completion _____   Instructor's Initials _____

Helping the Person to Walk (NNAAP®)

Name: _____   Date: _____

Quality of Life	S	U	Comments

Quality of Life

Remembered to:
- Knock before entering the person's room
- Address the person by name
- Introduce yourself by name and title
- Explain the procedure to the person before beginning and during the procedure
- Protect the person's rights during the procedure
- Handle the person gently during the procedure

Pre-Procedure

1. Followed *Delegation Guidelines: Ambulation.* Reviewed *Promoting Safety and Comfort: Ambulation.*
2. Practiced hand hygiene.
3. Collected the following:
   - Robe and non-skid shoes
   - Paper or sheet to protect bottom linens
   - Gait (transfer) belt
4. Identified the person. Checked the ID bracelet against the assignment sheet. Called the person by name.
5. Provided for privacy.

Procedure

6. Lowered the bed to its lowest position. Locked the bed wheels. Lowered the bed rail near you if up.
7. Fan-folded top linens to the foot of the bed.
8. Placed the paper or sheet under the person's feet. Put the shoes on the person. Fastened the shoes.
9. Helped the person sit on the side of the bed.
10. Made sure the person's feet were flat on the floor.
11. Helped the person put on the robe.
12. Applied the gait (transfer) belt at the waist and over clothing.
13. Helped the person stand. Grasped the gait (transfer) belt at each side. If no gait (transfer) belt, placed your arms under the person's arms around to the shoulder blades.
14. Stood at the person's weak side while the person gained balance. Held the belt at the side and back. If no gait belt, had one arm around the back and the other at the elbow to support the person.
15. Encouraged the person to stand erect with the head up and back straight.
16. Helped the person walk. Walked to the side and slightly behind the person on the person's weak side. Provided support with the gait belt. If did not use a gait belt, had one arm around the back and the other at the elbow to support the person. Encouraged the person to use the hand rail on the person's strong side.
17. Encouraged the person to walk normally. The heel struck the floor first. Discouraged shuffling, sliding, or walking on tiptoes.
18. Walked the required distance if the person tolerated the activity. Did not rush the person.
19. Helped the person return to bed. Removed the gait belt.
20. Lowered the head of the bed. Helped the person to the center of the bed.
21. Removed the shoes. Removed the paper or sheet over the bottom sheet.

Date of Satisfactory Completion _____   Instructor's Initials _____

Post-Procedure

22. Provided for comfort.
23. Placed the signal light within reach.
24. Raised or lowered bed rails. Followed the care plan.
25. Returned the robe and shoes to their proper place.
26. Unscreened the person.
27. Completed a safety check of the room.
28. Practiced hand hygiene.
29. Reported and recorded your observations.

Date of Satisfactory Completion _____   Instructor's Initials _____

Preparing the Person's Room

Name: _____   Date: _____

Procedure	S	U	Comments
1. Followed *Delegation Guidelines: Admitting, Transferring, and Discharging Residents.*	_____	_____	_____
2. Practiced hand hygiene.	_____	_____	_____
3. Collected the following:			
• Admission kit—wash basin, soap, toothpaste, toothbrush, water pitcher, cup, and so on	_____	_____	_____
• Bedpan and urinal (for a man)	_____	_____	_____
• Admission form	_____	_____	_____
• Thermometer	_____	_____	_____
• Sphygmomanometer	_____	_____	_____
• Stethoscope	_____	_____	_____
• Gown or pajamas (if needed)	_____	_____	_____
• Towels and washcloth	_____	_____	_____
• IV pole (if needed)	_____	_____	_____
• Other items requested by the nurse	_____	_____	_____
4. Placed the following on the overbed table:			
• Thermometer	_____	_____	_____
• Sphygmomanometer	_____	_____	_____
• Stethoscope	_____	_____	_____
• Admission form	_____	_____	_____
5. Placed the water pitcher and cup one the bedside stand or overbed table.	_____	_____	_____
6. Placed the following in the bedside stand:			
a. Admission kit	_____	_____	_____
b. Bedpan and urinal	_____	_____	_____
c. Gown or pajamas	_____	_____	_____
d. Towels and washcloth	_____	_____	_____
7. If the *person arrived by stretcher:*			
a. Made a surgical bed.	_____	_____	_____
b. Raised the bed it its highest level.	_____	_____	_____
8. If the person was ambulatory or arrived by wheelchair:			
a. Left the bed closed.	_____	_____	_____
b. Lowered the bed to its lowest position.	_____	_____	_____
9. Attached the signal light to the bed linens.	_____	_____	_____
10. Practiced hand hygiene.	_____	_____	_____

Date of Satisfactory Completion _____   Instructor's Initials _____

Admitting the Person

Name: _____   Date: _____

Quality of Life	S	U	Comments
Remembered to:			
• Knock before entering the person's room	_____	_____	_____
• Address the person by name	_____	_____	_____
• Introduce yourself by name and title	_____	_____	_____
• Explain the procedure to the person before beginning and during the procedure	_____	_____	_____
• Protect the person's rights during the procedure	_____	_____	_____
• Handle the person gently during the procedure	_____	_____	_____

Pre-Procedure

	S	U	Comments
1. Followed *Delegation Guidelines: Admissions, Transfers, and Discharges.* Reviewed *Promoting Safety and Comfort: Admissions, Transfers, and Discharges.*	_____	_____	_____
2. Practiced hand hygiene.	_____	_____	_____
3. Prepared the room.	_____	_____	_____

Procedure

	S	U	Comments
4. Checked the person's name on the admission form and ID bracelet.	_____	_____	_____
5. Greeted the person by name. Asked if he or she preferred a certain name.	_____	_____	_____
6. Introduced yourself to the person and others present. Gave your name and title. Explained that you assist the nurse in giving care.	_____	_____	_____
7. Introduced the roommate.	_____	_____	_____
8. Provided for privacy. Asked family or friends to leave the room. Told them how much time you needed, and directed them to the waiting area. Allowed a family member or friend to stay if the person preferred.	_____	_____	_____
9. Allowed the person to stay dressed if his or her condition permitted. Or helped the person change into a gown or pajamas.	_____	_____	_____
10. Provided for comfort. The person was in bed or in a chair as directed by the nurse.	_____	_____	_____
11. Assisted the nurse with assessments:			
a. Measured vital signs.	_____	_____	_____
b. Measured weight and height.	_____	_____	_____
c. Collected information for the admission form as requested by the nurse.	_____	_____	_____
12. Explained ordered activity limits.	_____	_____	_____
13. Oriented the person and family to the area:			
a. Gave names of the nurses and nursing assistants.	_____	_____	_____
b. Identified items in the bedside stand. Explained the purpose of each.	_____	_____	_____
c. Explained how to use the overbed table.	_____	_____	_____
d. Showed how to use the signal light.	_____	_____	_____
e. Showed how to use the bed, TV, and light controls.	_____	_____	_____
f. Explained how to make phone calls. Placed the phone within reach.	_____	_____	_____
g. Showed the person the bathroom. Also showed how to use the signal light in the bathroom.	_____	_____	_____
h. Explained visiting hours and policies.	_____	_____	_____

Date of Satisfactory Completion _____   Instructor's Initials _____

Procedure—cont'd	S	U	Comments
i. Explained where to find the nurses' station, lounge, chapel, dining room, and other areas.	_____	_____	_____
j. Identified staff—housekeeping, dietary, physical therapy, and others. Identified students in the agency.	_____	_____	_____
k. Explained when meals and nourishments are served.	_____	_____	_____
14. Filled the water pitcher and cup if oral fluids were allowed.	_____	_____	_____
15. Placed the signal light within reach.	_____	_____	_____
16. Placed other controls and needed items within reach.	_____	_____	_____
17. Provided a denture container if needed. Labeled it with the person's name, room, and bed number.	_____	_____	_____
18. Labeled the person's property and personal care items his or her name (if not done by family).	_____	_____	_____
19. Completed a clothing and personal belongings list.	_____	_____	_____
20. Helped the person put away clothes and personal items. Put them in the closet, drawers, and bedside stand. (The family may have wanted to help with this step.)	_____	_____	_____

Post-Procedure

	S	U	Comments
21. Provided for comfort.	_____	_____	_____
22. Lowered the bed to its lowest position.	_____	_____	_____
23. Raised or lowered bed rails. Followed the care plan.	_____	_____	_____
24. Completed a safety check of the room.	_____	_____	_____
25. Practiced hand hygiene.	_____	_____	_____
26. Reported and recorded your observations.	_____	_____	_____

Date of Satisfactory Completion _____   Instructor's Initials _____

Measuring Weight and Height (NNAAP®)

Name: _____   Date: _____

Quality of Life	S	U	Comments
Remembered to:			
• Knock before entering the person's room	___	___	_____
• Address the person by name	___	___	_____
• Introduce yourself by name and title	___	___	_____
• Explain the procedure to the person before beginning and during the procedure	___	___	_____
• Protect the person's rights during the procedure	___	___	_____
• Handle the person gently during the procedure	___	___	_____

Pre-Procedure

1. Followed *Delegation Guidelines: Measuring Weight and Height*. Reviewed *Promoting Safety and Comfort: Measuring Weight and Height*.   ___ ___ _____
2. Asked the person to void.   ___ ___ _____
3. Practiced hand hygiene.   ___ ___ _____
4. Brought the scale and paper towels (for standing scale) to the person's room.   ___ ___ _____
5. Practiced hand hygiene.   ___ ___ _____
6. Identified the person. Checked the ID bracelet against the assignment sheet. Called the person by name.   ___ ___ _____
7. Provided for privacy.   ___ ___ _____

Procedure

8. Placed the paper towels on the scale platform.   ___ ___ _____
9. Raised the height rod.   ___ ___ _____
10. Moved the weights to zero (0). The pointer was in the middle.   ___ ___ _____
11. Had the person remove the robe and footwear. Assisted as needed. (NOTE: For some state competency tests, shoes are worn.)   ___ ___ _____
12. Helped the person stand on the scale. The person stood in the center of the scale. Arms were at the sides.   ___ ___ _____
13. Moved the lower and upper weights until the balance pointer was in the middle.   ___ ___ _____
14. Noted the weight on your notepad or assignment sheet.   ___ ___ _____
15. Asked the person to stand very straight.   ___ ___ _____
16. Lowered the height rod until it rested on the person's head.   ___ ___ _____
17. Read the height at the movable part of the height rod. Recorded the height in feet and inches to the nearest ¼ inch.   ___ ___ _____
18. Noted the height on your notepad or assignment sheet.   ___ ___ _____
19. Raised the height rod. Helped the person step off of the scale.   ___ ___ _____
20. Helped the person put on a robe and non-skid footwear if he or she was to be up. Or helped the person back to bed.   ___ ___ _____
21. Lowered the height rod. Adjusted the weights to zero (0) if this was agency policy.   ___ ___ _____

Post-Procedure

22. Provided for comfort.   ___ ___ _____
23. Placed the signal light within reach.   ___ ___ _____
24. Raised or lowered bed rails. Followed the care plan.   ___ ___ _____
25. Unscreened the person.   ___ ___ _____
26. Completed a safety check of the room.   ___ ___ _____
27. Discarded the paper towels.   ___ ___ _____
28. Returned the scale to its proper place.   ___ ___ _____
29. Practiced hand hygiene.   ___ ___ _____
30. Reported and recorded the measurements.   ___ ___ _____

Date of Satisfactory Completion _____   Instructor's Initials _____

Measuring the Height—The Person is in Bed

Name: _____   Date: _____

Quality of Life	S	U	Comments
Remembered to:			
• Knock before entering the person's room	___	___	_____
• Address the person by name	___	___	_____
• Introduce yourself by name and title	___	___	_____
• Explain the procedure to the person before beginning and during the procedure	___	___	_____
• Protect the person's rights during the procedure	___	___	_____
• Handle the person gently during the procedure	___	___	_____

Pre-Procedure

	S	U	Comments
1. Followed *Delegation Guidelines: Measuring Weight and Height.* Reviewed *Promoting Safety and Comfort: Measuring Weight and Height.*	___	___	_____
2. Practiced hand hygiene.	___	___	_____
3. Asked a co-worker to help you.	___	___	_____
4. Collected a measuring tape and ruler.	___	___	_____
5. Practiced hand hygiene.	___	___	_____
6. Identified the person. Checked the ID bracelet against the assignment sheet. Called the person by name.	___	___	_____
7. Provided for privacy.	___	___	_____
8. Raised the bed for body mechanics. Bed rails were up if used.	___	___	_____

Procedure

	S	U	Comments
9. Lowered the bed rails if up.	___	___	_____
10. Positioned the person supine if the position is allowed.	___	___	_____
11. Had your co-worker place and hold the beginning of the tape measure at the person's heel.	___	___	_____
12. Pulled the other end of tape measure along the person's body. Pulled it until it extended a few inches past the person's head.	___	___	_____
13. Placed a ruler flat across the top of the person's head. The ruler was extended from the person's head to over the tape measure. Made sure the ruler was level.	___	___	_____
14. Read the height measurement. Noted that this was the point where the lower edge of the ruler touched the tape measure.	___	___	_____
15. Noted the height measurement on your notepad or assignment sheet.	___	___	_____

Post-Procedure

	S	U	Comments
16. Provided for comfort.	___	___	_____
17. Placed the signal light within reach.	___	___	_____
18. Lowered the bed to its lowest position.	___	___	_____
19. Raised or lowered bed rails. Followed the care plan.	___	___	_____
20. Completed a safety check of the room.	___	___	_____
21. Returned equipment to its proper place.	___	___	_____
22. Practiced hand hygiene.	___	___	_____
23. Reported and recorded the height.	___	___	_____

Date of Satisfactory Completion _____   Instructor's Initials _____

Moving the Person to a New Room

Name: _____   Date: _____

Quality of Life	S	U	Comments

Remembered to:
- Knock before entering the person's room
- Address the person by name
- Introduce yourself by name and title
- Explain the procedure to the person before beginning and during the procedure
- Protect the person's rights during the procedure
- Handle the person gently during the procedure

Pre-Procedure

1. Followed *Delegation Guidelines: Admissions, Transfers, and Discharges.* Reviewed *Promoting Safety and Comfort: Admissions, Transfers, and Discharges.*
2. Asked a co-worker to help you.
3. Practiced hand hygiene.
4. Collected the following:
   - Wheelchair or stretcher
   - Utility cart
   - Bath blanket
5. Practiced hand hygiene.
6. Identified the person. Checked the ID bracelet against the assignment sheet. Called the person by name.
7. Provided for privacy.

Procedure

8. Collected the person's belongings and care equipment. Placed them on the utility cart.
9. Transferred the person to a wheelchair or a stretcher. Covered the person with a blanket.
10. Transported the person to the new room. Your co-worker brought the utility cart.
11. Helped transfer the person to the bed or chair. Helped position the person.
12. Helped arrange the person's belongings and equipment.
13. Reported the following to the receiving nurse:
    a. How the person tolerated the transfer.
    b. Any observations made during the transfer.
    c. That the nurse will bring the medical record, care plan, Kardex, and drugs.

Post-Procedure

14. Returned the wheelchair or stretcher and the utility cart to the storage area.
15. Practiced hand hygiene.
16. Reported and recorded the following:
    a. The time of the transfer.
    b. Who helped you with the transfer.
    c. Where the person was taken.
    d. How the person was transferred (bed, wheelchair, or stretcher).
    e. How the person tolerated the transfer.
    f. Who received the person.
    g. Any other observations.

Date of Satisfactory Completion _____   Instructor's Initials _____

Post-Procedure—cont'd	**S**	**U**	**Comments**
17. Stripped the bed, and cleaned the unit. Practiced hand hygiene and put on gloves for this step. (The housekeeping staff may have done this step.)	————	————	————————————
18. Removed and discarded the gloves. Practiced hand hygiene.	————	————	————————————
19. Followed agency policy for dirty linen.	————	————	————————————
20. Made a closed bed.	————	————	————————————
21. Practiced hand hygiene.	————	————	————————————

Date of Satisfactory Completion _____   Instructor's Initials _____

Transferring or Discharging the Person

Name: _____ Date: _____

Quality of Life	S	U	Comments

Remembered to:
- Knock before entering the person's room
- Address the person by name
- Introduce yourself by name and title
- Explain the procedure to the person before beginning and during the procedure
- Protect the person's rights during the procedure
- Handle the person gently during the procedure

Pre-Procedure

1. Followed *Delegation Guidelines: Admissions, Transfers, and Discharges.* Reviewed *Promoting Safety and Comfort: Admissions, Transfers, and Discharges.*
2. Asked a co-worker to help you.
3. Practiced hand hygiene.
4. Identified the person. Checked the ID bracelet against the assignment sheet. Called the person by name.
5. Provided for privacy.

Procedure

6. Helped the person dress as needed.
7. Helped the person pack. Checked all drawers and closets. Made sure all items were collected.
8. Checked off the clothing list and personal belongings list. Gave the lists to the nurse.
9. Told the nurse that the person was ready for the final visit. The nurse:
    a. Gave prescriptions written by the doctor.
    b. Provided discharge instructions.
    c. Got valuables from the safe.
    d. Had the person sign the clothing and personal belongings lists.
10. *If the person left by wheelchair:*
    a. Got a wheelchair and a utility cart for the person's items. Asked a co-worker to help you.
    b. Helped the person into the wheelchair.
    c. Took the person to the exit area.
    d. Locked the wheelchair wheels.
    e. Helped the person out of the wheelchair and into the car.
    f. Helped put the person's items into the car.
11. *If the person left by ambulance:*
    a. Raised the bed rails.
    b. Placed the signal light within reach.
    c. Waited for the ambulance attendants.
    d. Raised the bed to its highest level when the ambulance attendants arrived.

Post-Procedure

12. Returned the wheelchair and cart to the storage area.
13. Practiced hand hygiene.
14. Reported and recorded the following:
    a. The time of the discharge
    b. Who helped you with the procedure
    c. How the person was transported
    d. Who was with the person
    e. The person's destination
    f. Any other observations

Date of Satisfactory Completion _____   Instructor's Initials _____

Post-Procedure—cont'd	S	U	Comments
15. Stripped the bed, and cleaned the unit. Practiced hand hygiene and put on gloves for this step. (The housekeeping staff may have done this step.)	————	————	————————
16. Removed and discarded the gloves. Practiced hand hygiene.	————	————	————————
17. Followed agency policy for dirty linen.	————	————	————————
18. Made a closed bed.	————	————	————————
19. Practiced hand hygiene.	————	————	————————

Date of Satisfactory Completion ————————————————   Instructor's Initials ————————————————

Preparing the Person for an Examination

Name: _____   Date: _____

Quality of Life	S	U	Comments

Remembered to:
- Knock before entering the person's room
- Address the person by name
- Introduce yourself by name and title
- Explain the procedure to the person before beginning and during the procedure
- Protect the person's rights during the procedure
- Handle the person gently during the procedure

Pre-Procedure

1. Followed *Delegation Guidelines: Preparing the Person*. Reviewed *Promoting Safety and Comfort: Preparing the Person*.
2. Practiced hand hygiene.
3. Collected the following:
   - Flashlight
   - Sphygmomanometer
   - Stethoscope
   - Thermometer
   - Tongue depressors (blades)
   - Laryngeal mirror
   - Ophthalmoscope
   - Otoscope
   - Nasal speculum
   - Percussion (reflex) hammer
   - Tuning fork
   - Tape measure
   - Gloves
   - Water-soluble lubricant
   - Vaginal speculum
   - Cotton-tipped applicators
   - Specimen containers and labels
   - Disposable bag
   - Kidney basin
   - Towel
   - Bath blanket
   - Tissues
   - Drape (sheet, bath blanket, drawsheet, or paper drape)
   - Paper towels
   - Cotton balls
   - Waterproof pad
   - Eye chart (Snellen chart)
   - Slides
   - Gown
   - Alcohol wipes
   - Wastebasket
   - Container for soiled instruments
   - Marking pencils or pens
4. Practiced hand hygiene.
5. Identified the person. Checked the ID bracelet against the assignment sheet. Called the person by name.
6. Provided for privacy.

Date of Satisfactory Completion _____   Instructor's Initials _____

Procedure

7. Had the person put on the gown. Told the person to remove all clothes. Assisted as needed.   _____ _____ _____
8. Asked the person to void. Collected a urine specimen if needed. Provided for privacy.   _____ _____ _____
9. Transported the person to the exam room. (This was not done for an exam in the person's room.)   _____ _____ _____
10. Measured weight and height. Recorded the measurements on the exam form.   _____ _____ _____
11. Helped the person onto the exam table. Provided a step stool if necessary. (Omitted this step for an exam in person's room.)   _____ _____ _____
12. Raised the far bed rail (if used). Raised the bed to its highest level. (Omitted this step if an exam table used.)   _____ _____ _____
13. Measured vital signs. Recorded them on the exam form.   _____ _____ _____
14. Positioned the person as directed.   _____ _____ _____
15. Draped the person.   _____ _____ _____
16. Placed a waterproof pad under the buttocks.   _____ _____ _____
17. Raised the bed rail near you if used.   _____ _____ _____
18. Provided adequate lighting.   _____ _____ _____
19. Put the signal light on for the examiner. Did not leave the person alone.   _____ _____ _____

Date of Satisfactory Completion _____   Instructor's Initials _____

Collecting a Random Urine Specimen

Name: _____   Date: _____

Quality of Life	S	U	Comments
Remembered to:			
• Knock before entering the person's room	___	___	_____
• Address the person by name	___	___	_____
• Introduce yourself by name and title	___	___	_____
• Explain the procedure to the person before beginning and during the procedure	___	___	_____
• Protect the person's rights during the procedure	___	___	_____
• Handle the person gently during the procedure	___	___	_____

Pre-Procedure

	S	U	Comments
1. Followed *Delegation Guidelines: Urine Specimens.* Reviewed *Promoting Safety and Comfort: Urine Specimens.*	___	___	_____
2. Practiced hand hygiene.	___	___	_____
3. Collected the following before going to the person's room:			
• Laboratory requisition slip	___	___	_____
• Specimen container and lid	___	___	_____
• New voiding receptacle—bedpan and cover, urinal, commode, or specimen pan	___	___	_____
• Specimen label	___	___	_____
• Plastic bag	___	___	_____
• BIOHAZARD label (if needed)	___	___	_____
• Gloves	___	___	_____
4. Arranged collected items in the person's bathroom.	___	___	_____
5. Practiced hand hygiene.	___	___	_____
6. Identified the person. Checked the ID bracelet against the assignment sheet. Called the person by name.	___	___	_____
7. Labeled the container in the person's presence.	___	___	_____
8. Put on gloves.	___	___	_____
9. Collected a graduate to measure output	___	___	_____
10. Provided for privacy.	___	___	_____

Procedure

	S	U	Comments
11. Asked the person to void into the device. Reminded the person to put toilet tissue into the wastebasket or toilet. Toilet tissue was not put in the bedpan or specimen pan.	___	___	_____
12. Took the voiding device to the bathroom.	___	___	_____
13. Poured about 120 mL (milliliters) (4 oz [ounces]) into the specimen container.	___	___	_____
14. Placed the lid on the specimen container. Put the container in the plastic bag. Did not let the container touch the outside of the bag. Applied a BIOHAZARD label.	___	___	_____
15. Measured urine if I&O was ordered. Included the specimen amount.	___	___	_____
16. Emptied, rinsed, cleaned, and disinfected equipment. Returned equipment to its proper place.	___	___	_____
17. Removed and discarded the gloves. Practiced hand hygiene. Put on clean gloves.	___	___	_____
18. Assisted with hand washing.	___	___	_____
19. Removed and discarded the gloves. Practiced hand hygiene.	___	___	_____

Date of Satisfactory Completion _____   Instructor's Initials _____

Post-Procedure

20. Provided for comfort.
21. Placed the signal light within reach.
22. Raised or lowered bed rails. Followed the care plan.
23. Unscreened the person.
24. Completed a safety check of the room.
25. Practiced hand hygiene.
26. Took the specimen and the requisition slip to the
    storage area. Wore gloves.
27. Removed and discarded the gloves. Practiced hand hygiene.
28. Reported and recorded your observations.

Date of Satisfactory Completion _____ Instructor's Initials _____

Collecting a Midstream Specimen

Name: _____   Date: _____

Quality of Life	S	U	Comments

Remembered to:
- Knock before entering the person's room
- Address the person by name
- Introduce yourself by name and title
- Explain the procedure to the person before beginning and during the procedure
- Protect the person's rights during the procedure
- Handle the person gently during the procedure

Pre-Procedure

1. Followed *Delegation Guidelines: Urine Specimens.* Reviewed *Promoting Safety and Comfort: Urine Specimens.*
2. Practiced hand hygiene.
3. Collected the following before going to the person's room:
   - Laboratory requisition slip
   - Midstream specimen kit—includes specimen container, label, towelettes, sterile gloves
   - Plastic bag
   - Sterile gloves (if not part of kit)
   - Disposable gloves
   - BIOHAZARD label (if needed)
4. Arranged your work area.
5. Practiced hand hygiene.
6. Identified the person. Checked the ID bracelet against the assignment sheet. Called the person by name.
7. Put on disposable gloves.
8. Collected the following:
   - Voiding device—bedpan and cover, urinal, commode, or specimen pan if needed
   - Supplies for perineal care
   - Graduate to measure output
   - Paper towel
9. Provided for privacy.

Procedure

10. Provided perineal care. (Wore gloves for this step. Practiced hand hygiene after removing and discarding gloves.)
11. Opened the sterile kit.
12. Put on the sterile gloves.
13. Opened the packet of towelettes.
14. Opened the sterile specimen container. Did not touch the inside of the container or the lid. Sat the lid down so the inside faced up.
15. *For a female:* cleaned the perineal area with the towelettes.
    a. Spread the labia with your thumb and index finger. Used your non-dominant hand. (This hand was contaminated and did not touch anything sterile.)
    b. Cleaned down the urethral area from front to back. Used a clean towelette for each stroke.
    c. Kept the labia separated to collect the urine specimen.

Date of Satisfactory Completion _____   Instructor's Initials _____

Procedure—cont'd   S   U   **Comments**

16. *For a male:* cleaned the penis with towelettes.
    a. Held the penis with your non-dominant hand.
       (This hand was contaminated and did not touch
       anything sterile.)   _____   _____   _____
    b. Cleaned the penis starting at the meatus. Retracted the foreskin
       if the male was uncircumcised. Cleaned in a circular motion.
       Started at the center and worked outward.   _____   _____   _____
    c. Kept holding the penis and kept the foreskin retracted in
       the uncircumcised male until the specimen was collected. _____   _____   _____
17. Asked the person to void into a device.   _____   _____   _____
18. Passed the specimen container into the urine stream.
    (If female, kept the labia separated.)   _____   _____   _____
19. Collected about 30 to 60 mL (1 to 2 oz) of urine.   _____   _____   _____
20. Removed the specimen container before the person stopped
    voiding. Released the retracted foreskin of the uncircumcised male. _____   _____   _____
21. Released the labia or penis. Allowed the person to finish
    voiding into the device.   _____   _____   _____
22. Put the lid on the specimen container. Touched only the
    outside of the container and lid. Wiped the outside of the
    container. Placed the container on a paper towel.   _____   _____   _____
23. Provided toilet tissue after the person was done voiding. _____   _____   _____
24. Took the voiding device to the bathroom.   _____   _____   _____
25. Measured urine if I&O was ordered. Included the
    specimen amount.   _____   _____   _____
26. Emptied, rinsed, cleaned, disinfected, and dried equipment.
    Returned equipment to its proper place.   _____   _____   _____
27. Removed and discarded the gloves. Practiced hand hygiene.
    Put on clean disposable gloves.   _____   _____   _____
28. Labeled the specimen container. Placed the container in
    the plastic bag. Did not let the container touch the outside
    of the bag. Applied a *BIOHAZARD* label.   _____   _____   _____
29. Assisted with hand washing.   _____   _____   _____
30. Removed and discarded the gloves. Practiced hand hygiene. _____   _____   _____

Post-Procedure
31. Provided for comfort.   _____   _____   _____
32. Placed the signal light within reach.   _____   _____   _____
33. Raised or lowered bed rails. Followed the care plan.   _____   _____   _____
34. Unscreened the person.   _____   _____   _____
35. Completed a safety check of the room.   _____   _____   _____
36. Practiced hand hygiene.   _____   _____   _____
37. Took the specimen and the requisition slip to the
    storage area. Wore gloves.   _____   _____   _____
38. Removed and discarded the gloves. Practiced hand hygiene. _____   _____   _____
39. Reported and recorded your observations.   _____   _____   _____

Date of Satisfactory Completion _____   Instructor's Initials _____

Collecting a 24-hour Urine Specimen

Name: _____   Date: _____

Quality of Life	S	U	Comments

Remembered to:
- Knock before entering the person's room
- Address the person by name
- Introduce yourself by name and title
- Explain the procedure to the person before beginning and during the procedure
- Protect the person's rights during the procedure
- Handle the person gently during the procedure

Pre-Procedure

1. Followed *Delegation Guidelines: Urine Specimens*.
   Reviewed *Promoting Safety and Comfort*:
   a. *Urine Specimens*
   b. *The 24-Hour Urine Specimen*
2. Practiced hand hygiene.
3. Collected the following before going to the person's room:
   - Laboratory requisition slip
   - Urine container for a 24-hour collection
   - Specimen label
   - Preservative if needed
   - Bucket with ice if needed
   - Two "24-hour Urine" labels
   - Funnel
   - *BIOHAZARD* label
   - Gloves
4. Arranged collected items in the person's bathroom.
5. Placed one "24-hour urine" label in the bathroom. Placed the other near the bed.
6. Practiced hand hygiene.
7. Identified the person. Checked the ID bracelet against the assignment sheet. Called the person by name.
8. Labeled the urine container in the person's presence. Applied the *BIOHAZARD* label. Placed the labeled urine container in the person's bathroom.
9. Put on gloves.
10. Collected the following:
    - Voiding device—bedpan and cover, urinal, commode, or specimen pan
    - Graduate for output
11. Provided for privacy.

Procedure

12. Asked the person to void. Provided a voiding device.
13. Measured and discarded the urine. Noted the time. This started the 24-hour urine period.
14. Marked the time on the urine container.
15. Emptied, rinsed, cleaned, disinfected, and dried equipment. Returned equipment to its proper place.
16. Removed the gloves, and practiced hand hygiene. Put on clean gloves.
17. Assisted with hand washing.
18. Removed the gloves. Practiced hand hygiene.
19. Marked the time the test began and the end time on the room and bathroom labels.

Date of Satisfactory Completion _____   Instructor's Initials _____

Procedure—cont'd	S	U	Comments
20. Reminded the person to:			
a. Use the voiding device when voiding during the next 24 hours.	___	___	_____
b. Not have a BM when voiding.	___	___	_____
c. Put toilet tissue in the toilet or wastebasket.	___	___	_____
d. Turn on the signal light after voiding.	___	___	_____
21. Returned to the room when the person signaled for you. Knocked before entering the room.	___	___	_____
22. Did the following after every voiding:			
a. Practiced hand hygiene. Put on gloves.	___	___	_____
b. Measured urine if I&O was ordered.	___	___	_____
c. Poured urine into the urine container using the funnel. Did not spill any urine. Restarted the test if you spilled or discarded the urine.	___	___	_____
d. Emptied, rinsed, cleaned, disinfected, and dried equipment. Returned equipment to its proper place.	___	___	_____
e. Removed and discarded the gloves. Practiced hand hygiene. Put on clean gloves.	___	___	_____
f. Assisted with hand washing.	___	___	_____
g. Removed and discarded the gloves. Practiced hand hygiene.	___	___	_____
h. Did the following after each voiding:			
• Provided for comfort.	___	___	_____
• Placed the signal light within reach.	___	___	_____
• Raised or lowered bed rails. Followed the care plan.	___	___	_____
• Put on gloves.	___	___	_____
• Cleaned and returned equipment to its proper place. Discarded disposable items.	___	___	_____
• Removed the gloves. Practiced hand hygiene.	___	___	_____
• Unscreened the person.	___	___	_____
• Completed safety check of the room.	___	___	_____
23. Asked the person to void at the end of the 24-hour period and did the following:			

Post-Procedure

	S	U	Comments
24. Provided for comfort.	___	___	_____
25. Placed the signal light within reach.	___	___	_____
26. Raised or lowered bed rails. Followed the care plan.	___	___	_____
27. Put on gloves.	___	___	_____
28. Removed the labels from the room and bathroom.	___	___	_____
29. Cleaned, dried, and returned equipment to its proper place. Discarded disposable items.	___	___	_____
30. Removed and discarded the gloves. Practiced hand hygiene.	___	___	_____
31. Unscreened the person.	___	___	_____
32. Completed a safety check of the room.	___	___	_____
33. Took the specimen (labeled urine container) and the requisition slip to the storage area. Wore gloves.	___	___	_____
34. Removed and discarded gloves. Practiced hand hygiene.	___	___	_____
35. Reported and recorded your observations.	___	___	_____

Date of Satisfactory Completion _____   Instructor's Initials _____

Collecting a Urine Specimen From an Infant or Child

Name: _____   Date: _____

Quality of Life   **S**   **U**   **Comments**
Remembered to:
- Knock before entering the child's room   ____   ____   _____
- Address the child by name   ____   ____   _____
- Introduce yourself by name and title   ____   ____   _____
- Explain the procedure to the person before beginning and
  during the procedure   ____   ____   _____
- Protect the child's rights during the procedure   ____   ____   _____
- Handle the child gently during the procedure   ____   ____   _____

Pre-Procedure
1. Followed *Delegation Guidelines: Urine Specimens.*
   Reviewed *Promoting Safety and Comfort: Urine Specimens.*   ____   ____   _____
2. Practiced hand hygiene.   ____   ____   _____
3. Collected the following:
   - Collection bag ("wee" bag)   ____   ____   _____
   - BIOHAZARD label (if needed)   ____   ____   _____
   - Cotton balls   ____   ____   _____
   - Specimen container   ____   ____   _____
   - Plastic bag   ____   ____   _____
   - Scissors   ____   ____   _____
   - Wash basin   ____   ____   _____
   - Bath towel   ____   ____   _____
   - Two diapers   ____   ____   _____
   - Gloves   ____   ____   _____
4. Arranged your work area.   ____   ____   _____
5. Practiced hand hygiene.   ____   ____   _____
6. Identified the child. Checked the ID bracelet against the
   assignment sheet. Called the child by name.   ____   ____   _____
7. Provided for privacy.   ____   ____   _____

Procedure
8. Practiced hand hygiene. Put on gloves.   ____   ____   _____
9. Positioned the child on his or her back.   ____   ____   _____
10. Removed and set aside the diaper.   ____   ____   _____
11. Cleaned the perineal area with cotton balls. Used a new
    cotton ball for each stroke. Rinsed and dried the area.   ____   ____   _____
12. Removed and discarded the gloves. Practiced hand hygiene. ____   ____   _____
13. Put on clean gloves.   ____   ____   _____
14. Flexed the child's knees. Spread the legs.   ____   ____   _____
15. Removed the adhesive backing from the collection bag.   ____   ____   _____
16. Applied the bag to the perineum.   ____   ____   _____
17. Cut a slit in the bottom of a new diaper.   ____   ____   _____
18. Diapered the child.   ____   ____   _____
19. Pulled the collection bag through the slit in the diaper.   ____   ____   _____
20. Removed and discarded the gloves. Practiced hand hygiene.   ____   ____   _____
21. Raised the head of the crib if allowed. This helped the
    urine to collect in the bottom of the bag.   ____   ____   _____
22. Made sure the crib rails were raised and locked before
    leaving the bedside.   ____   ____   _____
23. Unscreened the child.   ____   ____   _____
24. Disposed of the removed diaper. Followed agency policy.
    (Wore gloves for this step.)   ____   ____   _____
25. Practiced hand hygiene.   ____   ____   _____
26. Checked the child often. Checked the bag for urine.
    (Provided for privacy and wore gloves for this step.)   ____   ____   _____

Date of Satisfactory Completion _____   Instructor's Initials _____

Procedure—cont'd	**S**	**U**	**Comments**
27. Did the following if the child voided:			
a. Provided for privacy.	_____	_____	_____
b. Practiced hand hygiene. Put on clean gloves.	_____	_____	_____
c. Removed the diaper.	_____	_____	_____
d. Removed the collection bag gently.	_____	_____	_____
e. Pressed the adhesive surfaces of the bag together. Made sure the seal was tight and there were no leaks. Or transferred the urine to the specimen container using the drainage tab.	_____	_____	_____
f. Cleaned the perineal area. Rinsed and dried well.	_____	_____	_____
g. Diapered the child.	_____	_____	_____
h. Removed and discarded the gloves. Practiced hand hygiene.	_____	_____	_____
28. Put on clean gloves.	_____	_____	_____
29. Labeled the collection bag or specimen container in the child's presence. Placed it in the plastic bag. Applied the BIOHAZARD label (if needed).	_____	_____	_____

Post-Procedure

	S	**U**	**Comments**
30. Provided for comfort.	_____	_____	_____
31. Made sure the crib rail was raised and locked before leaving the bedside.	_____	_____	_____
32. Unscreened the child.	_____	_____	_____
33. Cleaned, rinsed, and returned equipment to its proper place. Discarded disposable items. (Wore gloves for this step.)	_____	_____	_____
34. Completed a safety check of the room.	_____	_____	_____
35. Removed and discarded the gloves. Practiced hand hygiene.	_____	_____	_____
36. Took the specimen and the requisition slip to the storage area. Wore gloves.	_____	_____	_____
37. Removed and discarded the gloves. Practiced hand hygiene.	_____	_____	_____
38. Reported and recorded your observations.	_____	_____	_____

Date of Satisfactory Completion _____   Instructor's Initials _____

Testing Urine With Reagent Strips

Name: _____   Date: _____

	S	U	Comments
Quality of Life			

Quality of Life
Remembered to:
- Knock before entering the person's room
- Address the person by name
- Introduce yourself by name and title
- Explain the procedure to the person before beginning and during the procedure
- Protect the person's rights during the procedure
- Handle the person gently during the procedure

Pre-Procedure
1. Followed *Delegation Guidelines: Testing Urine*. Reviewed *Promoting Safety and Comfort: Testing Urine*.
2. Practiced hand hygiene.
3. Collected gloves and the reagent strips ordered.
4. Practiced hand hygiene.
5. Identified the person. Checked the ID bracelet against the assignment sheet. Called the person by name.
6. Put on gloves.
7. Collected the following:
   - Specimen container and lid
   - Gloves
8. Provided for privacy.

Procedure
9. Collected the urine specimen.
10. Removed the strip from the bottle. Put the cap on the bottle at once. It was on tight.
11. Dipped the test strip areas into the urine.
12. Removed the strip after the correct amount of time. Followed the manufacturer's instructions.
13. Tapped the strip gently against the urine container. This removed excess urine.
14. Waited the required amount of time. Followed the manufacturer's instructions.
15. Compared the strip with the color chart on the bottle. Read the results.
16. Discarded disposable items and the specimen.
17. Emptied, rinsed, cleaned, disinfected, and dried equipment. Returned equipment to its proper place.
18. Removed and discarded the gloves. Practiced hand hygiene.

Post-Procedure
19. Provided for comfort.
20. Placed the signal light within reach.
21. Raised or lowered bed rails. Followed the care plan.
22. Unscreened the person.
23. Completed a safety check of the room.
24. Practiced hand hygiene.
25. Reported and recorded the results and other observations.

Date of Satisfactory Completion _____   Instructor's Initials _____

Straining Urine

Name: _____   Date: _____

	S	U	Comments

Quality of Life

Remembered to:
- Knock before entering the person's room
- Address the person by name
- Introduce yourself by name and title
- Explain the procedure to the person before beginning and during the procedure
- Protect the person's rights during the procedure
- Handle the person gently during the procedure

Pre-Procedure

1. Followed *Delegation Guidelines: Testing Urine.* Reviewed *Promoting Safety and Comfort: Testing Urine.*
2. Practiced hand hygiene.
3. Collected the following before going to the person's room:
   - Laboratory requisition slip
   - Gauze or strainer
   - Specimen container
   - Specimen label
   - Two STRAIN ALL URINE labels
   - Plastic bag
   - BIOHAZARD label (if needed)
   - Gloves
4. Arranged collected items in the person's bathroom.
5. Placed one STRAIN ALL URINE label in the bathroom. Placed the other near the bed.
6. Practiced hand hygiene.
7. Identified the person. Checked the ID bracelet against the assignment sheet. Called the person by name.
8. Labeled the specimen container in the person's presence.
9. Put on gloves.
10. Collected the following:
    - Voiding device—bedpan and cover, urinal, commode, or specimen pan
    - Graduate
11. Provided for privacy.

Procedure

12. Asked the person to use the voiding device for urinating. Asked the person to turn on the signal light after voiding.
13. Removed and discarded the gloves. Practiced hand hygiene.
14. Returned to the room when the person signaled for you. Knocked before entering the room.
15. Practiced hand hygiene. Put on gloves.
16. Placed the gauze or strainer into the graduate.
17. Poured urine into the graduate. Urine passed through the gauze or strainer.
18. Placed the gauze or strainer in the specimen container if any crystals, stones, or particles appeared.
19. Placed the specimen container in the plastic bag. Did not let the container touch the outside of the bag. Applied a BIOHAZARD label.
20. Measured urine if I&O was ordered.
21. Emptied, rinsed, cleaned, disinfected, and dried equipment. Returned equipment to its proper place.

Date of Satisfactory Completion _____   Instructor's Initials _____

Procedure—cont'd	S	U	Comments

Procedure—cont'd

22. Removed and discarded the gloves. Practiced hand hygiene. Put on clean gloves.
23. Assisted with hand washing.
24. Removed and discarded the gloves. Practiced hand hygiene.

Post-Procedure

25. Provided for comfort.
26. Placed the signal light within reach.
27. Raised or lowered bed rails. Followed the care plan.
28. Unscreened the person.
29. Completed a safety check of the room.
30. Practiced hand hygiene.
31. Took the specimen container and requisition slip to the storage area. Wore gloves.
32. Removed and discarded the gloves. Practiced hand hygiene.
33. Reported and recorded your observations.

Date of Satisfactory Completion _____   Instructor's Initials _____

Collecting and Testing a Stool Specimen

Name: _____   Date: _____

Quality of Life	S	U	Comments

Remembered to:
- Knock before entering the person's room
- Address the person by name
- Introduce yourself by name and title
- Explain the procedure to the person before beginning and during the procedure
- Protect the person's rights during the procedure
- Handle the person gently during the procedure

Pre-Procedure

1. Followed *Delegation Guidelines: Stool Specimens.*
   Reviewed *Promoting Safety and Comfort: Stool Specimens.*
2. Practiced hand hygiene.
3. Collected the following before going to the person's room:
   - Laboratory requisition slip
   - Occult blood test kit (if needed)
   - Specimen pan for the toilet
   - Specimen container and lid
   - Specimen label
   - Tongue blade
   - Disposable bag
   - Plastic bag
   - *BIOHAZARD* label (if needed)
   - Gloves
4. Arranged collected items in the person's bathroom.
5. Practiced hand hygiene.
6. Identified the person. Checked the ID bracelet against the requisition slip. Called the person by name.
7. Labeled the specimen container in the person's presence.
8. Put on gloves.
9. Collected the following:
   - Device for voiding—bedpan and cover, urinal, commode, or specimen pan
   - Toilet tissue
10. Provided for privacy.

Procedure

11. Asked the person to void. Provided the voiding device if the person did not use the bathroom. Emptied, rinsed, cleaned, disinfected, and dried the device. Returned it to its proper place.
12. Put the specimen pan on the toilet if the person used the bathroom. Placed it at the back of the toilet. Or provided a bedpan or commode.
13. Asked the person not to put toilet tissue into the bedpan, commode, or specimen pan. Provided a bag for toilet tissue.
14. Placed the signal light and toilet tissue within reach. Raised or lowered bed rails. Followed the care plan.
15. Removed and discarded the gloves. Practiced hand hygiene. Left the room if the person could be left alone.
16. Returned when the person signaled. Or checked on the person every 5 minutes. Knocked before entering.
17. Practiced hand hygiene. Put on clean gloves.
18. Lowered the bed rail near you if up.
19. Removed the bedpan (if used). Noted the color, amount, consistency, and odor of stools.

Date of Satisfactory Completion _____   Instructor's Initials _____

Procedure—cont'd   S   U   **Comments**

20. Provided perineal care if needed.   ____   ____   _____
21. Collected the specimen:
    - Used a tongue blade to take about 2 tablespoons of stool to the
      specimen container. Took the sample from the middle of a
      formed stool.   ____   ____   _____
    - Included pus, mucus, or blood present in the stool.   ____   ____   _____
    - Took stool from 2 different places in the BM if required by
      agency policy.   ____   ____   _____
    - Put the lid on the specimen container.   ____   ____   _____
    - Placed the container in the plastic bag. Did not let the
      container touch the outside of the bag. Applied a BIOHAZARD
      label according to agency policy.   ____   ____   _____
    - Wrapped the tongue blade in toilet tissue. Discarded it into
      the disposable bag.   ____   ____   _____
22. Removed and discarded the gloves. Practiced hand hygiene.
    Put on clean gloves.   ____   ____   _____
23. Tested the specimen (if ordered):
    - Opened the test kit.   ____   ____   _____
    - Used a tongue blade to obtain a small amount of stool.   ____   ____   _____
    - Applied a thin smear of stool on *box A* on the test paper.   ____   ____   _____
    - Used another tongue blade to obtain stool from another
      part of the specimen.   ____   ____   _____
    - Applied a thin smear of stool on *box B* on the test paper.   ____   ____   _____
    - Closed the packet.   ____   ____   _____
    - Turned the test packet to the other side. Opened the flap.
      Applied developer (from the kit) to *boxes A* and *B*.
      Followed the manufacturer's instructions.   ____   ____   _____
    - Waited 10 to 60 seconds as required by the manufacturer.   ____   ____   _____
    - Noted the color changes on your assignment sheet.   ____   ____   _____
    - Disposed of the test packet.   ____   ____   _____
    - Wrapped the tongue blades with toilet tissue.
      Put on clean gloves.   ____   ____   _____
24. Emptied, rinsed, cleaned, disinfected, and dried equipment.
    Returned equipment to its proper place.   ____   ____   _____
25. Removed and discarded the gloves. Practiced hand hygiene.
    Put on clean gloves.   ____   ____   _____
26. Assisted with hand washing.   ____   ____   _____
27. Removed and discarded the gloves. Practiced hand hygiene.   ____   ____   _____

Post-Procedure

28. Provided for comfort.   ____   ____   _____
29. Placed the signal light within reach.   ____   ____   _____
30. Raised or lowered bed rails. Followed the care plan.   ____   ____   _____
31. Unscreened the person.   ____   ____   _____
32. Completed a safety check of the room.   ____   ____   _____
33. Delivered the specimen and requisition slip to the
    laboratory or storage area. Wore gloves.   ____   ____   _____
34. Removed and discarded the gloves. Practiced hand hygiene.   ____   ____   _____
35. Reported and recorded your observations.   ____   ____   _____

Date of Satisfactory Completion _____   Instructor's Initials _____

Collecting a Sputum Specimen

Name: _____   Date: _____

	S	U	Comments

Quality of Life

Remembered to:
- Knock before entering the person's room
- Address the person by name
- Introduce yourself by name and title
- Explain the procedure to the person before beginning and during the procedure
- Protect the person's rights during the procedure
- Handle the person gently during the procedure

Pre-Procedure

1. Followed *Delegation Guidelines: Sputum Specimens*. Reviewed *Promoting Safety and Comfort: Sputum Specimens*.
2. Practiced hand hygiene.
3. Collected the following before going to the person's room:
   - Laboratory requisition slip
   - Sputum specimen container and lid
   - Specimen label
   - Plastic bag
   - *BIOHAZARD* label (if needed)
4. Arranged collected items in the person's bathroom.
5. Practiced hand hygiene.
6. Identified the person. Checked the ID bracelet against the assignment sheet. Called the person by name.
7. Labeled the specimen container in the person's presence.
8. Collected gloves and tissues.
9. Provided for privacy. If able, the person used the bathroom for this procedure.

Procedure

10. Put on gloves.
11. Asked the person to rinse the mouth out with clear water.
12. Had the person hold the container. Touched only the outside.
13. Asked the person to cover the mouth and nose with tissues when coughing. Followed agency policy for used tissues.
14. Asked the person to take 2 or 3 deep breaths and cough up sputum.
15. Had the person expectorate directly into the container. Sputum did not touch the outside of the container.
16. Collected 1 to 2 tablespoons of sputum unless told to collect more.
17. Put the lid on the container.
18. Placed the container in the plastic bag. Did not let the container touch the outside of the bag. Applied a *BIOHAZARD* label according to agency policy.
19. Removed and discarded gloves. Practiced hand hygiene. Put on clean gloves.
20. Assisted with hand washing.
21. Removed and discarded the gloves. Practiced hand hygiene.

Date of Satisfactory Completion _____   Instructor's Initials _____

Post-Procedure

22. Provided for comfort.
23. Placed the signal light within reach.
24. Raised or lowered bed rails. Followed the care plan.
25. Unscreened the person.
26. Completed a safety check of the room.
27. Decontaminated you hands.
28. Delivered the specimen and requisition slip to the storage area. Followed agency policy. Wore gloves.
29. Removed and discarded gloves. Practiced hand hygiene.
30. Reported and recorded your observations.

Date of Satisfactory Completion _____   Instructor's Initials _____

Measuring Blood Glucose

Name: _____   Date: _____

Quality of Life	S	U	Comments

Remembered to:
- Knock before entering the person's room
- Address the person by name
- Introduce yourself by name and title
- Explain the procedure to the person before beginning and during the procedure
- Protect the person's rights during the procedure
- Handle the person gently during the procedure

Pre-Procedure

1. Followed *Delegation Guidelines: Blood Glucose Testing.* Reviewed *Promoting Safety and Comfort: Blood Glucose Testing.*
2. Practiced hand hygiene.
3. Collected the following:
    - Sterile lancet
    - Antiseptic wipes
    - Gloves
    - 2 × 2 cotton squares
    - Glucometer
    - Reagent strips (Used correct ones for the meter. Checked expiration date.)
    - Disinfectant
    - Paper towels
    - Warm washcloth
4. Read the manufacturer's instructions for the lancet and glucometer.
5. Disinfected the glucometer. Followed manufacturer's instructions for the disinfectant.
6. Arranged your work area.
7. Identified the person. Checked the ID bracelet against the assignment sheet. Called the person by name.
8. Provided for privacy.
9. Raised the bed for good body mechanics. The far bed rail was up if used.

Procedure

10. Helped the person to a comfortable position.
11. Put on gloves.
12. Prepared the supplies:
    a. Opened the antiseptic wipes.
    b. Removed a reagent strip from the bottle. Placed it on the paper towel. Placed the cap securely on the bottle.
    c. Prepared the lancet.
    d. Turned on the glucometer.
    e. Followed the prompts. You entered a user ID and the person's ID number, if needed. Scanned the bar code on the bottle of reagents strips, if needed.
    f. Inserted reagent strip into the glucose meter.
13. Performed a skin puncture to obtain a drop of blood:
    a. Inspected the person's fingers. Selected a puncture site.
    b. Warmed the finger. Rubbed it gently or applied a warm washcloth.
    c. Massaged the hand and finger toward the puncture site. Lowered the finger below the person's waist. These actions increased blood flow to the site.

Date of Satisfactory Completion _____   Instructor's Initials _____

Procedure—cont'd   S   U   **Comments**

    d. Held the finger with your thumb and forefinger. Used your
       non-dominant hand. Held the finger until first blood drop.   _____ _____ _____

    e. Cleaned the site with an antiseptic wipe. *Did not touch the site*
       after cleaning.   _____ _____ _____

    f. Let the site dry.   _____ _____ _____

    g. Picked up the sterile lancet.   _____ _____ _____

    h. Placed the lancet against the puncture site.   _____ _____ _____

    i. Pushed the button on the lancet to puncture the skin.
       (Followed manufacturer's instructions.)   _____ _____ _____

    j. Wiped away the first blood drop. Used a gauze square.   _____ _____ _____

    k. Applied gentle pressure below the puncture site.   _____ _____ _____

    l. Allowed a large drop of blood to form.   _____ _____ _____

14. Collected and tested the specimen. Followed the manufacturer's
    instructions and agency procedures for the glucometer used:

    a. Held the test area of the reagent strip close to the
       drop of blood.   _____ _____ _____

    b. Lightly touched the reagent strip to the blood drop.
       Did not smear the blood. The glucometer tested the sample
       when enough blood was applied.   _____ _____ _____

    c. Applied pressure to the puncture site until bleeding stopped.
       Used a gauze square. Allowed the person to apply pressure to
       the site, if able.   _____ _____ _____

    d. Read the result on the display. Noted the result on your
       notepad or assignment sheet. Told the person the result.   _____ _____ _____

    e. Turned off the glucometer.   _____ _____ _____

15. Discarded the lancet into the sharps container.   _____ _____ _____

16. Discarded the gauze squares and reagent strip. Followed
    agency policy.   _____ _____ _____

17. Removed and discarded the gloves. Practiced
    hand hygiene.   _____ _____ _____

Post-Procedure

18. Provided for comfort.   _____ _____ _____

19. Placed the signal light within reach.   _____ _____ _____

20. Lowered the bed to its lowest position.   _____ _____ _____

21. Raised or lowered bed rails. Followed the care plan.   _____ _____ _____

22. Unscreened the person.   _____ _____ _____

23. Discarded used supplies.   _____ _____ _____

24. Completed a safety check of the room.   _____ _____ _____

25. Followed agency policy for soiled linen.   _____ _____ _____

26. Disinfected the glucometer (wore gloves). Followed the
    manufacturer's instructions. Returned the device to its proper
    place.   _____ _____ _____

27. Removed and discarded gloves. Practiced hand hygiene.   _____ _____ _____

28. Reported and recorded the test result and your observations.   _____ _____ _____

Date of Satisfactory Completion _____   Instructor's Initials _____

The Surgical Skin Prep—Shaving the Skin

Name: _____   Date: _____

Quality of Life	S	U	Comments
Remembered to:			
• Knock before entering the person's room	___	___	_____
• Address the person by name	___	___	_____
• Introduce yourself by name and title	___	___	_____
• Explain the procedure to the person before beginning and during the procedure	___	___	_____
• Protect the person's rights during the procedure	___	___	_____
• Handle the person gently during the procedure	___	___	_____

Pre-Procedure

1. Followed *Delegation Guidelines: Skin Preparation.* Reviewed *Promoting Safety and Comfort: Skin Preparation.*
2. Practiced hand hygiene.
3. Collected the following:
   - Skin prep kit
   - Bath blanket
   - Warm water
   - Gloves
   - Waterproof pad
   - Bath towel
4. Identified the person. Checked the ID bracelet against the assignment sheet. Called the person by name.
5. Provided for privacy.

Procedure

6. Made sure you had good lighting.
7. Raised the bed for body mechanics. Lowered bed rail near you (if up).
8. Covered the person with a bath blanket. Fan-folded top linens to the foot of the bed.
9. Placed the waterproof pad under the area you will shave.
10. Opened the skin prep kit.
11. Positioned the person for the skin prep.
12. Draped the person with the drape.
13. Added warm water to the basin. Bed rails (if used) were up before you left the bedside.
14. Put on gloves.
15. Lathered the skin with the sponge.
16. Held the skin taut. Shaved in the direction of hair growth.
17. Shaved outward from the center; used short strokes.
18. Rinsed the razor often.
19. Made sure the entire area was free of hair. Checked for cuts, scratches, or nicks.
20. Rinsed the skin thoroughly. Patted dry.
21. Removed the drape and waterproof pad.
22. Removed and discarded the gloves. Practiced hand hygiene.
23. Returned top linens. Removed the bath blanket.

Post-Procedure

24. Provided for comfort.
25. Placed the signal light within reach.
26. Lowered the bed to its lowest position. Locked the bed wheels.
27. Raised or lowered bed rails. Followed the care plan.
28. Unscreened the person.

Date of Satisfactory Completion _____   Instructor's Initials _____

	S	U	Comments

Post-Procedure—cont'd
29. Returned equipment to its proper place.
30. Discarded supplies.
31. Completed a safety check of the room.
32. Followed agency policy for dirty linen.
33. Practiced hand hygiene.

Date of Satisfactory Completion _____   Instructor's Initials _____

Applying Elastic Stockings (NNAAP®)

Name: _____   Date: _____

Quality of Life	S	U	Comments

Remembered to:

- Knock before entering the person's room   _____ _____ _____
- Address the person by name   _____ _____ _____
- Introduce yourself by name and title   _____ _____ _____
- Explain the procedure to the person before beginning and
  during the procedure   _____ _____ _____
- Protect the person's rights during the procedure   _____ _____ _____
- Handle the person gently during the procedure _____ _____ _____

Pre-Procedure

1. Followed *Delegation Guidelines: Elastic Stockings.*
   Reviewed *Promoting Safety and Comfort: Elastic Stockings.*   _____ _____ _____
2. Practiced hand hygiene.   _____ _____ _____
3. Obtained elastic stockings in the correct size and length.
   Noted the location of the toe opening.   _____ _____ _____
4. Identified the person. Checked the ID bracelet against the
   assignment sheet. Called the person by name.   _____ _____ _____
5. Provided for privacy.   _____ _____ _____
6. Raised the bed for body mechanics. Bed rails were up if used.   _____ _____ _____

Procedure

7. Lowered the bed rail near you if up.   _____ _____ _____
8. Positioned the person supine.   _____ _____ _____
9. Exposed the legs. Fan-folded top linens toward the thighs.   _____ _____ _____
10. Turned the stocking inside out down to the heel.   _____ _____ _____
11. Slipped the foot of the stocking over the toes, foot, and heel.
    Made sure the heel pocket was properly positioned on the
    person's heel. The toe opening was over or under the toes.   _____ _____ _____
12. Grasped the stocking top. Pulled the stocking up the leg.
    It turned right side out as it was pulled up. The stocking was
    even and snug.   _____ _____ _____
13. Removed twists, creases, or wrinkles.   _____ _____ _____
14. Repeated for the other leg:
    a. Turned the stocking inside out down to the heel.   _____ _____ _____
    b. Slipped the foot of the stocking over the toes, foot, and heel.
       Made sure the stocking heel was properly positioned on the
       person's heel.   _____ _____ _____
    c. Grasped the stocking top. Pulled the stocking up the leg.
       It turned right side out as it was pulled up. The stocking was
       even and snug.   _____ _____ _____
    d. Removed twists, creases, or wrinkles.   _____ _____ _____

Post-Procedure

15. Covered the person.   _____ _____ _____
16. Provided for comfort.   _____ _____ _____
17. Placed the signal light within reach.   _____ _____ _____
18. Lowered the bed to its lowest position.   _____ _____ _____
19. Raised or lowered bed rails. Followed the care plan.   _____ _____ _____
20. Unscreened the person.   _____ _____ _____
21. Completed a safety check of the room.   _____ _____ _____
22. Practiced hand hygiene.   _____ _____ _____
23. Reported and recorded your observations.   _____ _____ _____

Date of Satisfactory Completion _____   Instructor's Initials _____

Applying Elastic Bandages

Name: _____   Date: _____

Quality of Life	S	U	Comments

Remembered to:
- Knock before entering the person's room   _____ _____ _____
- Address the person by name   _____ _____ _____
- Introduce yourself by name and title   _____ _____ _____
- Explain the procedure to the person before beginning and during the procedure   _____ _____ _____
- Protect the person's rights during the procedure   _____ _____ _____
- Handle the person gently during the procedure   _____ _____ _____

Pre-Procedure
1. Followed *Delegation Guidelines: Elastic Bandages.* Reviewed *Promoting Safety and Comfort: Elastic Bandages.*   _____ _____ _____
2. Practiced hand hygiene.   _____ _____ _____
3. Collected the following:
   - Elastic bandage as directed by the nurse   _____ _____ _____
   - Tape or clips (unless the bandage was Velcro)   _____ _____ _____
4. Identified the person. Checked the ID bracelet against the assignment sheet. Called the person by name.   _____ _____ _____
5. Provided for privacy.   _____ _____ _____
6. Raised the bed for body mechanics. Bed rails were up if used.   _____ _____ _____

Procedure
7. Lowered the bed rail near you if up.   _____ _____ _____
8. Helped the person to a comfortable position. Exposed the part you bandaged.   _____ _____ _____
9. Made sure the area was clean and dry.   _____ _____ _____
10. Held the bandage so the roll was up. The loose end was on the bottom.   _____ _____ _____
11. Applied the bandage to the smallest part of the wrist, foot, ankle, or knee.   _____ _____ _____
12. Made two circular turns around the part.   _____ _____ _____
13. Made overlapping spiral turns in an upward direction. Each turn overlapped about ½ to ⅔ of the previous turn. Made sure the overlap was equal.   _____ _____ _____
14. Applied the bandage smoothly with firm, even pressure. It was not tight.   _____ _____ _____
15. Ended the bandage with two circular turns.   _____ _____ _____
16. Secured the bandage in place with Velcro, tape, or clips. The clips were not under the body part.   _____ _____ _____
17. Checked the fingers or toes for coldness or cyanosis (bluish color). Asked about pain, itching, numbness, or tingling. Removed the bandage if any were noted. Reported your observations to the nurse.   _____ _____ _____

Post-Procedure
18. Provided for comfort.   _____ _____ _____
19. Placed the signal light within reach.   _____ _____ _____
20. Lowered the bed to its lowest position.   _____ _____ _____
21. Raised or lowered bed rails. Followed the care plan.   _____ _____ _____
22. Unscreened the person.   _____ _____ _____
23. Completed a safety check of the room.   _____ _____ _____
24. Practiced hand hygiene.   _____ _____ _____
25. Reported and recorded your observations.   _____ _____ _____

Date of Satisfactory Completion _____   Instructor's Initials _____

[VIDEO] Applying a Dry, Non-Sterile Dressing

Name: _____   Date: _____

	S	U	Comments

Quality of Life
Remembered to:
- Knock before entering the person's room
- Address the person by name
- Introduce yourself by name and title
- Explain the procedure to the person before beginning and during the procedure
- Protect the person's rights during the procedure
- Handle the person gently during the procedure

Pre-Procedure
1. Followed *Delegation Guidelines: Applying Dressings.* Reviewed *Promoting Safety and Comfort: Applying Dressings.*
2. Practiced hand hygiene.
3. Collected the following:
   - Gloves
   - Personal protective equipment (PPE) as needed
   - Tape or Montgomery ties
   - Dressings as directed by the nurse
   - Saline solution as directed by the nurse
   - Cleansing solution as directed by the nurse
   - Adhesive remover
   - Dressing set with scissors and forceps
   - Plastic bag
   - Bath blanket
4. Practiced hand hygiene.
5. Identified the person. Checked the ID bracelet against the assignment sheet. Called the person by name.
6. Provided for privacy.
7. Arranged your work area. You did not have to reach over or turn your back on your work area.
8. Raised the bed for body mechanics. Bed rails were up if used.

Procedure
9. Lowered the bed rail near you if up.
10. Helped the person to a comfortable position.
11. Covered the person with a bath blanket. Fan-folded top linens to the foot of the bed.
12. Exposed the affected body part.
13. Made a cuff on the plastic bag. Placed it within reach.
14. Practiced hand hygiene.
15. Put on needed personal protection equipment (PPE). Put on gloves.
16. Removed tape or undid Montgomery ties:
    a. Tape: held the skin down. Gently pulled the tape toward the wound.
    b. Montgomery ties: folded ties away from the wound.
17. Removed any adhesive from the skin. Wet a 4 × 4 gauze dressing with adhesive remover. Cleaned away from the wound.
18. Removed gauze dressings. Started with the top dressing, and removed each layer. Kept the soiled side of each dressing away from the person's sight. Put dressings in the plastic bag. They did not touch the outside of the bag.
19. Removed the dressing over the wound very gently. If it stuck to the wound or drain site, moistened the dressing with saline.

Date of Satisfactory Completion _____   Instructor's Initials _____

Procedure—cont'd   S   U   Comments

20. Observed the wound, drain site, and wound drainage. _____ _____ _____
21. Removed the gloves, and put them in a plastic bag.
    Practiced hand hygiene.   _____ _____ _____
22. Opened the new dressings.   _____ _____ _____
23. Cut the length of tape needed.   _____ _____ _____
24. Put on clean gloves.   _____ _____ _____
25. Cleaned the wound with saline as directed by the nurse. _____ _____ _____
26. Applied dressings as directed by the nurse.   _____ _____ _____
27. Secured the dressings in place. Used tape or Montgomery ties. _____ _____ _____
28. Removed the gloves. Put them in the bag.   _____ _____ _____
29. Removed and discarded personal protective equipment (PPE). _____ _____ _____
30. Practiced hand hygiene.   _____ _____ _____
31. Covered the person. Removed the bath blanket.   _____ _____ _____

Post-Procedure

32. Provided for comfort.   _____ _____ _____
33. Placed the signal light within reach.   _____ _____ _____
34. Lowered the bed to its lowest position.   _____ _____ _____
35. Raised or lowered bed rails. Followed the care plan. _____ _____ _____
36. Returned equipment and supplies to the proper place.
    Left extra dressings and tape in the room.   _____ _____ _____
37. Discarded used supplies into the bag. Tied the bag closed.
    Discarded the bag following agency policy. (Wore gloves
    for this step.)   _____ _____ _____
38. Cleaned your work area. Followed the Bloodborne
    Pathogen Standard.   _____ _____ _____
39. Unscreened the person.   _____ _____ _____
40. Completed a safety check of the room.   _____ _____ _____
41. Removed and discarded the gloves. Practiced hand hygiene. _____ _____ _____
42. Reported and recorded your observations.   _____ _____ _____

Date of Satisfactory Completion _____   Instructor's Initials _____

▣ **Applying Heat and Cold Applications**

Name: _____   Date: _____

Quality of Life	S	U	Comments

Remembered to:
- Knock before entering the person's room
- Address the person by name
- Introduce yourself by name and title
- Explain the procedure to the person before beginning and during the procedure
- Protect the person's rights during the procedure
- Handle the person gently during the procedure

Pre-Procedure
1. Followed *Delegation Guidelines: Heat and Cold Applications.* Reviewed *Promoting Safety and Comfort: Heat and Cold Applications.*
2. Practiced hand hygiene.
3. Collected the following:
   a. For a *hot compress:*
      - Basin
      - Bath thermometer
      - Small towel, washcloth, or gauze squares
      - Plastic wrap or aquathermia pad
      - Ties, tape, or rolled gauze
      - Bath towel
      - Waterproof pad
   b. For a *hot soak:*
      - Water basin or arm or foot bath
      - Bath thermometer
      - Waterproof pad
      - Bath blanket
      - Towel
   c. For a *sitz bath:*
      - Disposable sitz bath
      - Bath thermometer
      - Two bath blankets, bath towels, and a clean gown
   d. For a *hot or cold pack:*
      - Commercial pack
      - Pack cover
      - Ties, tape, or rolled gauze (if needed)
      - Waterproof pad
   e. For an *aquathermia pad:*
      - Aquathermia pad and heating unit
      - Distilled water
      - Flannel cover or other cover as directed by the nurse
      - Ties, tape, or rolled gauze
   f. For an *ice bag, ice collar, ice glove, or dry cold pack:*
      - Ice bag, collar, glove, or cold pack
      - Crushed ice (except for a cold pack)
      - Flannel cover or other cover as directed by the nurse
      - Paper towels
   g. For a *cold compress:*
      - Large basin with ice
      - Small basin with cold water
      - Gauze squares, washcloths, or small towels
      - Waterproof pad
4. Identified the person. Checked the ID bracelet against the assignment sheet. Called the person by name.
5. Provided for privacy.

Date of Satisfactory Completion _____   Instructor's Initials _____

Procedure

6. Positioned the person for the procedure.
7. Placed the waterproof pad (if needed) under the body part.
8. For a *hot compress*:
   a. Filled the basin ½ to ⅔ full with hot water as directed by the nurse. Measured water temperature.
   b. Placed the compress in the water.
   c. Wrung out the compress.
   d. Applied the compress over the area. Noted the time.
   e. Covered the compress quickly. Used one of the following as directed by the nurse:
      (1) Applied plastic wrap and then a bath towel. Secured the towel in place with ties, tape, or rolled gauze.
      (2) Applied an aquathermia pad.
9. For a *hot soak*:
   a. Filled a container ½ full with hot water. Measured water temperature.
   b. Placed the part into the water. Padded the edge of the container with a towel. Noted the time.
   c. Covered the person with a bath blanket for warmth.
10. For a *sitz bath*:
    a. Placed the disposable sitz bath on the toilet seat.
    b. Filled the sitz bath ⅔ full with water. Measured water temperature.
    c. Secured the gown above the waist.
    d. Helped the person sit on the sitz bath. Noted the time.
    e. Provided for warmth. Placed a bath blanket around the shoulders. Placed another over the legs.
    f. Stayed with the person if he or she was weak or unsteady.
11. For a *hot or cold pack*:
    a. Squeezed, kneaded, or struck the pack as directed by the manufacturer's instructions.
    b. Placed the pack in the cover.
    c. Applied the pack. Noted the time.
    d. Secured the pack in place with ties, tape, or rolled gauze. Some packs are secured with Velcro straps.
12. For an *aquathermia pad*:
    a. Filled the heating unit to the fill line with distilled water.
    b. Removed the bubbles. Placed the pad and tubing below the heating unit. Tilted the heating unit from side to side.
    c. Set the temperature as the nurse directed (usually 105° F [40.5° C]). Removed the key.
    d. Placed the pad in the cover.
    e. Plugged in the unit. Allowed water to warm to the desired temperature.
    f. Set the heating unit on the bedside stand. Kept the pad and connecting hoses level with the unit. Hoses did not have kinks.
    g. Applied the pad to the part. Noted the time.
    h. Secured the pad in place with ties, tape, or rolled gauze. Did not use pins.
13. For an *ice bag, collar, or glove*:
    a. Filled the device with water. Put in the stopper. Turned the device upside down; checked for leaks.
    b. Emptied the device.
    c. Filled the device ½ to ⅔ full with crushed ice or ice chips.
    d. Removed excess air. Bent, twisted, or squeezed the device. Or pressed it against a firm surface.
    e. Placed the cap or stopper on securely.
    f. Dried the device with paper towels.

Date of Satisfactory Completion _____   Instructor's Initials _____

Procedure—cont'd	**S**	**U**	**Comments**
g. Placed the device in the cover.	___	___	_____
h. Applied the device. Noted the time.	___	___	_____
i. Secured the device in place with ties, tape, or rolled gauze.	___	___	_____
14. For a *cold compress:*			
a. Placed the small basin with cold water into the large basin with ice.	___	___	_____
b. Placed the compress into the cold water.	___	___	_____
c. Wrung out the compress.	___	___	_____
d. Applied the compress to the part. Noted the time.	___	___	_____
15. Placed the signal light within reach. Unscreened the person.	___	___	_____
16. Raised or lowered bed rails. Followed the care plan.	___	___	_____
17. Checked the person every 5 minutes. Checked for signs and symptoms of complications. Removed the application if complications occurred. Told the nurse at once.	___	___	_____
18. Checked the application every 5 minutes. Changed the application if cooling (hot applications) or warming (cold applications) occurred.	___	___	_____
19. Removed the application at the specified time. Heat and cold applications usually left on for 15 to 20 minutes.	___	___	_____

Post-Procedure

	S	**U**	**Comments**
20. Provided for comfort.	___	___	_____
21. Placed the signal light within reach.	___	___	_____
22. Raised or lowered bed rails. Followed the care plan.	___	___	_____
23. Unscreened the person.	___	___	_____
24. Cleaned, rinsed, dried, and returned re-usable items to the proper place. Followed agency policy for soiled linen. Wore gloves for this step.	___	___	_____
25. Completed a safety check of the room.	___	___	_____
26. Removed and discarded the gloves. Practiced hand hygiene.	___	___	_____
27. Reported and recorded your observations.	___	___	_____

Date of Satisfactory Completion _____   Instructor's Initials _____

Using a Pulse Oximeter

Name: _____   Date: _____

Quality of Life	S	U	Comments

Remembered to:
- Knock before entering the person's room
- Address the person by name
- Introduce yourself by name and title
- Explain the procedure to the person before beginning and during the procedure
- Protect the person's rights during the procedure
- Handle the person gently during the procedure

Pre-Procedure

1. Followed *Delegation Guidelines: Pulse Oximetry*. Reviewed *Promoting Safety and Comfort: Pulse Oximetry*.
2. Practiced hand hygiene.
3. Collected the following:
   - Oximeter and sensor
   - Tape
   - Towel
4. Arranged your work area.
5. Practiced hand hygiene.
6. Identified the person. Checked the ID bracelet against the assignment sheet. Called the person by name.
7. Provided for privacy.

Procedure

8. Provided for comfort.
9. Dried the site with a towel.
10. Clipped or taped the sensor to the site.
11. Turned on the oximeter.
12. Set the high and low alarm limits for SpO_2 and pulse rate. Turned on audio and visual alarms. (This step is for continuous monitoring.)
13. Checked the person's pulse (apical or radial) with the pulse on the display. The pulse rates should have been about the same. Noted both pulses on your assignment sheet.
14. Read the SpO_2 on the display. Noted the value on the flow sheet and your assignment sheet.
15. Left the sensor in place for continuous monitoring. Otherwise, turned off the device and removed the sensor.

Post-Procedure

16. Provided for comfort.
17. Placed the signal light within reach.
18. Unscreened the person.
19. Completed a safety check of the room.
20. Returned the device to its proper place (unless monitoring was continuous).
21. Practiced hand hygiene.
23. Reported and recorded the SpO_2, the pulse rate, and your other observations.

Date of Satisfactory Completion _____   Instructor's Initials _____

Assisting With Deep-Breathing and Coughing Exercises

Name: _____   Date: _____

Quality of Life	S	U	Comments

Remembered to:
- Knock before entering the person's room   _____ _____ _____
- Address the person by name   _____ _____ _____
- Introduce yourself by name and title   _____ _____ _____
- Explain the procedure to the person before beginning and during
  the procedure   _____ _____ _____
- Protect the person's rights during the procedure _____ _____ _____
- Handle the person gently during the procedure   _____ _____ _____

Pre-Procedure
1. Followed *Delegation Guidelines: Deep Breathing and Coughing.*
   Reviewed *Promoting Safety and Comfort: Deep Breathing and Coughing.* _____ _____ _____
2. Practiced hand hygiene.   _____ _____ _____
3. Identified the person. Checked the ID bracelet against the
   assignment sheet. Called the person by name.   _____ _____ _____
4. Provided for privacy.   _____ _____ _____

Procedure
5. Lowered the bed rail if up.   _____ _____ _____
6. Helped the person to a comfortable sitting position: sitting on the
   side of the bed, semi-Fowler, or Fowler.   _____ _____ _____
7. Had the person deep breathe:
   a. Had the person place the hands over the rib cage.
   b. Had the person take a deep breath. It should have been as deep
      as possible. Reminded the person to inhale through the nose. _____ _____ _____
   c. Asked the person to hold the breath for 2 to 3 seconds.   _____ _____ _____
   d. Asked the person to exhale slowly through pursed lips. Asked
      the person to exhale until the ribs moved as far down as possible. _____ _____ _____
   e. Repeated 4 more times:
      (1) Deep breath in through the nose.   _____ _____ _____
      (2) Held 2 to 3 seconds.   _____ _____ _____
      (3) Exhaled slowly with pursed lips until the ribs moved as far
          down as possible.   _____ _____ _____
8. Asked the person to cough:
   a. Had the person place both hands over the incision. One hand
      on top of the other. The person could have held a pillow or
      folded towel over the incision.   _____ _____ _____
   b. Had the person take a deep breath through the nose.   _____ _____ _____
   c. Asked the person to cough strongly twice with the mouth open. _____ _____ _____

Post-Procedure
9. Provided for comfort.   _____ _____ _____
10. Placed the signal light within reach.   _____ _____ _____
11. Raised or lowered bed rails. Followed care plan. _____ _____ _____
12. Unscreened the person.   _____ _____ _____
13. Completed a safety check of the room.   _____ _____ _____
14. Practiced hand hygiene.   _____ _____ _____
15. Reported and recorded your observations.   _____ _____ _____

Date of Satisfactory Completion _____   Instructor's Initials _____

Setting Up for Oxygen Administration

Name: _____   Date: _____

	S	U	Comments
Quality of Life			

Remembered to:
- Knock before entering the person's room
- Address the person by name
- Introduce yourself by name and title
- Explain the procedure to the person before beginning and during the procedure
- Protect the person's rights during the procedure
- Handle the person gently during the procedure

Pre-Procedure

1. Followed *Delegation Guidelines: Oxygen Administration Set-Up*. Reviewed *Promoting Safety and Comfort: Oxygen Administration Set-Up*.
2. Practiced hand hygiene.
3. Collected the following before going to the person's room:
   - Oxygen device with connection tubing
   - Flowmeter
   - Humidifier (if ordered)
   - Distilled water (if used humidifier)
4. Arranged your work area.
5. Practiced hand hygiene.
6. Identified the person. Checked the ID bracelet against the assignment sheet. Called the person by name.

Procedure

7. Made sure the flowmeter was in the *OFF* position.
8. Attached the flowmeter to the wall outlet or to the tank.
9. Filled the humidifier with distilled water.
10. Attached the humidifier to the bottom of the flowmeter.
11. Attached the oxygen device and connecting tubing to the humidifier. *Did not set the flowmeter. Did not apply the oxygen device on the person.*
12. Placed the cap securely on the distilled water. Stored the water according to agency policy.
13. Discarded the packaging from the oxygen device and connecting tubing.

Post-Procedure

14. Provided for comfort.
15. Placed the signal light within reach.
16. Completed a safety check of the room.
17. Practiced hand hygiene.
18. Told the nurse when you were done.
    The nurse:
    a. Turned on the oxygen and set the flow rate.
    b. Applied the oxygen device on the person.

Date of Satisfactory Completion _____   Instructor's Initials _____

Caring for Eyeglasses

Name: _____   Date: _____

Quality of Life	S	U	Comments

Remembered to:
- Knock before entering the person's room
- Address the person by name
- Introduce yourself by name and title
- Explain the procedure to the person before beginning and during the procedure
- Protect the person's rights during the procedure
- Handle the person gently during the procedure

Pre-Procedure
1. Followed *Delegation Guidelines: Eyeglasses.*
   Reviewed *Promoting Safety and Comfort: Eyeglasses.*
2. Practiced hand hygiene.
3. Collected the following:
   - Eyeglass case
   - Cleaning solution or warm water
   - Disposable lens cloth or cotton cloth

Procedure
4. Removed the eyeglasses:
   a. Held the frames in front of the ear on both sides.
   b. Lifted the frames from the ears. Brought the eyeglasses down away from the face.
5. Cleaned the lenses with cleaning solution or warm water. Cleaned in a circular motion. Dried the lenses with the cloth.
6. If the person did not wear the glasses:
   a. Opened the eyeglass case.
   b. Folded the eyeglasses. Put them in the case. Did not touch the clean lenses.
   c. Placed the eyeglass case in the top drawer of the bedside stand.
7. If the person wore the eyeglasses:
   a. Unfolded the eyeglasses.
   b. Held the frames at each side. Placed them over the ears.
   c. Adjusted the eyeglasses so the nosepiece rested on the nose.
   d. Returned the eyeglass case to the top drawer in the bedside stand.

Post-Procedure
8. Provided for comfort.
9. Placed the signal light within reach.
10. Returned the cleaning solution to its proper place.
11. Discarded the disposable cloth.
12. Completed a safety check of the room.
13. Practiced hand hygiene.
14. Reported and recorded your observations.

Date of Satisfactory Completion _____   Instructor's Initials _____

Cleaning Baby Bottles

Name: _____   Date: _____

	S	U	Comments
Pre-Procedure			
1. Reviewed *Promoting Safety and Comfort: Cleaning Baby Bottles*.	___	___	_____
2. Practiced hand hygiene.	___	___	_____
3. Collected the following:			
a. Bottles, nipples, and caps	___	___	_____
b. Funnel	___	___	_____
c. Can opener	___	___	_____
d. Bottle brush	___	___	_____
e. Dishwashing soap	___	___	_____
f. Other items used to prepare formula	___	___	_____
g. Towel	___	___	_____
Procedure			
4. Washed the bottles, nipples, caps, funnel, and can opener in hot, soapy water. Washed other items used to prepare formula.	___	___	_____
5. Cleaned inside baby bottles with the bottle brush.	___	___	_____
6. Squeezed hot, soapy water through the nipples. This removed formula.	___	___	_____
7. Rinsed all items thoroughly in hot water. Squeezed hot water through the nipples to remove soap.	___	___	_____
8. Placed a clean towel on the counter.	___	___	_____
9. Stood bottles upside down to drain. Placed nipples, caps, and other items on the towel. Allowed items to dry.	___	___	_____

Date of Satisfactory Completion _____   Instructor's Initials _____

Diapering a Baby

Name: _____   Date: _____

	S	U	Comments

Quality of Life

Remembered to:
- Knock before entering the baby's room
- Address the baby and the parents by name
- Introduce yourself by name and title
- Explain the procedure to the parents before beginning and during the procedure
- Protect the baby's rights during the procedure
- Handle the baby gently during the procedure

Pre-Procedure

1. Followed *Delegation Guidelines: Diapering a Baby.* Reviewed *Promoting Safety and Comfort: Diapering a Baby.*
2. Practiced hand hygiene.
3. Collected the following:
   - Gloves
   - Clean diaper
   - Waterproof changing pad
   - Washcloth
   - Disposable wipes or cotton balls
   - Basin of warm water
   - Baby soap
   - Baby lotion or cream

Procedure

4. Put on gloves.
5. Placed the changing pad under the baby.
6. Unfastened the dirty diaper. Placed diaper pins out of the baby's reach.
7. Wiped the genital area with the front of the diaper. Wiped from the front to the back.
8. Folded the diaper so urine and feces were inside. Set the diaper aside.
9. Cleaned the genital area from front to back. Used a wet washcloth, disposable wipes, or cotton balls. Washed with mild soap and water for a large amount of feces or if the baby had a rash. Rinsed thoroughly and patted the area dry.
10. Cleaned the circumcision. Gave cord care.
11. Applied cream or lotion to the genital area and the buttocks. Did not use too much. Caking did not occur.
12. Raised the baby's legs. Slid a clean diaper under the buttocks.
13. Folded a cloth diaper as follows:
    a. For a boy: the extra thickness was in the front.
    b. For a girl: the extra thickness was in the back.
    c. Brought the diaper between the baby's legs.
14. Made sure the diaper was snug around the hips and abdomen.
    a. It was loose near the penis if the circumcision had not healed.
    b. It was below the umbilicus if the cord stump had not healed.
15. Secured the diaper in place. Used the tape strips or Velcro on disposable diapers. Made sure the tabs stuck in place. Used baby pins or Velcro for cloth diapers. Pins pointed away from the abdomen.
16. Applied a diaper cover or plastic pants if cloth diaper was worn.
17. Placed the baby in the crib, infant seat, or other safe location.

Date of Satisfactory Completion _____   Instructor's Initials _____

Post-Procedure

18. Rinsed feces from the cloth diaper in the toilet.   _____ _____ _____
19. Stored used cloth diapers in a covered pail. Placed disposable
    diaper and paper tabs in the trash.   _____ _____ _____
20. Removed and discarded the gloves. Practiced hand hygiene.   _____ _____ _____
21. Put on clean gloves.   _____ _____ _____
22. Cleaned, rinsed, dried, and returned other items to their
    proper location.   _____ _____ _____
23. Removed and discarded the gloves. Practiced hand hygiene.   _____ _____ _____
24. Reported and recorded your observations.   _____ _____ _____

Giving a Baby a Sponge Bath

Name: _____   Date: _____

Quality of Life	S	U	Comments
Remembered to:			
• Knock before entering the baby's room	____	____	_____
• Address the baby and the parents by name	____	____	_____
• Introduce yourself by name and title	____	____	_____
• Explain the procedure to the parents before beginning and during the procedure	____	____	_____
• Protect the baby's rights during the procedure	____	____	_____
• Handle the baby gently during the procedure	____	____	_____

Pre-Procedure

	S	U	Comments
1. Followed *Delegation Guidelines: Bathing an Infant.* Reviewed *Promoting Safety and Comfort: Bathing an Infant.*	____	____	_____
2. Practiced hand hygiene.	____	____	_____
3. Placed the following items in your work area:			
• Bath basin	____	____	_____
• Bath thermometer	____	____	_____
• Bath towel	____	____	_____
• Two hand towels	____	____	_____
• Receiving blanket	____	____	_____
• Washcloth	____	____	_____
• Clean diaper	____	____	_____
• Clean clothing for the baby	____	____	_____
• Cotton balls	____	____	_____
• Baby soap (if needed)	____	____	_____
• Baby shampoo	____	____	_____
• Baby lotion	____	____	_____
• Gloves	____	____	_____

Procedure

	S	U	Comments
4. Filled the bath basin with warm water. Water temperature was 100° F to 105° F (37.7° C to 40.5° C). Measured water temperature with the bath thermometer or used the inside of your wrist. The water felt warm and comfortable.	____	____	_____
5. Provided for privacy.	____	____	_____
6. Identified the baby following agency policy.	____	____	_____
7. Put on gloves.	____	____	_____
8. Undressed the baby. Left the diaper on.	____	____	_____
9. Washed the baby's eyelids:			
a. Dipped a cotton ball into the water.	____	____	_____
b. Squeezed out excess water.	____	____	_____
c. Washed one eyelid from the inner part to the outer part.	____	____	_____
d. Repeated for the other eyelid:			
(1) Dipped new cotton ball into water.	____	____	_____
(2) Squeezed out excess water.	____	____	_____
(3) Washed eyelid from the inner part to the outer part.	____	____	_____
10. Moistened the washcloth and made a mitt. Cleaned the outside of the ear and then behind the ear. Repeated for the other ear. Was gentle.	____	____	_____
11. Rinsed and squeezed out the washcloth. Made a mitt with the washcloth.	____	____	_____
12. Washed the baby's face. Cleaned inside the nostrils with the washcloth. *Did not use cotton swabs to clean inside the nose.* Patted the face dry.	____	____	_____
13. Picked up the baby. Held the baby over the basin; used the football hold. Supported the baby's head and neck with your wrist and hand.	____	____	_____

Date of Satisfactory Completion _____   Instructor's Initials _____

Procedure—cont'd	S	U	Comments

14. Washed the baby's head.
   a. Squeezed a small amount of water from the washcloth onto the baby's head. Or brought water to the baby's head using a cupped hand.
   b. Applied a small amount of baby shampoo to the head.
   c. Washed the head with circular motions.
   d. Rinsed the head by squeezing water from a washcloth over the baby's head. Or brought water to the baby's head using a cupped hand. Rinsed thoroughly. Did not get soap in the baby's eyes.
   e. Used a small hand towel to dry the head.

15. Laid the baby on the table.

16. Removed the diaper.

17. Washed the front of the body. Also washed the arms, hands, fingers, legs, feet, and toes. Used a washcloth. Or washed the baby with your hands. Did not get the cord wet. Rinsed thoroughly. Patted dry. Was sure to wash and dry all creases and folds.

18. Turned the baby to the prone position. Washed the back and buttocks. Used a washcloth or your hands. Rinsed thoroughly. Patted dry.

19. Gave cord care. Cleaned the circumcision.

20. Applied baby lotion as directed by the nurse.

21. Removed and discarded the gloves. Practiced hand hygiene.

22. Put a clean diaper and clean clothes on the baby.

23. Wrapped the baby in the receiving blanket. Placed the baby in the crib or other safe area.

Post-Procedure

24. Practiced hand hygiene. Put on gloves.

25. Cleaned, rinsed, dried, and returned equipment and supplies to the proper place. Did this when the baby was settled.

26. Removed and discarded the gloves. Practiced hand hygiene.

27. Completed a safety check of the room.

28. Reported and recorded your observations.

Date of Satisfactory Completion _____   Instructor's Initials _____

Giving a Baby a Tub Bath

Name: _____   Date: _____

	S	U	Comments

Quality of Life

Remembered to:
- Knock before entering the baby's room   _____ _____ _____
- Address the baby and the parents by name   _____ _____ _____
- Introduce yourself by name and title   _____ _____ _____
- Explain the procedure to the parents before beginning and during the procedure   _____ _____ _____
- Protect the baby's rights during the procedure   _____ _____ _____
- Handle the baby gently during the procedure   _____ _____ _____

Procedure

1. Followed steps 1 through 16 in procedure: *Giving a Baby a Sponge Bath.*
   a. *Delegation Guidelines: Bathing an Infant.*
   Reviewed *Promoting Safety and Comfort: Bathing an Infant.*   _____ _____ _____
   b. Practiced hand hygiene.   _____ _____ _____
   c. Placed the following items in your work area:
   - Bath basin   _____ _____ _____
   - Bath thermometer   _____ _____ _____
   - Bath towel   _____ _____ _____
   - Two hand towels   _____ _____ _____
   - Receiving blanket   _____ _____ _____
   - Washcloth   _____ _____ _____
   - Clean diaper   _____ _____ _____
   - Clean clothing for the baby   _____ _____ _____
   - Cotton balls   _____ _____ _____
   - Baby soap (if needed)   _____ _____ _____
   - Baby shampoo   _____ _____ _____
   - Baby lotion   _____ _____ _____
   - Gloves   _____ _____ _____
   d. Filled the bath basin with warm water. Water temperature was 100° F to 105° F (37.7° C to 40.5° C). Measured water temperature with the bath thermometer or used the inside of your wrist. The water felt warm and comfortable.   _____ _____ _____
   e. Provided for privacy.   _____ _____ _____
   f. Identified the baby following agency policy.   _____ _____ _____
   g. Put on gloves.   _____ _____ _____
   h. Undressed the baby. Left the diaper on.   _____ _____ _____
   i. Washed the baby's eyelids:
      (1) Dipped a cotton ball into the water.   _____ _____ _____
      (2) Squeezed out excess water.   _____ _____ _____
      (3) Washed one eyelid from the inner part to the outer part.   _____ _____ _____
      (4) Repeated for the other eyelid:
         i. Dipped new cotton ball into water.   _____ _____ _____
         ii. Squeezed out excess water.   _____ _____ _____
         iii. Washed eyelid from the inner part to the outer part.   _____ _____ _____
   j. Moistened the washcloth and made a mitt. Cleaned the outside of the ear and then behind the ear. Repeated for the other ear. Was gentle.   _____ _____ _____
   k. Rinsed and squeezed out the washcloth. Made a mitt with the washcloth.   _____ _____ _____
   l. Washed the baby's face. Cleaned inside the nostrils with the washcloth. *Did not use cotton swabs to clean inside the nose.* Patted the face dry.   _____ _____ _____
   m. Picked up the baby. Held the baby over the basin; used the football hold. Supported the baby's head and neck with your wrist and hand.   _____ _____ _____

Date of Satisfactory Completion _____   Instructor's Initials _____

Procedure—cont'd   **S**   **U**   **Comments**

    n. Washed the baby's head:
      (1) Squeezed a small amount of water from the washcloth
         onto the baby's head.   _____ _____ _____
      (2) Applied a small amount of baby shampoo to the head. _____ _____ _____
      (3) Washed the head with circular motions. _____ _____ _____
      (4) Rinsed the head by squeezing water from a washcloth
         over the baby's head. Rinsed thoroughly. Did not get soap
         in the baby's eyes. _____ _____ _____
      (5) Used a small hand towel to dry the head. _____ _____ _____
    o. Laid the baby on the table. _____ _____ _____
    p. Removed the diaper. _____ _____ _____
 2. Held the baby as follows:
    a. Placed one hand under the baby's shoulders. Your thumb was
      over the baby's shoulder. Your fingers were under the arm. _____ _____ _____
    b. Supported the buttocks with your other hand. Slid your hand
      under the thighs. Held the far thigh with your other hand. _____ _____ _____
 3. Lowered the baby into the water feet first. _____ _____ _____
 4. Washed the front of the baby's body. Also washed the arms, hands,
    fingers, legs, feet, and toes. Washed all folds and creases. _____ _____ _____
 5. Washed the genital area. Rinsed thoroughly. _____ _____ _____
 6. Reversed your hold. Used your other hand to hold the baby. _____ _____ _____
 7. Washed the baby's back and buttocks. Rinsed thoroughly. _____ _____ _____
 8. Reversed your hold again. Held the baby with your other hand. _____ _____ _____
 9. Lifted the baby out of the water and onto a towel. _____ _____ _____
10. Wrapped the baby in the towel. Also covered the baby's head. _____ _____ _____
11. Patted the baby dry. Dried all folds and creases. _____ _____ _____
12. Followed steps 20–23 in procedure: *Giving a Baby a Sponge Bath.*
    a. Applied baby lotion as directed by the nurse. _____ _____ _____
    b. Removed and discarded the gloves. Practiced hand hygiene. _____ _____ _____
    c. Put a clean diaper and clean clothes on the baby. _____ _____ _____
    d. Wrapped the baby in the receiving blanket. Placed the baby in
      the crib or other safe area. _____ _____ _____

Post-Procedure

13. Practiced hand hygiene. _____ _____ _____
14. Cleaned, rinsed, dried, and returned equipment and supplies
    to the proper place. Did this when the baby was settled. _____ _____ _____
15. Removed and discarded the gloves. Practiced hand hygiene. _____ _____ _____
16. Completed a safety check of the room. _____ _____ _____
17. Reported and recorded your observations. _____ _____ _____

Date of Satisfactory Completion _____   Instructor's Initials _____

Weighing an Infant

Name: _____   Date: _____

Quality of Life	S	U	Comments

Remembered to:
- Knock before entering the baby's room
- Address the baby and the parents by name
- Introduce yourself by name and title
- Explain the procedure to the parents before beginning and during the procedure
- Protect the baby's rights during the procedure
- Handle the baby gently during the procedure

Pre-Procedure

1. Followed *Delegation Guidelines: Weighing Infants.* Reviewed *Promoting Safety and Comfort: Weighing Infants.*
2. Practiced hand hygiene.
3. Collected the following:
   - Baby scale
   - Paper for scale
   - Items for diaper change
   - Gloves

Procedure

4. Identified the baby followed agency policy.
5. Placed the paper on the scale. Adjusted the scale to zero (0).
6. Put on gloves.
7. Undressed the baby and removed the diaper. Cleaned the genital area.
8. Removed and discarded gloves. Practiced hand hygiene. Put on clean gloves.
9. Laid the baby on the scale. Kept one hand over the baby. Prevented falling.
10. Read the digital display or moved the weights until the scale was balanced.
11. Noted the measurement.
12. Took the baby off the scale.
13. Diapered and dressed the baby. Laid the baby in the crib.
14. Discarded the paper and soiled diaper.
15. Disinfected the scale following agency policy.
16. Removed and discarded the gloves. Practiced hand hygiene.

Post-Procedure

17. Returned the scale to its proper place.
18. Practiced hand hygiene.
19. Reported and recorded your observations.

Date of Satisfactory Completion _____   Instructor's Initials _____

Adult CPR—One Rescuer

Name: _____   Date: _____

Procedure	S	U	Comments
1. Made sure the scene was safe.	____	____	_____
2. Took 5 to 10 seconds to check for a response and breathing:			
a. Checked if the person was responding. Tapped or gently shook the person. Called the person by name, if known. Shouted, "Are you OK?"	____	____	_____
b. Checked for no breathing or no normal breathing (gasping).	____	____	_____
3. Called for help. Activated the EMS system or agency's rapid response team if the person was not responding and not breathing or not breathing normally (gasping).	____	____	_____
4. Got or asked someone to bring an (AED) if available.	____	____	_____
5. Positioned the person supine on a hard, flat surface. Logrolled the person so there was no twisting of the spine. Placed the arms alongside the body.	____	____	_____
6. Checked for a carotid pulse. This took 5 to 10 seconds. Started chest compressios if you did not feel a pulse.	____	____	_____
7. Exposed the person's chest.	____	____	_____
8. Gave chest compressions at a rate of 100 per minute. Pushed hard and fast. Established a regular rhythm. Counted out loud. Pressed down at least 2 inches. Allowed the chest to recoil between compressions. Gave 30 chest compressions.	____	____	_____
9. Opened the airway. Used the head tilt–chin lift method.	____	____	_____
10. Gave 2 breaths. Each breath took only 1 second. Each breath made the chest rise. (If the first breath did not make the chest rise, tried to open the airway again. Used the head tilt–chin lift method.)	____	____	_____
11. Continued the cycle of 30 compressions followed by 2 breaths. Limited interruptions in compressions to less than 10 seconds. Continued cycles until the AED arrived. Or continued until help arrived or the person began to move. If movement occurred, placed the person in the recovery position.	____	____	_____

Date of Satisfactory Completion _____   Instructor's Initials _____

Adult CPR With AED—Two Rescuers

Name: _____   Date: _____

Procedure	S	U	Comments
1. Made sure the scene was safe.	___	___	_____
2. *Rescuer 1:* Took 5 to 10 seconds to check for a response and breathing:			
a. Checked if the person was responding. Tapped or gently shook the person. Called the person by name, if known. Shouted, "Are you OK?"	___	___	_____
b. Checked for no breathing or no normal breathing (gasping).	___	___	_____
3. *Rescuer 2:*			
a. Activated the EMS system or agency's rapid response team, if the person was not responding and not breathing or not breathing normally (gasping).	___	___	_____
b. Got the defibrillator (AED) if available.	___	___	_____
4. *Rescuer 1:*			
a. Positioned the person supine on a hard, flat surface. Logrolled the person so there was no twisting of the spine. Placed the arms along side the body.	___	___	_____
b. Checked for a carotid pulse. This took 5 to 10 seconds. Started chest compressions, if you did not feel a pulse.	___	___	_____
c. Exposed the person's chest.	___	___	_____
d. Gave chest compressions at a rate of at least 100 per minute. Pushed hard and fast. Established a regular rhythm. Counted out loud. Pressed down at least 2 inches. Allowed the chest to recoil between compressions. Gave 30 compressions.	___	___	_____
e. Opened the airway. Used the head tilt–chin lift method.	___	___	_____
f. Gave 2 breaths. Each breath took only 1 second. Each breath made the chest rise. (If the first breath did not make the chest rise, tried opening the airway again. Used the head tilt–chin lift method.)	___	___	_____
5. *Rescuer 2:*			
a. Opened the case with the AED.	___	___	_____
b. Turned on the AED.	___	___	_____
c. Applied adult electrode pads to the person's chest. Followed the instructions and diagram provided with the AED.	___	___	_____
d. Attached the connected cables to the AED.	___	___	_____
e. Cleared away from the person. Made sure no one was touching the person.	___	___	_____
f. Allowed the AED to check the person's heart rhythm.	___	___	_____
g. Made sure everyone was clear of the person if the AED advised a "shock." Loudly instructed others not to touch the person. Said: "I am clear, you are clear, everyone is clear!" Looked to make sure no one was touching the person.	___	___	_____
h. Pressed the "SHOCK" button if the AED advised a "shock."	___	___	_____
6. *Rescuers 1 and 2:*			
a. Performed 2-person CPR:			
(1) Began with compressions. One rescuer gave chest compressions at a rate of at least 100 per minute. Pushed hard and fast. Established a regular rhythm. Counted out loud. Allowed the chest to recoil between compressions. Gave 30 chest compressions. Paused to allow the other rescuer to give 2 breaths.	___	___	_____
7. After 2 minutes of CPR (5 cycles of 30 compression and 2 breaths), repeated:			
a. Cleared away from the person. Made sure no one was touching the person.	___	___	_____
b. Allowed the AED to check the person's heart rhythm.	___	___	_____

Date of Satisfactory Completion _____   Instructor's Initials _____

Procedure—cont'd   S   U   **Comments**

   c. Made sure everyone was clear of the person if the AED
      advised a "shock." Loudly instructed others not to touch
      the person. Said: "I am clear, you are clear, everyone is clear!"
      Looked to make sure no one was touching the person.   _____ _____ _____

   d. Pressed the "SHOCK" button if the AED advised a "shock."   _____ _____ _____

   e. Changed positions and continued CPR began with
      compressions.   _____ _____ _____

8. Continued until help took over or the person began to move.
   If movement occurred, placed the person in the recovery position. _____ _____ _____

Date of Satisfactory Completion _____   Instructor's Initials _____

Child CPR—One Rescuer

Name: _____   Date: _____

Procedure	S	U	Comments
1. Made sure the scene was safe.	___	___	_____
2. Took 5 to 10 seconds to check for a response and breathing:			
a. Checked if the child was responding. Tapped or gently shook the child. Called the child by name, if known. Shouted, "Are you OK?"	___	___	_____
b. Checked for no breathing or no normal breathing (gasping).	___	___	_____
3. Called for help if the child was not responding and not breathing or not breathing normally (gasping). If someone responded, asked the person to. Do the following before beginning CPR if the arrest was sudden and witnessed:			
a. Activate the EMS system or agency's rapid response team.	___	___	_____
b. Got an AED.	___	___	_____
4. Positioned the child supine on a hard, flat surface. Logrolled the child so there was no twisting of the spine. Placed the arms alongside the body.	___	___	_____
5. Checked for a carotid pulse. This took 5 to 10 seconds. Started CPR if you did not feel a pulse or if the pulse was less than 60 with signs of poor circulation.	___	___	_____
6. Exposed the child's chest.	___	___	_____
7. Gave chest compressions at a rate of at least 100 per minute. Pushed hard and fast. Established a regular rhythm. Counted out loud. Pressed down at least ⅓ the depth of the chest (about 2 inches). Allowed the chest to recoil between compressions. Gave 30 chest compressions.	___	___	_____
8. Opened the airway. Used the head tilt–chin lift method.	___	___	_____
9. Gave 2 breaths. Each breath took only 1 second. Each breath made the chest rise. If the first breath did not make the chest rise:			
a. Opened the airway again. Used the head tilt–chin lift method.	___	___	_____
b. Gave another breath.	___	___	_____
10. Continued the cycle of 30 chest compressions followed by 2 breaths. Limited interruptions in compressions to less than 10 seconds.	___	___	_____
11. Did the following after 5 cycles (2 minutes) of CPR if not already done:			
a. Activated the EMS system or the agency rapid response team.	___	___	_____
b. Got a defibrillator (AED).	___	___	_____
c. Used the AED.	___	___	_____
12. Rescuer did the following:			
a. Opened the case with the AED.	___	___	_____
b. Turned on the AED.	___	___	_____
c. Applied child electrode pads if available. Or used the key or switch to change to the child setting. If neither was available, used the adult pads and settings. The pads did not touch or overlap. Followed the instructions provided with the AED.	___	___	_____
d. Attached the connecting cables to the AED.	___	___	_____
e. Cleared away from the child. Made sure no one was touching the child.	___	___	_____
f. Allowed the AED to check the child's heart rhythm.	___	___	_____
g. Made sure everyone was clear of the child if the AED advised a "shock." Loudly instructed others not to touch the child. Said: "I am clear, you are clear, everyone is clear!" Looked to make sure no one was touching the child.	___	___	_____
h. Pressed the "SHOCK" button if the AED advised a "shock."	___	___	_____
i. Gave one shock if advised. Then started CPR beginning with compressions.	___	___	_____
j. If the rhythm was not shockable, started CPR beginning with compressions.	___	___	_____

Date of Satisfactory Completion _____   Instructor's Initials _____

Procedure—cont'd   S   U   **Comments**

13. Checked the rhythm after every 5 cycles of CPR.   _____   _____   _____

14. Continued CPR and used the AED until helped arrived or the
    child started to move.   _____   _____   _____

Date of Satisfactory Completion _____   Instructor's Initials _____

Child CPR With AED—Two Rescuers

Name: _____   Date: _____

Procedure	S	U	Comments
1. Made sure the scene was safe.	_____	_____	_____
2. *Rescuer 1:* Took 5 to 10 seconds to check for a response and breathing:			
a. Checked if the child was responding. Tapped or shook the child. Called the child by name. Shouted, "Are you OK?"	_____	_____	_____
b. Checked for no breathing or no normal breathing (gasping).	_____	_____	_____
3. *Rescuer 2:*			
a. Activated the EMS system or the agency's rapid response team, if the child was not responding and not breathing or not breathing normally (gasping).	_____	_____	_____
b. Got a defibrillator (AED), if one available.	_____	_____	_____
4. *Rescuer 1:* Positioned the child supine on a hard, flat surface. Logrolled the child so there was no twisting of the spine. Placed the arms alongside the body.	_____	_____	_____
5. *Rescuer 2:*			
a. Opened the case with the AED.	_____	_____	_____
b. Turned on the AED.	_____	_____	_____
c. Applied child electrode pads if available. Or used the key or switch to change to the child setting. If neither was available, used the adult pads and settings. The pads did not touch or overlap. Followed the instructions and diagram provided with the AED.	_____	_____	_____
d. Attached the connecting cables to the AED.	_____	_____	_____
e. Cleared away from the child. Made sure no one was touching the child.	_____	_____	_____
f. Allowed the AED to check the child's heart rhythm.	_____	_____	_____
g. Made sure everyone was clear of the child if AED advised a "shock." Loudly instructed others not to touch the child. Said: "I am clear, you are clear, everyone is clear!" Looked to make sure no one touching the child.	_____	_____	_____
h. Pressed the "SHOCK" button if the AED advised a "shock."	_____	_____	_____
6. *Rescuers 1 and 2:*			
a. Performed 2-rescuer CPR:			
(1) Began chest compressions. One rescuer gave chest compressions at a rate of at least 100 per minute. Pushed hard and fast. Established a regular rhythm. Counted out loud. Allowed the chest to recoil between compressions. Gave 15 chest compressions. Paused to allow the other rescuer to give 2 breaths.	_____	_____	_____
(2) The other rescuer gave 2 breaths after every 15 chest compressions	_____	_____	_____
7. Repeated these steps after 2 minutes of CPR (10 cycles of 15 compressions and 2 breaths). Changed positions and continued CPR beginning with compressions.	_____	_____	_____
a. Cleared away from the child. Made sure no one was touching the child.	_____	_____	_____
b. Allowed the AED to check the child's heart rhythm.	_____	_____	_____
c. Made sure everyone was clear of the child if AED advised a "shock." Loudly instructed others not to touch the child. Said: "I am clear, you are clear, everyone is clear!" Looked to make sure no one was touching the child.	_____	_____	_____
d. Pressed the "SHOCK" button if the AED advised a "shock."	_____	_____	_____

Date of Satisfactory Completion _____   Instructor's Initials _____

Procedure—cont'd	**S**	**U**	**Comments**
8. *Rescuers 1 and 2:*			
a. Performed 2-person CPR.	_____	_____	_____
b. One rescuer gave chest compressions at the rate of 100 per minute—30 chest compressions followed by 2 breaths. Established a regular rhythm, and counted out loud—tried "1 and, 2 and, 3 and, 4 and," so on to 15.	_____	_____	_____
c. The other rescuer gave 2 breaths after every 15 chest compressions.	_____	_____	_____
9. After 2 minutes of CPR (5 cycles of 15 compressions and 2 breaths) repeated these steps. Then continued CPR.			
a. Cleared away from the child. Made sure no one was touching the child.	_____	_____	_____
b. Let the AED check the child's heart rhythm.	_____	_____	_____
c. Made sure everyone was clear of the child if the AED advised a "shock."	_____	_____	_____
d. Pressed the "SHOCK" button when the AED advised a "shock."	_____	_____	_____
10. Continued CPR and used the AED until help arrived or the child started to move.	_____	_____	_____

Date of Satisfactory Completion _____   Instructor's Initials _____

Infant CPR—One Rescuer

Name: _____   Date: _____

Procedure	S	U	Comments
1. Made sure the scene was safe.	___	___	_____
2. Took 5 to 10 seconds to check for a response and breathing:			
a. Checked if the infant was responding. Tapped the infant's foot, and shouted, "Are you OK?" (NOTE: Infants could not answer you. However, shouting startled the responsive infant.)	___	___	_____
b. Checked for no breathing or no normal breathing (gasping).	___	___	_____
3. Called for help, if the infant did not respond and not breathing or not breathing normally (gasping). If someone responded, asked the person to do the following. You did the following before beginning CPR if the arrest was sudden and witnessed:			
a. Activate the EMS system or the agency's rapid response team.	___	___	_____
b. Got a defibrillator (AED) if one available.	___	___	_____
4. Positioned the infant supine on a hard, flat surface.	___	___	_____
5. Checked for a brachial pulse. This took 5 to 10 seconds. Started CPR if you did not feel a pulse or if the pulse was less than 60 with signs of poor circulation.	___	___	_____
6. Exposed the infant's chest.	___	___	_____
7. Placed 2 fingers on the sternum just below the nipple line. Gave chest compressions at a rate of 100 per minute. Pushed hard and fast. Established a regular rhythm. Counted out loud. Pressed down at least ⅓ the depth of the chest. Allowed chest to recoil between compressions. Gave 30 chest compressions.	___	___	_____
8. Opened the airway. Used the head tilt–chin lift method. The head was in a neutral ("sniffing") position.	___	___	_____
9. Gave 2 breaths. Each breath took only 1 second. Each breath made the chest rise. If the first breat did not make the chest rise:			
a. Opened the airway again. Used the head tilt–chin lift method.	___	___	_____
b. Gave another breath.	___	___	_____
10. Completed the cycle of 30 chest compressions followed by 2 breaths. Limited interruptions in compressions to less than 10 seconds.	___	___	_____
11. Did the following after 5 cycles (2 minutes) of CPR if not already done:			
a. Activated the EMS system or agency's rapid response team.	___	___	_____
b. Got a defibrillator (AED).	___	___	_____
c. Used the AED.	___	___	_____
12. Did the following:			
a. Opened the case with the AED.	___	___	_____
b. Turned on the AED.	___	___	_____
c. Applied child electrode pads if available. Or used the key or switch to change to the child setting. If neither was available, used the adult pads and settings. The pads did not touch or overlap. Followed the instructions and diagram provided with the AED.	___	___	_____
d. Attached the connecting cables to the AED.	___	___	_____
e. Cleared away from the child. Made sure no one was touching the child.	___	___	_____
f. Allowed the AED to check the child's heart rhythm.	___	___	_____
g. Made sure everyone was clear of the child if AED advised a "shock." Loudly instructed others not to touch the child. Said: "I am clear, you are clear, everyone is clear!" Looked to make sure no one was touching the child.	___	___	_____
h. Pressed the "SHOCK" button if the AED advised a "shock."	___	___	_____
i. Gave 1 shock if advised. Then started CPR beginning with compressions.	___	___	_____
j. If the rhythm was not shockable, started CPR beginning with compressions.	___	___	_____

Date of Satisfactory Completion _____   Instructor's Initials _____

Procedure—cont'd

	S	U	Comments
13. Checked the rhythm after 5 cycles of CPR.	_____	_____	_____
14. Continued CPR and used the AED until help arrived or the infant started to move.	_____	_____	_____

Date of Satisfactory Completion _____   Instructor's Initials _____

Infant CPR With AED—Two Rescuers

Name: _____   Date: _____

Procedure	S	U	Comments
1. Made sure the scene was safe.			
2. *Rescuer 1:* Took 5 to 10 seconds to check for a response and breathing:			
a. Checked if the infant was responding. Tapped the infant's foot. Shouted "Are you OK?" (Note: Infant did not answer you. However, shouting startled the responsive infant.)			
b. Checked for no breathing or no normal breathing (gasping).			
3. *Rescuer 2:*			
a. Activated the EMS system or agency's rapid response team. If the infant was not responding and not breathing or not breathing normally (gasping).			
4. *Rescuer 1:* Positioned the infant supine on a hard, flat surface. Began 1-rescuer CPR until the second rescuer returned.			
5. *Rescuer 2:*			
a. Opened the case with the AED.			
b. Turned on the AED.			
c. Applied child electrode pads if available. Or used the key or switch to change to the child setting. If neither was available, used the adult pads and settings. The pads did not touch or overlap. Followed the instructions and diagram provided with the AED.			
d. Attached the connecting cables to the AED.			
e. Cleared away from the infant. Made sure no one was touching the infant.			
f. Allowed the AED to check the infant's heart rhythm.			
g. Made sure everyone was clear of the infant if the AED advised a "shock." Loudly instructed others not to touch the infant. Said: "I am clear, you are clear, everyone is clear!" Looked to make sure no one was touching the infant.			
h. Pressed the "SHOCK" button if the AED advised a "shock."			
6. *Rescuers 1 and 2:*			
a. Performed 2-person CPR:			
(1) Began with compressions. One rescuer used the 2 thumb-encircling hands method and gave chest compressions at a rate of 100 per minute. Pushed hard and fast. Established a regular rhythm. Counted out loud. Allowed the chest to recoil between compressions. Gave 15 chest compressions. Paused to allow the other rescuer to give 2 breaths.			
(2) The other rescuer gave 2 breaths after every 15 compressions.			
7. After 2 minutes of CPR (10 cycles of 15 compressions and 2 breaths), repeated the following and changed positions and continued CPR beginning with compressions.			
a. Opened the case with the AED.			
b. Turned on the AED.			
c. Applied child electrode pads if available. Or used the key or switch to change to the child setting. If neither was available, used the adult pads and settings. The pads did not touch or overlap. Followed the instructions and diagram provided with the AED.			
d. Attached the connecting cables to the AED.			
e. Cleared away from the infant. Made sure no was touching the infant.			
f. Allowed the AED to check the infant's heart rhythm.			

Date of Satisfactory Completion _____   Instructor's Initials _____

Procedure—cont'd	**S**	**U**	**Comments**
g. Made sure everyone was clear of the infant if the AED advised a "shock." Loudly instructed others not to touch the infant. Said: "I am clear, you are clear, everyone is clear!" Looked to make sure no one was touching the infant.	_____	_____	_____
h. Pressed the "SHOCK" button if the AED advised a "shock."	_____	_____	_____
8. Continued CPR and used the AED until help arrived or the child started to move.	_____	_____	_____

Date of Satisfactory Completion _____   Instructor's Initials _____

Assisting With Post-Mortem Care

Name: _____   Date: _____

Pre-Procedure	S	U	Comments
1. Followed *Delegation Guidelines: Post-mortem Care.* Reviewed *Promoting Safety and Comfort: Post-mortem Care.*	____	____	_____
2. Practiced hand hygiene.	____	____	_____
3. Collected the following:			
• Post-mortem kit (shroud or body bag, gown, ID tags, gauze squares, safety pins)	____	____	_____
• Bed protectors	____	____	_____
• Wash basin	____	____	_____
• Bath towel and washcloths	____	____	_____
• Denture cup	____	____	_____
• Tape	____	____	_____
• Dressings	____	____	_____
• Gloves	____	____	_____
• Cotton balls	____	____	_____
• Valuables envelope	____	____	_____
4. Provided for privacy.	____	____	_____
5. Raised the bed for body mechanics.	____	____	_____
6. Made sure the bed was flat.	____	____	_____

Procedure	S	U	Comments
7. Put on gloves.	____	____	_____
8. Positioned the body supine. Arms and legs were straight. A pillow was under the head and shoulders. Or raised the head of the bed 15 to 20 degrees, if agency policy.	____	____	_____
9. Closed the eyes. Gently pulled the eyelids over the eyes. Applied moist cotton balls gently over the eyelids if the eyes did not stay closed.	____	____	_____
10. Inserted dentures if it is agency policy to do so. If not, placed them in a labeled denture cup.	____	____	_____
11. Closed the mouth. If necessary, placed a rolled towel under the chin to keep the mouth closed.	____	____	_____
12. Followed agency policy for jewelry. Removed all jewelry, except for wedding rings if this was agency policy. Listed the jewelry that you removed. Placed the jewelry and the list in a valuables envelope.	____	____	_____
13. Placed cotton balls over the rings. Taped them in place.	____	____	_____
14. Removed drainage containers.	____	____	_____
15. Removed tubes and catheters. Used the gauze squares as needed.	____	____	_____
16. Bathed soiled areas with plain water. Dried thoroughly.	____	____	_____
17. Placed a bed protector under the buttocks.	____	____	_____
18. Removed soiled dressings. Replaced them with clean ones.	____	____	_____
19. Put a clean gown on the body. Positioned the body supine. Arms and legs were straight. A pillow was under the head and shoulders. Or the head of the bed was raised 15 to 20 degrees if agency policy.	____	____	_____
20. Brushed and combed the hair if necessary.	____	____	_____
21. Covered the body to the shoulders with a sheet if the family viewed the person.	____	____	_____
22. Gathered the person's belongings. Put them in a bag labeled with the person's name. Made sure you included eyeglasses, hearing aids, and other valuables.	____	____	_____
23. Removed supplies, equipment, and linens. Straightened the room. Provided soft lighting.	____	____	_____
24. Removed and discarded the gloves. Practiced hand hygiene.	____	____	_____
25. Let the family view the body. Provided for privacy. Returned to the room after they left.	____	____	_____

Date of Satisfactory Completion _____   Instructor's Initials _____

Procedure—cont'd	S	U	Comments
26. Practiced hand hygiene. Put on gloves.			
27. Filled out the ID tags. Tied one to the ankle or to the right big toe.			
28. Placed the body in the body bag or covered it with a sheet. Or applied the shroud.			
a. Positioned the shroud under the body.			
b. Brought the top down over the head.			
c. Folded the bottom up over the feet.			
d. Folded the sides over the body.			
e. Pinned or taped the shroud in place.			
29. Attached the second ID tag to the shroud, sheet, or body bag.			
30. Left the denture cup with the body.			
31. Pulled the privacy curtain around the bed. Or closed the door.			

Post-Procedure

	S	U	Comments
32. Removed and discarded the gloves. Practiced hand hygiene.			
33. Stripped the unit after the body had been removed. Wore gloves.			
34. Removed and discarded the gloves. Practiced hand hygiene.			
35. Reported the following:			
a. The time the body was taken by the funeral director			
b. What was done with jewelry, other valuables, and personal items			
c. What was done with dentures			

Date of Satisfactory Completion _____   Instructor's Initials _____

Preparing for the Competency Evaluation

After completing your state's training program, you need to pass the competency evaluation. The purpose of the competency evaluation is to make sure you can safely do your job. This section will help you prepare for the test.

Competency Evaluation

The competency evaluation has a written test and a skills test. The number of questions varies with each state. Each question has four answer choices. Although some questions may appear to have more than one possible answer, there is only one best answer. You will have about 1 minute to read and answer each question. Some questions take less time to read and answer. Other questions take longer. You should have enough time to take the test without feeling rushed.

The content of the written test varies depending on your state. Content may include:

- Activities of Daily Living—hygiene, dressing and grooming, nutrition and hydration, elimination, rest/sleep/comfort
- Basic Nursing Skills—infection control, safety/emergency, therapeutic/technical procedures (e.g., vital signs, bedmaking), data collection and reporting
- Restorative Skills—prevention, self-care/independence
- Emotional and Mental Health Needs
- Spiritual and Cultural Needs
- The Person's Rights
- Legal and Ethical Behavior
- Being a member of the Health Care Team
- Communication

The written test is given as a paper and pencil test in most states. Some test sites may use computers. You do not need computer experience to take the test on the computer. If you have difficulty reading English, you may request to take an oral test. Talk with your instructor or employer about details for computer testing or oral testing.

The skills test involves performing five nursing skills that you learned in your training program. These skills are randomly chosen. You do not select the skills. You are allowed about 30 minutes to do the skills. See p. 509 for more information about the skills test.

Taking the Competency Evaluation

To register for the test, you need to complete an application. Your instructor or employer tells you when and where the tests are given. There is a fee for the evaluation. If you work in a nursing center, the employer may pay this fee. If you pay the fee, you may need to purchase a money order or certified check. Make sure your name is on the money order or certified check. Cash and personal checks may not be accepted.

Plan to arrive at the test site about 15 to 30 minutes before the evaluation begins. Most centers do not admit you if you are late. Know the exact location of the test site and room. Actually drive or take transportation to the test site a few days or a week before the test. Making a "dry run" lets you know how much time you need to travel, park, and get to the test site. It will also help decrease your anxiety level on the test day.

To be admitted to the test, you need two pieces of identification (ID). The first form of ID is a government-issued document such as a driver's license or passport. It must have a current photo and your signature. The name on the ID must be the same as the name on your application form. If your name has changed and you have not been able to have the name changed on your identification documents, ask your instructor or employer what to do. The second form of ID must include your name and signature. Examples include a library card, hunting license, or credit card.

Take several sharpened Number 2 pencils to the test. For the skills test you will need a watch with a second hand. You may need a person to play the role of the patient or resident. Ask your instructor or employer how this is done in your state.

Taking the written test and skills test may take several hours. You may want to bring snacks or lunch and a beverage to the testing site. Eating and drinking are not allowed during the test. However, you may be told where you can eat while waiting for the test.

You cannot bring textbooks, study notes, or other materials into the testing room. The only exception may be a language translation dictionary that you show to the proctor (a person who monitors the test) before the test begins. Cell phones, pagers, calculators, or other electronic devices are not permitted during testing. Children and pets are not allowed in the testing areas.

Studying for the Competency Evaluation

You began to prepare for the written and skills test during your training program. You learned the basic nursing content and skills needed to provide safe, quality care. The following suggestions can help you study for the competency evaluation:

- Begin to study at least 2 to 3 weeks before the test. Plan to study for 1 to 2 hours each day.
- Decide on a specific time to study. Choose a study time that is best for you. This may be early in the morning before others are awake. It may be in the evening after others go to sleep. Try to choose a time when you are mentally alert.
- Choose a specific area to study in. This area should be quiet, well lit and comfortable. You should have enough room to write and to spread out your books, notes, and other study aids—CD, DVD. The area does not need to be noise-free. The testing site is not absolutely quiet. You want to concentrate and not be distracted by the noise around you.
- Collect everything you need before settling down to study. This includes your textbook, notes, paper, highlighters, pens or pencils, CD, and DVD.
- Take short breaks when you need them. Take a break when your mind begins to wander or if you feel sleepy.
- Develop a study plan. Write your plan down so you can refer to it. Study one content area before going on to the next. For example, study personal hygiene before going on to vital signs. Do not jump from one subject to another.
- Use a variety of ways to study:

  Use index cards to help you review abbreviations and terminology. Put the abbreviation or term on the front of the card and place the meaning on the back. Take the cards with you and review them whenever you have a break or are waiting.

  Record key points. You can listen to the recording while cooking or while riding in the car.

  Study groups are another way to prepare for a test. Group members can quiz each other.

- To remember what you are learning, try these ideas:
  - Relax when you study. When relaxed, you learn information quickly and recall it with greater ease.
  - Repeat what you are learning. Say it out loud. This helps you remember the idea.
  - Make the information you are learning meaningful. Think about how the information will help you be a good nursing assistant.
  - Write down what you are learning. Writing helps you remember information. Prepare study sheets.
  - Be positive about what you are learning. You remember what you find interesting.
- Suggestions for studying if you have children:
  - When you first come home from work or school, spend time with your children. Then plan study time.
  - Select educational programs on TV that your children can watch as you study. Or get a CD-ROM from the library.
  - When you take your study breaks, spend time with your children.
  - Ask other adults to take care of the children while you study.

- Take the two 75-question practice tests in this section. Each question has the correct answer and the reason why an answer is correct or incorrect. If you practice taking tests, you are more likely to pass them. Take the practice tests under conditions similar to the real test. Work within time limits.
- If your state has a practice test and a candidate handbook, study the content. Some states have practice tests on-line.

Managing Anxiety

Almost everyone dreads taking tests. It is common and normal to experience anxiety before taking a test. If used wisely, anxiety can actually help you do well. When you are anxious, that means you are concerned. You may be concerned about how prepared you are to take the test. Or you may be concerned about how you will feel about yourself if you do not pass the test. Being concerned usually results in some action. To overcome anxiety before the test:

- Study and prepare for the test. That helps increase your confidence as you recall or clarify what you have learned. Anxiety decreases as confidence increases. When you think you know the information, keep studying. This reinforces your learning.
- Develop a positive mental attitude. You can pass this test. You took tests in your training program and passed them. Praise yourself. Talk to yourself in a positive way. If a negative thought enters your mind, stop it at once. Challenge the mental thought and tell yourself you will pass the test.
- Visualize success. Think about how wonderful you will feel when you are notified that you have passed the test.
- Perform breathing exercises. Breathe slowly and deeply.
- Perform regular exercise. Exercise helps you stay physically fit. It also helps keep you calm.
- Good nourishment helps you think clearly. Eat a nourishing meal before the test. Do not skip breakfast. Vitamin C helps fight short-term stress. Protein and calcium help overcome the effects of long-term stress. Complex carbohydrates (pasta, nuts, yogurt) can help settle your nerves. Eat familiar foods the day before and the day of the test. Do not eat foods that could cause stomach or intestinal upset.
- Maintain a normal routine the day before the test.
- Get a good night's sleep before the test. Go to bed early enough so you do not oversleep or are too tired to get up. Set your alarm clock properly. You may want to set two alarm clocks.
- Do not "cram" the evening before or the day of the test. Last minute cramming increases your anxiety. Do something relaxing with family and friends.
- Avoid drinking large amounts of coffee, colas, water, or other beverages. You do not want to be uncomfortable with a full bladder when you take the test.
- Wear comfortable clothes. Dress in layers so that you are prepared for a cold or warm room.
- If you are a woman, remember that worry and anxiety can affect your menstrual cycle. Wear a panty liner, sanitary napkin, or tampon if you think your period

may start. This eliminates worry about soiling your clothing during the test.
- Allow plenty of time for travel, traffic, and parking.
- Arrive early enough to use the restroom before the test begins.
- Do not talk about the test with others. Their panic or anxiety may affect your self-confidence.

Taking the Test

Follow these guidelines for taking the test:
- Listen carefully, and follow the instructions given by the proctor (person administering the test).
- When you receive the test, make certain you have all the test pages.
- Read and follow all directions carefully.
- You are not allowed to ask questions about the content of the test questions.
- Do deep-breathing and muscle-relaxation exercises as needed.
- Cheating of any kind is not allowed. If the proctor sees you giving or receiving any type of assistance, your test booklet is taken and you must leave the testing site.
- If using a computer answer sheet, completely fill in the bubble.
- If you make a mistake, erase the wrong answer completely. Do not make any stray marks on the paper. Not erasing completely or leaving stray marks could cause the computer to misread your answer.
- Do not worry or get anxious if people finish the test before you do. Persons who finish a test early do not necessarily have a better score than those who finish later.
- You cannot take any evaluation materials or notes out of the testing room.

Answering Multiple-Choice Questions

Pace yourself during the test. First, answer all the questions that you know. Then go back and answer skipped questions. Sometimes you will remember the answer later. Or another test question may give you a clue to the one you skipped. Spending too much time on a question can cost you valuable time later. To help you answer the questions or statements:
- Always read the questions or statements carefully. Do not scan or glance at questions. Scanning or glancing can cause you to miss important key words. Read each word of the question.
- Before reading the answers, decide what the answer is in your own words. Then read all four answers to the question. Select the one best answer.

- Do not read into a question. Take the question as it is asked. Do not add your own thoughts and ideas to the question. Do not assume or suppose "what if." Just respond to the information provided.
- Trust your common sense. If unsure of an answer, select your first choice. Do not change your answer unless you are absolutely sure of the correct answer. Your first reaction is usually correct.
- Look for key words in every question. Sometimes key words are in italics, highlighted, or underlined. Common key words are: *always, never, first, except, best, not, correct, incorrect, true,* or *false.*
- Know which words can make a statement correct (e.g., *may, can, usually, most, at least, sometimes*). The word "except" can make a question a false statement.
- Be careful of answers with these key words or phrases: *always, never, every, only, all, none, at all times,* or *at no time.* These words and phrases do not allow for exceptions. In nursing, exceptions are generally present. However, sometimes answers containing these words are correct. For example, which of the following is correct and which are incorrect?
  a. Always use a turning sheet.
  b. Never shake linens.
  c. Soap is used for all baths.
  d. The signal light must always be attached to the bed.
  The correct answer is b. Incorrect answers are a, c, and d.
- Omit answers that are obviously wrong. Then choose the best of the remaining answers.
- Go back to the questions you skipped. Answer all questions by eliminating or narrowing your choices. Always mark an answer even if you are not sure.
- Review the test a second time for completeness and accuracy before turning it in.
- Make sure you have answered each question. Also check that you have given only one answer for each question.
- Remember, the test is not designed to trick or confuse you. The written competency evaluation tests what you know, not what you do not know. You know more than you are asked.

On-Line Testing

The test may be given by computer at the test site. Ask your instructor what computer skills you will need. You usually do not need keyboard or typing skills. You will use a computer mouse to select answers. Also, you will usually receive instruction before the test begins. This will let you practice using the computer before starting the test.

Textbook Chapters Review

NOTE: This review covers selected chapters based on Competency Evaluation requirements.

CHAPTER 1 INTRODUCTION TO HEALTH CARE AGENCIES

Rehabilitation and Subacute Care Agencies
- Provide medical and nursing care for people who do not need hospital care but are too sick to go home.

Long-Term Care Centers
- Provide medical and nursing, dietary, recreational, rehabilitative, and social services. Housekeeping and laundry services are also provided.
- Residents are older or disabled.
- Some residents are recovering from illness, injury, or surgery.
- Some residents return home when well enough. Some residents need nursing care until death.
- Long-term care centers include board and care homes, assisted-living residences, nursing centers, hospices, Alzheimer's or dementia care units, and rehabilitation and subacute care units.

The Health Team
- Involves many health care workers whose skills and knowledge focus on total care.
- Works together to provide coordinated care to meet each person's needs.
- Follows the direction of the RN leading the team.

The Nursing Team
- Provides quality care to people.
- Care is coordinated by an RN.

Nursing Assistants
- Report to the nurse supervising their work.
- Provide basic nursing care under the supervision of a licensed nurse.
- Need formal training and must pass a competency test.

Meeting Standards

Survey Process
- Surveys are done to see if agencies meet standards for licensure, certification, and accreditation.
  - A license is issued by the state. A center must have a license to operate and provide care.
  - Certification is required to receive Medicare and Medicaid funds.
  - Accreditation is voluntary. It signals quality and excellence.

Your Role
- Provide quality care.
- Protect the person's rights.
- Provide for the person's and your own safety.
- Help keep the center clean and safe.
- Conduct yourself in a professional manner.
- Have good work ethics.
- Follow agency policies and procedures.
- Answer questions honestly and completely.

CHAPTER 1 REVIEW QUESTIONS
Circle the BEST answer.
1. Nursing assistants do all the following *except*
   a. Provide quality care
   b. Follow agency policies and procedures
   c. Conduct themselves in an unprofessional manner
   d. Help keep the agency clean and safe
2. Nursing assistants report to
   a. Other nursing assistants
   b. Licensed nurses
   c. The administrator
   d. The medical director
3. The health team do all the following *except*
   a. Involves many health care workers.
   b. Follows the direction of the physician.
   c. Works together to provide coordinated care.
   d. Follows the direction of the RN.
Answers to these questions are on p. 521.

CHAPTER 2 THE PERSON'S RIGHTS
- Centers must protect and promote residents' rights. Residents must be free to exercise their rights without interference. If residents are not able to exercise their rights, legal representatives do so for them.

The Omnibus Budget Reconciliation Act of 1987 (OBRA)
- OBRA is a federal law.
- OBRA requires that nursing centers provide care in a manner and in a setting that maintains or improves each person's quality of life, health, and safety.
- OBRA requires nursing assistant training and competency evaluation.
- Resident rights are a major part of OBRA.

Information
- The right to information includes:
  - Access to all records about the person, including medical records, incident reports, contracts, and financial records.
  - Information about his or her health condition.
  - Information about his or her doctor including name, specialty and contact information.
- Report any request for information to the nurse.

Refusing Treatment

- The person has the right to refuse treatment.
- A person who does not give consent or refuses treatment cannot be treated against his or her wishes
- The center must find out what the person is refusing and why.
- Advance directives are part of the right to refuse treatment.
- Report any treatment refusal to the nurse.

Privacy and Confidentiality

- Residents have the right to:
  - Personal privacy. The person's body is not exposed unnecessarily. Only staff directly involved in care and treatments are present. The person must give consent for others to be present. A person has the right to use the bathroom in private. Privacy is maintained for all personal care measures.
  - Visit with others in private—in areas where others cannot see or hear them. This includes phone calls.
  - Send and receive mail without others interfering. No one can open mail the person sends or receives without his or her consent. Unopened mail is given to the person within 24 hours of delivery to the center.
- Information about the person's care, treatment, and condition is kept confidential. So are medical and financial records. Consent is needed to release information to other agencies or persons.

Personal Choice

- Residents have the right to make their own choices. They can:
  - Choose their own doctors.
  - Take part in planning and deciding their care and treatment.
  - Choose activities, schedules, and care based on their preferences.
  - Choose when to get up and go to bed, what to wear, how to spend their time, and what to eat.
  - Choose friends and visitors inside and outside the center.

Grievances

- Residents have the right to voice concerns, questions, and complaints about treatment or care.
- The center must promptly try to correct the matter.
- No one can punish the person in any way for voicing the grievance.

Work

- The person is not required to work or perform services for the center.
- The person has the right to work or perform services if he or she wants to.
- Residents volunteer or are paid for their services

Taking Part in Resident Groups

- The person has the right to:
  - Form and take part in resident and family groups.
  - Take part in social, cultural, religious, and community events. The resident has the right to help in getting to and from events of their choice.

Personal Items

- The resident has the right to:
  - Keep and use personal items, such as clothing and some furnishings.
  - Have his or her property treated with care and respect. Items are labeled with the person's name.
- Protect yourself and the center from being accused of stealing a person's property. Do not go through a person's closet, drawers, purse, or other space without the person's knowledge and consent. If you have to inspect closets and drawers, follow center policy for reporting and recording the inspection.

Freedom From Abuse, Mistreatment, and Neglect

- Residents have the right to be free from:
  - Verbal, sexual, physical, or mental abuse.
  - Involuntary seclusion—separating a person from others against his or her will, confining a person to a certain area, keeping the person away from his or her room without consent.
- No one can abuse, neglect, or mistreat a resident. This includes center staff, volunteers, staff from other agencies or groups, other residents, family members, friends, visitors, and legal representatives.
- Nursing centers must investigate suspected or reported cases of abuse.

Freedom From Restraint

- Residents have the right to residents have the right not to have body movements restricted by restraints or drugs.
- Restraints are used only if required to treat the person's medical symptoms or if necessary to protect the person or others from harm. If a restraint is required, a doctor's order is needed.

Quality of Life

- Residents must be cared for in a manner that promotes dignity and self-esteem. Physical, psychological, and mental well-being must be promoted. Review Box 2-3, OBRA-Required Actions to Promote Dignity and Privacy, in the Textbook.
- Centers must provide activity programs that promote physical, intellectual, social, spiritual, and emotional well-being. Many centers provide religious services for spiritual health. You assist residents to and from activity programs. You may need to help them with activities.
- Residents have a right to a safe, clean, comfortable, and home-like setting. The center must provide a setting and services that meet the person's needs and preferences. The setting and staff must promote the person's independence, dignity, and well-being.

Ombudsman Program

- The Older Americans Act requires a long-term care ombudsman program in every state.
- Ombudsmen are employed by a state agency. They are not nursing center employees. Some are volunteers.
- **Ombudsmen** protect the health, safety, welfare, and rights of residents. They also may investigate and resolve complaints, provide support to resident and family groups, and help the center manage difficult problems.
- OBRA requires that nursing centers post the names, addresses, and phone numbers of local and state ombudsmen where the residents can easily see it.
- Because a family or resident may share a concern with you, you must know the state and center policies and procedures for contacting an ombudsman.

CHAPTER 2 REVIEW QUESTIONS

Circle the BEST answer.

1. Residents have all the following rights *except*
   a. Refusing a treatment
   b. Making a telephone call in private
   c. Choosing activities to attend
   d. Being punished for voicing a grievance
2. OBRA does not require nursing assistant training and competency evaluation.
   a. True
   b. False
3. The person has a right to take part in planning and deciding their care and treatment.
   a. True
   b. False
4. The person is required to work for the center.
   a. True
   b. False

Answers to these questions are on p. 521.

CHAPTER 3 THE NURSING ASSISTANT
Federal and State Laws

Nurse Practice Acts
- Each state has a nurse practice act. It regulates nursing practice in that state.

Nursing Assistants
- A state's nurse practice act is used to decide what nursing assistants can do. Some nurse practice acts also regulate nursing assistant roles, functions, education, and certification requirements. Some states have separate laws for nursing assistants.
- Nursing assistants must be able to function with skill and safety. They can have their certification, license, or registration denied, revoked, or suspended.

Reasons for Losing Certification, a License or Registration
- The National Council of State Boards of Nursing (NCSBN) lists these reasons (see Box 3-1 in the Textbook):
  - Substance abuse or dependency.
  - Abandoning, abusing, or neglecting a resident.

- Fraud or deceit. Examples include:
  - Filing false personal information
  - Providing false information when applying for initial certification or re-instatement.
- Violating professional boundaries.
- Giving unsafe care.
- Performing acts beyond the nursing assistant role.
- Misappropriation (stealing, theft) or mis-using property.
- Obtaining money or property from a resident through fraud, falsely representing oneself, and force are examples.
- Being convicted of a crime. Examples include murder, assault, kidnapping, rape or sexual assault, robbery, sexual crimes involving children, criminal mistreatment of children or a vulnerable adult, drug trafficking, embezzlement, theft, and arson.
- Failing to conform to the standards of nursing assistants.
- Putting patients and residents at risk for harm.
- Violating resident's privacy.
- Failing to maintain the confidentiality of patient or resident information.

The Omnibus Budget Reconciliation Act of 1987 (OBRA)
- The purpose of OBRA, a federal law, is to improve the quality of life of nursing center residents.
- OBRA sets minimum training and competency evaluation requirements for nursing assistants. Each state must have a nursing assistant training and competency evaluation program (NATCEP). A nursing assistant must successfully complete a NATCEP to work in a nursing center, hospital, long-term care unit, or home care agency receiving Medicare funds.
- OBRA requires at least 75 hours of instruction. Some states have more hours. At least 16 hours of supervised training in a laboratory or clinical setting are required.
- OBRA requires a nursing assistant registry in each state. It is an official record that lists persons who have successfully completed the NATCEP.
- Retraining and a new competency evaluation program are required for nursing assistants who have not worked for 24 months.
- Each state's NATCEP must meet OBRA Requirements

Roles, Limits, and Standards
- OBRA, state laws, and legal and advisory opinions direct what you can do.
- Rules for you to follow (see Box 3-2 in the Textbook):
  - You are an assistant to the nurse.
  - A nurse assigns and supervises your work.
  - You report observations about the person's physical and mental status to the nurse. Report changes in the person's condition or behavior at once.
  - The nurse decides what should be done for a person. You do not make these decisions.

○ Review directions and the care plan with the nurse before going to the person.

○ Perform only those nursing tasks that you are trained to do.

○ Ask a nurse to supervise you if you are not comfortable performing a nursing task.

○ Perform only the nursing tasks that your state and job description allow.

- Role limits for nursing assistants (see Box 3-3 in the Textbook):

○ Never give drugs.

○ Never insert tubes or objects into body openings. Do not remove tubes from the body.

○ Never take oral or telephone orders from doctors.

○ Never perform procedures that require sterile technique.

○ Never tell the person or family the person's diagnosis or treatment plans.

○ Never diagnose or prescribe treatments or drugs for anyone.

○ Never supervise others, including other nursing assistants.

○ Never ignore an order or request to do something. This includes nursing tasks that you can do, those you cannot do, and those that are beyond your legal limits.

- Review Box 3-4, Nursing Assistant Standards, in the Textbook.

- Always obtain a written job description when you apply for a job. Do not take a job that requires you to:

○ Act beyond the legal limits of your role.

○ Function beyond your training limits.

○ Perform acts that are against your morals or religion.

Delegation

- RNs can delegate tasks to you. In some states, LPNs/LVNs can delegate tasks to you.

- Nursing assistants cannot delegate. You cannot delegate any task to other nursing assistants or to any other worker.

- Delegation decisions must protect the person's health and safety. The delegating nurse is legally responsible for his or her actions and the actions of others who performed the delegated tasks.

- If you perform a task that places the person at risk, you may face serious legal problems.

The Five Rights of Delegation

- *The right task.* Does your state allow you to perform the task? Were you trained to do the task? Do you have experience performing the task? Is the task in your job description?

- *The right circumstances.* Do you have experience performing the task given the person's condition and needs? Do you understand the purposes of the task for the person? Can you perform the task safely under the current circumstances? Do you have the equipment and supplies to safely complete the task? Do you know how to use the equipment and supplies?

- *The right person.* Are you comfortable performing the task? Do you have concerns about performing the task?

- *The right directions and communication.* Did the nurse give clear directions and instructions? Did you review the task with the nurse? Do you understand what the nurse expects?

- *The right supervision.* Is a nurse available to answer questions? Is a nurse available if the person's condition changes or if problems occur?

Your Role in Delegation

- When you agree to perform a task, you are responsible for your own actions. You must complete the task safely. Report to the nurse what you did and the observations you made.

- You should refuse to perform a task when:

○ The task is beyond the legal limits of your role.

○ The task is not in your job description.

○ You were not prepared to perform the task.

○ The task could harm the person.

○ The person's condition has changed.

○ You do not know how to use the supplies or equipment.

○ Directions are not ethical or legal.

○ Directions are against agency policies.

○ Directions are unclear or incomplete.

○ A nurse is not available for supervision.

- Never ignore an order or request to do something. Tell the nurse about your concerns.

CHAPTER 3 REVIEW QUESTIONS

Circle the BEST answer.

1. Nursing assistants perform nursing tasks delegated to them by an RN or LPN/LVN.
   a. True
   b. False

2. A resident asks you about his or her medical condition. You
   a. Tell the nurse about the resident's request
   b. Tell the resident what is in his or her medical record
   c. Ignore the question
   d. Tell another nursing assistant about the resident's request

3. You answer the telephone. The doctor starts to give you an order. You
   a. Take the order from the doctor
   b. Politely give your name and title, and ask the doctor to wait for the nurse. Promptly find the nurse
   c. Politely ask the doctor to call back later
   d. Ask the doctor if the nurse may call him back

4. You can have your certification revoked for all the following *except*
   a. Substance abuse or dependency
   b. Abandoning a patient or resident
   c. Performing acts beyond the nursing assistant role
   d. Giving safe care

5. When should you refuse a task?
   a. The task is not in your job description.
   b. The task is within the legal limits of your role.
   c. The directions for the task are clear.
   d. A nurse is available for questions and supervision.

6. A nurse delegates a task that you did not learn in your training. The task is in your job description. What is your appropriate response to the nurse?
   a. "I cannot do that task."
   b. "I did not learn that task in my training. Can you show me how to do it?"
   c. "I will ask the other nursing assistant to watch me do the task."
   d. "I will ask the other nursing assistant to do the task for me."
7. You are busy with a new resident. It is time for another resident's bath. You may delegate the bath to another nursing assistant.
   a. True
   b. False

Answers to these questions are on p. 521.

CHAPTER 4   ETHICS AND LAWS

Ethical Aspects

- Ethics is the knowledge of what is right conduct and wrong conduct. It also deals with choices or judgments about what should or should not be done. An ethical person does not cause a person harm.
- Ethical behavior involves not being prejudiced or biased. To be prejudiced or biased means to make judgments and have views before knowing the facts. You should not judge a person by your values and standards. Also, do not avoid persons whose standards and values differ from your own.
- Ethical problems involve making choices. You must decide what is the right thing to do.

Boundaries

- **Professional boundaries** separate helpful behaviors from behaviors that are not helpful.
- A **boundary violation** is an act or behavior that meets your needs, not the person's. The act or behavior is unethical. Boundary violations include abuse, keeping secrets with a person, or giving a lot of personal information about yourself to another. Review Box 4-1, Code of Conduct for Nursing Assistants, in the Textbook.
- **Professional sexual misconduct** is an act, behavior, or comment that is sexual in nature. It is sexual misconduct even if the person consents or makes the first move.
- To maintain professional boundaries, review Box 4-2, Rules for Maintaining Professional Boundaries. Be alert to **boundary signs** (acts, behaviors, or thoughts that warn of a boundary crossing or violation).

Legal Aspects

- **Negligence** is an unintentional wrong. The negligent person did not act in a reasonable and careful manner. As a result, the person or person's property was harmed. The person causing harm did not mean to cause harm.
- **Malpractice** is negligence by a professional person.
- You are legally responsible (liable) for your own actions. The nurse is liable as your supervisor.
- **Defamation** is injuring a person's name and reputation by making false statements to a third person. **Libel** is making false statements in print, writing, or through pictures or drawings. **Slander** is making false statements orally. Never make false statements about a patient, resident, family member, co-worker, or any other person.
- **False imprisonment** is the unlawful restraint or restriction of a person's freedom of movement. It involves threatening to restrain a person, restraining a person, and preventing a person from leaving the agency.
- **Invasion of privacy** is violating a person's right not to have his or her name, photo, or private affairs exposed or made public without giving consent. Review Box 4-4, Protecting the Right to Privacy, in the Textbook.
- The Health Insurance Portability and Accountability Act (HIPAA) of 1996 protects the privacy and security of a person's health information. **Protected health information** refers to identifying information and information about the person's health care that is maintained or sent in any form (paper, electronic, oral). Direct any questions about the person or the person's care to the nurse.
- **Fraud** is saying or doing something to trick, fool, or deceive a person. The act is fraud if it does or could cause harm to a person or the person's property.
- **Assault** is intentionally attempting or threatening to touch a person's body without the person's consent. The person fears bodily harm. **Battery** is touching a person's body without his or her consent. Protect yourself from being accused of assault and battery. Explain to the person what you are going to do and get the person's consent.

Informed Consent

- A person has the right to decide what will be done to his or her body and who can touch his or her body. Consent is informed when the person clearly understands all aspects of treatment.
- Persons who cannot give consent are persons who are under the legal age or are mentally incompetent. Unconscious, sedated, or confused persons cannot give consent. Informed consent is given by a responsible party—wife, husband, daughter, son, legal representative.
- You are never responsible for obtaining written consent.

Reporting Abuse

- **Abuse** is
  ○ The willful infliction of injury, unreasonable confinement, intimidation, or punishment that results in physical harm, pain, or mental anguish. Intimidation means to make afraid with threats of force or violence.
  ○ Depriving the person (or the person's caregiver) of the goods or services needed to attain or maintain well-being.
- Abuse also includes involuntary seclusion.
- **Vulnerable adults** are persons 18 years old or older who have disabilities or conditions that make them at risk to be wounded, attacked, or damaged. They have problems caring for or protecting themselves due to:
  ○ A mental, emotional, physical, or developmental disability
  ○ Brain damage
  ○ Changes from aging
  ○ All residents are vulnerable. Older persons and children are at risk for abuse.

- **Elder abuse** is any knowing, intentional, or negligent act by a caregiver or another person to an older adult. It may include physical abuse, neglect, verbal abuse, involuntary seclusion, financial exploitation or misappropriation, emotional or mental abuse, sexual abuse, or abandonment. Review Box 4-5, Signs of Elder Abuse, in the Textbook.
- Child abuse and neglect involve a child 18 years old or younger. Child abuse and neglect have many forms. Review Box 4-7, Signs and Symptoms of Child Abuse and Neglect, in the Textbook.
- If you suspect a person is being abused, report your observations to the nurse.

CHAPTER 4 REVIEW QUESTIONS

Circle the BEST answer.

1. A resident offers you a gift certificate for being kind to her. You should
   a. Say "thank you" and accept the gift
   b. Accept the gift and give it to charity
   c. Thank the resident for thinking of you, then explain it is against policy for you to accept the gift
   d. Accept the gift and give it to your daughter
2. To protect a person's privacy, you should do the following *except*
   a. Keep all information about the person confidential
   b. Discuss the person's treatment or diagnosis with the nurse supervising your work
   c. Open the person's mail
   d. Allow the person to visit with others in private
3. What should you do if you suspect an older person is being abused?
   a. Report the situation to the health department.
   b. Notify the nurse and discuss the observations with him or her.
   c. Notify the doctor about the suspected abuse.
   d. Ask the family why they are abusing the person.
4. A resident needs help going to the bathroom. You do not answer her signal light promptly. She gets up without help, falls, and breaks a leg. This is an example of
   a. Negligence
   b. Defamation
   c. False imprisonment
   d. Slander
5. Examples of defamation include all the following *except*
   a. Implying or suggesting that a person uses drugs
   b. Saying that a person is insane or mentally ill
   c. Implying that a person steals money from staff
   d. Burning a resident with water that is too hot
6. Which statement about ethics is *false*?
   a. An ethical person does not judge others by his or her values and standards.
   b. An ethical person avoids persons whose standards and values differ from his or her own.
   c. An ethical person is not prejudiced or biased.
   d. An ethical person does not cause harm to another person.
7. Examples of false imprisonment include all of the following *except*
   a. Threatening to restrain a resident
   b. Restraining a resident without a doctor's order

   c. Treating the resident with respect
   d. Preventing a resident from leaving the agency
8. To protect yourself from being accused of assault and battery, you should explain to the resident what you plan to do before touching him or her and get consent.
   a. True
   b. False

Answers to these questions are on p. 521.

CHAPTER 5 WORK ETHICS

Health, Hygiene, and Appearance

- To give safe and effective care, you must be physically and mentally healthy. You need a balanced diet, sleep and rest, good body mechanics, and exercise on a regular basis.
- Personal hygiene needs careful attention. Bathe daily, use deodorant or antiperspirant, and brush your teeth often. Shampoo often. Keep fingernails clean, short, and neatly shaped.
- Review Box 5-1, Practices for a Professional Appearance, in the Textbook.

Teamwork

- Practice good work ethics—work when scheduled, be cheerful and friendly, perform delegated tasks, be kind to others, be available to help others.
- Be ready to work when your shift starts. Arrive on your nursing unit a few minutes early. Stay the entire shift. When it is time to leave, report off-duty to the nurse.
- A good attitude is needed. Review Box 5-2, Qualities and Traits for Good Work Ethics, in the Textbook.
- Gossiping is unprofessional and hurtful. To avoid being a part of **gossip:**
  ○ Remove yourself from a group or setting where people are gossiping.
  ○ Do not make or repeat any comment that can hurt another person or the agency.
  ○ Do not make or repeat any comment that you do not know is true.
  ○ Do not talk about residents, family members, patients, visitors, co-workers, or the agency at home or in social settings.
- **Confidentiality** means trusting others with personal and private information. The person's information is shared only among staff involved in his or her care. Agency, family and co-worker information also is confidential.
- Your speech and language must be professional:
  ○ Do not swear or use foul, vulgar, or abusive language.
  ○ Do not use slang.
  ○ Speak softly, gently, and clearly.
  ○ Do not shout or yell.
  ○ Do not fight or argue with a person, family member, visitor, or co-worker.
- A courtesy is a polite, considerate, or helpful comment or act.
  ○ Address others by Miss, Mrs., Ms., Mr., or Doctor. Use a first name only if the person asks you to do so.

- Say "please" and "thank you." Say "I'm sorry" when you make a mistake or hurt someone.
- Let residents, families, and visitors enter elevators first.
- Be thoughtful—compliment others, give praise.
- Wish the person and family well when they leave the center.
- Hold doors open for others.
- Help others willingly when asked.
- Do not take credit for another person's deeds. Give the person credit for the action.
- Keep personal matters out of the workplace:
  - Make personal phone calls during meals and breaks.
  - Do not let family and friends visit you on the unit.
  - Do not use the agency's computers and other equipment for personal use.
  - Do not take agency supplies for personal use.
  - Do not discuss personal problems at work.
  - Control your emotions.
  - Do not borrow money from or lend money to co-workers.
  - Do not sell things or engage in fund-raising at work.
  - Do not have wireless phones or personal pagers on while at work.
  - Do not text message.
- Leave for and return from breaks and meals on time. Tell the nurse when you leave and return to the unit.

Managing Stress

- These guidelines can help you reduce or cope with stress:
  - Exercise regularly.
  - Get enough sleep or rest.
  - Eat healthy.
  - Plan personal and quiet time for yourself.
  - Use common sense about what you can do.
  - Do one thing at a time.
  - Do not judge yourself harshly.
  - Give yourself praise.
  - Have a sense of humor.
  - Talk to the nurse if your work or a person is causing too much stress.

Harassment

- **Harassment** means to trouble, torment, offend, or worry a person by one's behavior or comments. Harassment can be sexual. Or it can involve age, race, ethnic background, religion, or disability. You must respect others. Do not offend others by your gestures, remarks, or use of touch. Do not offend others with jokes, photos, or other pictures.

CHAPTER 5 REVIEW QUESTIONS

Circle the BEST answer.

1. You believe you have good work ethics. This means you do the following *except*
   a. Work when scheduled
   b. Act cheerful and friendly
   c. Refuse to help others
   d. Perform tasks assigned by the nurse

2. A nursing assistant is gossiping about a co-worker. You should
   a. Stay with the group and listen to what is being said
   b. Repeat the comment to your family
   c. Remove yourself from the group where gossip is occurring
   d. Repeat the comment to another co-worker

3. You want to maintain confidentiality about others. You do the following *except*
   a. Share information about a resident with a nurse who is on another unit
   b. Avoid talking about a resident in the elevator, hallway, or dining area
   c. Avoid talking about co-workers and residents when others are present
   d. Avoid eavesdropping

4. When you are at work, you should do which of the following?
   a. Swear and use foul language.
   b. Use slang.
   c. Argue with a visitor.
   d. Speak clearly and softly.

5. To give safe and effective care, you do all the following *except*
   a. Eat a balanced diet
   b. Get enough sleep and rest
   c. Exercise on a regular basis
   d. Drink too much alcohol

6. While at work, you should do all of the following *except*
   a. Be courteous to others
   b. Make personal phone calls
   c. Admit when you are wrong or make mistakes
   d. Respect others

Answers to these questions are on p. 521.

CHAPTER 6   COMMUNICATING WITH THE HEALTH TEAM

Communication

- For good communication:
  - Use words that mean the same thing to you and the receiver of the message.
  - Use familiar words.
  - Be brief and concise.
  - Give information in a logical and orderly manner.
  - Give facts and be specific.

The Medical Record

- The **medical record, chart, clinical record** is a written or electronic account of a person's condition and response to treatment and care. It is a permanent legal document.
- The medical record is a way for the health team to share information about the person. If you know a person in the agency, but you do not give care to that person, you have no right to review the person's chart. To do so is an invasion of privacy.
- Only staff involved in person's care can review charts.
- A person or legal representative may ask you for the chart. Report the request to the nurse.
- Follow your agency's policies about recording in the medical record.

Reporting and Recording
- The health team communicates by reporting and recording.

Reporting
- You report care and observations to the nurse. Follow these rules:
  - Be prompt, thorough, and accurate.
  - Give the person's name, and room and bed numbers.
  - Give the time your observations were made or the care was given.
  - Report only what you observed or did yourself.
  - Report care measures that you expect the person to need.
  - Report expected changes in the person's condition.
  - Give reports as often as the person's condition requires or when the nurse asks you to.
  - Report any changes from normal or changes in the person's condition at once.
  - Use your written notes to give a specific, concise, and clear report.

Recording
- Rules for recording are:
  - Always use ink. Use the color required by the center.
  - Include the date and time for every recording.
  - Make sure writing is readable and neat.
  - Use only agency-approved abbreviations.
  - Use correct spelling, grammar, and punctuation.
  - Do not use ditto marks.
  - Never erase or use correction fluid. Follow agency procedure for correcting errors.
  - Sign all entries with your name and title as required by agency policy.
  - Do not skip lines.
  - Make sure each form has the person's name and other identifying information.
  - Record only what you observed and did yourself.
  - Never chart a procedure, treatment, or care measure until after it is completed.
  - Be accurate, concise, and factual. Do not record judgments or interpretations.
  - Record in a logical and sequential manner.
  - Be descriptive. Avoid terms with more than one meaning.
  - Use the person's exact words whenever possible. Use quotation marks to show that the statement is a direct quote.
  - Chart any changes from normal or changes in the person's condition. Also chart that you informed the nurse (include the nurse's name), what you told the nurse, and the time you made the report.
  - Do not omit information.
  - Record safety measures. Example: Reminding a person not to get out of bed.
- Review the 24-hour clock, Figure 6-6, and Box 6-1 in the Textbook.

Medical Terminology and Abbreviations
- Medical terminology and abbreviations are used in health care. Someone may use a word or phrase that you do not understand. If so, ask the nurse to explain its meaning.
- Review Box 6-3, Medical Terminology, and Box 6-4, Common Health Care Terms and Phrases, in the Textbook.

- Use only the abbreviations accepted by the center. If you are not sure that an abbreviation is acceptable, write the term out in full. See the inside back cover of the Textbook for common abbreviations.

Computers and Other Electronic Devices
- Computers contain vast amounts of information about a person. Therefore the right to privacy must be protected. If allowed access, you must follow the agency's policies. Review Box 6-5, Using the Agency's Computer and Other Electronic Devices, in the Textbook.

Phone Communications
- Guidelines for answering phones:
  - Answer the call after the first ring if possible.
  - Do not answer the phone in a rushed or hasty manner.
  - Give a courteous greeting. Identify the nursing unit and your name and title.
  - When taking a message, write down the caller's name, phone number, date and time, and message.
  - Repeat the message and phone number back to the caller.
  - Ask the caller to "Please hold" if necessary.
  - Do not lay the phone down or cover the receiver with your hand when not speaking to the caller. The caller may hear confidential information.
  - Return to a caller on hold within 30 seconds.
  - Do not give confidential information to any caller.
  - Transfer a call if appropriate. Tell the caller you are going to transfer the call. Give the name and phone number in case the call gets disconnected or line is busy.
  - End the conversation politely.
  - Give the message to the appropriate person.

Dealing With Conflict
- These guidelines can help you deal with conflict:
  - Ask your supervisor for some time to talk privately about the problem.
  - Approach the person with whom you have the conflict. Ask to talk privately. Be polite and professional.
  - Agree on a time and place to talk.
  - Talk in a private setting. No one should hear you or the other person.
  - Explain the problem and what is bothering you. Give facts and specific behaviors. Focus on the problem. Do not focus on the person.
  - Listen to the person. Do not interrupt.
  - Identify ways to solve the problem. Offer your thoughts. Ask for the co-worker's ideas.
  - Set a date and time to review the matter.
  - Thank the person for meeting with you.
  - Carry out the solution.
  - Review the matter as scheduled.

CHAPTER 6 REVIEW QUESTIONS

Circle the BEST answer.

1. For good communication, you should do the following *except*
   a. Use words with more than one meaning
   b. Use familiar words to the person or family
   c. Give facts in a brief and concise manner
   d. Give information in a logical and orderly manner

2. When you record in a person's chart, you do the following *except*
   a. Record what you observed and did
   b. Record the person's response to the treatment or procedure
   c. Use abbreviations that are not on the accepted list for the center
   d. Record the time the observation was made or the treatment performed
3. When reporting care and observations to the nurse, you do the following *except*
   a. Give the person's name and room and bed numbers
   b. Report only what you observed or did yourself
   c. Report any changes from normal or changes in the person's condition at once
   d. Report any changes from normal or changes in the person's condition at the end of the shift

Answers to these questions are on p. 521.

CHAPTER 7 ASSISTING WITH THE NURSING PROCESS

- The **nursing process** is the method nurses use to plan and deliver nursing care. It has five steps: assessment, nursing diagnosis, planning, implementation, and evaluation.
- You play a key role by making observations as you care and talk with the person.
- **Assessment** involves collecting information about the person. Nurses use many sources. A health history is taken. An RN assesses the person's body systems and mental systems. You play a key role in assessment. You make many observation as you give care and talk to the person.
- **Observation** is using the senses of sight, hearing, touch, and smell to collect information. Box 7-1, Basic Observations, in the Textbook lists the basic observations you need to make and report to the nurse. Examples are:
  - Can the person give his or her name, the time, and location when asked?
  - Can the person move the arms and legs?
  - Is the skin pale or flushed?
  - Is there drainage from the eyes? What color is the drainage?
  - Does the person like the food served?
  - Can the person bathe without help?
- Observations you need to report to the nurse at once are (see Box 7-1 in the Textbook):
  - A change in the person's ability to respond
    - A responsive person no longer responds
    - A non-responsive person now responds
  - A change in the person's mobility
    - The person cannot move a body part.
    - The person can now move a body part.
  - Complaints of sudden, severe pain
  - A sore or reddened area on the person's skin
  - Complaints of a sudden change in vision
  - Complaints of pain or difficulty breathing
  - Abnormal respirations
  - Complaints of or signs of difficulty swallowing
  - Vomiting
  - Bleeding
  - Vital signs outside their normal ranges

- **Objective data (signs)** are seen, heard, felt, or smelled by an observer. For example, you can feel a pulse.
- **Subjective data (symptoms)** are things a person tells you about that you cannot observe through your senses. For example, you cannot see the person's nausea.
- The nurse communicates delegated tasks to you. This is the purpose of an assignment sheet. An assignment sheet tells you about each person's care, what measures and tasks need to be done and which nursing unit tasks to do. Talk to the nurse about any unclear assignment.

Resident Care Conferences

- The RN may conduct a care conference to share information and ideas about the person's care. The RN, nursing assistants, and other health team members take part in the conference. The person has the right to take part in care planning conferences. Sometimes the family is involved. The person may refuse actions suggested by the health team.

CHAPTER 7 REVIEW QUESTIONS

Circle the BEST answer.
1. Which statement about observations is *false*?
   a. You make observations as you care and talk with people.
   b. Observation uses the senses of smell, sight, touch, and hearing.
   c. A reddened area on the person's skin is reported to the nurse at once.
   d. You report observations to the doctor.
2. Objective data include all the following *except*
   a. The person has pain in his abdomen
   b. The person's pulse is 76
   c. The person's urine is dark amber
   d. The person's breath has an odor

Answers to these questions are on p. 521.

CHAPTER 8 UNDERSTANDING THE PERSON

Caring for the Person

- The whole person needs to be considered when you provide care—physical, social, psychological, and spiritual parts. These parts are woven together and cannot be separated.
- Follow these rules to address persons with dignity and respect:
  - Call persons by their titles—Mrs. Dennison, Mr. Smith, Miss Turner, or Dr. Gonzalez.
  - Do not call persons by their first names unless they ask you to.
  - Do not call persons by any other name unless they ask you to.
  - Do not call persons Grandma, Papa, Sweetheart, Honey, or other name.

Basic Needs

- A **need** is something necessary or desired for maintaining life and mental well-being.

- According to Maslow, basic needs must be met for a person to survive and function. Needs are arranged in order of importance, lower-level to higher level:
  - *Physiological or physical needs*—are required for life. They are oxygen, food, water, elimination, rest, and shelter.
  - *Safety and security needs*—relate to feeling safe from harm, danger, and fear.
  - *Love and belonging needs*—relate to love, closeness, affection, and meaningful relationships with others. Family, friends, and the health team can meet love and belonging needs.
  - *Self-esteem needs*—relate to thinking well of oneself and to seeing oneself as useful and having value. People often lack self-esteem when ill, injured, older, or disabled.
  - *The need for self-actualization*—involves learning, understanding, and creating to the limit of a person's capacity. Rarely, if ever, is it totally met.

Culture and Religion

- **Culture** is the characteristics of a group of people. People come from many cultures, races, and nationalities. Family practices, food choices, hygiene habits, clothing styles, and language are part of their culture. The person's culture also influences health beliefs and practices.
- **Religion** relates to spiritual beliefs, needs, and practices. A person's religion influences health and illness practices. Many may want to pray and observe religious practices. Assist residents to attend religious services as needed. If a person wants to see a spiritual leader or advisor, tell the nurse. Provide privacy during the visit.
- A person may not follow all the beliefs and practices of his or her culture or religion. Some people do not practice a religion.
- Respect and accept the person's culture and religion. Learn about practices and beliefs different from your own. Do not judge a person by your standards.

Communicating With the Person

- For effective communication between you and the person, you must:
  - Follow the rules of communication in Chapter 6.
  - Understand and respect the patient or resident as a person.
  - View the person as a physical, psychological, social, and spiritual human being.
  - Appreciate the person's problems and frustrations.
  - Respect the person's rights.
  - Respect the person's religion and culture.
  - Give the person time to understand the information that you give.
  - Repeat information as often as needed.
  - Ask questions to see if the person understood you.
  - Be patient. People with memory problems may ask the same question many times.
  - Include the person in conversations when others are present.

Verbal Communication

- When talking with a person follow these rules:
  - Face the person. Look directly at the person.
  - Position yourself at the person's eye level.
  - Control the loudness and tone of your voice.
  - Speak clearly, slowly, and distinctly.
  - Do not use slang or vulgar words.
  - Repeat information as needed.
  - Ask one question at a time, and wait for an answer.
  - Do not shout, whisper, or mumble.
  - Be kind, courteous, and friendly.
- Use written words if the person cannot speak or hear but can read. Keep written messages brief and concise. Use a black felt pen on white paper, and print in large letters.
- Some persons cannot speak or read. Ask questions that have "yes" and "no" answers. A picture board may be helpful.

Nonverbal Communication

- Messages are sent with gestures, facial expressions, posture, body movements, touch, and smell. Nonverbal messages more accurately reflect a person's feelings than words do. A person may say one thing but act another way. Watch the person's eyes, hand movements, gestures, posture, and other actions.
- Touch conveys comfort, caring, love, affection, interest, trust, concern, and reassurance. Touch should be gentle. Touch means different things to different people. Some people do not like to be touched. To use touch, follow the care plan. Maintain profession boundaries.
- People send messages through their **body language**—facial expressions, gestures, posture, hand and body movements, gait, eye contact, and appearance. Your body language should show interest, enthusiasm, caring, and respect for the person. Often you need to control your body language. Control reactions to odors from body fluids, secretions, or excretions.

Communication Methods

- *Listening* means to focus on verbal and nonverbal communication. You use sight, hearing, touch, and smell. To be a good listener:
  - Face the person.
  - Have good eye contact with the person.
  - Lean toward the person. Do not sit back with your arms crossed.
  - Respond to the person. Nod your head, and ask questions.
  - Avoid communication barriers.
- *Paraphrasing* is restating the person's message in your own words.
- *Direct questions* focus on certain information. You ask the person something you need to know.
- *Open-ended questions* lead or invite the person to share thoughts, feelings, or ideas. The person chooses what to talk about.
- *Clarifying* lets you make sure that you understand the message. You can ask the person to repeat the message, say you do not understand, or restate the message.
- *Focusing* deals with a certain topic. It is useful when a person wanders in thought.

- *Silence* is a very powerful way to communicate. Silence gives time to think, organize thoughts, choose words, make decisions, and gain control. Silence on your part shows caring and respect for the person's situation and feelings.

Communication Barriers

- *Language.* You and the person must use and understand the same language.
- *Cultural differences.* A person from another country may attach different meanings to verbal and nonverbal communication from what you intended.
- *Changing the subject.* Avoid changing the subject whenever possible.
- *Giving your opinions.* Opinions involve judging values, behaviors, or feelings. Let others express feelings and concerns without adding your opinion. Do not make judgments or jump to conclusions.
- *Talking a lot when others are silent.* Talking too much is usually because of nervousness and discomfort with silence.
- *Failure to listen.* Do not pretend to listen. It shows lack of caring and interest. You may miss complaints of pain, discomfort, or other symptoms that you must report to the nurse.
- *Pat answers.* "Don't worry." "Everything will be okay." These make the person feel that you do not care about his or her concerns, feelings, and fears.
- *Illness and disability.* Speech, hearing, vision, cognitive function, and body movements may be affected. Verbal and nonverbal communication is affected.
- *Age.* Values and communication styles vary among age-groups.

Persons With Disabilities

- Common courtesies and manners apply to any person with a disability. Review Box 8-1, Disability Etiquette, in the Textbook.
- The person who is comatose is unconscious and cannot respond to others. Often the person can hear, feel touch and pain. Assume that the person hears and understands you. Use touch and give care gently. Practice these measures:
- Knock before entering the person's room.
- Tell the person your name, the time, and the place every time you enter the room.
- Give care on the same schedule every day.
- Explain what you are going to do.
- Tell the person when you are finishing care.
- Use touch to communicate care, concern, and comfort.
- Tell the person what time you will be back to check on him or her.
- Tell the person when you are leaving the room.

Family and Friends

- If you need to give care when visitors are there, protect the person's right to privacy. Politely ask the visitors to leave the room when you give care. A partner or family member may help you if the patient or resident consents.
- Treat family and visitors with courtesy and respect.
- Do not discuss the person's condition with family and friends. Refer questions to the nurse. A visitor may upset or tire a person. Report your observations to the nurse.

Behavior Issues

- Many people do not adjust well to illness, injury, and disability. They have some of the following behaviors:
  - *Anger.* Anger may be communicated verbally and nonverbally. Verbal outbursts, shouting, and rapid speech are common. Some people are silent. Others are uncooperative and may refuse to answer questions. Nonverbal signs include rapid movements, pacing, clenched fists, and a red face. Glaring and getting close to you when speaking are other signs. Violent behaviors can occur.
  - *Demanding behavior.* Nothing seems to please the person. The person is critical of others.
  - *Self-centered behavior.* The person cares only about his or her own needs. The needs of others are ignored. The person becomes impatient if needs are not met.
  - *Aggressive behavior.* The person may swear, bite, hit, pinch, scratch, or kick. Protect the person, others, and yourself from harm.
  - *Withdrawal.* The person has little or no contact with family, friends, and staff. Some people are generally not social and prefer to be alone.
    - *Inappropriate sexual behavior.* Some people make inappropriate sexual remarks or touch others in the wrong way. These behaviors may be on purpose. Or they are caused by disease, confusion, dementia, or drug side effects.
- You cannot avoid persons with unpleasant behaviors or lose control. Review Box 8-2, Dealing With Behavior Issues, in the Textbook.

CHAPTER 8 REVIEW QUESTIONS

Circle the BEST answer.

1. While caring for a person, you need to
   a. Consider only the person's physical and social needs
   b. Consider the person's physical, social, psychological, and spiritual needs
   c. Consider only the person's cultural needs
   d. Ignore the person's spiritual needs
2. When referring to residents, you should
   a. Refer to them by their room number
   b. Call them "Honey"
   c. Call them by their first name
   d. Call them by their name and title
3. Based on Maslow's theory of basic needs, which person's needs must be met first?
   a. The person who wants to talk about her granddaughter's wedding
   b. The person who is uncomfortable in the dining room
   c. The person who wants mail opened
   d. The person who asks for more water
4. Which statement about culture is *false*?
   a. A person's culture influences health beliefs and practices.
   b. You must respect a person's culture.
   c. You should ignore the person's culture while you give his or her care.
   d. You should learn about another person's culture that is different from yours.

5. Which statement about religion and spiritual beliefs is *false?*
   a. A person's religion influences health and illness practices.
   b. You should assist a person to attend services in the nursing center.
   c. Many people find comfort and strength from religion during illness.
   d. A person must follow all beliefs of his or her religion.

6. A person is angry and is shouting at you. You should do the following *except*
   a. Stay calm and professional
   b. Yell so the person will listen to you
   c. Listen to what the person is saying
   d. Report the person's behavior to the nurse

7. A person tries to scratch and kick you. You should
   a. Protect yourself from harm
   b. Argue with the person
   c. Become angry with the person
   d. Refuse to care for the person

8. When speaking with another person, you do the following *except*
   a. Position yourself at the person's eye level
   b. Speak slowly, clearly, and distinctly
   c. Shout, mumble, and whisper
   d. Ask one question at a time

9. Which statement about listening is *false?*
   a. You use sight, hearing, touch, and smell when you listen.
   b. You observe nonverbal cues.
   c. You have good eye contact with the person.
   d. You sit back with your arms crossed.

10. Which statement about silence is *false?*
    a. Silence is a powerful way to communicate.
    b. Silence gives people time to think.
    c. You should talk a lot when the other person is silent.
    d. Silence helps when the person is upset and needs to gain control.

11. A person speaks a foreign language. You should do the following *except*
    a. Keep messages short and simple
    b. Use gestures and pictures
    c. Shout or speak loudly
    d. Repeat the message in other words

12. When caring for a person who is comatose, you do the following *except*
    a. Tell the person your name when you enter the room
    b. Explain what you are doing
    c. Use touch to communicate care and comfort
    d. Make jokes about how sick the person is

13. A person is in a wheelchair. You should do all the following *except*
    a. Lean on a person's wheelchair
    b. Sit or squat to talk to a person in a wheelchair or chair
    c. Think about obstacles before giving directions to a person in a wheelchair
    d. Extend the same courtesies to the person as you would to anyone else

14. A person's daughter is visiting and you need to provide care to the person. You
    a. Expose the person's body in front of the visitor
    b. Politely ask the visitor to leave the room
    c. Decide to not provide the care at all
    d. Discuss the person's condition with the visitor

Answers to these questions are on p. 521.

CHAPTER 10 GROWTH AND DEVELOPMENT

- **Growth** is the physical changes that are measured and that occur in a steady and orderly manner.
- **Development** relates to changes in mental, emotional, and social function.
- Growth and development occur in a sequence, order, and pattern. Review the stages of growth and development detailed in the Textbook.
- Middle Adulthood (40 to 65 years old). At this stage, developmental tasks are: adjusting to physical changes, having grown children, developing leisure-time activities, adjusting to aging parents.
- Late Adulthood (65 years and older). At this stage, developmental tasks are: Adjusting to decreased strength and loss of health, adjusting to retirement and reduced income, coping with a partner's death, developing new friends and relationships, preparing for one's own death.

CHAPTER 10 REVIEW QUESTIONS

Circle the BEST answer.

1. Growth and development occur in a sequence, order, and pattern.
   a. True
   b. False

2. Growth relates to changes in mental, emotional, and social function.
   a. True
   b. False

3. Which is a developmental task of late adulthood?
   a. Accepting changes in appearance
   b. Adjusting to decreased strength
   c. Developing a satisfactory sex life
   d. Performing self-care

Answers to these questions are on p. 521.

CHAPTER 11 CARE OF THE OLDER PERSON

- Aging is normal. It is not a disease. Normal changes occur in body structure and function. Psychological and social changes also occur.

Social Changes

- Physical reminders of growing old affect self-esteem and may threaten self-image, feelings of self-worth, and independence.
- People cope with aging in their own way. How they cope depends on their health status, life experiences, finances, education, and social support systems.
- *Retirement.* Many people enjoy retirement. Others are in poor health and have medical bills that can make retirement hard.

- *Reduced income.* Retirement usually means reduced income. The retired person still has expenses. Reduced income may force life-style changes. One example is the person avoids health care or needed drugs.
- *Social relationships.* Social relationships change throughout life. Family time helps prevent loneliness. So do hobbies, religious and community events, and new friends.
- *Children as caregivers.* Some older persons feel more secure when children care for them. Others feel unwanted and useless. Some lose dignity and self-respect. Tensions may occur among the child, parent, and other household members.
- *Death of a partner.* When death occurs, the person loses a lover, friend, companion, and confidant. Grief may be great. The person's life will likely change.

Physical Changes

- Body processes slow down. Energy level and body efficiency decline.
- *The integumentary system.* The skin loses its elasticity, strength, and fatty tissue layer. Wrinkles appear. Dry skin occurs and may cause itching. The skin is fragile and easily injured. The person is more sensitive to cold. Nails become thick and tough. Feet may have poor circulation. White or gray hair is common. Hair thins. Facial hair may occur in women. Hair is drier. The risk of skin cancer increases.
- *The musculoskeletal system.* Muscle and bone strength are lost. Bones become brittle and break easily. Vertebrae shorten. Joints become stiff and painful. Mobility decreases. There is a gradual loss of height.
- *The nervous system.* Confusion, dizziness, and fatigue may occur. Responses are slower. The risk for falls increases. Forgetfulness increases. Memory is shorter. Events from long ago are remembered better than recent ones. Older persons have a harder time falling asleep. Sleep periods are shorter. Older persons wake often during the night and have less deep sleep. Less sleep is needed. They may rest or nap during the day. They may go to bed early and get up early.
- *The senses.* Hearing and vision losses occur. Taste and smell dull. Appetite decreases. Touch and sensitivity to pain, pressure, hot, and cold are reduced.
- *The circulatory system.* The heart muscle weakens. Arteries narrow and are less elastic. Poor circulation occurs in many body parts.
- *The respiratory system.* Respiratory muscles weaken. Lung tissue becomes less elastic. Difficult, labored, or painful breathing may occur with activity. The person may lack strength to cough and clear the airway of secretions. Respiratory infections and diseases may develop.
- *The digestive system.* Less saliva is produced. The person may have difficulty swallowing (dysphagia). Indigestion may occur. Loss of teeth and ill-fitting dentures cause chewing problems and digestion problems. Flatulence and constipation can occur. Fewer calories are needed as energy and activity levels decline. More fluids are needed.
- *The urinary system.* Urine is more concentrated. Bladder muscles weaken. Bladder size decreases. Urinary frequency or urgency may occur. Urinary tract infections are risks. Many older persons have to urinate at night. Urinary incontinence may occur. In men, the prostate gland enlarges. This may cause difficulty urinating or frequent urination.
- *The reproductive system.* In men, testosterone decreases. An erection takes longer. Orgasm is less forceful. Women experience menopause. Female hormones of estrogen and progesterone decrease. The uterus, vagina, and genitalia shrink (atrophy). Vaginal walls thin. There is vaginal dryness. Arousal takes longer. Orgasm is less intense.

Housing Options

- A person's home is more than a place to live. It holds memories, is a link to neighbors and communities and brings pride and self-esteem. Aging can lead to changes in a person's home setting.
- Most older people live in their own homes. Others need help from family or community agencies. Review Box 11-3, In-Home and Community-Based Services

Nursing Centers

- The person needing nursing center care may suffer some or all of these losses:
  - Loss of identity as a productive member of a family and community
  - Loss of possessions—home, household items, car, and so on
  - Loss of independence
  - Loss of real-world experiences—shopping, traveling, cooking, driving, hobbies
  - Loss of health and mobility
- The person may feel useless, powerless, and hopeless. The health team helps the person cope with loss and improve quality of life. Treat the person with dignity and respect. Also practice good communication skills. Follow the care plan.

CHAPTER 11 REVIEW QUESTIONS

Circle the BEST answer.

1. Which statement is *false?*
   a. Physical changes occur with aging.
   b. Energy level and body efficiency decline with age.
   c. Some people age faster than others.
   d. Normal aging means loss of health.
2. As a person ages, the integumentary system changes. Which statement is *false?*
   a. Dry skin and itching occur.
   b. Nails become thick and tough.
   c. The person is less sensitive to cold.
   d. Skin is injured more easily.
3. Which statement is *false* about the musculo-skeletal system and aging?
   a. Strength decreases.
   b. Vertebrae shorten.
   c. Mobility increases.
   d. Bone mass decreases.

4. Which statement about the nervous system and aging is *false*?
   a. Reflexes slow.
   b. Memory may be shorter.
   c. Sleep patterns change.
   d. Forgetfulness decreases.
5. Which statement about the digestive system and aging is *false*?
   a. Appetite decreases.
   b. Less saliva is produced.
   c. Flatulence and constipation may decrease.
   d. Teeth may be lost.
6. Which statement about the urinary system and aging is *false*?
   a. Urine becomes more concentrated.
   b. Urinary frequency may occur.
   c. Urinary urgency may occur.
   d. Bladder muscles become stronger.

Answers to these questions are on p. 521.

CHAPTER 12 SAFETY
Accident Risk Factors
- *Age*. Older persons are at risk for falls and other injuries.
- *Awareness of surroundings*. People need to know their surroundings to protect themselves from injury.
- *Agitated and aggressive behaviors*. Pain, confusion, fear, and decreased awareness of surroundings can cause these behaviors.
- *Vision loss*. Persons can fall or trip over items. Some have problems reading labels on containers.
- *Hearing loss*. Persons have problems hearing explanations and instructions. They may not hear warning signals or fire alarms. They do not know to move to safety.
- *Impaired smell and touch*. Illness and aging affect smell and touch. The person may not detect smoke or gas, or may be unaware of injury. Burns are a risk.
- *Impaired mobility*. Some diseases and injuries affect mobility. A person may know there is danger but cannot move to safety. Some persons are paralyzed. Some persons cannot walk or propel wheelchairs.
- *Drugs*. Drugs have side effects. Reduced awareness, confusion, and disorientation can occur. Report behavior changes and the person's complaints.

Identifying the Person
- You must give the right care to the right person. To identify the person:
   - Compare identifying information on the assignment sheet or treatment card with that on the identification (ID) bracelet.
   - Call the person by name when checking the ID bracelet. Just calling the person by name is not enough to identify him or her. Confused, disoriented, drowsy, hard-of-hearing, or distracted persons may answer to any name.
   - Some nursing centers have photo ID systems. Use this system safely.
   - Alert and oriented persons may choose not to wear ID bracelets. Follow center policy and the care plan to identify the person.
   - Use at least 2 identifiers. Agencies have different requirements. Some may require the person state and spell his or her name and give birth date. Others require using the person's ID number. Always follow agency policy.

Preventing Burns
- Smoking, spilled hot liquids, very hot water, and electrical devices are common causes of burns. See Box 12-2 in the Textbook for safety measures to prevent burns.

Preventing Poisoning
- Drugs and household products are common poisons. Poisoning in adults may be from carelessness, confusion, or poor vision when reading labels. To prevent poisoning:
   - Make sure patients and residents cannot reach hazardous materials.
   - Follow agency policy for storing personal care items.
- See Box 12-3 in the Textbook for safety measures to prevent poisoning.

Preventing Suffocation
- **Suffocation** is when breathing stops from the lack of oxygen. Death occurs if the person does not start breathing.
- To prevent suffocation, review Box 12-6, Safety Measures to Prevent Suffocation, in the Textbook.

Choking
- Choking or foreign-body airway obstruction (FBAO) occurs when a foreign body obstructs the airway. Air cannot pass through the air passages into the lungs. The body does not get enough oxygen. This can lead to cardiac arrest.
- Choking often occurs during eating. A large, poorly chewed piece of meat is the most common cause. Other common causes include laughing and talking while eating.
- With *mild airway obstruction*, some air moves in and out of the lungs. The person is conscious. Usually the person can speak. Often forceful coughing can remove the object.
- With *severe airway obstruction*, the conscious person clutches at the throat—the "universal sign of choking." The person has difficulty breathing. Some persons cannot breathe, speak, or cough. The person appears pale and cyanotic (bluish color). Air does not move in and out of the lungs. If the obstruction is not removed, the person will die. Severe airway obstruction is an emergency.
- Use abdominal thrusts to relieve FBAO. Chest thrusts are used for very obese persons and pregnant women.
- Call for help when a person has an obstructed airway. Report and record what happened, what you did, and the person's response.

Preventing Equipment Accidents
- All equipment is unsafe if broken, not used correctly, or not working properly. Inspect all equipment before use. Review Box 12-8, Safety Measures to Prevent Equipment Accidents, in the Textbook.

Wheelchair and Stretcher Safety

- Review Box 12-9, Wheelchair and Stretcher Safety, in the Textbook.

Handling Hazardous Substances

- A hazardous substance is any chemical in the workplace that can cause harm. Hazardous substances include oxygen, mercury, disinfectants, and cleaning agents.
- Hazardous substance containers must have a warning label. If a label is removed or damaged, do not use the substance. Take the container to the nurse. Do not leave the container unattended.
- Check the material safety data sheet (MSDS) before using a hazardous substance, cleaning up a leak or spill, or disposing of the substance. Tell the nurse about a leak or spill right away. Do not leave a leak or spill unattended. Review Box 12-10 in the Textbook.

Fire Safety

- Faulty electrical equipment and wiring, overloaded electrical circuits, and smoking are major causes of fires.
- Safety measures are needed where oxygen is used and stored:
  - "NO SMOKING" signs are placed on the door and near the person's bed.
  - The person and visitors are reminded not to smoke in the room.
  - Smoking materials are removed from the room.
  - Electrical items are turned off before being unplugged.
  - Wool blankets and fabrics that cause static electricity are not used.
  - The person wears a cotton gown or pajamas.
  - Electrical items are in good working order.
  - Lit candles and other open flames are not allowed.
  - Materials that ignite easily are removed from the room.
- Review Box 12-11, Fire Prevention Measures, in the Textbook.
- Know your center's policies and procedures for fire emergencies. Know where to find fire alarms, fire extinguishers, and emergency exits. Remember the word RACE:
  - R—*rescue*. Rescue persons in immediate danger. Move them to a safe place.
  - A—*alarm*. Sound the nearest fire alarm. Notify the telephone operator.
  - C—*confine*. Close doors and windows. Turn off oxygen or electrical items.
  - E—*extinguish*. Use a fire extinguisher on a small fire.
- Remember the word PASS for using a fire extinguisher:
  - P—*pull* the safety pin.
  - A—*aim* low. Aim at the base of the fire.
  - S—*squeeze* the lever. This starts the stream of water.
  - S—*sweep* back and forth. Sweep side to side at the base of the fire.
- Do not use elevators during a fire.

Disasters

- A **disaster** is a sudden catastrophic event. The agency has procedures for disasters that could occur in your

area. Follow them to keep patients, residents, visitors, staff, and yourself safe.

Workplace Violence

- **Workplace violence** is violent acts (including assault or threat of assault) directed toward persons at work or while on duty. Review Box 12-12, Measures to Prevent or Control Workplace Violence, in the Textbook.

CHAPTER 12 REVIEW QUESTIONS

Circle the BEST answer.

1. You see a water spill in the hallway. What will you do?
   a. Ask housekeeping to wipe up the spill right away.
   b. Wipe up the spill right away.
   c. Report the spill to the nurse.
   d. Ask the resident to walk around the spill.
2. An electrical outlet in a person's room does not work. What will you do?
   a. Tell the administrator about the problem.
   b. Tell another nursing assistant about the problem.
   c. Try to repair the electrical outlet.
   d. Follow the center's policy for reporting the problem.
3. Accident risk factors include all of the following *except*
   a. Walking without difficulty
   b. Hearing problems
   c. Dulled sense of smell
   d. Poor vision
4. To prevent a person from being burned, you should do the following *except*
   a. Supervise the smoking of persons who are confused
   b. Turn cold water on first; turn hot water off first
   c. Do not let the person sleep with a heating pad
   d. Allow smoking in bed
5. To prevent suffocation, you should do the following *except*
   a. Make sure dentures fit properly
   b. Check the care plan for swallowing problems before serving food or liquids
   c. Leave a person alone in a bathtub or shower
   d. Position the person in bed properly
6. Which statement about mild airway obstruction is *false*?
   a. Some air moves in and out of the lungs.
   b. The person is conscious.
   c. Usually the person cannot speak.
   d. Forceful coughing will often remove the object.
7. The "universal sign of choking" is
   a. Clutching at the chest
   b. Clutching at the throat
   c. Not being able to talk
   d. Not being able to breathe
8. Which statement about wheelchair safety is *false*?
   a. Lock the wheels before transferring a resident to or from a wheelchair.
   b. The person's feet should rest on the footplate when you are pushing the wheelchair.
   c. Let the footplates fall back onto a person's legs.
   d. Check for flat or loose tires.

9. Which of the following is *not* a safety measure with oxygen?
   a. "No Smoking" signs are placed on the resident's door and near the bed.
   b. Lit candles and other open flames are permitted in the room.
   c. Electrical items are turned off before being unplugged.
   d. The person wears a cotton gown or pajamas.
10. You have discovered a fire in the nursing center. You should do the following *except*
    a. Rescue persons in immediate danger
    b. Sound the nearest fire alarm
    c. Open doors and windows, and keep oxygen on
    d. Use a fire extinguisher on a small fire that has not spread to a larger area
11. When using a fire extinguisher, you do the following *except*
    a. Pull the safety pin on the fire extinguisher
    b. Aim at the top of the flames
    c. Squeeze the lever to start the stream
    d. Sweep the stream back and forth

Answers to these questions are on p. 521.

CHAPTER 13 PREVENTING FALLS

- Falls are a leading cause of injuries and deaths among older persons. A history of falls increases the risk of falling again.
- Most falls occur in resident rooms and bathrooms. Most occur between 1600 (4:00 PM) and 2000 (8:00 PM). Falls are more likely during shift changes.
- Causes for falls are poor lighting, cluttered floors, throwrugs, needing to use the bathroom, and out-of-place furniture. So are wet and slippery floors, bathtubs, and showers. Review Box 13-1, Factors Increasing the Risk of Falls, in the Textbook.
- Agencies have fall prevention programs. Review Box 13-2, Safety Measures to Prevent Falls, in the Textbook. The person's care plan also lists measures specific for the person.

Bed Rails

- A **bed rail** (*side rail*) is a device that serves as a guard or barrier along the side of the bed.
- The nurse and care plan tell you when to raise bed rails. They are needed by persons who are unconscious or sedated with drugs. Some confused and disoriented people need them. If a person needs bed rails, keep them up at all times except when giving bedside nursing care.
- Bed rails present hazards. The person can fall when trying to get out of bed. Or the person can get caught, trapped, entangled, or strangled.
- Bed rails are considered restraints if the person cannot get out of bed or lower them without help.
- Bed rails cannot be used unless they are needed to treat a person's medical symptoms. The person or legal representative must give consent for raised bed rails. The need for bed rails is carefully noted in the person's medical record and the care plan. If a person uses bed

rails, check the person often. Record when you checked the person and your observations.

- To prevent falls:
  ○ Never leave the person alone when the bed is raised.
  ○ Always lower the bed to its lowest position when you are done giving care.
  ○ If a person does not use bed rails and you need to raise the bed, ask a co-worker to stand on the far side of the bed to protect the person from falling.
  ○ If you raise the bed to give care, always raise the far bed rail if you are working alone.
  ○ Be sure the person who uses raised bed rails has access to items on the bedside stand and overbed table. The signal light, water pitcher and cup, tissues, phone, and TV and light controls should be within the person's reach.

Hand Rails and Grab Bars

- Hand rails give support to persons who are weak or unsteady when walking.
- Grab bars provide support for sitting down or getting up from a toilet. They also are used for getting in and out of the shower or tub.

Wheel Locks

- Bed wheels are locked at all times except when moving the bed.
- Wheelchair and stretcher wheels are locked when transferring a person.

Transfer/Gait Belts

- Use a **transfer belt (gait belt)** to support a person who is unsteady or disabled. Always follow the manufacturer's instructions. Apply the belt over clothing and under the breasts. The belt buckle is never positioned over the person's spine. Tighten the belt so it is snug. You should be able to slide your open, flat hand under the belt. Tuck the excess strap under the belt. Remove the belt after the procedure.
- Check with the nurse and care plan before using a transfer/gait belt if the person has:
  ○ A colostomy, ileostomy, gastrostomy, urostomy
  ○ A gastric tube
  ○ Chronic obstructive pulmonary disease
  ○ An abdominal wound, incision, or drainage tube
  ○ A chest wound, incision, or drainage tube
  ○ Monitoring equipment
  ○ A hernia
  ○ Other conditions or care equipment involving the chest or abdomen

The Falling Person

- If a person starts to fall, do not try to prevent the fall. You could injure yourself and the person. Ease the person to the floor, and protect the person's head. Do not let the person get up before the nurse checks for injuries. An incident report is completed after all falls.
- Review Box 13-4, *Helping the Falling Person*, in the Textbook.

CHAPTER 13 REVIEW QUESTIONS

Circle the BEST answer.

1. Most falls occur in
   a. Resident rooms and bathrooms
   b. Dining rooms
   c. Hallways
   d. Activity rooms
2. Which statement about falls is *false?*
   a. Poor lighting, cluttered floors, and throw rugs may cause falls.
   b. Improper shoes and needing to use the bathroom may cause falls.
   c. Most falls occur between 4:00 PM and 8:00 PM.
   d. Falls are less likely to occur during shift changes.
3. You note the following after a person got dressed. Which is unsafe?
   a. Non-skid footwear is worn.
   b. Pant cuffs are dragging on the floor.
   c. Clothing fits properly.
   d. The belt is fastened.
4. Which statement about bed rails is *false?*
   a. The nurse and care plan tell you when to raise bed rails.
   b. Bed rails are considered restraints.
   c. You may leave a person alone when the bed is raised and the bed rails are down.
   d. Bed rails can present hazards because people try to climb over them.
5. Which statement about transfer/gait belts is *false?*
   a. To use the belt safely, follow the manufacturer's instructions.
   b. Always apply the belt over clothing.
   c. Tighten the belt so it is very snug and breathing is impaired.
   d. Place the belt buckle off center so it is not over the spine.
6. A person becomes faint in the hallway and begins to fall. You should do the following *except*
   a. Ease the person to the floor
   b. Protect the person's head
   c. Let the person get up before the nurse checks him or her
   d. Help the nurse complete the incident report

Answers to these questions are on p. 521.

CHAPTER 14 RESTRAINT ALTERNATIVES AND SAFE RESTRAINT USE

- The Centers for Medicare & Medicaid Services (CMS) has rules for using restraints. These rules protect the person's rights and safety.
- Restraints may only be used to treat a medical symptom or for the immediate physical safety of the person or others. Restraints may only be used when less restrictive measures fail to protect the person or others. They must be discontinued at the earliest possible time.
- The CMS uses these to define restraints:
  - A **physical restraint** is any manual method or physical or mechanical device, material, or equipment attached to or near the person's body that he or she cannot remove easily and that restricts freedom of movement or normal access to one's body.
  - A **chemical restraint** is a drug that is used for discipline or convenience and not required to treat medical symptoms. The drug or dosage is not a standard treatment for the person's condition.
  - **Freedom of movement** is any change in place or position of the body or any part of the body that the person is able to control.
  - **Remove easily** is the manual method, device, material, or equipment used to restrain the person that can be removed intentionally by the person in the same manner it was applied by staff.
- Federal, state, and accrediting agencies have guidelines about restraint use. They do not forbid restraint use. They require considering or trying all other appropriate alternatives first.
- Every agency has policies and procedures about restraints. They include identifying persons at risk for harm, harmful behaviors, restraint alternatives, and proper restraint use. Staff training is required.

Restraint Alternatives

- Knowing and treating the cause for harmful behaviors can prevent restraint use. There are many alternatives to restraints, such as answering the signal light promptly. For other alternatives see Box 14-2, Alternatives to Restraint Use, in the Textbook.

Safe Restraint Use

- Restraints are used only when necessary to treat a person's medical symptoms—physical, emotional, or behavioral problems. Sometimes restraints are needed to protect the person or others.

Physical and Chemical Restraints

- *Physical restraints* are applied to the chest, waist, elbows, wrists, hands, or ankles. They confine the person to a bed or chair. Or they prevent movement of a body part.
- Some furniture or barriers prevent free movement:
  - Geriatric chairs or chairs with attached trays
  - Any chair placed so close to the wall that the person cannot move
  - Bed rails
  - Sheets tucked in so tightly that they restrict movement
  - Wheelchair locks if the person cannot release them
- Drugs or drug dosages are *chemical restraints* if they:
  - Control behavior or restrict movement
  - Are not standard treatment for the person's condition

Complications of Restraint Use

- Restraints can cause many complications. Injuries occur as the person tries to get free of the restraint. Injuries also occur from using the wrong restraint, applying it wrong, or keeping it on too long. Cuts, bruises, and fractures are common. The most serious risk is death from strangulation. Review Box 14-1, Risks of Restraint Use, in the Textbook.
- Restraints may also affect a person's dignity and self-esteem. Depression, anger, and agitation are common. So are embarrassment, humiliation, and mistrust.

Legal Aspects

- *Restraints must protect the person.* A restraint is used only when it is the best safety measure for the person.
- *A doctor's order is required.* The doctor gives the reason for the restraint, what body part to restrain, what to use, and how long to use it.
- *The least restrictive method is used.* It allows the greatest amount of movement or body access possible.
- *Restraints are used only after other measures fail to protect the person.* Box 14-2 lists alternatives to restraint use.
- *Unnecessary restraint is false imprisonment.* If you apply an unneeded restraint, you could face false imprisonment charges.
- *Consent is required.* The person must understand the reason for the restraint. If the person cannot give consent, his or her legal representative must give consent before a restraint can be used. The doctor or nurse provides the necessary information and obtains the consent.

Safety Guidelines

- Review Box 14-3, Safety Measures for Using Restraints, in the Textbook.
- *Observe for increased confusion and agitation.* Restraints can increase confusion and agitation. Restrained persons need repeated explanations and reassurance. Spending time with them has a calming effect.
- *Protect the person's quality of life.* Restraints are used for as short a time as possible. You must meet the person's physical, emotional, and social needs.
- *Follow the manufacturer's instructions.* The restraint must be snug and firm, but not tight. You could be negligent if you do not apply or secure a restraint properly.
- *Apply restraints with enough help to protect the person and staff from injury.*
- *Observe the person at least every 15 minutes or more often as noted in the care plan.* Injuries and deaths can result from improper restraint use and poor observation.
- *Remove or release the restraint, reposition the person, and meet basic needs at least every 2 hours or as often as noted in the care plan.* The restraint is removed for at least 10 minutes. Provide for food, fluid, comfort, safety, hygiene, and elimination needs and give skin care. Perform range-of-motion exercises or help the person walk.

Reporting and Recording

- Report and record the following:
  - Type of restraint applied.
  - Body part or parts restrained.
  - Reason for the application.
  - Safety measures taken.
  - Time you applied the restraint.
  - Time you removed or released the restraint.
  - Care given when restraint was removed.
  - Person's vital signs.
  - Skin color and condition.
  - Condition of the limbs.
  - Pulse felt in the restrained part.
  - Changes in the person's behavior.
  - Complaints of discomfort; a tight restraint; difficulty breathing; or pain, numbness, or tingling in the restrained part. Report these complaints to the nurse at once.

CHAPTER 14 REVIEW QUESTIONS

Circle the BEST answer.

1. A geriatric chair or a bed rail may be considered a restraint if free movement is restricted.
   a. True
   b. False
2. Which statement about the use of restraints is *false?*
   a. A person may be embarrassed and humiliated when restraints are on.
   b. A person may experience depression and agitation when restraints are on.
   c. Restraints can be used for staff convenience.
   d. Restraints can cause serious injury and death.
3. Restraints can increase a person's confusion and agitation.
   a. True
   b. False
4. The person with a restraint should be observed at least every
   a. 15 minutes
   b. 30 minutes
   c. Hour
   d. 2 hours
5. Restraints need to be removed at least every
   a. Hour
   b. 2 hours
   c. 3 hours
   d. 4 hours
6. You should record all the following *except*
   a. The type of restraint used
   b. The consent for the restraint
   c. The time you removed the restraint
   d. The care you gave when the restraint was removed

Answers to these questions are on p. 521.

CHAPTER 15 PREVENTING INFECTION

- An **infection** is a disease state resulting from the invasion and growth of microbes in the body. Infection is a major safety hazard.
- The health team follows certain practices and procedures to prevent the spread of infection (**infection control**).

Microorganisms

- A **microorganism (microbe)** is a small *(micro)* living plant or animal *(organism)*.
- Some microbes are harmful and can cause infections (**pathogens**). Others do not usually cause infection (**non-pathogens**).

Multidrug-Resistant Organisms

- *Multidrug-resistant organisms (MDROs)* can resist the effects of antibiotics. Such organisms are able to change their structures to survive in the presence of antibiotics. The infections they cause are harder to treat.
- MDROs are caused by doctors prescribing antibiotics when they are not needed (over-prescribing). Not taking antibiotics for the prescribed length of time is also a cause.
- Two common types of MDROs are resistant to many antibiotics:

○ *Methicillin-resistant Staphylococcus aureus (MRSA)*
○ *Vancomycin-resistant Enterococcus (VRE)*

Infection

- **A local infection** is in a body part.
- **A systemic infection** involves the whole body.
- Review Box 15-1, Signs and Symptoms of Infection, in the Textbook.

Healthcare-Associated Infection

- A **healthcare-associated infection (HAI)** is an infection that develops in a person cared for in any setting where health care is given. Review Box 15-2 in the Textbook. The infection is related to receiving healthcare. Hospitals, nursing centers, clinics, and home care settings are examples. HAIs also are called *nosocomial infections*.
- The health team must prevent the spread of HAIs by:
  ○ Medical asepsis. This includes hand hygiene.
  ○ Surgical asepsis.
  ○ Standard Precautions and Transmission-Based Precautions.
  ○ The Bloodborne Pathogen Standard.

Infection in Older Persons

- Older persons may not show the normal signs and symptoms of infection. The person may have only a slight fever or no fever at all. Redness and swelling may be very slight. The person may not complain of pain. Confusion and delirium may occur.
- Infections can become life-threatening before the older person has obvious signs and symptoms. Be alert to minor changes in the person's behavior or condition. Review Box 15-1, Signs and Symptoms of Infection, in the Textbook. Report any concerns to the nurse at once.

Medical Asepsis

- **Asepsis** is being free of disease-producing microbes.
- **Medical asepsis (clean technique)** refers to the practices used to:
  ○ Remove or destroy pathogens.
  ○ Prevent pathogens from spreading from one person or place to another person or place.

Common Aseptic Practices

- To prevent the spread of microbes, wash your hands:
  ○ After urinating or having a bowel movement.
  ○ After changing tampons or sanitary pads.
  ○ After contact with your own or another person's blood, body fluids, secretions, or excretions. This includes saliva, vomitus, urine, feces, vaginal discharge, mucus, semen, wound drainage, pus, and respiratory secretions.
  ○ After coughing, sneezing, or blowing your nose.
  ○ Before and after handling, preparing, or eating food.
  ○ After smoking a cigarette, cigar, or pipe.
- Also do the following:
  ○ Provide all persons with their own linens and personal care items.
  ○ Cover your nose and mouth when coughing, sneezing, or blowing your nose.
  ○ Bathe, wash hair, and brush your teeth regularly.
  ○ Wash fruits and raw vegetables before eating or serving them.

○ Wash cooking and eating utensils with soap and water after use.

Hand Hygiene

- *Hand hygiene is the easiest and most important way to prevent the spread of infection.* Practice hand hygiene before and after giving care. Review Box 15-3, Rules of Hand Hygiene, in the Textbook.

Supplies and Equipment

- Most health care equipment is disposable. Bedpans, urinals, wash basins, water pitchers, and drinking cups are multi-use items. Do not "borrow" them for another person.
- Non-disposable items are cleaned and then disinfected. Then they are sterilized.

Other Aseptic Measures

- Review Box 15-4, Aseptic Measures, in the Textbook.

Isolation Precautions

- Isolation Precautions prevent the spread of **communicable diseases (contagious diseases).** They are diseases caused by pathogens that spread easily.
- The Centers for Disease and Control and Prevention (CDC) isolation precautions guideline has two tiers of precautions:
  ○ Standard Precautions
  ○ Transmission-Based Precautions

Standard Precautions

- Standard Precautions reduce the risk of spreading pathogens and known and unknown infections. Standard Precautions are used for all persons whenever care is given. They prevent the spread of infection from:
  ○ Blood.
  ○ All body fluids, secretions, and excretions even if blood is not visible. Sweat is not known to spread infections.
  ○ Non-intact skin (skin with open breaks).
  ○ Mucous membranes.
- Review Box 15-5, Standard Precautions, in the Textbook.

Transmission-Based Precautions

- Some infections require Transmission-Based Precautions. Review Box 15-6, Transmission-Based Precautions, in the Textbook.
- Agency policies may differ from those in the Textbook. The rules in Box 15-7, Rules for Isolation Precautions, in the Textbook are a guide for giving safe care.

Protective Measures

- Isolation Precautions involve wearing PPE—gloves, a gown, a mask, and goggles or a face shield.
- Removing linens, trash, and equipment from the room may require double-bagging.
- Follow agency procedures when collecting specimens and transporting persons.
- Wear gloves whenever contact with blood, body fluids, secretions, excretions, mucous membranes, and non-intact skin is likely. Wearing gloves is the most common protective measure used with Standard Precautions and Transmission-Based Precautions. Remember the following when using gloves:

- ○ The outside of gloves is contaminated.
- ○ Gloves are easier to put on when your hands are dry.
- ○ Do not tear gloves when putting them on.
- ○ You need a new pair for every person.
- ○ Remove and discard torn, cut, or punctured gloves at once. Practice hand hygiene. Then put on a new pair.
- ○ Wear gloves once. Discard them after use.
- ○ Put on clean gloves just before touching mucous membranes or non-intact skin.
- ○ Put on new gloves whenever gloves become contaminated with blood, body fluids, secretions, or excretions. A task may require more than one pair of gloves.
- ○ Change gloves if interacting with the person involves touching portable computer keyboards or other mobile equipment that is transported from room to room.
- ○ Put on gloves last when worn with other PPE.
- ○ Change gloves whenever moving from a contaminated body site to a clean body site.
- ○ Make sure gloves cover your wrists. If you wear a gown, gloves cover the cuffs.
- ○ Remove gloves so the inside part is on the outside. The inside is clean.
- ○ Decontaminate your hands after removing gloves.
- Latex allergies are common and can cause skin rashes. Asthma and shock are more serious problems. Report skin rashes and breathing problems at once. If you or a resident has a latex allergy, wear latex-free gloves.
- Gowns must completely cover you from your neck to your knees. The gown front and sleeves are considered contaminated. A wet gown is contaminated. Gowns are used once. When removing a gown, roll it away from you. Keep it inside out.
- Masks are disposable. A wet or moist mask is contaminated. When removing a mask, touch only the ties or elastic bands. The front of the mask is contaminated.
- The front of goggles or a face shield is contaminated. Use the device's ties, headband, or ear pieces to remove the device.
- Contaminated items, linens, and trash are bagged to remove them from the person's room. Leak-proof plastic bags are used. They have the BIOHAZARD symbol. Double-bagging is not needed unless the outside of the bag is wet, soiled, or may be contaminated.

Meeting Basic Needs

- Love, belonging, and self-esteem needs are often unmet when Transmission-Based Precautions are used. Visitors and staff often avoid the person. The person may feel lonely, unwanted, and rejected. He or she may feel dirty and undesirable. The person may feel ashamed and guilty for having a contagious disease. You can help meet love, belonging, and self-esteem needs.

Bloodborne Pathogen Standard

- The health team is at risk for exposure to human immunodeficiency virus (HIV) and the hepatitis B virus (HBV). HIV and HBV are bloodborne pathogens found in the blood.
- The Bloodborne Pathogen Standard is intended to protect you from exposure.

- Staff at risk for exposure to HIV and HBV receive free training.
- *Hepatitis B vaccination.* You can receive the hepatitis B vaccination within 10 working days of being hired. The agency pays for it. If you refuse the vaccination, you must sign a statement. You can have the vaccination at a later date.

Engineering and Work Practice Controls

- *Engineering controls* reduce employee exposure in the workplace. There are special containers for contaminated sharps (needles, broken glass) and specimens. These containers are puncture-resistant, leak-proof, and color-coded in red. They have the BIOHAZARD symbol.
- *Work practice controls* reduce exposure risk. All tasks involving blood or other potentially infectious materials (OPIM) are done in ways to limit splatters, splashes, and sprays. OSHA requires these work practice controls:
  - ○ Do not eat, drink, smoke, apply cosmetics or lip balm, or handle contact lenses in areas of occupational exposure.
  - ○ Do not store food or drinks where blood or OPIM are kept.
  - ○ Practice hand hygiene after removing gloves.
  - ○ Wash hands as soon as possible after skin contact with blood or OPIM.
  - ○ Never recap, bend, or remove needles by hand.
  - ○ Never shear or break needles.
  - ○ Discard needles and sharp instruments (razors) in containers that are closable, puncture-resistant, and leak-proof. Containers are color-coded in red and have the BIOHAZARD symbol.

Personal Protective Equipment (PPE)

- This includes gloves, goggles, face shields, masks, laboratory coats, gowns, shoe covers, and surgical caps. OSHA requires these measures for PPE:
  - ○ Remove PPE before leaving the work area.
  - ○ Remove PPE when a garment becomes contaminated.
  - ○ Place used PPE in marked areas or containers when being stored, washed, decontaminated, or discarded.
  - ○ Wear gloves when you expect contact with blood or OPIM.
  - ○ Wear gloves when handling or touching contaminated items or surfaces.
  - ○ Replace worn, punctured, or contaminated gloves.
  - ○ Never wash or decontaminate disposable gloves for re-use.
  - ○ Discard utility gloves that show signs of cracking, peeling, tearing, or puncturing. Utility gloves are decontaminated for re-use if the process will not ruin them.

Equipment

- Contaminated equipment is cleaned and decontaminated. Decontaminate work surfaces with a proper disinfectant:
  - ○ Upon completing tasks
  - ○ At once when there is obvious contamination
  - ○ After any spill of blood or OPIM

○ At the end of the work shift when surfaces become contaminated since the last cleaning.

Laundry

- OSHA requires these measures for contaminated laundry:
  ○ Handle it as little as possible.
  ○ Wear gloves or other needed PPE.
  ○ Bag contaminated laundry where it is used.
  ○ Mark laundry bags or containers with the BIOHAZARD symbol for laundry sent off-site.
  ○ Place wet, contaminated laundry in leak-proof containers before transport. The containers are color-coded in red or have the BIOHAZARD symbol.

Exposure Incidents

- An **exposure incident** is any eye, mouth, other mucous membrane, non-intact skin, or parenteral contact with blood or OPIM (other potentially infectious materials).
- Report exposure incidents at once. Medical evaluation, follow-up, and required tests are free. Your blood is tested for HIV and HBV. Confidentiality is important.

CHAPTER 15 REVIEW QUESTIONS

Circle the BEST answer.

1. A healthcare-associated infection (nosocomial infection) is
   a. An infection free of disease-producing microbes
   b. An infection that develops in a person cared for in any setting where health care is given
   c. An infection acquired by health care workers
   d. An infection acquired only by older persons
2. Which statement about hand hygiene is *false?*
   a. Hand hygiene is the easiest way to prevent the spread of infection.
   b. Hand hygiene is the most important way to prevent the spread of infection.
   c. Hand hygiene is practiced before and after giving care to a person.
   d. If hands are visibly soiled, hand hygiene can be done with an alcohol-based hand rub.
3. When washing your hands, you should do the following *except*
   a. Stand away from the sink so your clothes do not touch the sink
   b. Keep your hands lower than your elbows
   c. Wash your hands for at least 15 seconds
   d. Dry your arms from the forearms to the fingertips
4. Which statement about wearing gloves is *false?*
   a. The insides of gloves are contaminated.
   b. You need a new pair of gloves for each person you care for.
   c. Change gloves when moving from a contaminated body site to a clean body site.
   d. Gloves need to cover your wrists.
5. Which statement is *false?*
   a. Gowns must cover you from your neck to your waist.
   b. A moist mask is contaminated.
   c. The outside of goggles is contaminated.
   d. You should wash your hands after removing a gown, mask, or goggles.
6. Which statement about PPE is *false?*
   a. Remove PPE when a garment becomes contaminated.
   b. Wear gloves when handling or touching contaminated items or surfaces.
   c. Wash or decontaminate disposable gloves for re-use.
   d. Remove PPE before leaving the work area.

Answers to these questions are on p. 521.

CHAPTER 16 BODY MECHANICS

Principles of Body Mechanics

- Your strongest and largest muscles are in the shoulders, upper arms, hips, and thighs. Use these muscles to lift and move persons and heavy objects.
- For good body mechanics:
- Bend your knees and squat to lift a heavy object. Do not bend from your waist.
- Hold items close to your body and base of support.
- Review Box 16-1, Rules for Body Mechanics, in the Textbook.

Ergonomics

- **Ergonomics** is the science of designing a job to fit the worker. The task, work station, equipment, and tools are changed to help reduce stress on the worker's body. The goal is to prevent injury and disorders of the muscles, tendons, ligaments, joints, cartilage, and nervous system (musculoskeletal disorders [MSD]).
- Early signs and symptoms of injury include pain, limited joint movement, or soft tissue swelling. Always report a work-related injury as soon as possible. Early attention can help prevent the problem from becoming worse.

Positioning the Person

- The person must be properly positioned at all times. Regular position changes and good alignment promote comfort and well-being. Breathing is easier. Circulation is promoted. Pressure ulcers and contractures are prevented.
- Whether in bed or in a chair, the person is repositioned at least every 2 hours. To safely position a person:
  ○ Use good body mechanics.
  ○ Ask a co-worker to help you if needed.
  ○ Explain the procedure to the person.
  ○ Be gentle when moving the person.
  ○ Provide for privacy.
  ○ Use pillows as directed by the nurse for support and alignment.
  ○ Provide for comfort after positioning.
  ○ Place the signal light within reach after positioning.
  ○ Complete a safety check before leaving the room.
  ○ Use pillows and positioning devices to support body parts and keep the person in good alignment.
- **Fowler's position** is a semi-sitting position. The head of the bed is raised between 45 and 60 degrees. The knees may be slightly elevated.
- The **supine position (dorsal recumbent position)** is the back-lying position.
- A person in the **prone position** lies on the abdomen with the head turned to one side.

- A person in the **lateral position (side-lying position)** lies on one side or the other.
- The **Sims' position (semi-prone side position)** is a left side-lying position.
- Persons who sit in chairs must hold their upper bodies and heads erect. For good alignment:
  - The person's back and buttocks are against the back of the chair.
  - Feet are flat on the floor or wheelchair footplates. Never leave feet unsupported.
  - Backs of the knees and calves are slightly away from the edge of the seat.

CHAPTER 16   REVIEW QUESTIONS

Circle the BEST answer.

1. To lift and move residents and heavy objects you should
   a. Use the muscles in your lower arms
   b. Use the muscles in your legs
   c. Use the muscles in your shoulders, upper arms, hips, and thighs
   d. Use the muscles in your abdomen
2. For good body mechanics, you should do all of the following *except*
   a. Bend your knees and squat to lift a heavy object
   b. Bend from your waist to lift a heavy object
   c. Hold items close to your body and base of support
   d. Bend your legs; do not bend your back
3. Which statement is *false?*
   a. A person must be properly positioned at all times.
   b. Regular position changes and good alignment promote comfort and well-being.
   c. Regular position changes and good alignment promote pressure ulcers and contractures.
   d. When a person is in good alignment, breathing is easier and circulation is promoted.
4. In Fowler's position
   a. The head of the bed is flat
   b. The head of the bed is raised to 90 degrees
   c. The head of the bed is raised between 45 and 60 degrees
   d. The head of the bed is raised between 30 and 35 degrees

Answers to these questions are on p. 521.

CHAPTER 17 SAFELY MOVING AND TRANSFERRING THE PERSON
Preventing Work-Related Injuries
- To prevent work-related injuries:
  - Wear shoes that provide good traction.
  - Use assistive equipment and devices whenever possible.
  - Get help from other staff.
  - Plan and prepare for the task. Know what equipment you will need and on what side of the bed to place the chair or wheelchair.
  - Schedule harder tasks early in your shift.
  - Tell the resident what he or she can do to help. Give clear, simple instructions.
  - Do not hold or grab the person under the underarms.
- For additional guidelines, review Box 17-1, Preventing Work-Related Injuries, in the Textbook.

Protecting the Skin
- Protect the person's skin from fiction and shearing. Both cause infection and pressure ulcers. To reduce friction and shearing:
  - Roll the person.
  - Use a lift sheet (turning sheet).
  - Use a turning pad, slide board, slide sheet, or a large incontinence product.

Moving Persons in Bed
- Before moving a person in bed, you need to know from the nurse and care plan:
  - What procedure to use
  - How many staff are needed to safely move the person
  - Position limits and restrictions
  - How far you can lower the head of the bed
  - Any limits in the person's ability to move or be repositioned
  - What equipment is needed—trapeze, lift sheet, slide sheet, mechanical lift
  - How to position the person
  - If the person uses bed rails
  - What observations to report and record:
    - Who helped you with the procedure
    - How much help the person needed
    - How the person tolerated the procedure
    - How you positioned the person
    - Complaints of pain or discomfort
  - When to report observations
  - What specific concerns to report at once

Moving the Person up in Bed
- You can sometimes move lightweight adults up in bed alone if they can assist using a trapeze. Two or more staff members are needed to move heavy, weak, and very old persons up in bed. Always protect the person and yourself from injury.
- Assist devices are used to reduce shearing and friction. Such assist devices include a drawsheet (lift sheet), flat sheet folded in half, turning pad, slide sheet, and large incontinence product.

Turning Persons
- Turning persons onto their sides helps prevent complications from bedrest. Certain procedures and care measures also require the side-lying position. After the person is turned, position him or her in good alignment. Use pillows as directed to support the person in the side-lying position.
- **Logrolling** is turning the person as a unit, in alignment, with one motion. The spine is kept straight.

Sitting on the Side of the Bed (Dangling)
- Many older persons become dizzy or faint when getting out of bed too fast. They may need to sit on the side of the bed for 1 to 5 minutes before walking or transferring. Some persons increase activity in stages—bedrest, to sitting on the side of the bed, to sitting in a chair, to walking.

- While dangling, the person coughs and deep breathes. He or she moves the legs back and forth in circles to stimulate circulation. Provide for warmth during dangling.
- Observations to report and record:
  - Pulse and respiratory rates
  - Pale or bluish skin color (cyanosis)
  - Complaints of light-headedness, dizziness, or difficulty breathing
  - Who helped you with the procedure.
  - How well the activity was tolerated
  - The length of time the person dangled
  - The amount of help needed
  - Other observations and complaints

Transferring Persons

- The rules of body mechanics apply during transfers.
- Arrange the room so there is enough space for a safe transfer. Correct placement of the chair, wheelchair, or other device also is needed for a safe transfer.
- Have the person wear non-skid footwear for transfers.
- Lock the wheels of the bed, wheelchair, stretcher, or other assist device.
- After the transfer, position the person in good alignment.
- Transfer belts (gait belts) are used to support persons during transfers and reposition persons in chairs and wheelchairs.

Bed to Chair or Wheelchair Transfers

- Safety is important for transfers. In transferring, the strong side moves first. Help the person out of bed on his or her strong side. Help the person from the wheelchair to the bed on his or her strong side.
- The person must not put his or her arms around your neck.

Mechanical Lifts

- Persons who cannot help themselves are transferred with mechanical lifts. So are persons who are too heavy for the staff to transfer.
- Before using a mechanical lift, you must be trained in its use. The sling, straps, hooks, and chains must be in good repair. The person's weight must not exceed the lift's capacity. At least two staff members are needed. Always follow the manufacturer's instructions for using the lift.
- Falling from the lift is a common fear. To promote the person's mental comfort, always explain the procedure before you begin. Also show the person how the lift works.

CHAPTER 17   REVIEW QUESTIONS

Circle the BEST answer.

1. Friction and shearing are reduced by doing the following *except*
   a. Rolling the person
   b. Using a lift sheet or turning pad
   c. Using a pillow
   d. Using a slide board or slide sheet
2. After a person is turned, you must position him or her in good alignment.
   a. True
   b. False

3. Which statement about dangling is *false?*
   a. Many older persons become dizzy or faint when they first dangle.
   b. The person should cough and deep breathe while dangling.
   c. The person moves his or her legs before dangling.
   d. You should cover the person's shoulders with a robe or blanket while dangling.
4. You are transferring a person from the bed to a wheelchair. Which statement is *false?*
   a. The person should wear non-skid footwear.
   b. The person may put his or her arm around your neck.
   c. You should use a gait/transfer belt.
   d. You should lock the wheelchair wheels.
5. A person has a weak left side and a strong right side. In transferring the person from the bed to the wheelchair, his or her strong (right) side moves first.
   a. True
   b. False
6. Before using a mechanical lift, you do all the following *except*
   a. Check the sling, straps, and chains to ensure good repair
   b. Check the person's weight to be sure it does not exceed the lift's capacity
   c. Follow the manufacturer's instructions for using the lift
   d. Operate the lift without a co-worker

Answers to these questions are on p. 521.

CHAPTER 18   THE PERSON'S UNIT

- A person's unit is the personal space, furniture, and equipment provided for the person by the agency. OBRA requires that resident units be as personal and home-like as possible.

Comfort

- Age, illness, and activity are factors that affect comfort.
- Temperature, ventilation, noise, odors, and lighting are factors that are controlled to meet the person's needs.

Temperature and Ventilation

- Older persons, and those who are ill, may need higher temperatures for comfort.
- To protect older and ill persons from cool areas and drafts:
  - Keep room temperatures warm.
  - Make sure they wear enough clothing.
  - Offer lap robes to cover the legs.
  - Provide enough blankets for warmth.
  - Cover them with bath blankets when giving care.
  - Move them from drafty areas.

Odors

- To reduce odors in nursing centers:
  - Empty, clean, and disinfect bedpans, urinals, commodes, and kidney basins promptly.
  - Check to make sure toilets are flushed.
  - Check incontinent people often.
  - Clean persons who are wet or soiled from urine, feces, vomitus, or wound drainage.
  - Change wet or soiled linens and clothing promptly.
  - Keep laundry containers closed.

- Follow agency policy for wet or soiled linens and clothing.
  - Dispose of incontinence and ostomy products promptly.
  - Provide good hygiene to prevent body and breath odors.
  - Use room deodorizers as needed and as allowed by agency policy.
- If you smoke, practice hand washing after handling smoking materials and before giving care. Give careful attention to your uniforms, hair, and breath because of smoke odors.

Noise

- To decrease noise:
  - Control your voice.
  - Handle equipment carefully.
  - Keep equipment in good working order.
  - Answer phones, signal lights, and intercoms promptly.

Lighting

- Adjust lighting to meet the person's needs. Glares, shadows, and dull lighting can cause falls, headaches, and eyestrain. A bright room is cheerful. Dim light is better for relaxing and rest. Persons with poor vision need bright light. Always keep light controls within the person's reach.

Room Furniture and Equipment

- Rooms are furnished and equipped to meet basic needs.

The Bed

- Beds are raised horizontally to give care. This reduces bending and reaching.
- Bed wheels are locked at all times except when moving the bed.
- Use bed rails as the nurse and care plan direct.
- Basic bed positions:
  - *Flat*—the usual sleeping position.
  - *Fowler's position*—a semi-sitting position. The head of the bed is raised between 45 and 60 degrees.
  - *High-Fowler's position*—a semi-sitting position. The head of the bed is raised 60 to 90 degrees.
  - *Semi-Fowler's position*—the head of the bed is raised 30 degrees. Some agencies define semi-Fowler's position as when the head of the bed is raised 30 degrees and the knee portion is raised 15 degrees. Know the definition used by your agency.
  - *Trendelenburg's position*—the head of the bed is lowered and the foot of the bed is raised. A doctor orders the position.
  - *Reverse Trendelenburg's position*—the head of the bed is raised and the foot of the bed is lowered. A doctor orders the position.

Bed Safety

- *Entrapment* means the person can get caught, trapped, or entangled in spaces created by bed rails, the mattress, the bed frame, or the headboard and footboard. Serious injuries and deaths have occurred from entrapment. If a person is at risk for entrapment, report your concerns to the nurse at once. If a person is caught, trapped, or entangled, try to release the person. Call for the nurse at once.

The Overbed Table

- Only clean and sterile items are placed on the table. Never place bedpans, urinals, or soiled linen on the overbed table or on top of the bedside stand.
- Clean the table and bedside stand after using them for a work surface and before serving meal trays.

Privacy Curtains

- Always pull the curtain completely around the bed before giving care. Privacy curtains do not block sound or conversations.

The Call System

- The signal light must always be kept within the person's reach—in the room, bathroom, and shower or tub room. You must:
  - Place the signal light on the person's strong side.
  - Remind the person to signal when help is needed.
  - Answer signal lights promptly.
  - Answer bathroom and shower or tub room signal lights at once.
- Persons with limited hand mobility may need special communication measures.
- Be careful when using the intercom. Remember confidentiality. Persons nearby can hear what you and the person say.

Closet and Drawer Space

- The person must have free access to the closet and its contents. You must have the person's permission to open or search closets or drawers.
- Agency staff can inspect a person's closet or drawers if hoarding is suspected. The person is informed of the inspection and is present when it takes place. Have a co-worker present when you inspect a person's closet.

General Rules

- Keep the person's room clean, neat safe, and comfortable. Follow the rules in Box 18-1, OBRA and CMS Requirements for Resident Rooms and Box 18-2, Maintaining the Person's Unit.

CHAPTER 18   REVIEW QUESTIONS

Circle the BEST answer.

1. Serious injuries and death have occurred from entrapment.
   a. True
   b. False
2. You should never place bedpans, urinals, or soiled linen on the overbed table.
   a. True
   b. False
3. You should clean the bedside stand if you use it for a work surface.
   a. True
   b. False
4. The following protect a person from drafts *except*
   a. Wearing enough clothing
   b. Lap robes
   c. Using a sheet when giving care
   d. Providing blankets

5. To reduce odors, you do the following *except*
   a. Empty bedpans and commodes promptly
   b. Keep laundry containers open
   c. Check to make sure toilets are flushed
   d. Clean persons who are wet or soiled from urine or feces
6. Which statement about the signal light is *false*?
   a. The signal light must always be within the person's reach.
   b. Place the signal light on the person's strong side.
   c. You have to answer the signal lights only for residents assigned to you.
   d. Answer signal lights promptly.
7. You suspect a person is hoarding food in her closet. Before you inspect the closet, what do you do?
   a. Tell another nursing assistant what you suspect
   b. Inspect the closet without telling the resident
   c. Tell the family
   d. Ask the resident if you can inspect the closet

Answers to these questions are on p. 521.

CHAPTER 19   BEDMAKING

- Clean, dry, and wrinkle-free linens promote comfort. Skin breakdown and pressure ulcers are prevented.
- To keep beds neat and clean:
  ○ Straighten linens whenever loose or wrinkled and at bedtime.
  ○ Check for and remove food and crumbs after meals and snacks.
  ○ Check linens for dentures, eyeglasses, hearing aids, sharp objects, and other items.
  ○ Change linens whenever they become wet, soiled, or damp.
  ○ Follow Standard Precautions and the Bloodborne Pathogen Standard.

Types of Beds

- Beds are made in these ways:
  ○ A closed bed is not in use. Or the bed is ready for a new resident. Top linens are not folded back.
  ○ An open bed is in use. Top linens are fan-folded back so the person can get into bed. A closed bed becomes an open bed by fan-folding back the top linens.
  ○ A occupied bed is made with the person in it.
  ○ A surgical bed is made to transfer a person from a stretcher. This bed is also made for persons who arrive by ambulance.

Linens

- When handling linens and making beds:
  ○ Practice medical asepsis.
  ○ Always hold linen away from your body and uniform. Your uniform is considered dirty.
  ○ Never shake linen.
  ○ Place clean linens on a clean surface.
  ○ Never put clean or dirty linen on the floor.
- Collect enough linens. Do not bring unneeded linens into the person's room. Once in the room, extra linen is considered contaminated. It cannot be used for another person.
- Roll each piece of dirty linen away from you. The side that touched the person is inside the roll and away from you.

Making Beds

- When making beds, safety and medical asepsis are important. Use good body mechanics. Follow the rules for safe resident handling, moving, and transfers. Practice hand hygiene before handling clean linen and after handling dirty linen. To save time and energy, make beds with a co-worker.
- Review Box 19-1, Rules for Bedmaking, in the Textbook.

The Occupied Bed

You make an occupied bed when the person stays in bed. Keep the person in good alignment. Follow restrictions or limits in the person's movement or position. Explain each procedure step to the person before it is done. This is important even if the person cannot respond to you.

CHAPTER 19   REVIEW QUESTIONS

Circle the BEST answer.

1. Once in the person's room, extra linen is considered contaminated. It can be used for another person.
   a. True
   b. False
2. Roll each piece of dirty linen away from you. The side that touched the person is inside the roll.
   a. True
   b. False
3. Wear gloves when removing linen from the person's bed.
   a. True
   b. False
4. To keep beds neat and clean, do the following *except*
   a. Straighten linens whenever loose or wrinkled
   b. Check for and remove food and crumbs after meals
   c. Check linens for dentures, eyeglasses, and hearing aids
   d. Change linen monthly
5. Which statement is *false*?
   a. Practice medical asepsis when handling linen.
   b. Always hold linens away from your body and uniform.
   c. Shake linens to remove crumbs.
   d. Put dirty linens in the dirty laundry bin.

Answers to these questions are on p. 521.

CHAPTER 20   PERSONAL HYGIENE

- Besides cleansing, good hygiene prevents body and breath odors. It is relaxing and increases circulation.
- Culture and personal choice affect hygiene.

Daily Care

- Most people have hygiene routines and habits. Hygiene measures are often done before and after meals and at bedtime. You assist with hygiene whenever it is needed. Protect the person's right to privacy and to personal choice.

Oral Hygiene

- Oral hygiene keeps the mouth and teeth clean. It prevents mouth odors and infections, increases comfort, and makes food taste better. Mouth care also reduces the risk for cavities and periodontal disease.
- Assist with oral hygiene after sleep, after meals, and at bedtime. Follow the care plan.
- Follow Standard Precautions and the Bloodborne Pathogen Standard.
- Report and record:
  - Dry, cracked, swollen, or blistered lips
  - Mouth or breath odor
  - Redness, swelling, irritation, sores, or white patches in the mouth or on the tongue
  - Bleeding, swelling, or redness of the gums
  - Loose teeth
  - Rough, sharp, or chipped areas on dentures

Brushing and Flossing Teeth

- Flossing removes plaque and tartar from the teeth as well as food from between the teeth. Flossing is usually done after brushing. If done once a day, bedtime is the best time to floss.
- Some persons need help gathering and setting up equipment for oral hygiene. You may have to perform oral care for persons who are weak, cannot move their arms, or are too confused to brush their teeth.

Mouth Care for the Unconscious Person

- Unconscious persons have dry mouths and crusting on the tongue and mucous membranes. Oral hygiene keeps the mouth clean and moist. It also helps prevent infection.
- Use sponge swabs to apply the cleaning agent. To prevent cracking of the lips, apply a lubricant to the lips. Check the care plan.
- To prevent aspiration on the unconscious person:
  - Position the person on one side with the head turned well to the side.
  - Use only a small amount of fluid to clean the mouth.
  - Do not insert dentures. Dentures are not worn when the person is unconscious.
- When giving oral hygiene, keep the person's mouth open with a padded tongue blade.
- Mouth care is given at least every 2 hours. Follow the nurse's direction and the care plan.

Denture Care

- Mouth care is given and dentures are cleaned as often as natural teeth. Dentures are usually removed at bedtime. Remind people not to wrap dentures in tissues or napkins.
- Dentures are slippery when wet. Hold them firmly. During cleaning, hold them over a basin of water lined with a towel. Use a cleaning agent, and follow the manufacturer's instructions.
- Hot water causes dentures to lose their shape. If dentures are not worn after cleaning, store them in a container with cool water or a denture soaking solution.
- Label the denture cup with the person's name, room number, and bed number. Report lost or damaged dentures to the nurse at once. Losing or damaging dentures is negligent conduct.
- Many people do not like being seen without their dentures. Privacy is important. If you clean dentures, return them to the person as quickly as possible.
- Persons with partial dentures have some natural teeth. They need to brush and floss the natural teeth.

Bathing

- Bathing cleans the skin. The mucous membranes of the genital and anal areas are cleaned as well. A bath is refreshing and relaxing. Circulation is stimulated and body parts exercised. You have time to talk to the person. You also can make observations.
- Review Box 20-1, Rules for Bathing, in the Textbook.
- Soap dries the skin. Therefore older persons usually need a complete bath or shower twice a week. Partial baths are taken the other days. Some bathe daily but not with soap. Thorough rinsing is needed when using soap. Lotions and oils keep the skin soft.
- Water temperature for complete bed baths and partial bed baths is between 110° F and 115° F. Older persons have fragile skin and need lower water temperatures. Measure water temperature according to agency policy.
- Report and record:
  - The color of the skin, lips, nail beds, and sclera (whites of the eyes)
  - If the skin appears pale, grayish, yellow (jaundice), or bluish (cyanotic)
  - The location and description of rashes
  - Skin texture—smooth, rough, scaly, flaky, dry, moist
  - Diaphoresis—profuse (excessive) sweating
  - Bruises or open areas
  - Pale or reddened areas, particularly over bony parts
  - Drainage or bleeding from wounds or body openings
  - Swelling of the feet and legs
  - Corns or calluses on the feet
  - Skin temperature
  - Complaints of pain or discomfort
- Use caution when applying powders. Do not use powders near persons with respiratory disorders. Do not sprinkle or shake powder onto the person. To safely apply powder:
- Turn away from the person.
- Sprinkle a small amount onto your hands or a cloth.
- Apply the powder in a thin layer.
- Make sure powder does not get on the floor. Powder is slippery and can cause falls.

The Complete Bed Bath

- The complete bed bath involves washing the person's entire body in bed. Wash around the person's eyes with water. Do not use soap. Gently wipe from the inner to the outer aspect of the eye. Use a clean part of the washcloth for each stroke. Ask the person if you should use soap to wash the face. Let the person wash the genital area if he or she is able.
- Give a back massage after the bath. Apply deodorant or antiperspirant, lotion, and powder as requested. Comb and brush the hair. Empty and clean the wash basin.

The Partial Bath
- The partial bath involves bathing the face, hands, axillae (underarms), back, buttocks, and perineal area. You assist the person as needed. Most need help washing the back.

Tub Baths and Showers
- Falls, burns, and chilling from water are risks. Review Box 20-1, Rules for Bathing and 20-2, Safety Measures for Tub Baths and Showers, in the Textbook.
- A tub bath can cause a person to feel faint, weak, or tired. The person may need a transfer bench, a tub with a side entry door, a wheelchair or stretcher lift, or a mechanical lift to get in and out of the tub.
- Some people can use a regular shower. Have the person use the grab bars for support during the shower. Use a bath mat if the shower does not have non-skid surfaces. Never let weak or unsteady persons stand in the shower. They may need to use shower chairs, shower stalls or cabinets, or shower trolleys. Some shower rooms have two or more stations. Protect the person's privacy. Properly screen and cover the person.
- Water temperature for tub baths and showers is usually 105° F. Report and record dizziness and light-headedness.
- Clean and disinfect the tub or shower before and after use.

The Back Massage
- The back massage relaxes muscles and stimulates circulation.
- Massages are given after the bath and with evening care. You also can give back massages at other times, such as after repositioning a person. Massages last 3 to 5 minutes.
- Observe the skin for breaks, bruises, reddened areas, and other signs of skin breakdown.
- Lotion reduces friction during the massage. It is warmed before applying.
- Use firm strokes. Keep your hands in contact with the person's skin.
- After the massage, apply some lotion to the elbows, knees, and heels.
- Back massages are dangerous for persons with certain heart diseases, back injuries, back and other surgeries, skin diseases, and some lung disorders. Check with the nurse and the care plan before giving back massages to persons with these conditions.
- Do not massage reddened bony areas. Reddened areas signal skin breakdown and pressure ulcers. Massage can lead to more tissue damage.
- Wear gloves if the person's skin is not intact. Always follow Standard Precautions and the Bloodborne Pathogen Standard.
- Report and record skin breakdown, redness, and bruising, and breaks in the skin.

Perineal Care
- Perineal care involves cleaning the genital and anal areas. It is done daily during the bath and whenever the area is soiled with urine or feces. The person does perineal care if able.
- Perineal and perineum are not common terms. Most people understand privates, private parts, crotch, genitals, or the area between the legs. Use terms the person understands.
- Standard Precautions, medical asepsis, and the Bloodborne Pathogen Standard are followed.
- Work from the cleanest area to the dirtiest—commonly called cleaning from "front to back." On a woman, clean from the urethra (cleanest) to the anal (dirtiest) area. On a male, start at the meatus of the urethra and work outward.
- Use warm water. Use washcloths, towelettes, cotton balls, or swabs according to agency policy. Rinse thoroughly. Pat dry. Water temperature is usually 105° F to 109° F.
- Report and record:
  - Bleeding, redness, swelling, irritation, discharge
  - Complaints of pain, burning, or other discomfort
  - Signs of urinary or fecal incontinence
  - Signs of skin breakdown
  - Discharge from the vagina or urinary tract
  - Odors

CHAPTER 20   REVIEW QUESTIONS

Circle the BEST answer.

1. Oral hygiene does the following *except*
   a. Keeps the mouth and teeth clean
   b. Prevents mouth odors and infections
   c. Decreases comfort
   d. Makes food taste better
2. When giving oral hygiene, you should report and record the following *except*
   a. Dry, cracked, swollen, or blistered lips
   b. Redness, sores, or white patches in the mouth
   c. Bleeding, swelling, or redness of the gums
   d. The number of fillings a person has
3. A person is unconscious. When you do mouth care, you do the following *except*
   a. Use only a small amount of fluid to clean the mouth
   b. Use your fingers to keep the mouth open
   c. Explain what you are doing
   d. Give mouth care at least every 2 hours
4. Which statement about dentures is *false?*
   a. Dentures are slippery when wet.
   b. During cleaning, hold dentures over a basin of water lined with a towel.
   c. Store dentures in cool water.
   d. Remind people to wrap their dentures in tissues or napkins.
5. Bathing does the following *except*
   a. Cleanses the skin
   b. Stimulates circulation
   c. Makes a person tense
   d. Permits you to observe the person's skin
6. The water temperature for a complete bed bath is
   a. 102° F to 108° F
   b. 110° F to 115° F
   c. 115° F to 120° F
   d. 120° F to 125° F

7. Which statement is *false?*
   a. Use powder near persons with respiratory disorders.
   b. Before applying powder, check with the nurse and the care plan.
   c. Before applying powder, sprinkle a small amount of powder onto your hands.
   d. Apply powder in a thin layer.
8. When washing a person's eyes, you should do the following *except*
   a. Use only water
   b. Gently wipe from the inner to the outer aspect of the eye
   c. Gently wipe from the outer to the inner aspect of the eye
   d. Use a clean part of the washcloth for each stroke
9. Which statement is *false?*
   a. A back massage relaxes and stimulates circulation.
   b. Massages are given after the bath and with evening care.
   c. You can observe the person's skin before beginning the massage.
   d. You should use cold lotion for the massage.
10. When giving female perineal care, you should work from the urethra to the anal area.
    a. True
    b. False
11. When giving male perineal care, start at the meatus and work outward.
    a. True
    b. False

Answers to these questions are on p. 521.

CHAPTER 21   GROOMING

- Hair care, shaving, and nail and foot care prevent infection and promote comfort. They also affect love, belonging, and self-esteem needs.

Hair Care

- You assist patients and residents with brushing and combing hair and with shampooing according to the care plan. The nursing process reflects the person's culture, personal choice, skin and scalp condition, health history, and self-care ability.

Brushing and Combing Hair

- Brushing and combing prevent tangled and matted hair.
- When brushing and combing hair, start at the scalp and brush or comb to the hair ends.
- Never cut hair for any reason. Tell the nurse if you think the person's hair needs to be cut.
- Special measures are needed for curly, coarse, and dry hair. Check the care plan.
- When giving hair care, place a towel across the person's back and shoulders to protect garments from falling hair. If the person is in bed, give hair care before changing the linens and pillowcase.

Shampooing

- Shampooing frequency depends on the person's needs and preferences. Usually shampooing is done weekly on the person's bath or shower day.
- Hair is dried and styled as quickly as possible after the shampoo.
- During shampooing, report and record:
  - Scalp sores
  - Flaking
  - Itching
  - Presence of nits or lice
  - Patches of hair loss
  - Very dry or very oily hair
  - Matted or tangled hair
  - How the person tolerated the procedure
- Keep shampoo away from and out of eyes. Have the person hold a washcloth over the eyes.
- Wear gloves if the person has scalp sores.
- Follow Standard Precautions and the Bloodborne Pathogen Standard.

Shaving

- Review Box 21-1, Rules for Shaving, in the Textbook.

Caring for Mustaches and Beards

- Wash and comb mustaches and beards daily and as needed. Ask the person how to groom his mustache or beard.
- Never trim a mustache or beard without the person's consent.

Shaving Legs and Underarms

- Many women shave their legs and underarms. This practice varies among cultures. Legs and underarms are shaved after bathing when the skin is soft.

Nail and Foot Care

- Nail and foot care prevent infection, injury, and odors.
- Nails are easier to trim and clean right after soaking or bathing.
- Use nail clippers to cut fingernails. Never use scissors. Use extreme caution to prevent damage to nearby tissues.
- Follow Standard Precautions and the Bloodborne Pathogen Standard.
- Report and record:
  - Reddened, irritated, or callused areas
  - Breaks in the skin
  - Corns on top of and between the toes
  - Very thick nails
  - Loose nails
- You do not cut or trim toenails if a person has diabetes or poor circulation to the legs and feet or takes drugs that affect blood clotting. Also, do not cut or trim toenails if the person has very thick nails or ingrown toenails. The nurse or podiatrist cuts toenails and provides foot care for these persons.
- When doing foot care, check between the toes for cracks and sores. If left untreated, a serious infection could occur.
- The feet of persons with decreased sensation or circulatory problems may easily burn because they do not feel hot temperatures.

- After soaking, apply lotion to the feet. Because the lotion can cause slippery feet, help the person put on non-skid footwear before you transfer the person or let the person walk.

Changing Clothing and Hospital Gowns

- Garments are changed after the bath and whenever wet or soiled.
- When changing clothing:
  - Provide for privacy.
  - Encourage the person to do as much as possible.
  - Make sure garments and footwear are the correct size.
  - Let the person choose what to wear. Make sure the right undergarments are chosen.
  - Remove clothing from the strong or "good" (unaffected) side first.
  - Put clothing on the weak (affected) side first.
  - Support the arm or leg when removing or putting on a garment.

CHAPTER 21   REVIEW QUESTIONS

Circle the BEST answer.

1. Hair care, shaving, and nail and foot care prevent infection and promote comfort.
   a. True
   b. False
2. If a person's hair is matted, you may cut the hair.
   a. True
   b. False
3. When giving hair care, place a towel across the person's back and shoulders to protect garments from falling hair.
   a. True
   b. False
4. You should wear gloves when shampooing a person who has scalp sores.
   a. True
   b. False
5. A person takes an anticoagulant. Therefore he shaves with a blade razor.
   a. True
   b. False
6. You should wear gloves when shaving a person.
   a. True
   b. False
7. Never trim a mustache or beard without the person's consent.
   a. True
   b. False
8. Mustaches and beards need daily care.
   a. True
   b. False
9. A person has diabetes. You can cut his or her toenails.
   a. True
   b. False
10. Fingernails are cut with
    a. Scissors
    b. Nail clippers
    c. An emery board
    d. A nail file

11. Which statement is *false?*
    a. Provide privacy when a person is changing clothes.
    b. Most residents wear street clothes during the day.
    c. Let the person choose what to wear.
    d. You may tear a person's clothing.

Answers to these questions are on p. 521.

CHAPTER 22   URINARY ELIMINATION

Normal Urination

- The healthy adult produces about 1500 mL of urine a day.
- The frequency of urination is affected by amount of fluid intake, habits, availability of toilet facilities, activity, work, and illness. People usually void at bedtime, after sleep, and before meals. Some people void every 2 to 3 hours. The need to void at night disturbs sleep. Review Box 22-1, Rules for Normal Urination, in the Textbook.

Observations

- Observe urine for color, clarity, odor, amount, particles, and blood. Normal urine is pale yellow, straw-colored, or amber. It is clear with no particles. A faint odor is normal.
- Some foods and drugs affect urine color. Ask the nurse to observe urine that looks or smells abnormal.
- Report the following urinary problems:
  - **Dysuria**—painful or difficult urination
  - **Hematuria**—blood in the urine
  - **Nocturia**—frequent urination at night
  - **Oliguria**—scant amount of urine; less than 500 mL in 24 hours
  - **Polyuria**—abnormally large amounts of urine
  - **Urinary frequency**—voiding at frequent intervals
  - **Urinary incontinence**—involuntary loss or leakage of urine
  - **Urinary urgency**—the need to void at once

Bedpans

- Follow Standard Precautions and the Bloodborne Pathogen Standard when handling bedpans, urinals, commodes, and their contents.
- Thoroughly clean and disinfect bedpans, urinals, and commodes after use.

Urinals

- Some men need support when standing to use the urinal.
- You may have to place and hold the urinal for some men. This may embarrass both the person and you. Act in a professional manner at all times.
- Remind men to hang urinals on bed rails and to signal after using them.

Urinary Incontinence

- **Urinary incontinence** is the involuntary loss or leakage of urine.
- If urinary incontinence is a new problem, tell the nurse at once.
- Incontinence is embarrassing. Garments are wet, and odors develop. Skin irritation, infection, and pressure ulcers are risks. The person's pride, dignity,

and self-esteem are affected. Social isolation, loss of independence, and depression are common.

- Good skin care and dry garments and linens are essential. Promoting normal urinary elimination prevents incontinence in some people. Other people may need bladder training.
- Review Box 22-2, Nursing Measures for Persons With Urinary Incontinence, in the Textbook.
- Caring for persons with incontinence is stressful. Remember, the person does not choose to be incontinent. If you find yourself becoming short-tempered and impatient, talk to the nurse at once. Kindness, empathy, understanding, and patience are needed.

Catheters

- An *indwelling catheter (retention or Foley catheter)* drains urine constantly into a drainage bag.
- The catheter must not pull at the insertion site. Hold the catheter securely during catheter care. Then properly secure the catheter. Also make sure the tubing is not under the person. Besides obstructing urine flow, lying on the tubing is uncomfortable. It can also cause skin breakdown.
- Follow Standard Precautions and the Bloodborne Pathogen Standard. Review Box 22-4, Caring for Persons With Indwelling Catheters, in the Textbook.
- Report and record:
  - Complaints of pain, burning, irritation, or the need to void (report at once)
  - Crusting, abnormal drainage, or secretions
  - The color, clarity, and odor of urine
  - Particles in the urine
  - Cloudy urine
  - Urine leaking at the insertion site
  - Drainage system leaks

Drainage Systems

- A closed drainage system is used for indwelling catheters. The drainage bag hangs from the bed frame, chair, or wheelchair. It must not touch the floor. The bag is always kept lower than the person's bladder. Do not hang the drainage bag on a bed rail.
- If the drainage system is disconnected accidentally, tell the nurse at once. Do not touch the ends of the catheter or tubing. Do the following:
  - Practice hand hygiene. Put on gloves.
  - Wipe the end of the tube with an antiseptic wipe.
  - Wipe the end of the catheter with another antiseptic wipe.
  - Do not put the ends down. Do not touch the ends after you clean them.
  - Connect the tubing to the catheter.
  - Discard the wipes into a BIOHAZARD bag.
  - Remove the gloves. Practice hand hygiene.
- Check with the nurse and care plan about when to empty and measure the urine in the drainage bag. Follow Standard Precautions and the Bloodborne Pathogen Standard.
- A leg bag is a drainage system that attaches to the thigh or calf. Empty and measure a leg bag when it is half full.

- Report and record:
  - The amount of urine measured
  - The color, clarity, and odor of urine
  - Particles in the urine
  - Complaints of pain, burning, irritation, or the need to urinate
  - Drainage system leaks

Condom Catheters

- Condom catheters are often used for incontinent men. They are also called external catheters, Texas catheters, and urinary sheaths.
- These catheters are changed daily after perineal care.
- To apply a condom catheter, follow the manufacturer's instructions. Thoroughly wash and dry the penis before applying the catheter.
- Some condom catheters are self-adhering. Other catheters are secured in place with elastic tape in a spiral manner. Never use adhesive tape to secure catheters. It does not expand. Blood flow to the penis is cut off, injuring the penis.
- When removing or applying a condom catheter, report and record the following observations:
  - Reddened or open areas on the penis
  - Swelling of the penis
  - Color, clarity, and odor of urine
  - Particles in the urine
  - Blood in urine
  - Cloudy urine
- Do not apply a condom catheter if the penis is red, is irritated, or shows signs of skin breakdown. Report your observations to the nurse at once.

Bladder Training

- Bladder training helps some persons with urinary incontinence. Control of urination is the goal. Bladder control promotes comfort and quality of life. It also increases self-esteem. You assist with bladder training as directed by the nurse and the care plan.

CHAPTER 22   REVIEW QUESTIONS

Circle the BEST answer.

1. Which statement is *false?*
   a. Normal urine is yellow, straw-colored, or amber.
   b. Urine with a strong odor is normal.
   c. A person normally voids 1500 mL a day.
   d. Observe urine for color, clarity, odor, amount, and particles.
2. Which observation does *not* need to be reported to the nurse promptly?
   a. Complaints of urgency
   b. Burning on urination
   c. Painful or difficult urination
   d. Clear amber urine
3. Which statement is *false?*
   a. Incontinence is embarrassing.
   b. Caring for persons with incontinence may be stressful.
   c. Incontinence is a personal choice.
   d. Be kind and patient to persons who are incontinent.

4. A person with a catheter complains of pain. You should notify the nurse at once.
   a. True
   b. False
5. Which statement is *false*?
   a. The urine drainage system should hang from the bed frame or chair.
   b. The urine drainage system should hang on a bed rail.
   c. The urine drainage system must be off the floor.
   d. The urine drainage system must be kept lower than the person's bladder.
6. Which statement is *false*?
   a. Condom catheters are changed daily.
   b. Follow the manufacturer's instructions when applying a condom catheter.
   c. Use adhesive tape to secure a condom catheter in place.
   d. Report and record open or reddened areas on the penis at once.
7. The goal of bladder training is to
   a. Allow the person to use the toilet
   b. Keep the catheter
   c. Gain control of urination
   d. Decrease self-esteem

Answers to these questions are on p. 521.

CHAPTER 23 BOWEL ELIMINATION
Normal Bowel Elimination

Observations
- Stools are normally brown, soft, formed, moist, and shaped like the rectum. They have a normal odor caused by bacterial action in the intestines. Certain foods and drugs cause odors.
- Carefully observe stools before disposing of them. Observe and report the color, amount, consistency, odor, and shape of stools. Also, observe and report the presence of blood or mucus, frequency of defecation, and any complaints of pain or discomfort.

Factors Affecting Bowel Elimination
- *Privacy*. Bowel elimination is a private act.
- *Habits*. Many people have a bowel movement after breakfast. Some read. Defecation is easier when a person is relaxed.
- *Diet—high-fiber foods*. Fiber helps prevent constipation.
- *Diet—other foods*. Some foods cause constipation. Other foods cause frequent stools or diarrhea.
- *Fluids*. Drinking 6 to 8 glasses of water daily promotes normal bowel elimination. Warm fluids—coffee, tea, hot cider, warm water—increase peristalsis.
- *Activity*. Exercise and activity maintain muscle tone and stimulate peristalsis.
- *Drugs*. Drugs can prevent constipation or control diarrhea. Some have diarrhea or constipation as side effects.
- *Disability*. Some people cannot control bowel movements. A bowel training program is needed.
- *Aging*. Older persons are at risk for constipation. Some older persons lose bowel control and have fecal incontinence.
- To provide comfort and safety during bowel elimination, review Box 18-1, Safety and Comfort During Bowel Elimination, in the Textbook. Follow Standard Precautions and the Bloodborne Pathogen Standard.

Common Problems
- Common problems include constipation, fecal impaction, diarrhea, fecal incontinence, and flatulence.

Constipation
- **Constipation** is the passage of a hard, dry stool.
- Common causes of constipation are a low-fiber diet and ignoring the urge to defecate. Other causes include decreased fluid intake, inactivity, drugs, aging, and certain diseases.
- Dietary changes, fluids, and activity prevent or relieve constipation. So do drugs, suppositories, and enemas.

Fecal Impaction
- A **fecal impaction** is the prolonged retention and buildup of feces in the rectum.
- Fecal impaction results if constipation is not relieved. The person cannot defecate. Liquid feces pass around the hardened fecal mass in the rectum. The liquid feces seep from the anus.
- Abdominal discomfort, abdominal distention, nausea, cramping, and rectal pain are common. Older persons have poor appetite or confusion. Some persons have a fever. Report these signs and symptoms to the nurse.

Diarrhea
- **Diarrhea** is the frequent passage of liquid stools.
- The need to have a bowel movement is urgent. Some people cannot get to a bathroom in time. Abdominal cramping, nausea, and vomiting may occur.
- Assist with elimination needs promptly, dispose of stools promptly, and give good skin care. Liquid stools irritate the skin. So does frequent wiping with toilet paper. Skin breakdown and pressure ulcers are risks.
- Follow Standard Precautions and the Bloodborne Pathogen Standard when in contact with stools.
- Report signs of diarrhea at once. Ask the nurse to observe the stool.

Fecal Incontinence
- **Fecal incontinence** is the inability to control the passage of feces and gas through the anus.
- Fecal incontinence affects the person emotionally. Frustration, embarrassment, anger, and humiliation are common. The person may need:
  - Bowel training
  - Help with elimination after meals and every 2 to 3 hours
  - Incontinence products to keep garments and linens clean
  - Good skin care

Flatulence
- **Flatulence** is the excessive formation of gas or air in the stomach and intestines.
- Causes include swallowing air while eating and drinking and bacterial action in the intestines. Other causes may be gas-forming foods, constipation, bowel and abdominal surgeries, and drugs that decrease peristalsis.

- If flatus is not expelled, the intestines distend (swell or enlarge from the pressure of gases). Abdominal cramping or pain, shortness of breath, and a swollen abdomen occur. "Bloating" is a common complaint. Exercise, walking, moving in bed, and the left side-lying position often produce flatus. Enemas and drugs may be ordered.

Bowel Training

- Bowel training has two goals:
  - To gain control of bowel movements.
  - To develop a regular pattern of elimination. Fecal impactions, constipation, and fecal incontinence are prevented.
- Factors that promote elimination are part of the care plan and bowel training program.

Enemas

- An **enema** is the introduction of fluid into the rectum and lower colon.
- Doctors order enemas:
  - To remove feces
  - To relieve constipation, fecal impaction, or flatulence
  - To clean the bowel of feces before certain surgeries and diagnostic procedures
- Review Box 23-2, Safety and Comfort Measures for Giving Enemas, in the Textbook.

The Person With an Ostomy

- Sometimes part of the intestines is removed surgically. An ostomy is sometimes necessary. An **ostomy** is a surgically created opening for the elimination of body wastes. The opening is called a **stoma.** The person wears a pouch over the stoma to collect stools and flatus.
- Stools irritate the skin. Skin care prevents skin breakdown around the stoma. The skin is washed and dried. Then a skin barrier is applied around the stoma. It prevents stools from having contact with the skin. The skin barrier is part of the pouch or a separate device.
- The pouch has an adhesive backing that is applied to the skin. Sometimes pouches are secured to ostomy belts.
- The pouch is changed every 3 to 7 days and when it leaks. Frequent pouch changes can damage the skin.
- Many pouches have a drain at the bottom that closes with a clip, clamp, or wire closure. The drain is opened to empty the pouch. The drain is wiped with toilet tissue before it is closed.

CHAPTER 23   REVIEW QUESTIONS

Circle the BEST answer.

1. Which statement is *false?*
   a. Lack of privacy can prevent defecation.
   b. Low-fiber foods promote defecation.
   c. Drinking 6 to 8 glasses of water daily promotes normal bowel elimination.
   d. Exercise stimulates peristalsis.
2. Which of the following does *not* prevent constipation?
   a. A high-fiber diet
   b. Increased fluid intake
   c. Exercise
   d. Ignoring the urge to defecate
3. A person has fecal incontinence. You should do the following *except*
   a. Be patient
   b. Help with elimination after meals
   c. Provide good skin care
   d. Scold the person for being incontinent
4. The preferred position for an enema is the
   a. Sims' position or the left side-lying position
   b. Prone position
   c. Supine position
   d. Trendelenburg's position

Answers to these questions are on p. 521.

CHAPTER 24   NUTRITION AND FLUIDS

- Food and water are necessary for life. A poor diet and poor eating habits:
  - Increase the risk for infection
  - Cause healing problems
  - Increase the risk of acute and chronic diseases
  - Cause chronic illnesses to become worse
  - Affect physical and mental function, increasing the risk for accidents and injuries

Basic Nutrition

- **Nutrition** is the process involved in the ingestion, digestion, absorption, and use of foods and fluids by the body. Good nutrition is needed for growth, healing, and body functions.
- A *nutrient* is a substance that is ingested, digested, absorbed, and used by the body.
- A *calorie* is the fuel or energy value of food.

Nutrients

- A well-balanced diet ensures an adequate intake of essential nutrients.
- *Protein*—is needed for tissue growth and repair. Sources include meat, fish, poultry, eggs, milk and milk products, cereals, beans, peas, and nuts.
- *Carbohydrates*—provide energy and fiber for bowel elimination. They are found in fruits, vegetables, breads, cereals, and sugar.
- *Fats*—provide energy, add flavor to food, and help the body use certain vitamins. Sources include meats, lard, butter, shortening, oils, milk, cheese, egg yolks, and nuts.
- *Vitamins*—are needed for certain body functions. The body stores vitamins A, D, E, and K. The vitamin C and the B complex vitamins are not stored and must be ingested daily.
- *Minerals*—are needed for bone and tooth formation, nerve and muscle function, fluid balance, and other body processes.
- *Water*—is needed for all body processes.
- Review Tables 24-2 and 24-3 in the Textbook.

Factors Affecting Eating and Nutrition

- *Age.* Many changes occur in the digestive system with aging.
- *Culture.* Culture influences dietary practices, food choices, and food preparation.

- *Religion*. Selecting, preparing, and eating food often involve religious practices. A person may follow all, some, or none of the dietary practices of his or her faith.
- *Finances*. People with limited incomes often buy the cheaper carbohydrate foods. Their diets often lack protein and certain vitamins and minerals.
- *Appetite*. Illness, drugs, anxiety, pain, and depression can cause loss of appetite. Unpleasant sights, thoughts, and smells are other causes.
- *Personal choice*. Food likes and dislikes are influenced by foods served in the home. Usually food likes expand with age and social experiences.
- *Body reactions*. People usually avoid foods that cause allergic reactions. They also avoid foods that cause nausea, vomiting, diarrhea, indigestion, gas, or headaches.
- *Illness*. Appetite usually decreases during illness and recovery from injuries. However, nutritional needs are increased.
- *Drugs*. Drugs can cause loss of appetite, confusion, nausea, constipation, impaired taste, or changes in GI function. They can cause inflammation of the mouth, throat, esophagus, and stomach.
- *Chewing problems*. Mouth, teeth, and gum problems can affect chewing. Examples include oral pain, dry or sore mouth, gum disease (Chapter 20), and dentures that fit poorly. Broken, decayed, or missing teeth also affect chewing, especially the meat group.
- *Swallowing problems*. Many health problems can affect swallowing. They include stroke, pain, confusion, dry mouth, and diseases of the mouth, throat, and esophagus.
- *Disability*. Disease or injury can affect the hands, wrists, and arms. Adaptive equipment lets the person eat independently.
- *Impaired cognitive function*. Impaired cognitive function may affect the person's ability to use eating utensils. And it may affect eating, chewing, and swallowing.

OBRA Dietary Requirements

- OBRA has requirements for food served in nursing centers:
  - Each person's nutritional and dietary needs are met.
  - The person's diet is well-balanced. It is nourishing and tastes good. Food is well-seasoned.
  - Food is appetizing. It has an appealing aroma and is attractive.
  - Hot food is served hot. Cold food is served cold.
  - Food is served promptly.
  - Food is prepared to meet each person's needs. Some people need food cut, ground, or chopped. Others have special diets ordered by the doctor.
  - Other foods are offered if the person refused the food served. Substituted food must have a similar nutritional value to the first foods served.
  - Each person receives at least 3 meals a day. A bedtime snack is offered.
  - The center provides needed adaptive equipment and utensils.

Special Diets

The Sodium-Controlled Diet

- A sodium-controlled diet decreases the amount of sodium in the body. The diet involves:
  - Omitting high-sodium foods. Review Box 24-4, High-Sodium Foods, in the Textbook.
  - Not adding salt when eating.
  - Limiting the amount of salt used in cooking.
  - Diet planning

Diabetes Meal Planning

- Diabetes meal planning is for people with diabetes. It involves the person's food preferences and calories needed. It also involves eating meals and snacks at regular times.
- Serve the person's meals and snacks on time to maintain a certain blood sugar level.
- Always check the tray to see what was eaten. Tell the nurse what the person did and did not eat. If not all the food was eaten, a between-meal nourishment is needed. The nurse tells you what to give. Tell the nurse about changes in the person's eating habits.

The Dysphagia Diet

- **Dysphagia** means difficulty swallowing. Food thickness is changed to meet the person's needs. Review Box 24-4, Dysphagia Diet, in the Textbook.
- You may need to feed a person with dysphagia. To promote the person's comfort:
  - Know the signs and symptoms of dysphagia. Review Box 24-5 in the Textbook.
  - Feed the person according to the care plan and swallow guide.
  - Follow aspiration precautions. Review Box 24-6 in the Textbook.
  - Report changes in how the person eats.
  - Report choking, coughing, or difficulty breathing during or after meals. Also report abnormal breathing or respiratory sounds. Report these observations at once.

Fluid Balance

- Fluid balance is needed for health. The amount of fluid taken in (**intake**) and the amount of fluid lost (**output**) must be equal. If fluid intake exceeds fluid output, body tissues swell with water (**edema**).
- **Dehydration** is a decrease in the amount of water in body tissues. Fluid output exceeds intake. Common causes are poor fluid intake, vomiting, diarrhea, bleeding, excess sweating, and increased urine production.

Normal Fluid Requirements

- An adult needs 1500 mL of water daily to survive. About 2000 to 2500 mL of fluid per day is needed for normal fluid balance. Water requirements increase with hot weather, exercise, fever, illness, and excess fluid loss.
- Older persons may have a decreased sense of thirst. Their bodies need water, but they may not feel thirsty. Offer fluids according to the care plan.

Special Fluid Orders

- The doctor may order the amount of fluid a person can have in 24 hours. Intake and output (I&O) measurements may be ordered by the doctor or nurse.

- *Encourage fluids*. The person drinks an increased amount of fluid.
- *Restrict fluids*. Fluids are limited to a certain amount.
- *Nothing by mouth (NPO)*. The person cannot eat or drink.
- *Thickened liquids*. All liquids are thickened, including water.

Intake and Output

- All fluids taken by mouth are measured and recorded—water, milk, and so forth. So are foods that melt at room temperature—ice cream, sherbet, custard, pudding, gelatin, and Popsicles.
- Output includes urine, vomitus, diarrhea, and wound drainage.

Measuring Intake and Output

- To measure intake and output, you need to know:
- 1 ounce (oz) equals 30 mL
- A pint is about 500 mL
- A quart is about 1000 mL
- The serving sizes of bowls, dishes, cups, pitchers, glasses, and other containers
- An I&O record is kept at the bedside. Record I&O measurements in the correct column. Amounts are totaled at the end of the shift. The totals are recorded in the person's chart. They are also shared during the end-of-shift report.
- The urinal, commode, bedpan, or specimen pan is used for voiding. Remind the person not to void in the toilet. Also remind the person not to put toilet tissue into the receptacle.

Meeting Food and Fluid Needs

Preparing for Meals

- Preparing residents for meals promotes their comfort:
  - Assist with elimination needs.
  - Provide oral hygiene. Make sure dentures are in place.
  - Make sure eyeglasses and hearing aids are in place.
  - Make sure incontinent persons are clean and dry.
  - Position the person in a comfortable position.
  - Assist with hand washing.

Serving Meals

- Food is served in containers that keep foods at the correct temperature. Hot food is kept hot. Cold food is kept cold.
- Prompt serving keeps food at the correct temperature.

Feeding the Person

- Serve food and fluid in the order the person prefers. Offer fluids during the meal.
- Use teaspoons to feed the person.
- Persons who need to be fed are often angry, humiliated, and embarrassed. Some are depressed or refuse to eat. Let them do as much as possible. If strong enough, let them hold milk or juice glasses. Never let them hold hot drinks.
- Tell the visually impaired person what is on the tray. Describe what you are offering. For persons who feed themselves, use the numbers on the clock for the location of foods.

- Many people pray before eating. Allow time and privacy for prayer.
- Meals provide social contact with others. Engage the person in pleasant conversations. Also, sit facing the person. Allow time for chewing and swallowing.
- Report and record:
  - The amount and kind of food eaten
  - Complaints of nausea or dysphagia
  - Signs and symptoms of dysphagia
  - Signs and symptoms of aspiration
  - The person will eat better if not rushed.
  - Wipe the person's hands, face, and mouth as needed during the meal.

Between-Meal Snacks

- Many special diets involve between-meal snacks. These snacks are served upon arrival on the nursing unit. Follow the same considerations and procedures for serving meal trays and feeding persons.

Calorie Counts

- Calorie records are kept for some people. On a flow sheet, note what the person ate and how much. A nurse or dietitian converts these portions into calories.

Providing Drinking Water

- Patients and residents need fresh drinking water each shift. Follow the agency's procedure for providing fresh water.
- Water glasses and pitchers can spread microbes. To prevent the spread of microbes:
  - Label the water pitcher with the person's name and room and bed numbers.
  - Do not touch the rim or inside of the water glass, cup, or pitcher.
  - Do not let the ice scoop touch the rim or inside of the water glass, cup, or pitcher.
  - Place the ice scoop in the holder or on a towel, not in the ice container or dispenser.
  - Make sure the person's water pitcher and cup are clean and free of cracks and chips.

CHAPTER 24   REVIEW QUESTIONS

Circle the BEST answer.

1. A person is on a sodium-controlled diet. Which statement is *true*?
   a. High-sodium foods are allowed.
   b. Salt is added at the table.
   c. Pretzels and potato chips are a good snack.
   d. The amount of salt used in cooking is limited.

2. A person is a diabetic. You should do the following *except*
   a. Serve his meals and snacks late
   b. Always check his tray to see what he ate
   c. Tell the nurse what he ate and did not eat
   d. Provide a between-meal snack as the nurse directs

3. A person has dysphagia. You should do the following *except*
   a. Report choking and coughing during a meal at once
   b. Report difficulty in breathing during a meal at the end of the shift
   c. Report changes in how the person eats
   d. Follow aspiration precautions

4. Older persons have a decreased sense of thirst.
   a. True
   b. False
5. When feeding a person, you do the following *except*
   a. Use a teaspoon to feed the person
   b. Offer fluids during the meal
   c. Let the person do as much as possible
   d. Stand so you can feed 2 people at once
6. A person is visually impaired. You do the following *except*
   a. Tell the person what is on the tray
   b. Use the numbers on a clock to tell the person the location of food
   c. If feeding the person, describe what you are offering
   d. Let the person guess what is served
7. A person is on intake and output. He just ate ice cream. This is recorded as intake.
   a. True
   b. False
8. A person drank a pint of milk at lunch. You know he drank
   a. 250 mL of milk
   b. 350 mL of milk
   c. 500 mL of milk
   d. 750 mL of milk
9. The soup bowl holds 6 ounces. A person ate all of the soup. You record his intake as
   a. 50 mL
   b. 120 mL
   c. 180 mL
   d. 200 mL

Answers to these questions are on p. 521.

CHAPTER 26   MEASURING VITAL SIGNS

Vital Signs

- Accuracy is essential when you measure, record, and report vital signs. If unsure of your measurements, promptly ask the nurse to take them again.
- Report the following at once:
  - Any vital sign that is changed from a prior measurement
  - Vital signs above or below the normal range

Body Temperature

- Thermometers are used to measure temperature. It is measured using the Fahrenheit (F) and centigrade or Celsius (C) scales.
- Temperature sites are the mouth, rectum, axilla (underarm), tympanic membrane (ear), and temporal artery (forehead).
- Review Box 26-2, Temperature Sites, in the Textbook.
- Normal range for body temperatures depends on the site:
  - Oral: 97.6° F to 99.6° F
  - Rectal: 98.6° F to 100.6° F
  - Axillary: 96.6° F to 98.6° F
  - Tympanic membrane: 98.6° F
  - Temporal artery: 99.6° F
- Older persons have lower body temperatures than younger persons.

Glass Thermometers

- Long- or slender-tip thermometers are used for oral and axillary temperatures. So are thermometers with stubby and pear-shaped tips. Rectal thermometers have stubby tips.
- Glass thermometers are color-coded:
  - Blue—oral and axillary thermometers
  - Red—rectal thermometers
- If a mercury-glass thermometer breaks, tell the nurse at once. Do not touch the mercury. The agency must follow special procedures for handling all hazardous materials.
- When using a glass thermometer:
- Use the person's thermometer.
- Use a rectal thermometer only for rectal temperatures.
- Rinse the thermometer under cold, running water if it was soaking in a disinfectant. Dry it from the stem to the bulb end with tissues.
- Discard the thermometer if broken, cracked, or chipped.
- Shake down the thermometer to below 94° F or 34° C before using it.
- Clean and store the thermometer following center policy.
- Use plastic covers following center policy.
- Practice medical asepsis.
- Follow Standard Precautions and the Bloodborne Pathogen Standard.

Taking Temperatures

- *The oral site.* The glass thermometer remains in place 2 to 3 minutes or as required by center policy.
- *The rectal site.* Lubricate the bulb end of the rectal thermometer. Insert the glass thermometer 1 inch into the rectum. Hold the thermometer in place for 2 minutes or as required by center policy. Privacy is important.
- *The axillary site.* The axilla must be dry. The glass thermometer stays in place for 5 to 10 minutes or as required by center policy.

Electronic Thermometers

- Tympanic membrane thermometers are gently inserted into the ear. The temperature is measured in 1 to 3 seconds. These thermometers are not used if there is ear drainage.
- Temporal artery thermometers measure body temperature at the temporal artery in the forehead. These thermometers measure body temperature in 3 to 4 seconds. Follow the manufacturer's instructions for using, cleaning, and storing the device.

Pulse

Pulse Rate

- The adult pulse rate is between 60 and 100 beats per minute. Report these abnormal rates to the nurse at once:
  - *Tachycardia*—the heart rate is more than 100 beats per minute.
  - *Bradycardia*—the heart rate is less than 60 beats per minute.

Rhythm and Force of the Pulse

- The rhythm of the pulse should be regular. Report and record an irregular pulse rhythm.
- Report and record if the pulse force is strong, full, bounding, weak, thready, or feeble.

Taking Pulses
- The radial pulse is used for routine vital signs. Do not use your thumb to take a pulse. Count the pulse for 30 seconds and multiply by 2 if the agency policy permits. If the pulse is irregular, count it for 1 minute. Report and record if the pulse is regular or irregular, strong or weak.
- The apical pulse is on the left side of the chest slightly below the nipple. Count the apical pulse for 1 minute.

Respirations
- The healthy adult has 12 to 20 respirations per minute. Respirations are normally quiet, effortless, and regular. Both sides of the chest rise and fall equally.
- Count respirations when the person is at rest. Count respirations right after taking a pulse.
- Count respirations for 30 seconds and multiply the number by 2 if the agency policy permits. If an abnormal pattern is noted, count the respirations for 1 minute.
- Report and record:
  - The respiratory rate
  - Equality and depth of respirations
  - If the respirations were regular or irregular
  - If the person has pain or difficulty breathing
  - Any respiratory noises
  - An abnormal respiratory pattern

Blood Pressure
- *Normal and Abnormal Blood Pressures*
- Blood pressure has normal ranges:
  - *Systolic pressure* (upper number)—less than 120 mm Hg
  - *Diastolic pressure* (lower number)—less than 80 mm Hg
- **Hypertension**—blood pressure measurements that remain above a systolic pressure of 140 mm Hg or a diastolic pressure of 90 mm Hg. Report any systolic measurement above 120 mm Hg. Also report a diastolic pressure above 80 mm Hg.
- **Hypotension**—when the systolic blood pressure is below 90 mm Hg and the diastolic pressure is below 60 mm Hg. Report a systolic pressure below 90 mm Hg. Also report a diastolic pressure below 60 mm Hg.
- Review Box 26-2, Guidelines for Measuring Blood Pressure, in the Textbook.

CHAPTER 26   REVIEW QUESTIONS

Circle the BEST answer.

1. Which statement about taking a rectal temperature is *false?*
   a. The bulb end of the thermometer needs to be lubricated.
   b. The thermometer is held in place for 5 minutes.
   c. Privacy is important.
   d. The normal range is 98.6° F to 100.6° F.
2. Which pulse rate should you report at once?
   a. A pulse rate of 52 beats per minute
   b. A pulse rate of 60 beats per minute
   c. A pulse rate of 76 beats per minute
   d. A pulse rate of 100 beats per minute

3. Which statement is *false?*
   a. An irregular pulse is counted for 1 minute.
   b. You may use your thumb to take a radial pulse rate.
   c. The radial pulse is usually used to count a pulse rate.
   d. Tachycardia is a fast pulse rate.
4. Which blood pressure should you report?
   a. 120/80 mm Hg
   b. 88/62 mm Hg
   c. 110/70 mm Hg
   d. 92/68 mm Hg

Answers to these questions are on p. 521.

CHAPTER 27   EXERCISE AND ACTIVITY
Bedrest
- The doctor may order bedrest to treat a health problem.
- Bedrest is ordered to:
  - Reduce physical activity
  - Reduce pain
  - Encourage rest
  - Regain strength
  - Promote healing

Complications of Bedrest
- Pressure ulcers, constipation, and fecal impactions can result. Urinary tract infections and renal calculi (kidney stones) can occur. So can blood clots and pneumonia.
- The musculoskeletal system is affected by lack of exercise and activity. These complications must be prevented to maintain normal movement:
  - A **contracture** is the lack of joint mobility caused by abnormal shortening of a muscle. Common sites are the fingers, wrists, elbows, toes, ankles, knees, and hips. The person is permanently deformed and disabled.
  - **Atrophy** is the decrease in size or the wasting away of tissue. Tissues shrink in size.
- **Orthostatic hypotension (postural hypotension)** is abnormally low blood pressure when the person suddenly stands up. The person is dizzy and weak and has spots before the eyes. Fainting can occur. To prevent orthostatic hypotension, have the person change slowly from a lying or sitting position to a standing position.

Positioning
- Supportive devices are often used to support and maintain the person in a certain position:
  - *Bedboards*—are placed under the mattress to prevent the mattress from sagging.
  - *Footboards*—are placed at the foot of mattresses to prevent plantar flexion that can lead to footdrop.
  - *Trochanter rolls*—prevent the hips and legs from turning outward (external rotation).
  - *Hip abduction wedges*—keep the hips abducted (apart).
  - *Handrolls or handgrips*—prevent contractures of the thumb, fingers, and wrist.
  - *Splints*—keep the elbows, wrists, thumbs, fingers, ankles, and knees in normal position.
  - *Bed cradles*—keep the weight of top linens off the feet and toes.

Range-of-Motion Exercises

- **Range-of-motion (ROM)** exercises involve moving the joints through their complete range of motion without causing pain. They are usually done at least 2 times a day.
- *Active ROM*—exercises are done by the person.
- *Passive ROM*—you move the joints through their range of motion.
- *Active-assistive ROM*—the person does the exercises with some help.
- Review Box 27-2, Range-of-Motion Exercises, in the Textbook.
- Range-of-motion exercises can cause injury if not done properly. Practice these rules:
  - Exercise only the joints the nurse tells you to exercise.
  - Expose only the body part being exercised.
  - Use good body mechanics.
  - Support the part being exercised.
  - Move the joint slowly, smoothly, and gently.
  - Do not force a joint beyond its present range of motion.
  - Do not force a joint to the point of pain.
  - Ask the person if he or she has pain or discomfort.
  - Perform ROM exercises to the neck only if allowed by your agency and if the nurse instructs you to do so.

Ambulation

- **Ambulation** is the act of walking.
- Follow the care plan when helping a person walk. Use a gait (transfer) belt if the person is weak or unsteady. The person uses hand rails along the wall. Always check the person for orthostatic hypotension.
- When you help the person walk, walk to the side and slightly behind the person on the person's weak side. Encourage the person to use the hand rail on his or her strong side.

Walking Aids

- A cane is held on the strong side of the body. The cane tip is about 6 to 10 inches to the side of the foot. It is about 6 to 10 inches in front of the foot on the strong side. The grip is level with the hip. To walk:
  - Step A: The cane is moved forward 6 to 10 inches.
  - Step B: The weak leg (opposite the cane) is moved forward even with the cane.
  - Step C: The strong leg is moved forward and ahead of the cane and the weak leg.
- A walker gives more support than a cane. Wheeled walkers are common. They have wheels on the front legs and rubber tips on the back legs. The person pushes the walker about 6 to 8 inches in front of his or her feet.
- Braces support weak body parts, prevent or correct deformities, or prevent joint movement. A brace is applied over the ankle, knee, or back. Skin and bony points under braces are kept clean and dry. Report redness or signs of skin breakdown at once. Also report complaints of pain or discomfort. The care plan tells you when to apply and remove a brace.

CHAPTER 27   REVIEW QUESTIONS

Circle the BEST answer.

1. To prevent orthostatic hypotension, you should
   a. Move a person from the lying position to the sitting position quickly
   b. Move a person from the sitting position to the standing position quickly
   c. Move a person from the lying or sitting position to a standing position slowly
   d. Keep the person in bed
2. Exercise helps prevent contractures and muscle atrophy.
   a. True
   b. False
3. When performing ROM exercises, you should force a joint to the point of pain.
   a. True
   b. False
4. A person's left leg is weaker than his right. The person holds the cane on his right side.
   a. True
   b. False

Answers to these questions are on p. 521.

CHAPTER 28   COMFORT, REST, AND SLEEP

- Comfort is a state of well-being. Many factors affect comfort.

Assisting With Pain Relief

- **Pain or discomfort** means to ache, hurt, or be sore. Pain is subjective. You cannot see, hear, touch, or smell pain or discomfort. You must rely on what the person says.
- Report the person's complaints of pain and your observations to the nurse.
- Review Box 28-3, Nursing Measures to Promote Comfort and Relieve Pain, in the Textbook.

Factors Affecting Pain

- *Past experience*. The severity of pain, its cause, how long it lasted, and if relief occurred all affect the person's current response to pain.
- *Anxiety*. Pain and anxiety are related. Pain can cause anxiety. Anxiety increases how much pain the person feels. Reducing anxiety helps lessen pain.
- *Rest and sleep*. Pain seems worse when a person is tired or restless. Pain often seems worse at night.
- *Attention*. The more a person thinks about pain, the worse it seems.
- *Personal and family duties*. Often pain is ignored when there are children to care for. Some deny pain if a serious illness is feared.
- *The value or meaning of pain*. To some people, pain is a sign of weakness. For some persons, pain means avoiding work, daily routines and people. Some people like doting and pampering by others. The person values pain and wants such attention.
- *Support from others*. Dealing with pain is often easier when family and friends offer comfort and support. Just being nearby helps. Facing pain alone is hard for persons.

- *Culture.* Culture affects pain responses. Non–English-speaking persons may have problems describing pain.
- *Illness.* Some diseases cause decreased pain sensations.
- *Age.* Older persons may have decreased pain sensations. They may not feel pain or it may not feel severe. The person is at risk for undetected disease or injury. Chronic pain may mask new pain.
- *Persons with dementia.* Persons with dementia may not be able to complain of pain. Changes in usual behavior may signal pain. Loss of appetite also signals pain. Report any changes in a person's usual behavior to the nurse.

Signs and Symptoms
- You cannot see, hear, touch, or smell the person's pain. Rely on what the person tells you. Promptly report any information you collect about pain. Use the person's exact words when reporting and recording pain. The nurse needs the following information:
  - *Location.* Where is the pain?
  - *Onset and duration.* When did the pain start? How long has it lasted?
  - *Intensity.* Ask the person to rate the pain. Use a pain scale.
  - *Description.* Ask the person to describe the pain.
  - *Factors causing pain.* Ask when the pain started and what the person was doing before the pain started and when it started.
  - *Factors affecting pain.* Ask what makes the pain better and what makes it worse.
  - *Vital signs.* Increases often occur with acute pain. They may be normal with chronic pain.
  - *Other signs and symptoms.* Dizziness, nausea, vomiting, weakness, numbness, and tingling.
- Review Box 28-2, Signs and Symptoms of Pain, in the Textbook.

Rest
- *Rest* means to be calm, at ease, and relaxed with no anxiety or stress. Rest may involve inactivity. Or the person does things that are calming and relaxing.
- Promote rest by meeting physical, safety and security needs.
  - Thirst, hunger, pain or discomfort, and elimination needs can affect rest. A comfortable position and good alignment are important. A quiet setting promotes rest.
  - The person must feel safe from falling or other injuries. The person is secure with the signal light within reach. Understanding the reasons for care and knowing how care is given also help the person feel safe.
- Many person have rituals or routines before resting. Follow them whenever possible.
- Love and belonging are important for rest. Visits or calls from family and friends may relax the person. Reading cards and letter may also help.
- Meet self-esteem needs.
- Some persons are refreshed after a 15- or 20-minute rest. Others need more time.
- Ill or injured persons need to rest more often. Do not push the person beyond his or her limits.

Sleep
- Sleep is a basic need. Tissue healing and repair occur during sleep. Sleep lowers stress, tension, and anxiety. It refreshes and renews the person. The person regains energy and mental alertness. The person thinks and functions better after sleep.

Factors Affecting Sleep
- *Illness.* Illness increases the need for sleep.
- *Nutrition.* Sleep needs increase with weight gain. Foods with caffeine prevent sleep.
- *Exercise.* People tire after exercise. Being tired helps people sleep well. Exercise before bedtime interferes with sleep. Exercise is avoided 2 hours before bedtime.
- *Environment.* People adjust to their usual sleep settings.
- *Drugs and other substances.* Sleeping pills promote sleep. Drugs for anxiety, depression, and pain may cause the person to sleep.
- *Emotional problems.* Fear, worry, depression, and anxiety affect sleep.

Sleep Disorders
- **Insomnia** is a chronic condition in which the person cannot sleep or stay asleep all night.
- **Sleep deprivation** means that the amount and quality of sleep are decreased. Sleep is interrupted.
- **Sleep-walking** is when the person leaves the bed and walks about. If a person is sleep-walking, protect the person from injury. Guide sleep-walkers back to bed. They startle easily. Awaken them gently.

Promoting Sleep
- To promote sleep, allow a flexible bedtime, provide a comfortable room temperature, and have the person void before going to bed. Review Box 28-6, Nursing Measures to Promote Sleep, in the Textbook for other measures.

CHAPTER 28   REVIEW QUESTIONS
Circle the BEST answer.
1. A person complains of pain. You will do the following *except*
   a. Ask where the pain is
   b. Ask when the pain started
   c. Ask what the intensity of the pain is on a scale of 1 to 10
   d. Ask why he or she is complaining about pain
2. Persons with dementia may not complain of pain. Which of the following might be a signal of pain for a person with dementia?
   a. Illness
   b. Mental alertness
   c. Loss of appetite
   d. Forgetfulness
3. You can promote rest for a person by doing the following *except*
   a. Ask the person if he or she would like coffee or tea
   b. Place the signal light within reach
   c. Provide a quiet setting
   d. Follow the person's routines and rituals before rest
4. To promote sleep for a person, you should do the following *except*
   a. Follow the person's wishes
   b. Follow the care plan

c. Follow the person's rituals and routines before bedtime
d. Tell the person when to go to bed
Answers to these questions are on p. 521.

CHAPTER 29   ADMISSIONS, TRANSFERS AND DISCHARGES

Admissions
- During the admission process:
  - Identifying information is obtained from the person or family.
  - A nurse or social worker explains the resident's rights to the person and family.
  - The person's photo is taken and the person receives an ID bracelet
    - The person signs admitting papers and a general consent form.
- You prepare the person's room before the person arrives.

Admitting the Person
- Admission is your first chance to make a good impression. You must:
  - Greet the person by name and title. Use the admission form to find out the person's name.
  - Introduce yourself by name and title to the person, family, and friends.
  - Make roommate introductions.
  - Act in a professional manner
  - Treat the person with dignity and respect.
- During the admission procedure the nurse may ask you to:
  - Collect some information for the admission form.
  - Measure the person's weight and height.
  - Measure the person's vital signs.
  - Obtain a urine specimen (if needed)
  - Complete a clothing and personal belongings list.
  - Orient the person to the room, nursing unit, and the agency.

Weight and Height
- When weighing a person, follow the manufacturer's instructions and center procedures for using the scales. Follow these guidelines when measuring weight and height:
  - The person wears only a gown or pajamas. No footwear is worn.
  - A dry incontinence product is worn.
  - The person voids before being weighed.
  - Weigh the person at the same time of day. Before breakfast is the best time.
  - Use the same scale for daily, weekly, and monthly weights.
  - Balance the scale at zero before weighing the person.

Transfers and Discharges
- When transferred or discharged, the person leaves the agency. He or she goes home or to another health care setting.
- Transfers and discharges are usually planned in advance by the health team.
- For discharges, the health team teaches the person and family about diet, exercise, and drugs. They also teach them about procedures and treatments and arrange for home care, equipment, and therapies as needed.

- The nurse tells you when to start the transfer or discharge procedure. The doctor must give the order before the person can leave. Usually a wheelchair is used. If leaving by ambulance, a stretcher is used.
- If a person wants to leave the agency without the doctor's permission, tell the nurse at once. The nurse or social worker handles the matter.

CHAPTER 29   REVIEW QUESTIONS
Circle the BEST answer.
1. When admitted, you explain the resident's rights to the person and family.
   a. True
   b. False
2. When a person is admitted, you do the following *except*
   a. Greet the person by name and title
   b. Treat the person with dignity and respect
   c. Introduce the person to his or her roommate
   d. Rush the admission procedure
3. Which statement is *false*?
   a. Have the person void before being weighed.
   b. Weigh the person at the same time of day.
   c. Balance the scale at zero before weighing the person
   d. Have the person wear shoes when being weighed.
4. A person wants to leave the nursing center without the doctor's permission. You should tell the nurse at once.
   a. True
   b. False
Answers to these questions are on p. 521.

CHAPTER 32   THE PERSON HAVING SURGERY

Elastic Stockings
- Elastic stockings exert pressure on the veins. The pressure promotes venous blood return to the heart. The stocking help prevent blood clots in the leg veins.
- Elastic stockings also are called AE stockings (anti-embolism or anti-embolic). They also are called TED hose. TED means thrombo-embolic disease.
- The nurse measures the person for the correct size of elastic stockings. Most stocking have an opening near the toes that is used to check circulation, skin color, and skin temperature.
- The person usually has two pairs of stockings. One pair is washed; the other pair is worn.
- Stockings should not have twists, creases, or wrinkles after you apply them. Twists can affect circulation. Creases and wrinkles can cause skin breakdown.
- Loose stocking do not promote venous blood return to the heart. Stocking that are too tight can affect circulation. Tell the nurse if the stockings are too loose or tight.

CHAPTER 32   REVIEW QUESTION
Circle the BEST answer.
1. Which statement about elastic stocking is true?
   a. Elastic stockings should be loose to promote venous blood return to the heart.
   b. Stockings should not have twists, creases, or wrinkles after you apply them.

c. The doctor measures the person for the correct size of elastic stockings.

d. The person should have only one pair of stockings.

The answer to this question is on p. 521.

CHAPTER 33 WOUND CARE

- A **wound** is a break in the skin or mucous membrane.
- The wound is a portal of entry for microbes. Infection is a major threat. Wound care involves preventing infection and further injury to the wound and nearby tissues.

Skin Tears

- A **skin tear** is a break or rip in the skin.
- Skin tears are caused by friction, shearing, pulling, or pressure on the skin. Bumping a hand, arm, or leg on any hard surface can cause a skin tear. Beds, bed rails, chairs, wheelchair footplates, and tables are dangers. So is holding the person's arm or leg too tight, removing tape or adhesives, bathing, dressing and other tasks. Buttons, zippers, jewelry or long or jagged finger or toe nails can also cause skin tears.
- Skin tears are painful. They are portals of entry for microbes. Wound complications can develop. Tell the nurse at once if you cause or find a skin tear.
- Review Box 33-2, Measures to Prevent Skin Tears, in the Textbook.

Circulatory Ulcers

- *Circulatory ulcers (vascular ulcers)* are open sores on the lower legs or feet. They are caused by decreased blood flow through the arteries or veins.
- Review Box 33-3, Measures to Prevent Circulatory Ulcers, in the Textbook.
- *Venous ulcers (stasis ulcers)* are open sores on the lower legs or feet. They are caused by poor blood flow through the veins. The heels and inner aspect of the ankles are common sites for venous ulcers.
- *Arterial ulcers* are open wounds on the lower legs or feet caused by poor arterial blood flow. They are found between the toes, on top of the toes, and on the outer side of the ankle.
- A *diabetic foot ulcer* is an open wound on the foot caused by complications from diabetes. When nerves are affected, the person can lose sensation in a foot or leg. The person may not feel pain, heat, or cold. Therefore the person may not feel a cut, blister, burn, or other trauma to the foot. Infection and a large sore can develop. When blood flow to the foot decreases, tissues and cells do not get needed oxygen and nutrients. A sore does not heal properly. Tissue death (gangrene) can occur. Review Box 33-4, Foot Problems Common in Persons With Diabetes.

Prevention and Treatment

- Check the person's feet and legs every day. Report any sign of a problem to the nurse at once. Follow the care plan to prevent and treat circulatory ulcers.

CHAPTER 33 REVIEW QUESTIONS

Circle the BEST answer.

1. The following can cause a skin tear *except*
   a. Friction and shearing
   b. Holding a person's arm or leg too tight
   c. Rings, watches, bracelets
   d. Trimmed, short nails
2. A person is diabetic. Which statement is *false?*
   a. The person may not feel pain in her feet.
   b. The person may not feel heat or cold in her feet.
   c. You need to check her feet weekly for foot problems.
   d. The person is at risk for diabetic foot ulcers.
3. Which statement about elastic stockings is *false?*
   a. Elastic stockings are also called anti-embolic stockings.
   b. Elastic stockings should be wrinkle-free after being applied.
   c. A person usually has two pairs of elastic stockings.
   d. Elastic stockings are applied after a person gets out of bed.

Answers to these questions are on p. 521.

CHAPTER 34 PRESSURE ULCERS

- A **pressure ulcer** is a localized injury to the skin and/or underlying tissue. Pressure ulcers usually occur over a bony prominence—the back of the head, shoulder blades, elbows, hips, spine, sacrum, knees, ankles, heels, and toes.
- *Decubitus ulcer, bed sore,* and *pressure sore* are other terms for pressure ulcer.
- Pressure, shearing, and friction are common causes of skin breakdown and pressure ulcers. Risk factors include breaks in the skin, poor circulation to an area, moisture, dry skin, and irritation by urine and feces.

Persons at Risk

- Persons at risk for pressure ulcers are those who:
  - Are confined to a bed or chair
  - Need some or total help in moving
  - Are agitated or have involuntary muscle movements
  - Have loss of bowel or bladder control
  - Are exposed to moisture
  - Have poor nutrition
  - Have poor fluid balance
  - Have lowered mental awareness
  - Have problems sensing pain or pressure
  - Have circulatory problems
  - Are obese or very thin
  - Have a healed pressure ulcer.

Pressure Ulcer Stages

- In persons with light skin, a reddened bony area is the first sign of a pressure ulcer. In persons with dark skin, a bony area may appear red, blue, or purple. The area may feel warm or cool. The person may complain of pain, burning, tingling, or itching in the area.
- Box 34-2 in the Textbook describes pressure ulcer stages.
- Figure 34-4 in the Textbook shows the stages of pressure ulcers.

Prevention and Treatment
- Preventing pressure ulcers is much easier than trying to heal them. Review Box 34-3, Measures to Prevent Pressure Ulcers, in the Textbook.
- The person at risk for pressure ulcers may be placed on a foam, air, alternating air, gel, or water mattress.
- Protective devices are often used to prevent and treat pressure ulcers and skin breakdown. Protective devices include:
  - Bed cradle
  - Heel and elbow protectors
  - Heel and foot elevators
  - Gel or fluid-filled pads and cushions
  - Eggcrate-type pads
  - Special beds
  - Other equipment—pillows, trochanter rolls, and footboards

CHAPTER 34   REVIEW QUESTIONS

Circle the BEST answer.
1. You may expect to find a pressure ulcer at all of the following sites *except*
   a. Back of the head
   b. Ears
   c. Top of the thigh
   d. Toes
2. Which of the following is not a protective device used to prevent and treat pressure ulcers?
   a. Heel elevator
   b. Bed cradle
   c. Draw sheet
   d. Elbow protector
3. In obese people, pressure ulcers can occur between abdominal folds.
   a. True
   b. False
4. Pressure ulcers never occur over a bony prominence.
   a. True
   b. False

Answers to these questions are on p. 521.

CHAPTER 35   HEAT AND COLD APPLICATIONS

Heat Applications
- Heat relieves pain, relaxes muscles, promotes healing, reduces tissue swelling, and decreases joint stiffness.

Complications
- High temperatures can cause burns. Report pain, excessive redness, and blisters at once. Also observe for pale skin.
- Metal implants pose risks. Pacemakers and joint replacements are made of metal. Do not apply heat to an implant area.
- Heat is not applied to a pregnant woman's abdomen. The heat can affect fetal growth.

Cold Applications
- Cold applications reduce pain, prevent swelling, and decrease circulation and bleeding.

Complications
- Complications include pain, burns, blisters, and poor circulation. Burns and blisters occur from intense cold. They also occur when dry cold is in direct contact with the skin.

Applying Heat and Cold
- Protect the person from injury during heat and cold applications. Review Box 35-1, Rules for Applying Heat and Cold, in the Textbook.

CHAPTER 35   REVIEW QUESTIONS

Circle the BEST answer.
1. Complications from a heat application include the following *except*
   a. Excessive redness
   b. Blisters
   c. Pale skin
   d. Cyanotic (bluish) nail beds
2. When applying heat or cold, you should do the following *except*
   a. Ask the nurse what the temperature of the application should be
   b. Cover dry heat or cold applications before applying them
   c. Observe the skin every 2 hours
   d. Know how long to leave the application in place

Answers to these questions are on p. 521.

CHAPTER 36   OXYGEN NEEDS

Altered Respiratory Function
- Hypoxia means that cells do not have enough oxygen.
- Restlessness, dizziness, and disorientation are signs of hypoxia.
- Review Box 36-1, Signs and Symptoms of Hypoxia, in the Textbook. Report signs and symptoms of hypoxia to the nurse at once. Hypoxia is life-threatening.
- Review Box 36-2, Signs and Symptoms of Altered Respiratory Function, in the Textbook.

Abnormal Respirations
- Adults normally have 12 to 20 respirations per minute. They are quiet, effortless, and regular. Both sides of the chest rise and fall equally. Report these observations at once:
  - **Tachypnea**—rapid breathing. Respirations are 20 or more per minute.
  - **Bradypnea**—slow breathing. Respirations are fewer than 12 per minute.
  - **Apnea**—lack or absence of breathing.
  - **Hypoventilation**—respirations are slow, shallow, and sometimes irregular.
  - **Hyperventilation**—respirations are rapid and deeper than normal.
  - **Dyspnea**—difficult, labored, painful breathing.
  - **Cheyne-Stokes respirations**—respirations gradually increase in rate and depth. Then they become shallow and slow. Breathing may stop for 10 to 20 seconds.
  - **Orthopnea**—breathing deeply and comfortably only when sitting.

○ **Biot's respirations**—rapid and deep respirations followed by 10–30 seconds of apnea.

○ **Kussmaul respirations**—very deep and rapid respirations.

Promoting Oxygenation

Positioning

- Breathing is usually easier in semi-Fowler's and Fowler's positions. Persons with difficulty breathing often prefer the **orthopneic position** (sitting up and leaning over a table to breathe).

Deep Breathing and Coughing

- Deep breathing moves air into most parts of the lungs. Coughing removes mucus. Deep breathing and coughing are usually done every 1 to 2 hours while the person is awake. They help prevent pneumonia and atelectasis (the collapse of a portion of the lung).

Oxygen Devices

- A nasal cannula allows eating and drinking. Tight prongs can irritate the nose. Pressure on the ears and cheekbones is possible.
- A simple face mask covers the nose and mouth. Talking and eating are hard to do with a mask. Listen carefully. Moisture can build up under the mask. Keep the face clean and dry. Masks are removed for eating. Usually oxygen is given by cannula during meals.

Oxygen Flow Rates

- When giving care and checking the person, always check the flow rate. Tell the nurse at once if it is too high or too low. A nurse or respiratory therapist will adjust the flow rate.

Oxygen Safety

- You do not give oxygen. You assist the nurse in providing safe care.
- Always check the oxygen level when you are with or near persons using oxygen systems that contain a limited amount of oxygen. Oxygen tanks and liquid oxygen systems are examples. Report a low oxygen level to the nurse at once.
- Follow the rules for fire and the use of oxygen in Chapter 12.
- Never remove the oxygen device. However, turn off the oxygen flow if there is a fire.
- Make sure the oxygen device is secure but not tight.
- Check for signs of irritation from the oxygen device— behind the ears, under the nose, around the face, and cheekbones.
- Keep the face clean and dry when a mask is used.
- Never shut off the oxygen flow.
- Do not adjust the flow rate unless allowed by your state and agency.
- Tell the nurse at once if the flow rate is too high or too low.
- Tell the nurse at once if the humidifier is not bubbling.
- Secure tubing to the person's garment. Follow agency policy.
- Make sure there are no kinks in the tubing.
- Make sure the person does not lie on any part of the tubing.
- Report signs of hypoxia, respiratory distress, or abnormal breathing to the nurse at once.

- Give oral hygiene as directed. Follow the care plan.
- Make sure the oxygen device is clean and free of mucus.
- Make sure the oxygen tank is secure in its holder.

CHAPTER 36   REVIEW QUESTIONS

Circle the BEST answer.

1. Which statement is *false*?
   a. Restlessness, dizziness, and disorientation are signs of hypoxia.
   b. Hypoxia is life-threatening.
   c. Report signs and symptoms of hypoxia at the end of the shift.
   d. Anything that affects respiratory function can cause hypoxia.
2. Adults normally have
   a. 8 to 10 respirations per minute
   b. 12 to 20 respirations per minute
   c. 10 to 12 respirations per minute
   d. 20 to 24 respirations per minute
3. Dyspnea is
   a. Difficult, labored, or painful breathing
   b. Slow breathing with fewer than 12 respirations per minute
   c. Rapid breathing with 24 or more respirations per minute
   d. Lack or absence of breathing
4. Which statement about positioning is *false*?
   a. Breathing is usually easier in semi-Fowler's or Fowler's position.
   b. Persons with difficulty breathing often prefer the orthopneic position.
   c. Position changes are needed at least every 4 hours.
   d. Follow the person's care plan for positioning preferences.
5. A person has a nasal cannula. Which statement is *false*?
   a. You will leave the nasal cannula on while the person is eating.
   b. You will watch the nose area for irritation.
   c. You will watch the ears and cheekbones for skin breakdown.
   d. You will take the nasal cannula off while the person is eating.

Answers to these questions are on p. 522.

CHAPTER 38   REHABILITATION AND RESTORATIVE NURSING CARE

- A **disability** is any lost, absent, or impaired physical or mental function.
- **Rehabilitation** is the process of restoring the person to his or her highest possible level of physical, psychological, social, and economic function. The focus is on improving abilities. This promotes function at the highest level of independence.

Rehabilitation and the Whole Person

- Rehabilitation takes longer in older persons. Changes from aging affect healing, mobility, vision, hearing, and other functions. Chronic health problems can slow recovery.

Physical Aspects

- Rehabilitation starts when the person first seeks health care. Complications, such as contractures and pressure ulcers, are prevented.
- *Self-care*. Self-care for activities of daily living (ADL) is a major goal. Self-help devices are often needed.
- *Elimination*. Bowel or bladder training may be needed. Fecal impaction, constipation, and fecal incontinence are prevented.
- *Mobility*. The person may need crutches, a walker, a cane, a brace, or a wheelchair.
- *Nutrition*. The person may need a dysphagia diet or enteral nutrition.
- *Communication*. Speech therapy and communication devices may be helpful.

Psychological and Social Aspects

- A disability can affect function and appearance. Self-esteem and relationships may suffer. The person may feel unwhole, useless, unattractive, unclean, or undesirable. The person may deny the disability. The person may expect therapy to correct the problem. He or she may be depressed, angry, and hostile.
- Successful rehabilitation depends on the person's attitude. The person must accept his or her limits and be motivated. The focus is on abilities and strengths. Despair and frustration are common. Progress may be slow. Old fears and emotions may recur.
- Remind persons of their progress. They need help accepting disabilities and limits. Give support, reassurance, and encouragement. Spiritual support helps some people. Psychological and social needs are part of the care plan.

The Rehabilitation Team

- Rehabilitation is a team effort. The person is the key member. The health team and family help the person set goals and plan care. All help the person regain function and independence.

Your Role

- Every part of your job focuses on promoting the person's independence. Preventing decline in function also is a goal. Review Box 38-2, Assisting With Rehabilitation and Restorative Care, in the Textbook.

Quality of Life

- To promote quality of life:
- *Protect the right to privacy*. The person relearns old or practices new skills in private. Others do not need to see mistakes, falls, spills, clumsiness, anger, or tears.
- *Encourage personal choice*. This gives the person control.
- *Protect the right to be free from abuse and mistreatment*. Sometimes improvement is not seen for weeks. Repeated explanations and demonstrations may have little or no results. You and other staff and family may become upset and short-tempered. However, no one can shout, scream, or yell at the person. Nor can they call the person names or hit or strike the person. Unkind remarks are not allowed. Report signs of abuse or mistreatment.
- *Learn to deal with your anger and frustration*. The person does not choose loss of function. If the process upsets you, discuss your feelings with the nurse.

- *Encourage activities*. Provide support and reassurance to the person with the disability. Remind the person that others with disabilities can give support and understanding.
- *Provide a safe setting*. The setting must meet the person's needs. The overbed table, bedside stand, and signal light are moved to the person's strong side.
- *Show patience, understanding, and sensitivity*. The person may be upset and discouraged. Give support, encouragement, and praise when needed. Stress the person's abilities and strengths. Do not give pity or sympathy.

CHAPTER 38   REVIEW QUESTIONS

Circle the BEST answer.

1. Successful rehabilitation depends on the person's attitude.
   a. True
   b. False
2. A person with a disability may be depressed, angry, and hostile.
   a. True
   b. False
3. A person needs rehabilitation. You should do the following *except*
   a. Let the person relearn old skills in private
   b. Let the person practice new skills in private
   c. Encourage the person to make choices
   d. Shout at the person
4. You saw a family member hit and scream at a person. You need to report your observations to the nurse.
   a. True
   b. False
5. A person has a weak left arm. You will
   a. Place the signal light on his left side
   b. Place the signal light on his right side
   c. Give him sympathy
   d. Give him pity

Answers to these questions are on p. 522.

CHAPTER 39   HEARING, SPEECH, AND VISION PROBLEMS

Hearing Loss

- Hearing loss is not being able to hear the normal range of sounds associated with normal hearing. Deafness is the most severe form of hearing loss.
- Obvious signs and symptoms of hearing loss include:
   - Speaking too loudly
   - Leaning forward to hear
   - Turning and cupping the better ear toward the speaker
   - Answering questions or responding inappropriately
   - Asking for words to be repeated
   - Asking others to speak louder or to speak more slowly and clearly
   - Having trouble hearing over the phone
   - Finding it hard to follow conversations when two or more people are talking
   - Turning up the TV, radio, or music volume so loud that others complain
- Persons with hearing loss may wear hearing aids or lip-read (speech-read). They watch facial expressions,

gestures, and body language. Some people learn American Sign Language (ASL). Others may have hearing assistance dogs.

- Review Box 39-2, Measures to Promote Hearing, in the Textbook.
- Hearing aids are battery-operated. If they do not seem to work properly:
  - Check if the hearing aid is on. It has an on and off switch.
  - Check the battery position.
  - Insert a new battery if needed.
  - Clean the hearing aid. Follow the nurse's direction and the manufacturer's instructions.
- Hearing aids are turned off when not in use. The battery is removed.
- Handle and care for hearing aids properly. If lost or damaged, report it to the nurse at once.

Speech Disorders

Aphasia

- **Aphasia** is the total or partial loss of the ability to use or understand language.
- *Expressive aphasia* relates to difficulty expressing or sending out thoughts. Thinking is clear. The person knows what to say but has difficulty or cannot speak the words.
- *Receptive aphasia* relates to difficulty understanding language. The person has trouble understanding what is said or read. People and common objects are not recognized.

Eye Disorders

- *Glaucoma.* Glaucoma results when fluid builds up in the eye and causes pressure on the optic nerve. The optic nerve is damaged. Vision loss with eventual blindness occurs. Drugs and surgery can control glaucoma and prevent further damage to the optic nerve. Prior damage cannot be reversed.
- *Cataract.* Cataract is a clouding of the lens in the eye. Signs and symptoms include cloudy, blurry, or dimmed vision. Persons may also be sensitive to light and glares or see halos around lights. Poor vision at night and double vision in one eye are other symptoms. Surgery is the only treatment. Review the list of post-operative care measures on p. 659 in the Textbook.

Impaired Vision and Blindness

- Birth defects, injuries, accidents, and eye diseases are among the many causes of impaired vision and blindness. They also are complications of some diseases.
- Review Box 39-5, Caring for Blind and Visually Impaired Persons, in the Textbook.

Corrective Lenses

- Clean eyeglasses daily and as needed.
- Protect eyeglasses from loss or damage. When not worn, put them in their case.
- Contact lenses are cleaned, removed, and stored according to the manufacturer's instructions.

CHAPTER 39   REVIEW QUESTIONS

Circle the BEST answer.

1. A person is hard-of-hearing. You do the following *except*
   a. Face the person when speaking
   b. Speak clearly, distinctly, and slowly
   c. Use facial expressions and gestures to give clues
   d. Use long sentences
2. A person has taken his hearing aid out for the evening. You do the following *except*
   a. Make sure the hearing aid is turned off
   b. Keep the battery in the hearing aid
   c. Place the hearing aid in a safe place
   d. Handle the hearing aid carefully
3. A person is blind. You do the following *except*
   a. Identify yourself when you enter his room
   b. Describe people, places, and things thoroughly
   c. Rearrange his furniture without telling him
   d. Encourage him to do as much for himself as possible
4. Fluid build up in the eye that causes pressure on the optic nerve is
   a. Cataract
   b. Cerumen
   c. Glaucoma
   d. Tinnitus

Answers to these questions are on p. 522.

CHAPTER 40   CANCER, IMMUNE SYSTEM, AND SKIN DISORDERS

Cancer

- Cancer is the second leading cause of death in the United States.
- Review Box 40-1, Some Signs and Symptoms of Cancer, in the Textbook.
- Surgery, radiation therapy, and chemotherapy are the most common treatments.
- Persons with cancer have many needs. They include:
  - Pain relief or control
  - Rest and exercise
  - Fluids and nutrition
  - Preventing skin breakdown
  - Preventing bowel problems (constipation, diarrhea)
  - Dealing with treatment side effects
  - Psychological and social needs
  - Spiritual needs
  - Sexual needs
- Anger, fear, and depression are common. Some surgeries are disfiguring. The person may feel unwhole, unattractive, or unclean. The person and family need support.
- Talk to the person. Do not avoid the person because you are uncomfortable. Use touch and listening to show that you care.
- Spiritual needs are important. A spiritual leader may provide comfort.

Immune System Disorders

- The immune system protects the body from microbes, cancer cells, and other harmful substances. It defends against threats inside and outside the body.

Acquired Immunodeficiency Syndrome

- Acquired immunodeficiency syndrome (AIDS) is caused by a virus. The virus is spread through body fluids—blood, semen, vaginal secretions, and breast milk. HIV is not spread by saliva, tears, sweat, sneezing, coughing, insects, or casual contact.
- Persons with AIDS are at risk for pneumonia, tuberculosis, Kaposi's sarcoma (a cancer), and nervous system damage.
- To protect yourself and others from the virus, follow Standard Precautions and the Bloodborne Pathogen Standard.
- Review Box 40-4, Caring for the Person With AIDS, in the Textbook.
- Older persons also get AIDS. They get and spread HIV through sexual contact and IV drug use. Aging and some diseases can mask the signs and symptoms of AIDS. Older persons are less likely to be tested for HIV/AIDS.

CHAPTER 40   REVIEW QUESTIONS

Circle the BEST answer.

1. A person with cancer may need all the following *except*
   a. Pain relief or control
   b. Avoidance from you
   c. Fluids and nutrition
   d. Psychological support
2. Which statement about HIV is *false*?
   a. HIV is spread through body fluids.
   b. Standard Precautions and the Bloodborne Pathogen Standard are followed.
   c. Older persons cannot get and spread HIV.
   d. Older persons are less likely to be tested for HIV/AIDS.
3. The immune system defends against threats inside and outside the body.
   a. True
   b. False

Answers to these questions are on p. 522.

CHAPTER 41   NERVOUS SYSTEM AND MUSCULO-SKELETAL DISORDERS

Nervous System Disorders

Stroke

- Stroke is also called a brain attack or cerebrovascular accident (CVA). It is the third leading cause of death in the United States. Review Box 26-6, Warning Signs of Stroke, in the Textbook.
- The effects of stroke include:
  - Loss of face, hand, arm, leg, or body control
  - **Hemiplegia**—paralysis on one side of the body
  - Changing emotions (crying easily or mood swings, sometimes for no reason)
  - Difficulty swallowing (dysphagia)
  - Aphasia or slowed or slurred speech
  - Changes in sight, touch, movement, and thought
  - Impaired memory
  - Urinary frequency, urgency, or incontinence
  - Loss of bowel control or constipation
  - Depression and frustration
- The health team helps the person regain the highest possible level of function. Review Box 39-2, Care of the Person With a Stroke, in the Textbook.

Parkinson's Disease

- Parkinson's disease is a slow, progressive disorder with no cure. Persons over the age of 50 are at risk. Signs and symptoms become worse over time. They include:
  - *Tremors*—often start in one finger and spread to the whole arm. Pill-rolling movements—rubbing the thumb and index finger—may occur. The person may have trembling in the hands, arms, legs, jaw, and face.
  - *Rigid, stiff muscles*—in the arms, legs, neck, and trunk.
  - *Slow movements*—the person has a slow, shuffling gait.
  - *Stooped posture and impaired balance*—it is hard to walk. Falls are a risk.
  - *Mask-like expression*—the person cannot blink and smile. A fixed stare is common.
- Other signs and symptoms that develop over time include swallowing and chewing problems, constipation, and bladder problems. Sleep problems, depression, and emotional changes (fear, insecurity) can occur. So can memory loss and slow thinking. The person may have slurred, monotone, and soft speech. Some people talk too fast or repeat what they say.
- Drugs are ordered to treat and control the disease. Exercise and physical therapy improve strength, posture, balance, and mobility. Therapy is needed for speech and swallowing problems. The person may need help with eating and self-care. Safety measures are needed to prevent falls and injury.

Multiple Sclerosis

- Multiple sclerosis (MS) is a chronic disease. The myelin (which covers nerve fibers) in the brain and spinal cord is destroyed. Nerve impulses are not sent to and from the brain in a normal manner. Functions are impaired or lost. There is no cure.
- Symptoms usually start between the ages of 20 and 40. Signs and symptoms depend on the damaged area. They may include vision problems, muscle weakness in the arms and legs, balance problems that affect standing and walking. Tingling, prickling, or numb sensations may occur. Also, partial or complete paralysis and pain may occur.
- Persons with MS are kept active as long as possible and as independent as possible. Skin care, hygiene, and range-of-motion exercises are important. So are turning, positioning, and deep breathing and coughing. Bowel and bladder elimination is promoted. Injuries and complications from bedrest are prevented.

Spinal Cord Injury

- Spinal cord injuries can permanently damage the nervous system. Common causes are stab or gunshot wounds, motor vehicle crashes, falls, and sports injuries.
- The higher the level of injury, the more functions lost:
- Lumbar injuries—sensory and muscle function in the legs is lost. The person has **paraplegia**—paralysis and loss of sensory function in legs and lower trunk.
- Thoracic injuries—sensory and muscle function below the chest is lost. The person has paraplegia.
- Cervical injuries—sensory and muscle function of the arms, legs, and trunk is lost. Paralysis in the arms, legs, and trunk is called **quadriplegia** or **tetraplegia.**
- Review Box 41-3, Care of Persons With Paralysis, in the Textbook.

Musculo-Skeletal Disorders

Arthritis

- Arthritis means joint inflammation.
- *Osteoarthritis (Degenerative Joint Disease)*. The fingers, spine (neck and lower back), and weight-bearing joints (hips, knees, and feet) are often affected. Treatment involves pain relief, heat applications, exercise, rest and joint care, weight control, and a healthy life-style. Falls are prevented. Help is given with ADL as needed. Toilet seat risers are helpful when hips and knees are affected. So are chairs with higher seats and armrests. Some people need joint replacement surgery.
- *Rheumatoid Arthritis*. Rheumatoid arthritis (RA) causes joint pain, swelling, stiffness, and loss of function. Joints are tender, warm, and swollen. Fatigue and fever are common. The person does not feel well. The person's care plan may include rest balanced with exercise, proper positioning, joint care, weight control, measures to reduce stress, and measures to prevent falls. Drugs are ordered for pain relief and to reduce inflammation. Heat and cold applications may be ordered. Some persons need joint replacement surgery. Emotional support is needed. Persons with RA need to stay as active as possible. Give encouragement and praise. Listen when the person needs to talk.

CHAPTER 41   REVIEW QUESTIONS

Circle the BEST answer.

1. The person had a stroke. Care includes all the following *except*
   a. Place the signal light on the person's strong side
   b. Reposition the person every 2 hours
   c. Perform ROM exercises as ordered
   d. Place objects on the affected side
2. The person with hemiplegia
   a. Is paralyzed on one side of the body
   b. Has both arms paralyzed
   c. Has both legs paralyzed
   d. Has all extremities paralyzed
3. The person with multiple sclerosis should be kept active as long as possible.
   a. True
   b. False
4. The person has paralysis in the legs and lower trunk. This is called
   a. Quadriplegia
   b. Paraplegia
   c. Hemiplegia
   d. Tetraplegia
5. Fever is a common symptom of osteoarthritis.
   a. True
   b. False

Answers to these questions are on p. 522.

CHAPTER 42   CARDIOVASCULAR AND RESPIRATORY DISORDERS

Cardiovascular Disorders

Angina

- Angina is chest pain. It is from reduced blood flow to part of the heart muscle. Chest pain is described as tightness, pressure, squeezing, or burning in the chest. Pain can occur in the shoulders, arms, neck, jaw, or back. The person may be pale, feel faint, and perspire. Dyspnea is common. Nausea, fatigue, and weakness may occur. Some persons complain of "gas" or indigestion.
- Rest often relieves symptoms in 3 to 15 minutes. Chest pain lasting longer than a few minutes and not relieved by rest and nitroglycerin may signal heart attack. The person needs emergency care.

Myocardial Infarction

- Myocardial infarction (MI) also is called *heart attack, acute myocardial infarction (AMI),* and *acute coronary syndrome (ACS).*
- Blood flow to the heart muscle is suddenly blocked. Part of the heart muscle dies. MI is an emergency. Sudden cardiac death *(sudden cardiac arrest)* can occur.
- Review Box 40-2, Signs and Symptoms of Myocardial Infarction, in the Textbook.

Heart Failure

- Heart failure or congestive heart failure (CHF) occurs when the heart is weakened and cannot pump normally. Blood backs up. Tissue congestion occurs.
- Drugs are given to strengthen the heart. They also reduce the amount of fluid in the body. A sodium-controlled diet is ordered. Oxygen is given. Semi-Fowler's position is preferred for breathing. I&O, daily weight, elastic stockings, and range-of-motion exercises are part of the care plan.

Respiratory Disorders

Chronic Obstructive Pulmonary Disease

- Two disorders are grouped under chronic obstructive pulmonary disease (COPD). They are chronic bronchitis and emphysema. These disorders obstruct airflow. Lung function is gradually lost.
- *Chronic Bronchitis*. Bronchitis means inflammation of the bronchi. Chronic bronchitis occurs after repeated episodes of bronchitis. Smoking is the major cause. Smoker's cough in the morning is often the first symptom of chronic bronchitis. Over time, the cough becomes more frequent. The person has difficulty breathing and tires easily. The person must stop smoking. Oxygen therapy and breathing exercises are often ordered. If a respiratory tract infection occurs, the person needs prompt treatment.
- *Emphysema*. In emphysema, the alveoli enlarge and become less elastic. They do not expand and shrink normally when breathing in and out. Air becomes trapped when exhaling. Smoking is the most common cause. The person has shortness of breath and a cough. Sputum may contain pus. Fatigue is common.
  The person works hard to breathe in and out. Breathing is easier when the person sits upright and slightly forward. The person must stop smoking. Respiratory therapy, breathing exercises, oxygen, and drug therapy are ordered.

Asthma

- In asthma, the airway becomes inflamed and narrow. Extra mucus is produced. Dyspnea results. Wheezing and coughing are common. So are pain and tightening in the chest. Asthma usually is triggered by allergies. Other triggers include air pollutants and irritants, smoking and second-hand smoke, respiratory tract infections, exertion, and cold air. Asthma is treated with drugs. Severe attacks may require emergency care.

Pneumonia

- Pneumonia is an inflammation and infection of lung tissue. Bacteria, viruses, and other microbes are causes.
- High fever, chills, painful cough, chest pain on breathing, and rapid pulse occur. Shortness of breath and rapid breathing also occur. Cyanosis may be present. Sputum is thick and white, green, yellow, or rust-colored. Other signs and symptoms are nausea, vomiting, headache, tiredness, and muscle aches.
- Drugs are ordered for infection and pain. Fluid intake is increased. Intravenous therapy and oxygen may be needed. Semi-Fowler's position eases breathing. Rest is important. Standard Precautions are followed. Isolation Precautions are used depending on the cause.

Tuberculosis

- Tuberculosis (TB) is a bacterial infection in the lungs. TB is spread by airborne droplets with coughing, sneezing, speaking, singing, or laughing. Those who have close, frequent contact with an infected person are at risk. TB is more likely to occur in close, crowded areas. Age, poor nutrition, and HIV infection are other risk factors.
- Signs and symptoms are tiredness, loss of appetite, weight loss, fever, and night sweats. Cough and sputum production increase over time. Sputum may contain blood. Chest pain occurs.
- Drugs for TB are given. Standard Precautions and Isolation Precautions are needed. The person must cover the mouth and nose with tissues when sneezing, coughing, or producing sputum. Tissues are flushed down the toilet, placed in a BIOHAZARD bag, or placed in a paper bag and burned. Hand washing after contact with sputum is essential.

CHAPTER 42   REVIEW QUESTIONS

Circle the BEST answer.

1. Which statement about angina is *false?*
   a. Angina is chest pain.
   b. The person may be pale and perspire.
   c. Rest often relieves the symptoms.
   d. You do not report angina to the nurse.
2. A person has heart failure. You do all the following *except*
   a. Measure intake and output
   b. Measure weight daily
   c. Promote a diet that is high in salt
   d. Restrict fluids as ordered
3. Which position is usually best for the person with pneumonia?
   a. Semi-Fowler's
   b. Prone
   c. Supine
   d. Trendelenburg's

4. A bacterial infection in the lungs is
   a. Asthma
   b. Bronchitis
   c. Tuberculosis
   d. Emphysema

Answers to these questions are on p. 522.

CHAPTER 43   DIGESTIVE AND ENDOCRINE DISORDERS

Digestive Disorders

Vomiting

- These measures are needed:
  - Follow Standard Precautions and the Bloodborne Pathogen Standard.
  - Turn the person's head well to one side. This prevents aspiration.
  - Place a kidney basin under the person's chin.
  - Move vomitus away from the person.
  - Provide oral hygiene.
  - Observe vomitus for color, odor, and undigested food. If it looks like coffee grounds, it contains undigested blood. This signals bleeding. Report your observations.
  - Measure, report, and record the amount of vomitus. Also record the amount on the I&O record.
  - Save a specimen for laboratory study.
  - Dispose of vomitus after the nurse observes it.
  - Eliminate odors.
  - Provide for comfort.

Hepatitis

- Hepatitis is an inflammation of the liver. It can be mild or cause death. Signs and symptoms are listed in Box 43-2 in the Textbook. Some people do not have symptoms.
- Protect yourself and others. Follow Standard Precautions and the Bloodborne Pathogen Standard. Isolation Precautions are ordered as necessary. Assist the person with hygiene and hand washing as needed.

The Endocrine System

Diabetes

- In this disorder the body cannot produce or use insulin properly. Insulin is needed for glucose to move from the blood into the cells. Sugar builds up in the blood. Cells do not have enough sugar for energy and cannot function.
- Diabetes must be controlled to prevent complications. Complications include blindness, renal failure, nerve damage, and damage to the gums and teeth. Heart and blood vessel diseases are other problems. They can lead to stroke, heart attack, and slow healing. Foot and leg wounds and ulcers are very serious.
- Good foot care is needed. Corns, blisters, calluses, and other foot problems can lead to an infection and amputation.
- Blood glucose is monitored for:
  - *Hypoglycemia*—low sugar in the blood.
  - *Hyperglycemia*—high sugar in the blood.
- Review Table 43-1 in the Textbook for the causes, signs, and symptoms of hypoglycemia and hyperglycemia. Both can lead to death if not corrected. You must call for the nurse at once.

CHAPTER 43   REVIEW QUESTIONS

Circle the BEST answer.

1. A person is vomiting. You should do all the following *except*
   a. Follow Standard Precautions and the Bloodborne Pathogen Standard
   b. Keep the person supine
   c. Provide oral hygiene
   d. Observe vomitus for color, odor, and undigested food
2. A person with diabetes is trembling, sweating, and feels faint. You
   a. Tell the nurse immediately
   b. Tell the nurse at the end of the shift
   c. Tell another nursing assistant
   d. Ignore the symptoms
3. All of the following are signs and symptons of hepatitis except
   a. Itching
   b. Diarrhea
   c. Skin rash
   d. Increased appetite

Answers to these questions are on p. 522.

CHAPTER 44   URINARY AND REPRODUCTIVE DISORDERS

Urinary System Disorders

Urinary Tract Infections (UTIs)
- UTIs are common. Catheters, poor perineal hygiene, immobility, and poor fluid intake are common causes.

Prostate Enlargement
- The prostate grows larger as a man grows older. This is called benign prostatic hyperplasia (BPH). The enlarged prostate presses against the urethra. This obstructs urine flow through the urethra. Bladder function is gradually lost. Most men in their 60s and older have some symptoms of BPH.

Kidney Stones
- Kidney stones (calculi) are most common in white men 40 years of age and older. Bedrest, immobility, and poor fluid intake are risk factors. Review the list of symptoms listed on p. 722 in the Textbook.
- Stones vary in size from grains of sand to golf ball size.

Kidney Failure
- In kidney failure (renal failure) the kidneys do not function or are severely impaired. Waste products are not removed from the blood. Fluid is retained.
- Acute kidney failure is sudden. Blood flow to the kidneys is severely decreased. Causes include severe injury or bleeding, heart attack, heart failure, burns, infection, and severe allergic reactions.
- With chronic kidney failure the kidneys cannot meet the body's needs. Hypertension and diabetes are common causes. Infections, urinary tract obstructions, and tumors are other causes. Review Box 44-1, Signs and Symptoms of Chronic Kidney Failure.

Reproductive Disorders

Sexually Transmitted Diseases
- A sexually transmitted disease (STD) is spread by oral, vaginal, or anal sex. Some people do not have signs and symptoms or are not aware of an infection. Others know but do not seek treatment because of embarrassment. Standard Precautions and the Bloodborne Pathogen Standard are followed.

CHAPTER 44   REVIEW QUESTIONS

Circle the BEST answer.

1. Which statement is *false*?
   a. Older persons are at high risk for urinary tract infections.
   b. Skin irritation and infection can occur if urine leaks onto the skin
   c. Benign prostatic hypertrophy may cause urinary problems in women.
   d. Some people may not be aware of having a sexually transmitted disease.
2. An STD is spread by oral, vaginal, or anal sex.
   a. True
   b. False
3. A person with an STD always has signs and symptoms.
   a. True
   b. False

Answers to these questions are on p. 522.

CHAPTER 45   MENTAL HEALTH PROBLEMS

- The whole person has physical, social, psychological, and spiritual parts. Each part affects the other.
- **Mental health** means the person copes with and adjusts to everyday stresses in ways accepted by society.
- **Mental disorder** is a disturbance in the ability to cope with or adjust to stress. Behavior and function are impaired. Mental illness, emotional illness, and psychiatric disorder also mean mental illness.

Anxiety Disorders

- **Anxiety** is a vague, uneasy feeling in response to stress. The person may not know why or the cause. The person senses danger or harm—real or imagined. Some anxiety is normal. Review Box 45-1, Signs and Symptoms of Anxiety, in the Textbook.
- Coping and defense mechanisms are used to relieve anxiety. Review Box 45-2, Defense Mechanisms, in the Textbook.
- Some common anxiety disorders include panic disorder, phobias, obsessive-compulsive disorder, and post-traumatic stress disorder.
- *Panic disorder.* **Panic** is an intense and sudden feeling of fear, anxiety, terror, or dread. Onset is sudden with no obvious reason. The person cannot function. Signs and symptoms of anxiety are severe.
- *Phobias.* **Phobia** means an intense fear. The person has an intense fear of an object, situation, or activity that has little or no actual danger. The person avoids what is feared. When faced with the fear, the person has high anxiety and cannot function.

- *Obsessive-compulsive disorder (OCD)*. An **obsession** is a recurrent, unwanted thought, idea, or image. **Compulsion** is repeating an act over and over again. The act may not make sense, but the person has much anxiety if the act is not done. Some persons with OCD also have depression, eating disorders, substance abuse, and other anxiety disorders.
- *Post-traumatic stress disorder (PTSD)*. PTSD occurs after a terrifying ordeal. The ordeal involved physical harm or the threat of physical harm. Review Box 45-3, Signs and Symptoms of Post-Traumatic Stress Disorder, in the Textbook. Flashbacks are common. A **flashback** is reliving the trauma in thoughts during the day and in nightmares during sleep. He or she may believe that the trauma is happening all over again. Signs and symptoms usually develop about 3 months after the harmful event. Or they may emerge years later. PTSD can develop at any age.

Schizophrenia

- *Schizophrenia* means split mind. It is a severe, chronic, disabling brain disorder that involves:
  - **Psychosis**—a state of severe mental impairment. The person does not view the real or unreal correctly.
  - **Delusion**—a false belief.
  - **Hallucination**—seeing, hearing, smelling, or feeling something that is not real.
  - **Paranoia**—a disorder of the mind. The person has false beliefs (delusions). He or she is suspicious about a person or situation.
  - **Delusion of grandeur**—an exaggerated belief about one's importance, wealth, power, or talents.
  - **Delusion of persecution**—the false belief that one is being mistreated, abused, or harassed.
- The person with schizophrenia has problems relating to others. He or she may be paranoid. The person may have difficulty organizing thoughts. Responses are inappropriate. Communication is disturbed. The person may withdraw. Some people regress to an earlier time or condition. Some persons with schizophrenia attempt suicide.

Mood Disorders

- Mood disorders involve feelings, emotions, and moods.

Bipolar Disorder

- The person with bipolar disorder has severe extremes in mood, energy, and ability to function. There are emotional lows (depression) and emotional highs (mania). This disorder is also called manic-depressive illness. This disorder must be managed throughout life. Review Box 45-4, Signs and Symptoms of Bipolar Disorder, in the Textbook. Bipolar disorder can damage relationships and affect school or work performance. Some people are suicidal.

Major Depression

- Depression involves the body, mood, and thoughts. Symptoms affect work, study, sleep, eating, and other activities. The person is very sad.
- Depression is common in older persons. They have many losses—death of family and friends, loss of

health, loss of body functions, loss of independence. Loneliness and the side effects of some drugs also are causes. Review Box 45-5, Signs and Symptoms of Depression in Older Persons, in the Textbook. Depression in older persons is often overlooked or a wrong diagnosis is made.

Substance Abuse and Addiction

Alcoholism

- Alcohol affects alertness, judgment, coordination, and reaction time. Over time, heavy drinking damages the brain, central nervous system, liver, heart, kidneys, and stomach. It causes changes in the heart and blood vessels. It also can cause forgetfulness and confusion. Alcoholism is a chronic disease. There is no cure. However, alcoholism can be treated. Counseling and drugs are used to help the person stop drinking. The person must avoid all alcohol to avoid a relapse.
- Alcohol effects vary with age. Even small amounts can make older persons feel "high." Older persons are at risk for falls, vehicle crashes, and other injuries from drinking. Mixing alcohol with some drugs can be harmful or fatal. Alcohol also makes some health problems worse.

Suicide

- **Suicide** means to kill oneself.
- Suicide is most often linked to depression, alcohol or substance abuse, or stressful events. Review Box 45-7, Risk Factors for Suicide, in the Textbook.
- If a person mentions or talks about suicide, take the person seriously. Call for the nurse at once. Do not leave the person alone.

Care and Treatment

- Treatment of mental health problems involves having the person explore his or her thoughts and feelings. This is done through psychotherapy and behavior, group, occupational, art, and family therapies. Often drugs are ordered.
- The care plan reflects the person's needs. The physical, safety and security, and emotional needs of the person must be met.
- Communication is important. Be alert to nonverbal communication.

CHAPTER 45   REVIEW QUESTIONS

Circle the BEST answer.

1. A person may not know why anxiety occurs.
   a. True
   b. False
2. Panic is an intense and sudden feeling of fear, anxiety, terror, or dread.
   a. True
   b. False
3. A person with an obsessive-compulsive disorder has a ritual that is repeated over and over again.
   a. True
   b. False

4. A person talks about suicide. You must do the following *except*
   a. Call the nurse at once
   b. Stay with the person
   c. Leave the person alone
   d. Take the person seriously
5. Which statement about depression in older persons is *false*?
   a. Depression is often overlooked in older persons.
   b. Depression rarely occurs in older persons.
   c. Loneliness may be a cause of depression in older persons.
   d. Side effects of some drugs may cause depression in older persons.
6. Which statement is *false*?
   a. Communication is important when caring for a person with a mental health problem.
   b. You should be alert to nonverbal communication when caring for a person with a mental health problem.
   c. The care plan reflects the needs of the person.
   d. The focus is only on the person's emotional needs.

Answers to these questions are on p. 522.

CHAPTER 46 CONFUSION AND DEMENTIA

- Changes in the brain and nervous system occur with aging. Review Box 46-1, Changes in the Nervous System From Aging, in the Textbook.
- Changes in the brain can affect **cognitive function**—memory, thinking, reasoning, ability to understand, judgment, and behavior.

Confusion

- Confusion has many causes. Diseases, infections, hearing and vision loss, brain injury, and drug side effects are some causes.
- When caring for the confused person:
  - Follow the person's care plan.
  - Provide for safety.
  - Face the person and speak clearly.
  - Call the person by name every time you are in contact with him or her.
  - State your name. Show your name tag.
  - Give the date and time each morning. Repeat as needed during the day and evening.
  - Explain what you are going to do and why.
  - Give clear, simple directions and answers to questions.
  - Ask clear, simple questions. Give the person time to respond.
  - Keep calendars and clocks with large numbers in the person's room. Remind the person of holidays, birthdays, and other events.
  - Have the person wear eyeglasses and hearing aids as needed.
  - Use touch to communicate.
  - Place familiar objects and pictures within the person's view.
  - Provide newspapers, magazines, TV, and radio. Read to the person if appropriate.
  - Discuss current events with the person.
  - Maintain the day-night cycle.
  - Provide a calm, relaxed, and peaceful setting.
  - Follow the person's routine.
  - Break tasks into small steps when helping the person.
  - Do not rearrange furniture or the person's belongings.
  - Encourage the person to take part in self-care.
  - Be consistent.

Dementia

- **Dementia** is the loss of cognitive function that interferes with routine personal, social, and occupational activities.
- Dementia is not a normal part of aging. Most older people do not have dementia.
- Some early warning signs include problems with language, dressing, cooking, personality changes, poor or decreased judgment, and driving as well as getting lost in familiar places and misplacing items.
- Alzheimer's disease is the most common type of permanent dementia.

Alzheimer's Disease

- Alzheimer's disease (AD) is a brain disease. Memory, thinking, reasoning, judgment, language, behavior, mood, and personality are affected.

Signs of AD

- The classic sign of AD is gradual loss of short-term memory. Warning signs include:
  - Asking the same questions over and over again.
  - Repeating the same story—word for word, again and again.
  - The person forgets activities that were once done regularly with ease.
  - Losing the ability to pay bills or balance a checkbook.
  - Getting lost in familiar places. Or misplacing household objects.
  - Neglecting to bathe or wearing the same clothes over and over again. Meanwhile, the person insists that a bath was taken or that clothes were changed.
  - Relying on someone else to make decisions or answer questions that he or she would have handled.
- Review Box 46-5, Signs of Alzheimer's Disease, in the Textbook for other signs of AD.

Behaviors

- The following behaviors are common with AD:
  - *Wandering.* Persons with AD are not oriented to person, place, and time. They may wander away from home and not find their way back. The person cannot tell what is safe or dangerous.
  - *Sundowning.* With sundowning, signs, symptoms, and behaviors of AD increase during hours of darkness. As daylight ends, confusion, restlessness, anxiety, agitation, and other symptoms increase.
  - *Hallucinations.* The person with AD may see, hear, or feel things that are not real.
  - *Delusions.* People with AD may think they are some other person. A person may believe that the caregiver is someone else.

- ○ *Catastrophic Reactions.* The person reacts as if there is a disaster or tragedy.
- ○ *Agitation and Restlessness.* The person may pace, hit, or yell.
- ○ *Aggression and Combativeness.* These behaviors include hitting, pinching, grabbing, biting, or swearing.
- ○ *Screaming.* Persons with AD may scream to communicate.
- ○ *Abnormal Sexual Behaviors.* Sexual behaviors may involve the wrong person, the wrong time, and the wrong place. Persons with AD cannot control behavior.
- ○ *Repetitive Behaviors.* Persons with AD repeat the same motions over and over again.
- ○ *Rummaging and Hiding Things.* The person may search for things by moving things around, turning things over, or looking through something such as a drawer or closet. The person my hide things, throw things away, or lose something.

Care of Persons With AD and Other Dementias

- People with AD do not choose to be forgetful, incontinent, agitated, or rude. Nor do they choose to have other behaviors, signs, and symptoms of the disease. The disease causes the behaviors.
- Safety, hygiene, nutrition and fluids, elimination, and activity needs must be met. So must comfort and sleep needs. Review Box 46-9, Care of Persons With AD and Other Dementias, in the Textbook.
- The person can have other health problems and injuries. However, the person may not recognize pain, fever, constipation, incontinence, or other signs and symptoms. Carefully observe the person. Report any change in the person's usual behavior to the nurse.
- Infection is a risk. Provide good skin care, oral hygiene, and perineal care after bowel and bladder elimination.
- Supervised activities meet the person's needs and cognitive abilities.
- Impaired communication is a common problem. Avoid giving orders, wanting the truth, and correcting the person's errors.
- Always look for dangers in the person's room and in the hallways, lounges, dining areas, and other areas on the nursing unit. Remove the danger if you can.
- Every staff member must be alert to persons who wander. Such persons are allowed to wander in safe areas.

The Family

- The family may have physical, emotional, social, and financial stresses. The family often feels hopeless. No matter what is done, the person only gets worse. Anger and resentment may result. Guilt feelings are common.
- The family is an important part of the health team. They may help plan the person's care. For many persons, family members provide comfort. The family also needs support and understanding from the health team.

CHAPTER 46   REVIEW QUESTIONS

Circle the BEST answer.

1. Cognitive function involves all of the following *except*
   - a. Memory and thinking
   - b. Reasoning and understanding
   - c. Personality and mood
   - d. Judgment and behavior
2. When caring for a confused person, you do the following *except*
   - a. Provide for safety
   - b. Maintain the day-night schedule
   - c. Keep calendars and clocks in the person's room
   - d. Ask difficult-to-understand questions and give complex directions
3. Which statement about dementia is *false?*
   - a. Dementia is a normal part of aging.
   - b. The person may have changes in personality.
   - c. Alzheimer's disease is the most common type of dementia.
   - d. The person may have changes in behavior.
4. When caring for persons with AD, you do the following *except*
   - a. Provide good skin care
   - b. Talk to them in a calm voice
   - c. Observe them closely for unusual behavior
   - d. Allow personal choice in wandering

Answers to these questions are on p. 522.

CHAPTER 48   SEXUALITY

Sex and Sexuality

- Sexuality involves the whole person. Illness, injury, and aging can affect sexuality.

Sexuality and Older Persons

- Reproductive organs change with aging. Frequency of sex decreases for many older persons.
- Sexual partners are lost through death, divorce, and relationship break-ups. Or a partner needs hospital or nursing center care.
- Love, affection, and intimacy are needed throughout life. Older persons love, fall in love, hold hands, and embrace. Many have intercourse.

Meeting Sexual Needs

- The nursing team promotes the meeting of sexual needs.
- Review Box 48-1, Promoting Sexuality, in the Textbook.

The Sexually Aggressive Person

- Some persons want the health team to meet their sexual needs. They flirt or make sexual advances or comments. Some expose themselves, masturbate, or touch the staff. This can anger and embarrass the staff member. These reactions are normal.
- Touch may have a sexual purpose. You must be professional about the matter.
   - ○ Ask the person not to touch you. State the places where you were touched.

○ Tell the person that you will not do what he or she wants.

○ Tell the person what behaviors make you uncomfortable. Politely ask the person not to act that way.

○ Allow privacy if the person is becoming aroused.

○ Discuss the matter with the nurse. The nurse can help you understand the behavior.

○ Follow the care plan. It has measures to deal with sexually aggressive behaviors. They are based on the cause of the behavior.

Protecting the Person

- The Person must be protected from unwanted sexual comments and advances. This is sexual abuse (Chapter 4). Tell the nurse right away.

- No one should be allowed to sexually abuse another person. This includes staff members, patients, residents, family members or other visitors, and volunteers.

CHAPTER 48   *REVIEW QUESTIONS*

Circle the BEST answer.

1. A resident touches you in a sexual way. You should do the following *except*
   a. Ask the person not to touch you
   b. Discuss the matter with the nurse
   c. Tell the person what behaviors make you uncomfortable
   d. Yell at the person immediately

2. Unwanted sexual comments and advances are forms of sexual abuse.
   a. True
   b. False

Answers to these questions are on p. 522.

CHAPTER 51   BASIC EMERGENCY CARE

Emergency Care

- Rules for emergency care include:
  ○ Know your limits. Do not do more than you are able.
  ○ Stay calm.
  ○ Know where to find emergency supplies.
  ○ Follow Standard Precautions and the Bloodborne Pathogen Standard to the extent possible.
  ○ Check for life-threatening problems. Check for breathing, a pulse, and bleeding.
  ○ Keep the person lying down or as you found him or her.
  ○ Move the person only if the setting is unsafe. If the scene is not safe enough for you to approach, wait for help to arrive.
  ○ Perform necessary emergency measures.
  ○ Call for help.
  ○ Do not remove clothes unless necessary.
  ○ Keep the person warm. Cover the person with a blanket, coat, or sweater.
  ○ Reassure the person. Explain what is happening and that help was called.
  ○ Do not give the person food or fluids.
  ○ Keep onlookers away. They invade privacy.

- Review Box 51-1, Rules of Emergency Care, in the Textbook for more information.

Basic Life Support for Adults

- Cardiopulmonary resuscitation (CPR) supports breathing and circulation. It provides blood and oxygen to the heart, brain, and other organs until advanced emergency care is given. CPR is done if the person does not respond, is not breathing, and has no pulse.

- CPR involves:
  ○ *Chest compressions*—the heart brain and other organs must receive blood. Chest compressions force blood through the circulatory system.
  ○ *Airway*—the airway must be open and clear of obstructions. The head tilt–chin lift method opens the airway.
  ○ *Breathing*—the person must get oxygen. Air is not inhaled when breathing stops. The person is given breaths. A rescuer inflates the person's lungs.
  ○ *Defibrillation*—ventricular fibrillation (VF, V-fib) is an abnormal heart rhythm. Rather than beating in a regular rhythm, the heart shakes and quivers. The heart does not pump blood. The heart, brain, and other organs do not receive blood and oxygen. A *defibrillator* is used to deliver a shock to the heart. This allows the return of a regular heart rhythm. Defibrillation as soon as possible after the onset of VF (V-fib) increases the person's chance of survival.

Seizures

- You cannot stop a seizure. However, you can protect the person from injury:
  ○ Follow the rules in Box 51-1 in the Textbook.
  ○ Do not leave the person alone.
  ○ Lower the person to the floor.
  ○ Note the time the seizure started.
  ○ Place something soft under the person's head.
  ○ Loosen tight jewelry and clothing around the person's neck.
  ○ Turn the person onto his or her side. Make sure the head is turned to the side.
  ○ Do not put any object or your fingers between the person's teeth.
  ○ Do not try to stop the seizure or control the person's movements.
  ○ Move furniture, equipment, and sharp objects away from the person.
  ○ Note the time when the seizure ends.
  ○ Make sure the mouth is clear of food, fluids, and saliva after the seizure.
  ○ Provide basic life support if the person is not breathing after the seizure.

Fainting

- **Fainting** is the sudden loss of consciousness from an inadequate blood supply to the brain.

- Warning signals are dizziness, perspiration, and blackness before the eyes. The person looks pale. The pulse is weak. Respirations are shallow if consciousness is lost. Emergency care includes:
  ○ Have the person sit or lie down before fainting occurs.
  ○ If sitting, the person bends forward and places the head between the knees.

- If the person is lying down, raise the legs.
- Loosen tight clothing.
- Keep the person lying down if fainting has occurred. Raise the legs.
- Do not let the person get up until symptoms have subsided for about 5 minutes.
- Help the person to a sitting position after recovery from fainting.

CHAPTER 51   REVIEW QUESTIONS

Circle the BEST answer.

1. During an emergency, you do all of the following *except*
   a. Perform only procedures you have been trained to do
   b. Keep the person lying down or as you found him or her
   c. Let the person become cold
   d. Reassure the person and explain what is happening
2. During an emergency, you keep onlookers away.
   a. True
   b. False
3. During a seizure, you do the following *except*
   a. Turn the person's body to the side
   b. Place your fingers in the person's mouth
   c. Note the time the seizure started and ended
   d. Turn the person's head to the side
4. Which statement about fainting is *false*?
   a. If standing, have the person sit down before fainting.
   b. If sitting, have the person bend forward and place his head between his knees before fainting occurs.
   c. Tighten the person's clothing.
   d. Raise the legs if the person is lying down.

Answers to these questions are on p. 522.

CHAPTER 52   END-OF-LIFE CARE

Attitudes About Death
- Attitudes about death often change as a person grows older and with changing circumstances.

Culture and Spiritual Needs
- Practices and attitudes about death differ among cultures.
- Attitudes about death are closely related to religion. Many religions practice rites and rituals during the dying process and at the time of death.

Age
- Adults fear pain and suffering, dying alone, and the invasion of privacy. They also fear loneliness and separation from loved ones. Adults often resent death because it affects plans, hopes, dreams, and ambitions.
- Older persons usually have fewer fears than younger adults. Some welcome death as freedom from pain, suffering, and disability. Death also means reunion with those who have died. Like younger adults, they often fear dying alone.

The Stages of Dying
- Dr. Kübler-Ross described five stages of dying. They are:
  - *Stage 1: Denial.* The person refuses to believe he or she is going to die.
  - *Stage 2: Anger.* There is anger and rage, often at family, friends, and the health team.
  - *Stage 3: Bargaining.* Often the person bargains with God or higher power for more time.
  - *Stage 4: Depression.* The person is sad and mourns things that were lost.
  - *Stage 5: Acceptance.* The person is calm and at peace. The person accepts death.
- Dying persons do not always pass through all five stages. A person may never get beyond a certain stage. Some move back and forth between stages.

Comfort Needs
- Comfort is a basic part of end-of-life care. It involves physical, mental and emotional, and spiritual needs. Comfort goals are to:
  - Prevent or relieve suffering to the extent possible
  - Respect and follow end-of-life wishes
- Dying persons may want to talk about their fears, worries, and anxieties. You need to listen and use touch.
  - *Listening.* Let the person express feelings and emotions in his or her own way. Do not worry about saying the wrong thing or finding the right words. You do not need to say anything.
  - *Touch.* Touch shows caring and concern. Sometimes the person does not want to talk but needs you nearby. Silence, along with touch, is a meaningful way to communicate.
- Some people may want to see a spiritual leader. Or they may want to take part in religious practices.

Physical Needs
- As the person weakens, basic needs are met. The person may depend on others for basic needs and activities of daily living. Every effort is made to promote physical and psychological comfort. The person is allowed to die in peace and with dignity.

Pain
- Some dying persons do not have pain. Others may have severe pain. Always report signs and symptoms of pain at once. Pain management is important. The nurse can give pain-relief drugs. Preventing and controlling pain is easier than relieving pain.

Breathing Problems
- Shortness of breath and difficulty breathing (dyspnea) are common end-of-life problems. Semi-Fowler's position and oxygen are helpful.
- Noisy breathing (death rattle) is common as death nears. This is due to mucus collecting in the airway. The side-lying position, suctioning by the nurse, and drugs to reduce the amount of mucus may help.

Vision, Hearing, and Speech
- Vision blurs and gradually fails. Explain what you are doing to the person or in the room. Provide good eye care.
- Hearing is one of the last functions lost. Always assume that the person can hear.
- Speech becomes difficult. Anticipate the person's needs. Do not ask questions that need long answers.

Mouth, Nose, and Skin

- Frequent oral hygiene is given as death nears.
- Crusting and irritation of the nostrils can occur. Carefully clean the nose.
- Skin care, bathing, and preventing pressure ulcers are necessary. Change linens and gowns whenever needed.

Nutrition

- Nausea, vomiting, and loss of appetite are common at the end of life. The doctor can order drugs for nausea and vomiting.
- Some persons are too tired or too weak to eat. You may need to feed them.
- As death nears, loss of appetite is common. The person may choose not to eat or drink. Do not force the person to eat or drink. Report refusal to eat or drink to the nurse.

Elimination

- Urinary and fecal incontinence may occur. Give perineal care as needed.

The Person's Room

- The person's room should be comfortable and pleasant. It should be well lit and well ventilated. Remove unnecessary equipment.
- Mementos, pictures, cards, flowers, and religious items provide comfort. The person and family arrange the room as they wish.

The Family

- This is a hard time for family. The family goes through stages like the dying person. Be available, courteous, and considerate.
- The person and family need time together. However, you cannot neglect care because the family is present. Most agencies let family members help give care.

Legal Issues

- *Living wills*. A living will is a document about measures that support or maintain life when death is likely. A living will may instruct doctors not to start measures that promote dying or to remove measures that prolong dying.
- *Durable power of attorney for health care*. This gives the power to make health care decisions to another person. When a person cannot make health care decisions, the person with durable power of attorney can do so.
- *"Do Not Resuscitate" (DNR) order*. This means the person will not be resuscitated. The person is allowed to die with peace and dignity. The orders are written after consulting with the person and family.
- You may not agree with care and resuscitation decisions. However, you must follow the person's or family's wishes and the doctor's orders. These may be against your personal, religious, and cultural values. If so, discuss the matter with the nurse. An assignment change may be needed.

Signs of Death

- There are signs that death is near:
  - Movement, muscle tone, and sensation are lost.
  - Abdominal distention, fecal incontinence, nausea, and vomiting are common.
  - Body temperature rises. The person feels cool, looks pale, and perspires heavily.
  - The pulse is fast or slow, weak, and irregular. Blood pressure starts to fall.
  - Slow or rapid, and shallow respirations are observed. Mucus collects in the airway. This causes the death rattle that is heard.
  - Pain decreases as the person loses consciousness. Some people are conscious until the moment of death.
- The signs of death include no pulse, no respirations, and no blood pressure. The pupils are dilated and fixed.

Care of the Body After Death

- Post-mortem care is done to maintain a good appearance of the body.
- Moving the body when giving post-mortem care can cause remaining air in the lungs, stomach, and intestines to be expelled. When air is expelled, sounds are produced.
- When giving post-mortem care, follow Standard Precautions and the Bloodborne Pathogen Standard.

CHAPTER 52   REVIEW QUESTIONS

Circle the BEST answer.

1. Which statement is *false*?
   a. Adults fear dying alone.
   b. Older persons usually have fewer fears about dying than younger adults.
   c. Adults often resent death.
   d. All adults welcome death.
2. Persons in the denial stage of dying
   a. Are angry
   b. Bargain with God
   c. Refuse to believe that they are dying
   d. Are calm and at peace
3. When caring for a person who is dying, you should do the following *except*
   a. Listen to the person
   b. Talk about your feelings about death
   c. Provide privacy during spiritual moments
   d. Use touch to show care and concern
4. When caring for a dying person, you provide all of the following *except*
   a. Eye care
   b. Oral hygiene
   c. Good skin care
   d. Physical exercise
5. When giving post-mortem care, you should wear gloves.
   a. True
   b. False

Answers to these questions are on p. 522.

Practice Examination 1

This test contains 75 questions. For each question, circle the BEST answer.

1. A nurse asks you to give a person his drug when he is done in the bathroom. Your response to the nurse is
   A. "I will give the drug for you."
   B. "I will ask the other nursing assistant to give the drug."
   C. "I am sorry, but I cannot give that drug. I will let you know when he is out of the bathroom."
   D. "I refuse to give that drug."

2. An ethical person
   A. Does not judge others
   B. Avoids persons whose standards and values are different from his or hers
   C. Is prejudiced and biased
   D. Causes harm to another person

3. You smell alcohol on the breath of a co-worker. You
   A. Ignore the situation
   B. Tell the co-worker to get counseling
   C. Take a break and drink some alcohol too
   D. Tell the nurse at once

4. A person's signal light goes unanswered. He gets out of bed and falls. His leg is broken. This is
   A. Neglect
   B. Emotional abuse
   C. Physical abuse
   D. Malpractice

5. Your mom asks you about a person on your unit. How should you respond?
   A. "She is walking better now that she is receiving physical therapy."
   B. "I'm sorry, but I cannot talk about her. It is unprofessional, and violates her privacy and confidentiality."
   C. "Don't tell anyone I told you, but she is getting worse."
   D. "She has been very sad recently and needs visitors."

6. You are going off duty. The nursing assistant coming on duty is on the unit with you. A person puts her light on. Your response is
   A. "I'm ready to go. I will let you answer that light."
   B. "I've been here all day so I am not answering that light."
   C. "No one helped me answer lights when I came on duty."
   D. "I will answer that light so you can get organized for the shift."

7. When recording in the medical record, you
   A. Write in pencil
   B. Spell words incorrectly
   C. Use only center-approved abbreviations
   D. Record what your co-worker did

8. You are answering the phone in the nurses' station. You
   A. Answer in a rushed manner
   B. Give a courteous greeting
   C. End the conversation and hang-up without saying good-bye
   D. Give confidential information about a resident to the caller

9. A person who was admitted to the nursing center yesterday does not feel safe. You
   A. Are rude as you care for the person
   B. Ignore the person's requests for information
   C. Show the person around the nursing center
   D. Act rushed as you care for the person

10. A person is angry and is shouting at you. You should
    A. Yell back at the person
    B. Stay calm and professional
    C. Put the person in a room away from others
    D. Call the family

11. When speaking with another person, you
    A. Use medical terms that may not be familiar to the person
    B. Mumble your words as you talk
    C. Ask several questions at a time
    D. Speak clearly and distinctly

12. To use a transfer or gait belt safely, you should
    A. Ignore the manufacturer's instructions
    B. Leave the excess strap dangling
    C. Apply the belt over bare skin
    D. Apply the belt under the breasts

13. When you are listening to a person, you
    A. Look around the room
    B. Sit with your arms crossed
    C. Act rushed and not interested in what the person is saying
    D. Have good eye contact with the person

14. When caring for a person who is comatose, you
    A. Make jokes about how sick the person is
    B. Care for the person without talking to him or her
    C. Explain what you are doing to him or her
    D. Discuss your problems with the other nursing assistant in the room with you

15. You need to give care to a person when a visitor is present. You
    A. Politely ask the visitor to leave the room
    B. Do the care in the presence of the visitor
    C. Expose the person's body in front of the visitor
    D. Rudely tell the visitor where to wait while you care for the person
16. A person tells you he wants to talk with a minister. You
    A. Ignore the request
    B. Tell the nurse
    C. Ask what the person wants to discuss with the minister
    D. Tell the person there is no need to talk with a minister
17. When you care for a person who has a restraint, you
    A. Observe the person every 15 minutes
    B. Remove the restraint and reposition the person every 4 hours
    C. Apply the restraint tightly
    D. Apply the restraint incorrectly
18. As a person ages
    A. The skin becomes less dry
    B. Muscle strength increases
    C. Reflexes are faster
    D. Bladder muscles weaken
19. A person you are caring for touches your buttocks several times. You
    A. Tell the person you like being touched
    B. Ask the person not to touch you again
    C. Tell the person's daughter
    D. Tell the person's girlfriend
20. You are transporting a person in a wheelchair. You
    A. Pull the chair backward
    B. Let the person's feet touch the floor
    C. Push the chair forward
    D. Rest the foot plates on the person's leg
21. You cannot read the person's name on the ID bracelet. You
    A. Tell the nurse so a new bracelet can be made
    B. Ignore the fact that you cannot read the name
    C. Ask another nursing assistant to identify the person
    D. Tell the family the person needs a new ID bracelet
22. The universal sign of choking is
    A. Holding your breath
    B. Clutching at the throat
    C. Having difficulty breathing
    D. Coughing
23. A person is on a diabetic diet. You
    A. Serve the person's meals late
    B. Let the person eat whenever he or she is hungry
    C. Sometimes check the tray to see what was eaten
    D. Tell the nurse about changes in the person's eating habits
24. With mild airway obstruction
    A. The person is usually unconscious
    B. The person cannot speak
    C. Forceful coughing often does not remove the object
    D. Forceful coughing often can remove the object

25. To relieve severe airway obstruction in a conscious adult, you do
    A. Abdominal thrusts
    B. Back thrusts
    C. Chest compressions
    D. A finger sweep
26. Faulty electrical equipment
    A. Can be used in a nursing center
    B. Should be given to the nurse
    C. Should be taken home by you for repair
    D. Should be used only with alert persons
27. A warning label has been removed from a hazardous substance container. You
    A. May use the substance if you know what is in the container
    B. Leave the container where it is
    C. Take the container to the nurse and explain the problem
    D. Tell another nursing assistant about the missing label
28. A person's beliefs and values are different from your views. What should you do?
    A. Refuse to care for the person.
    B. Delegate care to another nursing assistant.
    C. Tell the nurse about your concerns.
    D. Tell the person how you feel.
29. You find a person smoking in the nursing center. You should
    A. Ignore the situation
    B. Tell the person to leave
    C. Tell another nursing assistant
    D. Ask the person to put the cigarette out and show him or her where smoking is permitted
30. During a fire, the first thing you do is
    A. Rescue persons in immediate danger
    B. Sound the nearest fire alarm
    C. Close doors and windows to confine the fire
    D. Extinguish the fire
31. A person with Alzheimer's disease has increased restlessness and confusion as daylight ends. You
    A. Try to reason with the person
    B. Ask the person to tell you what is bothering him or her
    C. Provide a calm, quiet setting late in the day
    D. Complete his or her treatments and activities late in the day
32. To prevent suffocation, you should
    A. Make sure dentures fit loosely
    B. Cut food into large pieces
    C. Make sure the person can chew and swallow the food served
    D. Ignore loose teeth or dentures
33. When using a wheelchair, you should
    A. Lock both wheels before you transfer a person to and from the wheelchair
    B. Lock only one wheel before you transfer a person to and from the wheelchair
    C. Let the person's feet touch the floor when the chair is moving
    D. Let the person stand on the footplates

34. A person begins to fall while you are walking him or her. You should
    A. Try to prevent the fall
    B. Ease the person to the floor
    C. Yell at the person for falling
    D. Tell the nurse at the end of the shift
35. A person has a restraint on. You know that
    A. Restraints are used for staff convenience
    B. Death from strangulation is a risk factor to using a restraint
    C. Restraints may be used to punish a person
    D. A written nurse's order is required for a restraint
36. Before feeding a person, you
    A. Tell the other nursing assistant
    B. Go to the restroom
    C. Wash your hands
    D. Tell the nurse
37. When wearing gloves, you remember to
    A. Wear them several times before discarding them
    B. Wear the same ones from room to room
    C. Wear gloves with a tear or puncture
    D. Change gloves when they become contaminated with urine
38. When washing your hands, you
    A. Use hot water
    B. Let your uniform touch the sink
    C. Keep your watch at your wrist
    D. Keep your hands and forearms lower than your elbows
39. You need to move a box from the floor to the counter in the utility room. You
    A. Bend from your waist to pick up the box
    B. Hold the box away from your body as you pick it up
    C. Bend your knees and squat to lift the box
    D. Stand with your feet close together as you pick up the box
40. The nurse asks you to place a person in Fowler's position. You
    A. Put the bed flat
    B. Raise the head of the bed between 45 and 60 degrees
    C. Raise the head of the bed between 80 and 90 degrees
    D. Raise the head of the bed 15 degrees
41. You accidentally scratch a person. This is
    A. Neglect
    B. Negligence
    C. Malpractice
    D. Physical abuse
42. You positioned a person in a chair. For good body alignment, you
    A. Have the person's back and buttocks against the back of the chair
    B. Leave the person's feet unsupported
    C. Have the backs of the person's knees touch the edge of the chair
    D. Have the person sit on the edge of the chair

43. You need to transfer a person with a weak left leg from the bed to the wheelchair. You
    A. Get the person out of bed on the left side
    B. Get the person out of bed on the right side
    C. Keep the person in bed
    D. Ask the person what side moves first
44. A person tries to scratch and kick you. You should
    A. Protect yourself from harm
    B. Argue with the person
    C. Become angry with the person
    D. Ignore the person
45. When moving a person up in bed
    A. Window coverings may be left open so people can look in
    B. Body parts may be exposed
    C. Ask the person to help
    D. Ask the person to lie still
46. For comfort, most older persons prefer
    A. Rooms that are cold
    B. Restrooms that smell of urine
    C. Loud talking and laughter in the nurses' station
    D. Lighting that meets their needs
47. Signal lights are
    A. Placed on the person's strong side
    B. Answered when time permits
    C. Kept on the bedside table
    D. Kept on the person's weak side
48. A nurse asks you to inspect a person's closet. You
    A. Tell the nurse you cannot do this
    B. Inspect the closet when the person is in the dining room
    C. Ask the person if you can inspect his or her closet
    D. Tell the nurse to inspect the closet
49. When changing bed linens, you
    A. Hold the linen close to your uniform
    B. Shake the sheet when putting it on the bed
    C. Take only needed linen into the person's room
    D. Put dirty linen on the floor
50. To use a fire extinguisher, you
    A. Keep the safety pin in the extinguisher
    B. Direct the hose or nozzle at the top of the fire
    C. Squeeze the lever to start the stream
    D. Sweep the stream at the top of the fire
51. When doing mouth care for an unconscious person, you
    A. Do not need to wear gloves
    B. Give mouth care at least every 2 hours
    C. Place the person in a supine position
    D. Keep the mouth open with your fingers
52. A person is angry because he did not get to the activity room on time because a co-worker did not come to work. How should you respond to him?
    A. "It's not my fault. A co-worker called off today and we are short-staffed."
    B. "I'm sorry you were late for activities. I will try to plan better."
    C. "I am doing the best I can."
    D. "I'm just too busy."

53. You are asked to clean a person's dentures. You
    A. Use hot water
    B. Hold the dentures firmly and line the basin with a towel
    C. Wrap the dentures in tissues after cleaning
    D. Store the dentures in a denture cup with the person's room number on it
54. When bathing a person, you notice a rash that was not there before. You
    A. Do nothing
    B. Tell the person
    C. Tell the nurse and record it in the medical record
    D. Tell the person's daughter
55. When washing a person's eyes, you
    A. Use soap
    B. Clean the eye near you first
    C. Wipe from the inner to the outer aspect of the eye
    D. Wipe from the outer aspect to the inner aspect of the eye
56. When giving a back massage, you
    A. Use cold lotion
    B. Use light strokes
    C. Massage reddened bony areas
    D. Look for bruises and breaks in the skin
57. You need to give perineal care to a female. You
    A. Separate the labia and clean downward from front to back
    B. Separate the labia and clean upward from back to front
    C. Wear gloves only if there is drainage
    D. Only use water
58. When giving a person a tub bath or shower, you
    A. Do not give the person a signal light
    B. Turn the hot water on first, then the cold water
    C. Stay within hearing distance if the person can be left alone
    D. Direct water toward the person while adjusting the water temperature
59. A person is on an anticoagulant. You
    A. Use a safety razor
    B. Use an electric razor
    C. Let him grow a beard
    D. Let him choose which type of razor to use
60. A person with a weak left arm wants to remove his or her sweater. You
    A. Let the person do it without any assistance
    B. Help the person remove the sweater from his or her right arm first
    C. Help the person remove the sweater from his or her left arm first
    D. Tell the person to keep the sweater on
61. When talking with a person, you should call the person
    A. "Honey"
    B. By his or her first name
    C. By his or her title—Mr. or Mrs. or Miss
    D. "Grandpa" or "Grandma"

62. A person has an indwelling catheter. You
    A. Let the person lie on the tubing
    B. Disconnect the catheter from the drainage tubing every 8 hours
    C. Secure the catheter to the lower leg
    D. Measure and record the amount of urine in the drainage bag
63. A person needs to eat a diet that contains carbohydrates. Carbohydrates
    A. Are needed for tissue repair and growth
    B. Provide energy and fiber for bowel elimination
    C. Add flavor to food and help the body use certain vitamins
    D. Are needed for nerve and muscle function
64. You are taking a rectal temperature with a glass thermometer. You
    A. Insert the thermometer before lubricating it
    B. Leave the privacy curtain open
    C. Leave the thermometer in place for 10 minutes
    D. Hold the thermometer in place
65. A person has a blood pressure of 86/58. You
    A. Report the BP to the nurse at once
    B. Record the BP but do not tell the nurse
    C. Ask the unit secretary to tell the nurse
    D. Retake the BP in 30 minutes before telling the nurse
66. On which person would you take an oral temperature?
    A. An unconscious person
    B. The person receiving oxygen
    C. The person who breathes through his or her mouth
    D. A conscious person
67. When caring for a person who is blind or visually impaired, you
    A. Offer the person your arm and have the person walk a half step behind you
    B. Do as much for the person as possible
    C. Shout at the person when talking with him or her
    D. Touch the person before indicating your presence
68. You are caring for a person with dementia. You
    A. Misplace the person's clothes
    B. Choose the activities the person attends
    C. Send personal items home
    D. Let the family make choices if the person cannot
69. When providing rehabilitation and restorative care for a person, you
    A. Can shout or scream at the person
    B. Can hit or strike the person
    C. Can call the person names
    D. Discuss your anger with the nurse
70. While bathing a person, you
    A. Keep doors and windows open
    B. Wash from the dirtiest areas to cleanest areas
    C. Encourage the person to help as much as possible
    D. Rub the skin dry

71. When a person is dying
    A. Assume that the person can hear you
    B. Oral care is done every 5 hours
    C. Skin care is done weekly
    D. Reposition the person every 3 hours
72. A person is on intake and output. You
    A. Measure only liquids such as water and juice
    B. Measure ice cream and gelatin as part of intake
    C. Measure IV fluids
    D. Measure tube feedings
73. A person has been on bedrest. You need to have the person walk. What will you do first?
    A. Help the person move quickly.
    B. Have the person dangle before getting out of bed.
    C. Have the person sit in a chair.
    D. Walk with the person as soon as he or she gets out of bed.

74. Your ring accidentally causes a skin tear on an elderly person. You
    A. Tell yourself to be more careful the next time
    B. Tell the nurse at once
    C. Do nothing
    D. Hope no one finds out
75. To protect a person's privacy, you should
    A. Keep all information about the person confidential
    B. Discuss the person's treatment with another nursing assistant in the lunch room
    C. Open the person's mail
    D. Keep the privacy curtain open when providing care to the person

Practice Examination 2

This test contains 75 questions. For each question, circle the BEST answer.

1. You can refuse to do a delegated task when
   A. You are too busy
   B. You do not like the task
   C. The task is not in your job description
   D. It is the end of the shift
2. Mr. Smith does not want life-saving measures. You
   A. Explain to Mr. Smith why he should have life-saving measures
   B. Respect his decision
   C. Explain to Mr. Smith's family why life-saving measures are needed
   D. Tell your friend about Mr. Smith's decision
3. You are walking by a resident's room. You hear a nurse shouting at a person. This is
   A. Battery
   B. Malpractice
   C. Verbal abuse
   D. Neglect
4. When communicating with a foreign-speaking person, you
   A. Speak loudly or shout
   B. Use medical terms the person may not understand
   C. Use words the person seems to understand
   D. Speak quickly and mumble
5. To protect a person from getting burned, you
   A. Allow smoking in bed
   B. Turn hot water on first, then cold water
   C. Assist the person with drinking or eating hot food
   D. Let the person sleep with a heating pad
6. To prevent equipment accidents, you should
   A. Use two-pronged plugs on all electrical devices
   B. Follow the manufacturer's instructions
   C. Wipe up spills when you have time
   D. Use unfamiliar equipment without training
7. To prevent a person from falling, you should
   A. Ignore signal lights
   B. Use throw rugs on the floor
   C. Keep the bed in a high position
   D. Use grab bars in showers
8. You need to wash your hands
   A. Before you document a procedure
   B. After you remove gloves
   C. After you talk with a person
   D. After you talk with a co-worker
9. You need to move a person weighing 250 pounds in bed. You
   A. Do the procedure alone
   B. Keep the privacy curtain open
   C. Ask the person to lie still
   D. Ask for assistance from at least 2 other staff members
10. When transferring a person from a bed to a wheelchair, you never
    A. Ask a co-worker to help you
    B. Use a transfer or gait belt
    C. Have the person put his or her arms around your neck
    D. Lock the wheels on the wheelchair
11. When making a bed, you
    A. Keep the bed in the low position
    B. Wear gloves when removing linen
    C. Raise the head of the bed
    D. Raise the foot of the bed
12. To give perineal care to a male, you
    A. Use a circular motion and work toward the meatus
    B. Use a circular motion and start at the meatus and work outward
    C. Wear gloves only if there is drainage
    D. Use only water
13. A person with a weak left arm wants to put his or her sweater on. You
    A. Let the person do it without any assistance
    B. Help the person put the sweater on his or her right arm first
    C. Help the person put the sweater on his or her left arm first
    D. Tell the person to keep the sweater off
14. A person has an indwelling catheter. You
    A. Let the drainage bag touch the floor
    B. Keep the drainage bag higher than the bladder
    C. Hang the drainage bag on a bed rail
    D. Have the drainage bag hang from the bed frame or chair
15. A person needs to eat a diet that contains protein. Protein
    A. Is needed for tissue repair and growth
    B. Provides energy and fiber for bowel elimination
    C. Adds flavor to food and helps the body use certain vitamins
    D. Is needed for nerve and muscle function

16. Older persons
    A. Have an increased sense of thirst
    B. Need less water than younger persons
    C. May not feel thirsty
    D. Seldom need to have water offered to them
17. A person is NPO. You
    A. Post a sign in the bathroom
    B. Keep the water pitcher filled at the bedside
    C. Remove the water pitcher and glass from the room
    D. Provide oral hygiene every day
18. A person drank 3 oz of milk at lunch. He or she drank
    A. 30 mL
    B. 60 mL
    C. 90 mL
    D. 120 mL
19. When feeding a person, you
    A. Offer fluids at the end of the meal
    B. Use forks
    C. Do not talk to the person
    D. Allow time for chewing and swallowing
20. You need to do ROM to a person's right shoulder. You
    A. Force the joint beyond its present ROM
    B. Move the joint quickly
    C. Force the joint to the point of pain
    D. Support the part being exercised
21. A person has a weak left leg. The person should
    A. Hold the cane in his or her left hand
    B. Hold the cane in his or her right hand
    C. Hold the cane in either hand
    D. Use a walker
22. To promote comfort and relieve pain, you
    A. Keep wrinkles in the bed linens
    B. Position the person in good alignment
    C. Talk loudly to the person
    D. Use sudden and jarring movements of the bed or chair
23. A person is receiving oxygen through a nasal cannula. You
    A. Turn the oxygen higher when he or she is short of breath
    B. Fill the humidifier when it is not bubbling
    C. Check behind the ears and under the nose for signs of irritation
    D. Remove the cannula when the person goes to the dining room
24. You accidentally dropped a mercury glass thermometer. You
    A. Tell the nurse at once
    B. Put the mercury in your pocket
    C. Pick up the pieces of glass with your hands
    D. Touch the mercury
25. When taking a person's pulse, you
    A. Use the brachial pulse
    B. Take the pulse for 30 seconds if it is irregular
    C. Tell the nurse if the pulse is less than 60
    D. Use your thumb to take a pulse
26. You are counting respirations on a person. You
    A. Tell the person you are counting his or her respirations
    B. Count for 1 minute if an abnormal breathing pattern is noted
    C. Report a rate of 16 to the nurse at once
    D. Count for 30 seconds if an abnormal breathing pattern is noted

27. You are taking blood pressures on people assigned to you. An older person has a blood pressure of 158/96. You
    A. Report the BP to the nurse at once
    B. Finish taking all the blood pressures before telling the nurse
    C. Retake the BP in 30 minutes before telling the nurse
    D. Ask the unit secretary to tell the nurse about the BP
28. When would you take a rectal temperature?
    A. The person has diarrhea
    B. The person is confused
    C. The person is unconscious
    D. The person is agitated
29. A person has been admitted to the nursing center recently. You
    A. Look through his or her belongings
    B. Ignore his or her questions
    C. Speak in a gentle, calm voice
    D. Enter the person's room without knocking
30. When taking a person's height and weight, you
    A. Let the person wear shoes
    B. Have the person void before being weighed
    C. Weigh the person at different times of the day
    D. Balance the scale every 6 months
31. A person is bedfast. To prevent pressure ulcers, you
    A. Reposition the person at least every 3 hours
    B. Massage reddened areas
    C. Let heels and ankles touch the bed
    D. Keep the skin free of moisture from urine, stools, or perspiration
32. A person has a hearing problem. When talking with the person, you
    A. Keep the TV or radio on
    B. Shout
    C. Face the person
    D. Speak quickly
33. When caring for a person who is blind or visually impaired, you
    A. Place furniture and equipment where the person walks
    B. Keep the lights off
    C. Explain the location of food and beverages
    D. Rearrange furniture and equipment
34. You are caring for a person with dementia. You
    A. Share information about the person's care
    B. Share information about the person's condition
    C. Protect confidential information
    D. Expose the person's body when you provide care
35. When caring for a confused person, you
    A. Call the person "Honey"
    B. Do not need to explain what you are doing
    C. Ask clear, simple questions
    D. Remove the calendar from the person's room
36. A person with Alzheimer's disease likes to wander. You
    A. Keep the person in his or her room
    B. Restrain the person
    C. Argue with the person who wants to leave
    D. Exercise the person as ordered

37. Restorative nursing programs
    A. Help maintain the lowest level of function
    B. Promote self-care measures
    C. Focus on the disability, not the person
    D. Help the person lose strength and independence
38. When caring for a person with a disability, you
    A. Focus on his or her limitations
    B. Expect progress in a rehabilitation program to be fast
    C. Remind the person of his or her progress in the rehabilitation program
    D. Deny the disability
39. After a person dies, you
    A. Can expose his or her body unnecessarily
    B. Can discuss the person's diagnosis with your family
    C. Can talk about the family's reactions to your friends
    D. Respect the person's right to privacy
40. You enter a person's room and find a fire in the wastebasket. Your first action is to
    A. Remove the person from the room
    B. Close the door
    C. Call for help
    D. Activate the fire alarm
41. You leave a person lying in urine and he or she develops a bedsore. This is
    A. Fraud
    B. Neglect
    C. Assault
    D. Battery
42. A nurse asks you to place a drug and a sterile dressing on a small foot wound. You
    A. Agree to do the task
    B. Ask another nursing assistant to do the task
    C. Politely tell the nurse you cannot do that task
    D. Report the nurse to the director of nursing
43. You observe a person's urine is foul-smelling and dark amber. Your first action is to
    A. Tell the other nursing assistant
    B. Tell the person
    C. Tell the nurse
    D. Record the observation
44. A daughter asks you for water for her mom. Your response is
    A. "I am not caring for your mom. I will get her nursing assistant for you."
    B. "I do not have time to do that."
    C. "That's not my job."
    D. "I will be happy to do that."
45. A person has a restraint on. You
    A. Observe the person for breathing and circulation complications every 30 minutes
    B. Know that unnecessary restraint is false imprisonment
    C. Use the most restrictive type of restraint
    D. Know that restraints decrease confusion and agitation

46. The nurse asks you to place a person in the supine position. You
    A. Elevate the head of the bed 45 degrees
    B. Elevate the foot of the bed 15 degrees
    C. Place the person on his or her back with the bed flat
    D. Place the person on his or her abdomen
47. The most important way to prevent or avoid spreading infection is to
    A. Wash hands
    B. Cover your nose when coughing
    C. Use disposable gloves
    D. Wear a mask
48. You are eating lunch and a nursing assistant begins to gossip about another person. You
    A. Join the conversation and talk about the person
    B. Remove yourself from the group
    C. Tell your roommate about the gossip you heard at lunch
    D. Tell another nursing assistant about the gossip you heard
49. When moving a person up in bed, you should
    A. Raise the head of the bed
    B. Ask the person to keep his or her legs straight
    C. Cause friction and shearing
    D. Ask a co-worker to help you
50. A person is on a sodium-controlled diet. This means
    A. Canned vegetables are omitted from his or her diet
    B. Salt may be added to food at the table
    C. Large amounts of salt are used in cooking
    D. Ham is eaten regularly
51. Elastic stockings
    A. Are applied after a person gets out of bed
    B. Should not have wrinkles or creases after being applied
    C. Come in one size only
    D. Are forced on the person
52. While walking, the person begins to fall. You
    A. Call for help
    B. Reach for a chair
    C. Ease the person to the floor
    D. Ask a visitor to help
53. Before bathing a person, you should
    A. Offer the bedpan or urinal
    B. Partially undress the person
    C. Raise the head of the bed
    D. Open the privacy curtain
54. When taking a rectal temperature, you insert the thermometer
    A. 1 inch
    B. 1.5 inches
    C. 2 inches
    D. 2.5 inches
55. Touch
    A. Is a form of nonverbal communication
    B. Is a form of verbal communication
    C. Means the same thing to everyone
    D. Should be used for all persons

56. You may share information about a person's care and condition to
    A. The staff caring for the person
    B. The person's daughter
    C. Your family members
    D. The volunteer in the gift shop
57. A person tells you he or she has pain upon urination. You
    A. Tell the nurse
    B. Let the nurse document this information
    C. Ask the person to tell you if it happens again
    D. Tell the person's son
58. A person's culture and religion are different from yours. You
    A. Laugh about the person's customs
    B. Tell your family about the person's customs
    C. Ask the person to explain his or her beliefs and practices to you
    D. Tell the person his or her beliefs and customs are silly
59. You need to wear gloves when you
    A. Do range-of-motion exercises
    B. Feed a person
    C. Give perineal care
    D. Walk a person
60. An older person is normally alert. Today he or she is confused. What should you do?
    A. Ask the person why he or she is confused
    B. Ignore the confusion
    C. Check to see if the person is confused later in the day
    D. Tell the nurse
61. While walking with a person, he tells you he feels faint. What do you do first?
    A. Have the person sit down.
    B. Call for the nurse.
    C. Open the window.
    D. Ask the person to take a deep breath.
62. You are asked to encourage fluids for a person. You
    A. Increase the person's fluid intake
    B. Decrease the person's fluid intake
    C. Limit fluids to mealtimes
    D. Keep fluids where the person cannot reach them
63. Communication fails when you
    A. Use words the other person understands
    B. Talk too much
    C. Let others express their feelings and concerns
    D. Talk about a topic that is uncomfortable
64. During bathing, a person may
    A. Decide what products to use
    B. Be exposed in the shower room
    C. Have visitors present without his or her permission
    D. Have no personal choices
65. People in late adulthood need to
    A. Adjust to increased income
    B. Adjust to their health being better
    C. Develop new friends and relationships
    D. Adjust to increased strength

66. When measuring blood pressure, you should do the following except
    A. Apply the cuff to a bare upper arm
    B. Turn off the TV
    C. Locate the brachial artery
    D. Use the arm with an IV infusion
67. You find clean linen on the floor in a person's room. You
    A. Use the linen to make the bed
    B. Return the linen to the linen cart
    C. Put the linen in the laundry
    D. Tell the nurse
68. When doing mouth care on an unconscious person, you
    A. Use a large amount of fluid
    B. Position the person on his or her side
    C. Do the task without telling the person what you are doing
    D. Insert his or her dentures when done
69. When brushing or combing a person's hair, you
    A. Cut matted or tangled hair
    B. Encourage the person to do as much as possible
    C. Style the hair as you want
    D. Perform the task weekly
70. When providing nail and foot care, you
    A. Cut fingernails with scissors
    B. Trim toenails for a diabetic person
    C. Trim toenails for a person with poor circulation
    D. Check between the toes for cracks and sores
71. An indwelling catheter becomes disconnected from the drainage system. You
    A. Reconnect the tubing to the catheter quickly without gloves
    B. Tell the nurse at once
    C. Get a new drainage system
    D. Touch the ends of the catheter
72. Urinary drainage bags are
    A. Hung on the bed rail
    B. Emptied and measured at the end of each shift
    C. Kept on the floor
    D. Kept higher than the person's bladder
73. A person needs a condom catheter applied. You remember to
    A. Apply it to a penis that is red and irritated
    B. Use adhesive tape to secure the catheter
    C. Use elastic tape to secure the catheter
    D. Act in an unprofessional manner
74. For comfort during bowel elimination
    A. Have the person use the bedpan rather than the bathroom or commode if possible
    B. Permit visitors to stay
    C. Keep the door and privacy curtain open
    D. Leave the person alone if possible
75. You are transferring a person with a weak right side from the wheelchair to the bed. You
    A. Place the wheelchair on the left side of the bed
    B. Place the wheelchair on the right side of the bed
    C. Keep the person in the wheelchair
    D. Ask the person what side moves first

Skills Evaluation Review

Each state has its own policies and procedures for the skills test. The following information is an overview of what to expect:

- To pass the skills evaluation, you will need to perform all 5 skills correctly.
- A nurse evaluates your performance of certain skills. Having someone watch as you work is not a new experience. Your instructor evaluated your performance during your training program. While you are working, your supervisor evaluates your skills.
- Mannequins and people are used as "patients" or "residents," depending on the skills you are performing.
- If you make a mistake, tell the evaluator what you did wrong. Then perform the skill correctly. Do not panic.
- Take whatever equipment you normally take or use at work. Wear a watch with a second hand. You may need it to measure vital signs and check how much time you have left.

Before and During the Procedure

- Hand washing is evaluated at the beginning of the skills test. You are expected to know when to wash your hands. Therefore you may not be told to do so. Follow the rules for hand hygiene during the test.
- Before entering a person's room, knock on the door. Greet the person by name and introduce yourself before beginning a procedure. Check the ID or the photo ID to make certain you are giving care to the right person.
- Explain what you are going to do before beginning the procedure and as needed throughout the procedure.
- Always follow the rules of medical asepsis. For example, remove gloves and dispose of them properly. Keep clean linen separated from dirty linen.
- Always protect the person's rights throughout the skills test.
- Communicate with the person as you give care. Focus on the person's needs and interests. Always treat the person with respect. Do not talk about yourself or your personal problems.
- Provide privacy. This involves pulling the privacy curtain around the bed, closing doors, and asking visitors to leave the room.
- Promote safety for the person. For example, lock the wheelchair when you transfer a person to and from it. Place the bed in the lowest horizontal position when

the person must get out of bed or when you are done giving care.

- Make sure the signal light is within the person's reach. Attaching it to the bed or bed rail does not mean the person can reach it.
- Use good body mechanics. Raise the bed and overbed table to a good working height.
- Provide for comfort:
  - Make sure the person and linens are clean and dry. The person may have become incontinent during the procedure.
  - Change or straighten bed linens as needed.
  - Position the person for comfort and in good alignment.
  - Provide pillows as directed by the nurse and the care plan.
  - Raise the head of the bed as the person prefers and allowed by the nurse and the care plan.
  - Provide for warmth. The person may need an extra blanket, a lap blanket, a sweater, socks, and so on.
  - Adjust lighting to meet the person's needs.
  - Make sure eyeglasses, hearing aids, and other devices are in place as needed.
  - Ask the person if he or she is comfortable.
  - Ask the person if there is anything else you can do for him or her.
  - Make sure the person is covered for warmth and privacy.

Skills

Ask your instructor to tell you which of the following skills are tested in your state. Place a checkmark in the box in front of each tested skill so it will be easy for you to reference. The skills marked with an asterisk (*) are used with permission of National Council of State Boards of Nursing (NCSBN). These skills are offered as a study guide to you. The word "client" refers to the resident or person receiving care. You are responsible for following the most current standards, practices, and guidelines of your state.

The steps in boldface type are critical element steps. Critical element steps must be done correctly to pass the skill. If you miss a critical element step, you will not pass the skills evaluation. For example, you are to transfer a client from the bed to a wheelchair. You will fail if you do not lock the wheels on the wheelchair before transferring

*Reproduced and used with permission from the Nurse Assistant Candidate Handbook from National Council of State Boards of Nursing (NCSBN), Chicago, Ill, © 2011.

the person. An automatic failure is one that could potentially cause harm to a person. Your state may mark critical element steps in another way—underline or italics. If your state has one, review the candidate's handbook.

❑ *Hand Hygiene (Hand Washing) (Chapter 15)

1. Addresses client by name and introduces self to client by name
2. Turns on water at sink
3. Wets hands and wrists thoroughly
4. Applies soap to hands
5. **Lathers all surfaces of wrists, hands, and fingers, producing friction for at least 20 (twenty) seconds keeping hands lower than the elbows and the fingertips down.**
6. Cleans fingernails by rubbing fingertips against palms of the opposite hand
7. **Rinse all surfaces of wrists, hands, and fingers, keeping hands lower than the elbows and the fingertips down**
8. Uses clean, dry paper towel/towels to dry all surfaces of hands, wrists, and fingers then disposes of paper towel/towels into waste container
9. Uses clean, dry paper towel/towels to turn off faucet then disposes of paper towel/towels into waste container or uses knee/foot control to turn off faucet
10. Does not touch inside of sink at any time

❑ *Applies One Knee-High Elastic Stocking (Chapter 32)

1. Explains procedure, speaking clearly, slowly, and directly, maintaining face-to-face contact whenever possible
2. Privacy is provided with a curtain, screen, or door
3. Client is in supine position (lying down in bed) while stocking is applied
4. Turns stocking inside-out, at least to heel
5. Places foot of stocking over toes, foot, and heel
6. Pulls top of stocking over foot, heel, and leg
7. Moves foot and leg gently and naturally, avoiding force and over-extension of limb and joints
8. **Finishes procedure with no twists or wrinkles and heel of stocking (if present) is over heel and opening in toe area (if present) is either under or over toe area**
9. Signaling device is within reach and bed is in low position
10. After completing skill, washes hands

❑ *Assists to Ambulate Using a Transfer Belt (Chapter 27)

1. Explains procedure, speaking clearly, slowly, and directly, maintaining face-to-face contact whenever possible
2. **Before assisting to stand, client is wearing shoes**
3. Before assisting to stand, bed is at a safe level
4. Before assisting to stand, checks and/or locks bed wheels
5. **Before assisting to stand, client is assisted to sitting position with feet flat on the floor**
6. Before assisting to stand, applies transfer belt securely at the waist over clothing/gown
7. Before assisting to stand, provides instructions to enable client to assist in standing including prearranged signal to alert client to begin standing
8. Stands facing client positioning self to ensure safety of candidate and client during transfer. Counts to three (or says other prearranged signal) to alert client to begin standing
9. On signal, gradually assists client to stand by grasping transfer belt on both sides with an upward grasp (candidate's hands are in upward position), and maintaining stability of client's legs
10. Walks slightly behind and to one side of client for a distance of ten (10) feet, while holding onto the belt
11. After ambulation, assists client to bed and removes transfer belt
12. Signaling device is within reach and bed is in low position
13. After completing skill, washes hands

❑ *Assists With Use of Bedpan (Chapter 22)

1. Explains procedure speaking clearly, slowly, and directly, maintaining face-to-face contact whenever possible
2. Privacy is provided with a curtain, screen, or door
3. Before placing bedpan, lowers head of bed
4. Puts on clean gloves before handling bedpan
5. **Places bedpan correctly under client's buttocks**
6. Removes and disposes of gloves (without contaminating self) into waste container and washes hands
7. After positioning client on bedpan and removing gloves, raises head of bed
8. Toilet tissue is within reach
9. Hand wipe is within reach and client is instructed to clean hands with hand wipe when finished
10. Signaling device within reach and client is asked to signal when finished
11. Puts on clean gloves before removing bedpan
12. Head of bed is lowered before bedpan is removed
13. Avoids overexposure of client
14. Empties and rinses bedpan and pours rinse into toilet
15. After rinsing bedpan, places bedpan in designated dirty supply area
16. After placing bedpan in designated dirty supply area, removes and disposes of gloves (without contaminating self) into waste container and washes hands
17. Signaling device is within reach and bed is in low position

*Reproduced and used with permission from the Nurse Assistant Candidate Handbook from National Council of State Boards of Nursing (NCSBN), Chicago, Ill, © 2011.

❑ *Cleans Upper or Lower Denture
(Chapter 20)*

1. Puts on clean gloves before handling dentures
2. Bottom of sink is lined and/or sink is partially filled with water before denture is held over sink
3. Rinses denture in moderate temperature running water before brushing them
4. Applies toothpaste to toothbrush
5. Brushes surfaces of denture
6. Rinses surfaces of denture under moderate temperature running water
7. Before placing denture into cup, rinses denture cup and lid
8. Places denture in denture cup with moderate temperature water solution and places lid on cup
9. Rinses toothbrush and places in designated toothbrush basin/container
10. Maintains clean technique with placement of toothbrush and denture
11. Sink liner is removed and disposed of appropriately and/or sink is drained
12. After rinsing equipment and disposing of sink liner, removes and disposes of gloves (without contaminating self) into waste container and washes hands

❑ *Counts and Records Radial Pulse
(Chapter 26)***

1. Explains procedure, speaking clearly, slowly, and directly, maintaining face-to-face contact whenever possible
2. Places fingertips on thumb side of client's wrist to locate radial pulse
3. Counts beats for one full minute
4. Signaling device is within reach
5. Before recording, washes hands
6. **After obtaining pulse by palpating in radial artery position, records pulse rate within plus or minus 4 beats of evaluator's reading**

❑ *Counts and Records Respirations
(Chapter 26)†*

1. Explains procedure (for testing purposes), speaking clearly, slowly, and directly, maintaining face-to-face contact whenever possible
2. Counts respirations for one full minute
3. Signaling device is within reach
4. Washes hands
5. **Records respiration rate within plus or minus 2 breaths of evaluator's reading**

❑ *Dresses Client With Affected (Weak) Right
Arm (Chapter 21)*

1. Explains procedure, speaking clearly, slowly, and directly, maintaining face-to-face contact whenever possible
2. Privacy is provided with a curtain, screen, or door
3. Asks which shirt he/she would like to wear and dresses him/her in shirt of choice
4. While avoiding overexposure of client, removes gown from the unaffected side first, then removes gown from the affected side and disposes of gown into soiled linen container
5. **Assists to put the right (affected/weak) arm through the right sleeve of the shirt before placing garment on left (unaffected) arm**
6. While putting on shirt, moves body gently and naturally, avoiding force and over-extension of limbs and joints
7. Finishes with clothing in place
8. Signaling device is within reach and bed is in low position
9. After completing skill, washes hands

❑ *Feeds Client Who Cannot Feed Self
(Chapter 24)*

1. Explains procedure to client, speaking clearly, slowly, and directly, maintaining face-to-face contact whenever possible
2. Before feeding, candidate looks at name card on tray and asks client to state name
3. **Before feeding client, client is in an upright sitting position (75–90 degrees)**
4. Places tray where the food can be easily seen by client
5. Candidate cleans client's hands with hand wipe before beginning feeding
6. Candidate sits facing client during feeding
7. Tells client what foods are on tray and asks what client would like to eat first
8. Using spoon, offers client one bite of each type of food on tray, telling client the content of each spoonful
9. Offers beverage at least once during meal
10. Candidate asks client if they are ready for next bite of food or sip of beverage
11. At end of meal, candiate cleans client's mouth and hands with wipes
12. Removes food tray and places tray in designated dirty supply area
13. Signaling device is within client's reach
14. After completing skill, washes hands

*Reproduced and used with permission from the Nurse Assistant Candidate Handbook from National Council of State Boards of Nursing (NCSBN), Chicago, Ill, © 2011.
**Count for one full minute
†Count for one full minute. For testing purposes you may explain to the client that you will be counting the respirations

❏ *Gives Modified Bed Bath (Face and One Arm, Hand, and Underarm) (Chapter 20)*

1. Explains procedure, speaking clearly, slowly, and directly, maintaining face-to-face contact whenever possible
2. Privacy is provided with a curtain, screen, or door
3. Removes gown and places in soiled linen container while avoiding over exposure of the client
4. Before washing, checks water temperature for safety and comfort and asks client to verify comfort of water
5. Puts on clean gloves before washing client
6. **Beginning with eyes, washes eyes with wet washcloth (no soap), using a different area of the washcloth for each stroke, washing inner aspect to outer aspect, then proceeds to wash face**
7. Dries face with towel
8. Exposes one arm and places towel underneath arm
9. Applies soap to wet washcloth
10. Washes arm, hand, and underarm, keeping rest of body covered
11. Rinses and dries arm, hand, and underarm
12. Moves body gently and naturally, avoiding force and over-extension of limbs and joints
13. Puts clean gown on client
14. Empties, rinses, and dries basin
15. After rinsing and drying basin, places basin in designated dirty supply area
16. Disposes of linen into soiled linen container
17. Avoids contact between candidate clothing and used linens
18. After placing basin in designated dirty supply area, and disposing of used linen, removes and disposes of gloves (without contaminating self) into waste container and washes hands
19. Signaling device is within reach and bed is in low position

❏ *Makes an Occupied Bed (Client Does Not Need Assistance to Turn) (Chapter 19)*

1. Explains procedure, speaking clearly, slowly, and directly, maintaining face-to-face contact whenever possible
2. Privacy is provided with a curtain, screen, or door
3. Lowers head of bed before moving client
4. Client is covered while linens are changed
5. Loosens top linen from the end of the bed
6. Raises side rail on side to which client will move and client moves toward raised side rail
7. Loosens bottom used linen on working side and moves bottom used linen toward center of bed
8. Places and tucks in clean bottom linen or fitted bottom sheet on working side and tucks under client
9. Before going to other side, client moves back onto clean bottom linen

10. Raises side rail then goes to other side of bed
11. Removes used bottom linen
12. Pulls and tucks in clean bottom linen, finishing with bottom sheet free of wrinkles
13. Client is covered with clean top sheet and bath blanket/used top sheet has been removed
14. Changes pillowcase
15. Linen is centered and tucked at foot of bed
16. Avoids contact between candidate's clothing and used linen
17. Disposes of used linen into soiled linen container and avoids putting linen on floor
18. Signaling device is within reach and bed is in low position
19. Washes hands

❏ *Measures and Records Blood Pressure (Chapter 26)*

1. Explains procedure, speaking clearly, slowly, and directly, maintaining face-to-face contact whenever possible
2. Before using stethoscope, wipes bell/diaphragm and earpieces of stethoscope with alcohol
3. Client's arm is positioned with palm up and upper arm is exposed
4. Feels for brachial artery on inner aspect of arm, at bend of elbow
5. Places blood pressure cuff snugly on client's upper arm with sensor/arrow over brachial artery site
6. Earpieces of stethoscope are in ears and bell/diaphragm is over brachial artery site
7. Candidate inflates cuff between 160 mm Hg to 180 mm Hg. (If beat heard immediately upon cuff deflation, completely deflate cuff). Re-inflate cuff to no more than 200 mm Hg.
8. Deflates cuff slowly and notes the **first sound** (systolic reading), and **last sound** (diastolic reading) (If rounding needed, measurements are rounded **UP** to the nearest 2 mm of mercury)
9. Removes cuff
10. Signaling device is within reach
11. Before recording, washes hands
12. **After obtaining reading using BP cuff and stethoscope, records both systolic and diastolic pressures each within plus or minus 8 mm of evaluator's reading**

❏ *Measures and Records Urinary Output (Chapter 24)*

1. Puts on clean gloves before handling bedpan
2. Pours the contents of the bedpan into measuring container without spilling or splashing urine outside of container

*Reproduced and used with permission from the Nurse Assistant Candidate Handbook from National Council of State Boards of Nursing (NCSBN), Chicago, Ill, © 2011.

3. Measures the amount of urine at eye level with container on flat surface
4. After measuring urine, empties contents of measuring container into toilet
5. Rinses measuring container and pours rinse water into toilet
6. Rinses bedpan and pours rinse into toilet
7. After rinsing equipment, and before recording output, removes and disposes of gloves (without contaminating self) into waste container and washes hands
8. **Records contents of container within plus or minus 25 mL/cc of evaluator's reading**

❑ *Measures and Records Weight of Ambulatory Client (Chapter 29)*
1. Explains procedure, speaking clearly, slowly, and directly, maintaining face-to-face contact whenever possible
2. Client has shoes on before walking to scale
3. Before client steps on scale, candidate sets scale to zero then obtains client's weight
4. While client steps onto scale, candidate stands next to scale and assists client (if needed) onto center of the scale
5. While client steps off scale, candidate stands next to scale and assists client, if needed, off scale before recording weight
6. Before recording, washes hands
7. **Records weight based on indicator on scale. Weight is within plus or minus 2 lbs of evaluator's reading (If weight recorded in kg weight is within plus or minus 0.9 kg of evaluator's reading)**

❑ *Positions on Side (Chapter 17)*
1. Explains procedure, speaking clearly, slowly, and directly, maintaining face-to-face contact whenever possible
2. Privacy is provided with a curtain, screen, or door
3. Before turning, lowers head of bed
4. Raises side rail on side to which body will be turned
5. Slowly rolls onto side as one unit toward raised side rail
6. Places or adjusts pillow under head for support
7. Candidate positions client so that client is not lying on arm
8. Supports top arm with supportive device
9. Places supportive device behind client's back
10. Places supportive device between legs with top knee flexed; knee and ankle supported
11. Signaling device is within reach and bed is in low position
12. After completing skill, washes hands

❑ *Provides Catheter Care for Female (Chapter 22)*
1. Explains procedure, speaking clearly, slowly, and directly, maintaining face-to-face contact whenever possible
2. Privacy is provided with a curtain, screen, or door
3. Before washing checks water temperature for safety and comfort and asks client to verify comfort of water
4. Puts on clean gloves before washing
5. Places linen protector under perineal area before washing
6. Exposes area surrounding catheter while avoiding overexposure of client
7. Applies soap to wet washcloth
8. **While holding catheter at meatus without tugging, cleans at least four inches of catheter from meatus, moving in only one direction (i.e., away from meatus) using a clean area of the cloth for each stroke**
9. **While holding catheter at meatus without tugging, rinses at least four inches of catheter from meatus, moving only in one direction, away from meatus, using a clean area of the cloth for each stroke**
10. While holding catheter at meatus without tugging, dries at least four inches of catheter moving away from meatus
11. Empties, rinses, and dries basin
12. After rinsing and drying basin, places basin in designated dirty supply area
13. Disposes of used linen into soiled linen container and disposes of linen protector appropriately
14. Avoids contact between candidate clothing and used linen
15. After disposing of used linen and cleaning equipment, removes and disposes of gloves (without contaminating self) into waste container and washes hands
16. Signaling device is within reach and bed is in low position

❑ *Provides Fingernail Care on One Hand (Chapter 20)*
1. Explains procedure, speaking clearly, slowly, and directly, maintaining face-to-face contact whenever possible
2. Before immersing fingernails, checks water temperature for safety and comfort and asks client to verify comfort of water
3. Basin is in a comfortable position for client
4. Puts on clean gloves before cleaning fingernails
5. Fingernails are immersed in basin of water
6. Cleans under each fingernail with orange stick
7. Wipes orange stick on towel after each nail
8. Dries fingernail area
9. Candidate feels each nail and files as needed

*Reproduced and used with permission from the Nurse Assistant Candidate Handbook from National Council of State Boards of Nursing (NCSBN), Chicago, Ill, © 2011.

10. Disposes of orange stick and emery board into waste container (for testing purposes)
11. Empties, rinses, and dries basin
12. After rinsing basin, places basin in designated dirty supply area
13. Disposes of used linen into soiled linen container
14. After cleaning nails and equipment, and disposing of used linen, removes and disposes of gloves (without contaminating self) into waste container and washes hands
15. Signaling device is within reach

☐ *Provides Foot Care on One Foot (Chapter 20)

1. Explains procedure, speaking clearly, slowly, and directly, maintaining face-to-face contact whenever possible
2. Privacy is provided with a curtain, screen, or door
3. Before washing, checks water temperature for safety and comfort and asks client to verify comfort of water
4. Basin is in a comfortable position for client and on protective barrier
5. Puts on clean gloves before washing foot
6. Client's bare foot is placed into the water
7. Applies soap to wet washcloth
8. Lifts foot from water and washes foot (including between the toes)
9. Foot is rinsed (including between the toes)
10. Dries foot (including between the toes)
11. Applies lotion to top and bottom of foot, removing excess (if any) with a towel
12. Supports foot and ankle during procedure
13. Empties, rinses, and dries basin
14. After rinsing and drying basin, places basin in designated dirty supply area
15. Disposes of used linen into soiled linen container
16. After cleaning foot and equipment, and disposing of used linen, removes and disposes of gloves (without contaminating self) into waste container and washes hands
17. Signaling device is within reach

☐ *Provides Mouth Care (Chapter 20)

1. Explains procedure, speaking clearly, slowly, and directly, maintaining face-to-face contact whenever possible
2. Privacy is provided with a curtain, screen, or door
3. Before providing mouth care, client is in upright sitting position (75–90 degrees)
4. Puts on clean gloves before cleaning mouth
5. Places clothing protector across chest before providing mouth care
6. Secures cup of water and moistens toothbrush
7. Before cleaning mouth applies toothpaste to moistened toothbrush
8. **Cleans mouth (including tongue and surfaces of teeth) using gentle motions**

9. Maintains clean technique with placement of toothbrush
10. Candidate holds emesis basin to chin while client rinses mouth
11. Candidate wipes mouth and removes clothing protector
12. After rinsing toothbrush, empty, rinse, and dry the basin and place used toothbrush in designated basin/container
13. Places basin and toothbrush in designated dirty supply area
14. Disposes of used linen into soiled linen container
15. After placing basin and toothbrush in designated dirty supply area, and disposing of used linen, removes and disposes of gloves (without contaminating self) into waste container and washes hands
16. Signaling device is within reach and bed is in low position

☐ *Provides Perineal Care (Peri-Care) for Female (Chapter 20)

1. Explains procedure, speaking clearly, slowly, and directly, maintaining face-to-face contact whenever possible
2. Privacy is provided with a curtain, screen, or door
3. Before washing checks water temperature for safety and comfort and asks client to verify comfort of water
4. Puts on clean gloves before washing perineal area
5. Places pad/linen protector under perineal area before washing
6. Exposes perineal area while avoiding overexposure of client
7. Applies soap to wet washcloth
8. **Washes genital area, moving from front to back, while using a clean area of the washcloth for each stroke**
9. **Using clean washcloth, rinses soap from genital area, moving from front to back, while using a clean area of the washcloth for each stroke**
10. Dries genital area moving from front to back with towel
11. **After washing genital area, turns to side, then washes and rinses rectal area moving from front to back using a clean area of washcloth for each stroke. Dries with towel**
12. Repositions client
13. Empties, rinses, and dries basin
14. After rinsing and drying basin, places basin in designated dirty supply area
15. Disposes of used linen into soiled linen container and disposes of linen protector appropriately
16. Avoids contact between candidate clothing and used linen
17. After disposing of used linen, and placing used equipment in designated dirty supply area, removes and disposes of gloves (without contaminating self) into waste container and washes hands
18. Signaling device is within reach and bed is in low position

*Reproduced and used with permission from the Nurse Assistant Candidate Handbook from National Council of State Boards of Nursing (NCSBN), Chicago, Ill, © 2011.

❑ *Transfers From Bed to Wheelchair Using Transfer Belt (Chapter 17)*

1. Explains procedure, speaking clearly, slowly, and directly, maintaining face-to-face contact whenever possible
2. Privacy is provided with a curtain, screen, or door
3. Before assisting to stand, wheelchair is positioned along side of bed, at head of bed, facing the foot, or foot of bed facing head
4. Before assisting to stand, footrests are folded up or removed
5. Before assisting to stand, bed is at a safe level
6. **Before assisting to stand, locks wheels on wheelchair**
7. Before assisting to stand, checks and/or locks bed wheels
8. **Before assisting to stand, client is assisted to a sitting position with feet flat on the floor**
9. Before assisting to stand, client is wearing shoes
10. Before assisting to stand, applies transfer belt securely at the waist over clothing/gown
11. Before assisting to stand, provides instructions to enable client to assist in transfer including prearranged signal to alert when to begin standing
12. Stands facing client, positioning self to ensure safety of candidate and client during transfer. Counts to three (or says other prearranged signal) to alert client to begin standing
13. On signal, gradually assists client to stand by grasping transfer belt on both sides with an upward grasp (candidates hands are in upward position) and maintaining stability of client's legs
14. Assists client to turn to stand in front of wheelchair with back of client's legs against wheelchair
15. Lowers client into wheelchair
16. Positions client with hips touching back of wheelchair and transfer belt is removed
17. Positions feet on footrests
18. Signaling device is within reach
19. After completing skill, washes hands

❑ *Performs Modified Passive Range-of-Motion (PROM) for One Knee and One Ankle (Chapter 27)*

1. Explains procedure, speaking clearly, slowly, and directly, maintaining face-to-face contact whenever possible
2. Privacy is provided with a curtain, screen, or door
3. Instructs client to inform candidate if pain is experienced during exercise
4. Supports leg at knee and ankle while performing range of motion for knee
5. Bends the knee then returns leg to client's normal position (extension/flexion) (AT LEAST 3 TIMES unless pain is verbalized)

6. Supports foot and ankle close to the bed while performing range of motion for ankle
7. Pushes/pulls foot toward head (dorsiflexion), and pushes/pulls foot down, toes point down (plantar flexion) (AT LEAST 3 TIMES unless pain is verbalized)
8. **While supporting the limb, moves joints gently, slowly, and smoothly through the range of motion, discontinuing exercise if client verbalizes pain**
9. Signaling device is within reach and bed is in low position
10. After completing skill, washes hands

❑ *Performs Modified Passive Range-of-Motion (PROM) for One Shoulder (Chapter 27)*

1. Explains procedure, speaking clearly, slowly, and directly, maintaining face-to-face contact whenever possible
2. Privacy is provided with a curtain, screen, or door
3. Instructs client to inform candidate if pain is experienced during exercise
4. Supports client's upper and lower arm while performing range of motion for shoulder
5. **Raises client's straightened arm from side position upward toward head to ear level and returns arm down to side of body (flexion/extension) (AT LEAST 3 TIMES unless pain is verbalized) supporting the limb, moves joint gently, slowly, and smoothly through the range of motion, discontinuing exercise if client verbalizes pain**
6. **Moves client's straightened arm away from the side of body to shoulder level and returns to side of body (abduction/adduction) (AT LEAST 3 TIMES unless pain is verbalized) supporting the limb, moves joint gently, slowly, and smoothly through the range of motion, discontinuing exercise if client verbalizes pain**
7. Signaling device is within reach and bed is in low position
8. After completing skill, washes hands

❑ *Passive Range-of-Motion of Lower Extremity (Hip, Knee, Ankle) (Chapter 27)*

1. Washes hands before contact with client
2. Identifies self to client by name and addresses client by name
3. Explains procedure to client, speaking clearly, slowly, and directly, maintaining face-to-face contact whenever possible
4. Provides for client's privacy during procedure with curtain, screen, or door
5. Positions client supine and in good body alignment
6. Supports client's leg by placing one hand under knee and other hand under heel

---

*Reproduced and used with permission from the Nurse Assistant Candidate Handbook from National Council of State Boards of Nursing (NCSBN), Chicago, Ill, © 2011.

7. Moves entire leg away from body (Performs AT LEAST 3 TIMES unless pain occurs)
8. Moves entire leg toward body (Performs AT LEAST 3 TIMES unless pain occurs)
9. Bends client's knee and hip toward client's trunk (Performs AT LEAST 3 TIMES unless pain occurs)
10. Straightens knee and hip (Performs AT LEAST 3 TIMES unless pain occurs)
11. Flexes and extends ankle through range-of-motion exercises (Performs AT LEAST 3 TIMES unless pain occurs)
12. Rotates ankle through range-of-motion exercises (Performs AT LEAST 3 TIMES unless pain occurs)
13. **While supporting limb, moves joints gently, slowly, and smoothly through range-of-motion to point of resistance, discontinuing exercise if pain occurs**
14. Provides for comfort
15. Before leaving client, places signaling device within client's reach
16. Washes hands

❏ *Passive Range-of-Motion of Upper Extremity (Shoulder, Elbow, Wrist, Finger) (Chapter 27)*

1. Washes hands before contact with client
2. Identifies self to client by name and addresses client by name
3. Explains procedure to client, speaking clearly, slowly, and directly, maintaining face-to-face contact whenever possible
4. Provides for client's privacy during procedure with curtain, screen, or door
5. Supports client's extremity above and below joints while performing range-of-motion
6. Raises client's straightened arm toward ceiling and back toward head of bed and returns to flat position (flexion/extension) (Performs AT LEAST 3 TIMES unless pain occurs)
7. Moves client's straightened arm away from client's side of body toward head of bed, and returns client's straightened arm to midline of client's body (abduction/adduction) (Performs AT LEAST 3 TIMES unless pain occurs)
8. Moves client's shoulder through rotation range-of-motion exercises (Performs AT LEAST 3 TIMES unless pain occurs)
9. Flexes and extends elbow through range-of-motion exercises (Performs AT LEAST 3 TIMES unless pain occurs)
10. Provides range-of-motion exercises to wrist (Performs AT LEAST 3 TIMES unless pain occurs)
11. Moves finger and thumb joints through range-of-motion exercises (Performs AT LEAST 3 TIMES unless pain occurs)
12. **While supporting body part, moves joint gently, slowly, and smoothly through range-of-motion to point of resistance, discontinuing exercise if pain occurs**

13. Before leaving client, places signaling device within client's reach
14. Washes hands

❏ *Makes a Unoccupied (Closed) Bed (Chapter 19)*

1. Washes hands
2. Collects clean linen
3. Places clean linen on a clean surface
4. Raises the bed for good body mechanics
5. Puts on gloves
6. Removes linen without contaminating uniform. Rolls each piece away from self
7. Discards linen into laundry bag
8. Moves the mattress to the head of the bed
9. Applies mattress pad
10. Applies bottom sheet, keeping it smooth and free of wrinkles
11. Places the top sheet and bedspread on the bed, keeping them smooth and free of wrinkles
12. Tucks in top linens at the foot of the bed. Makes mitered corners
13. Applies clean pillowcase with zippers and/or tags to inside of pillowcase
14. Lowers the bed to its lowest position. Locks the bed wheels
15. Washes hands

❏ **Donning and Removing PPE (Gown and Gloves) (Chapter 15)*

1. Picks up gown and unfolds
2. Facing the back opening of gown, places arms through each sleeve
3. Fastens the neck opening
4. Secures gown at waist making sure that back of clothing is covered by gown (as much as possible)
5. Puts on gloves
6. Cuffs of gloves overlap cuffs of gown
7. **Before removing gown, with one gloved hand, grasps the other glove at the palm, remove glove**
8. **Slips fingers from ungloved hand underneath cuff of remaining glove at wrist, and removes glove turning it inside out as it is removed**
9. Disposes of gloves into designated waste container without contaminating self
10. After removing gloves, unfastens gown at neck and, at waist
11. After removing gloves, removes gown without touching outside of gown
12. While removing gown, holds gown away from body, without touching the floor turns gown inward and keeps it inside out
13. Disposes of gown in designated container without contaminating self
14. After completing skill, washes hands

*Reproduced and used with permission from the Nurse Assistant Candidate Handbook from National Council of State Boards of Nursing (NCSBN), Chicago, Ill, © 2011.

❑ *Performs Abdominal Thrusts (Chapter 12)*

1. Asks client if he or she is choking
2. Stands behind the client
3. Wraps arms around client's waist
4. Makes a fist with one hand
5. Places thumb side of fist against the client's abdomen
6. Positions fist in middle above navel and well below sternum (breastbone)
7. Grasps fist with other hand
8. Presses fist and other hand into client's abdomen with quick upward thrusts
9. Repeats thrusts until object is expelled or client becomes unresponsive

❑ *Ambulation With Cane or Walker (Chapter 27)*

1. Explains procedure to client, speaking clearly, slowly, and directly, maintaining face-to-face contact whenever possible
2. Locks bed wheels or wheelchair brakes
3. Assists client to a sitting position
4. **Before ambulating, puts on and properly fastens non-skid footwear**
5. Positions cane or walker correctly. Cane is on the client's strong side
6. Assists client to stand, using correct body mechanics
7. Stabilizes cane or walker and ensures client stabilizes cane or walker
8. Stands behind and slightly to the side of client on the person's weak side
9. Ambulates client
10. Assists client to pivot and sit, using correct body mechanics
11. Before leaving client, places signaling device within client's reach
12. Washes hands

❑ *Fluid Intake (Chapter 24)*

1. Observes dinner tray
2. Determines, in milliliters (mL), the amount of fluid consumed from each container
3. Determines total fluid consumed in mL
4. Records total fluid consumed on I&O sheet
5. Calculated total is within required range of evaluator's reading

❑ *Brushes or Combs Client's Hair (Chapter 21)*

1. Explains procedure to client, speaking clearly, slowly, and directly, maintaining face-to-face contact whenever possible
2. Collects brush or comb and bath towel
3. Places towel across the person's back and shoulders or across the pillow
4. Asks client how he or she wants his or her hair styled
5. Combs/brushes hair gently and completely
6. Leaves hair neatly brushed, combed, and/or styled
7. Removes towel

8. Removes hair from comb or brush
9. Before leaving client, places signaling device within client's reach
10. Washes hands

❑ *Transfers a Client Using a Mechanical Lift (Chapter 17)*

1. Assembles required equipment; performs safety check of slings, straps, hooks, and chains
2. Checks client's weight to ensure it does not exceed the lift's capacity
3. Asks a co-worker to help
4. Explains procedure to client, speaking clearly, slowly, and directly, maintaining face-to-face contact whenever possible
5. Provides for privacy during procedure with curtain, screen, or door
6. Locks the bed wheels
7. Raises the bed for proper body mechanics
8. Lowers the head of the bed to a level appropriate for the client
9. Stands on one side of the bed; co-worker stands on the other side
10. Lowers the bed rails if up
11. Centers the sling under the client following the manufacturer's instructions
12. Ensures that the sling is smooth
13. Positions the client in semi-Fowler's position
14. Positions a chair to lower the client into it
15. Lowers the bed to its lowest position
16. Raises the lift to position it over the client
17. Positions the lift over the client
18. Attaches the sling to the sling hooks checks fasteners for security
19. Crosses the client's arms over the chest
20. Raises the lift high enough until the client and sling are free of the bed
21. Instructs co-worker to support the client's legs as candidate moves the lift and the client away from the bed
22. Positions the lift so the client's back is toward the chair
23. Slowly lowers the client into the chair
24. Places client in comfortable position, in correct body alignment
25. Lowers the sling hooks and unhooks the sling
26. Removes the sling from under the client unless otherwise indicated. Moves lift away from client
27. Puts footwear on the client
28. Covers the client's lap and legs with a lap blanket
29. Positions the chair as the client prefers
30. Places signaling device within client's reach
31. Washes hands

❑ *Provides Mouth Care for an Unconscious Client (Chapter 20)*

1. Explains procedure to client, speaking clearly, slowly, and directly, maintaining face-to-face contact whenever possible

2. Provides for privacy during procedure with curtain, screen, or door
3. Washes hands
4. Positions client on side with head turned well to one side
5. Puts on gloves
6. Places the towel under the client's face
7. Places the kidney basin under the chin
8. Uses swabs or toothbrush and toothpaste or other cleaning solution
9. Cleans inside of mouth including the gums, tongue, and teeth
10. Cleans and dries face
11. Removes the towel, kidney basin
12. Applies lubricant to the lips
13. Positions client for comfort and safety
14. Removes and discards the gloves
15. Places signal light within the client's reach
16. Washes hands

❏ Providing Drinking Water (Chapter 24)

1. Washes hands
2. Assembles equipment—ice, scoop, pitcher, cup, straw
3. Explains procedure to client, speaking clearly, slowly, and directly, maintaining face-to-face contact whenever possible
4. Uses the scoop to fill the pitcher with ice; does not let the scoop touch the rim or inside of the pitcher
5. Places scoop in appropriate receptacle after each use
6. Adds water to pitcher
7. Places the pitcher, disposable cup, and straw (if used) on the overbed table, within the person's reach
8. Before leaving, places signaling device within client's reach
9. Washes hands

❏ Provides Perineal Care for Uncircumcised Male (Chapter 20)

1. Explains procedure to client, speaking clearly, slowly, and directly, maintaining face-to-face contact whenever possible
2. Provides for privacy during procedure with curtain, screen, or door
3. Washes hands
4. Fills basin with comfortably warm water
5. Puts on gloves
6. Elevates bed to working height
7. Places waterproof pad under buttocks
8. Gently grasps penis
9. Retracts the foreskin
10. Using a circular motion, cleans the tip by starting at the meatus of the urethra and working outward
11. Rinses the area with another washcloth
12. Returns the foreskin to its natural position
13. Cleans the shaft of the penis with firm, downward strokes and rinses the area
14. Cleans the scrotum

15. Pats dry the penis and the scrotum
16. Cleans the rectal area
17. Removes the waterproof pad
18. Lowers the bed
19. Removes and discards the gloves
20. Washes hands
21. Before leaving, places signaling device within client's reach

❏ Empties and Records Content of Urinary Drainage Bag (Chapter 22)

1. Explains procedure to client, speaking clearly, slowly, and directly, maintaining face-to-face contact whenever possible
2. Washes hands
3. Puts on gloves
4. Places a paper towel on the floor
5. Places the graduate on the paper towel
6. Places the graduate under the collection bag
7. Ensures the bag is below the bladder and the drainage tube is not kinked
8. Opens the clamp on the drain
9. Lets all urine drain into the graduate—does not let the drain touch the graduate
10. Closes and positions the clamp
11. Measures urine
12. Removes and discards the paper towel
13. Empties the contents of the graduate into the toilet and flushes
14. Rinses the graduate
15. Returns the graduate to its proper place
16. Removes the gloves
17. Washes hands
18. Records the time and amount on the intake and output (I&O) record
19. Provides for client comfort
20. Places the signal light within reach of client

❏ Applying a Vest Restraint (Chapter 14)

1. Obtains the correct type and size of restraint
2. Checks straps for tears or frays
3. Washes hands
4. Explains procedure to client, speaking clearly, slowly, and directly, maintaining face-to-face contact whenever possible
5. Provides for privacy during procedure with curtain, screen, or door
6. Makes sure the client is comfortable and in good alignment
7. Assists the person to a sitting position
8. Applies the restraint following the manufacturer's instructions—the "V" part of the vest crosses in front
9. Makes sure the vest is free of wrinkles in the front and back
10. Brings the straps through the slots
11. Makes sure the client is comfortable and in good alignment

*Reproduced and used with permission from the Nurse Assistant Candidate Handbook from National Council of State Boards of Nursing (NCSBN), Chicago, Ill, © 2011.

12. Secures the straps to the chair or to the movable part of the bed frame
13. Uses a secure knot that can be released with one pull
14. Makes sure the vest is snug—slide an open hand between the restraint and the client
15. Places the signal light within the client's reach
16. Washes hands

❏ *Performs a Back Rub (Massage) (Chapter 20)*

1. Washes hands
2. Explains procedure to client, speaking clearly, slowly, and directly, maintaining face-to-face contact whenever possible
3. Provides for privacy during procedure with curtain, screen, or door
4. Raises the bed for good body mechanics
5. Lowers the bed rail near the candidate, if up
6. Positions the person in the prone or side-lying position
7. Exposes the back, shoulders, upper arms, and buttocks
8. Warms the lotion
9. Rubs entire back in upward, outward motion for approximately 2 to 3 minutes; does not massage reddened bony areas
10. Straightens and secures clothing or sleepwear
11. Returns client to comfortable and safe position
12. Places the signal light within reach
13. Lowers the bed to its lowest position
14. Washes hands

❏ *Position Foley Catheter (Chapter 22)*

1. Explains procedure to client, speaking clearly, slowly, and directly, maintaining face-to-face contact whenever possible
2. Washes hands
3. Puts on gloves
4. Secures catheter and drainage tubing according to facility procedure
5. Places tubing over leg
6. Positions drainage tubing so urine flows freely into drainage bag and has no kinks
7. Attaches bag to bed frame, below level of bladder
8. Washes hands

❏ *Apply Cold Pack or Warm Compress (Chapter 35)*

1. Washes hands
2. Collects needed equipment
3. Explains procedure to client, speaking clearly, slowly, and directly, maintaining face-to-face contact whenever possible
4. Provides for privacy during procedure with curtain, screen, or door
5. Positions the client for the procedure
6. Covers cold pack or warm compress with towel or other protective cover

7. Properly places cold pack or warm compress on site
8. Checks the client for complications every 5 minutes
9. Checks the cold pack or warm compress every 5 minutes
10. Removes the application at the specified time—usually after 15 to 20 minutes
11. Provides for comfort
12. Places the signal light within reach
13. Washes hands

❏ *Position for an Enema (Chapter 23)*

1. Washes hands
2. Explains procedure to client, speaking clearly, slowly, and directly, maintaining face-to-face contact whenever possible
3. Provides for privacy
4. Positions the client in Sims' position or in a left side-lying position
5. Covers client appropriately
6. Provides for comfort
7. Places the signal light within reach
8. Washes hands

❏ *Position Client for Meals (Chapter 24)*

1. Washes hands
2. Explains procedure to client, speaking clearly, slowly, and directly, maintaining face-to-face contact whenever possible
3. If the person will eat in bed:
   a. Raises the head of the bed to a comfortable position—usually Fowler's or high Fowler's position is preferred
   b. Removes items from the overbed table and cleans the overbed table
   c. Adjusts the overbed table in front of the person
   d. Places the client in proper body alignment
4. If the person will sit in a chair:
   a. Positions the person in a chair or wheelchair
   b. Provides support for the client's feet
   c. Removes items from the overbed table and cleans the table
   d. Adjusts the overbed table in front of the person
   e. Places the client in proper body alignment
5. Places the signal light within reach
6. Washes hands

❏ *Takes and Records Axillary Temperature, Pulse, and Respirations (Chapter 26)*

1. Washes hands before contact with client
2. Identifies self to client by name and addresses client by name
3. Explains procedure to client, speaking clearly, slowly, and directly, maintaining face-to-face contact whenever possible
4. Provides for client's privacy during procedure with curtain, screen, or door

*Reproduced and used with permission from the Nurse Assistant Candidate Handbook from National Council of State Boards of Nursing (NCSBN), Chicago, Ill, © 2011.

5. Turns on digital oral thermometer
6. Dries axilla and places thermometer in the center of the axilla
7. Holds thermometer in place for appropriate length of time
8. Removes and reads thermometer
9. Records temperature on pad of paper
10. **Recorded temperature is within required range**
11. Discards sheath from thermometer
12. Places fingertips on thumb side of client's wrist to locate radial pulse
13. Counts beats for 1 full minute
14. Records pulse rate on pad of paper
15. **Recorded pulse is within required range**
16. Counts respirations for 1 full minute
17. Records respirations on pad of paper
18. **Recorded respirations are within required range**
19. Before leaving client, places signaling device within client's reach
20. Washes hands

❑ *Transfers Client From Wheelchair to Bed (Chapter 17)*

1. Washes hands before contact with client
2. Identifies self to client by name and addresses client by name
3. Explains procedure to client, speaking clearly, slowly, and directly, maintaining face-to-face contact whenever possible
4. Provides for client's privacy during procedure with curtain, screen, or door
5. Positions wheelchair close to bed with arm of wheelchair almost touching bed
6. Before transferring client, ensures client is wearing non-skid footwear
7. Before transferring client, folds up footplates
8. Before transferring client, places bed at safe and appropriate level for client
9. **Before transferring client, locks wheels on wheelchair and locks bed brakes**
10. With transfer (gait) belt: Stands in front of client, positioning self to ensure safety of candidate and client during transfer (for example, knees bent, feet apart, back straight), places belt around client's waist, and grasps belt. Tightens belt so that fingers of candidate's hand can be slipped between transfer/gait belt and client
    Without transfer belt: Stands in front of client, positioning self to ensure safety of candidate and client during transfer (for example, knees bent, feet apart, back straight, arms around client's torso under arms)
11. Provides instructions to enable client to assist in transfer, including prearranged signal to alert client to begin standing
12. Braces client's lower extremities to prevent slipping
13. Counts to three (or says other prearranged signal) to alert client to begin transfer

14. On signal, gradually assists client to stand
15. Assists client to pivot and sit on bed in manner that ensures safety
16. Removes transfer belt, if used
17. Assists client to remove non-skid footwear
18. Assists client to move to center of bed
19. Provides for comfort and good body alignment
20. Before leaving client, places signaling device within client's reach
21. Washes hands

❑ *Weighing and Measuring Height of an Ambulatory Client (Chapter 29)*

1. Washes hands before contact with client
2. Identifies self to client by name and addresses client by name
3. Explains procedure to client, speaking clearly, slowly, and directly, maintaining face-to-face contact whenever possible
4. Starts with scale balanced at zero before weighing client
5. Assists client to step up onto center of scale
6. Determines client's weight and height
7. Assists client off scale before recording weight and height
8. Before leaving client, places signaling device within client's reach
9. Records weight and height within required range
10. Washes hands

After a Procedure

- After you demonstrate a skill, complete a safety check of the room:
- The person is wearing eyeglasses, hearing aids, and other devices as needed.
- The signal light is plugged in and within reach.
- Bed rails are up or down according to the care plan.
- The bed is in the lowest horizontal position.
- The bed position is locked if needed.
- Manual bed cranks are in the down position.
- Bed wheels are locked.
- Assistive devices are within reach. Walker, cane, and wheelchair are examples.
- The overbed table, filled water pitcher and cup, tissues, phone, TV controls, and other needed items are within reach.
- Unneeded equipment is unplugged or turned off.
- Harmful substances are stored properly. Lotion, mouthwash, shampoo, after-shave, and other personal care products are examples.

After the Test

- Celebrate—you have completed the competency evaluation! The length of time for you to get your test results varies with each state. In the meantime, try to relax. Continue your daily routine, and be the best nursing assistant you can be.

*Reproduced and used with permission from the Nurse Assistant Candidate Handbook from National Council of State Boards of Nursing (NCSBN), Chicago, Ill, © 2011.

Answers to Review Questions in Textbook Chapters Review

Chapter 1
1. c
2. b
3. a

Chapter 2
1. d
2. b
3. a
4. b

Chapter 3
1. a
2. a
3. b
4. d
5. a
6. b
7. b

Chapter 4
1. c
2. c
3. b
4. a
5. d
6. b
7. c
8. a

Chapter 5
1. c
2. c
3. a
4. d
5. d
6. b

Chapter 6
1. a
2. c
3. d

Chapter 7
1. d
2. a

Chapter 8
1. b
2. d
3. d
4. c
5. d
6. b
7. a
8. c
9. d
10. c
11. c
12. d
13. a
14. b

Chapter 10
1. a
2. b
3. b

Chapter 11
1. d
2. c
3. c
4. d
5. c
6. d

Chapter 12
1. b
2. d
3. a
4. d
5. c
6. c
7. b
8. c
9. b
10. c
11. b

Chapter 13
1. a
2. d
3. b
4. c
5. c
6. c

Chapter 14
1. a
2. c
3. a
4. a
5. b
6. b

Chapter 15
1. b
2. d
3. d
4. a
5. a
6. c

Chapter 16
1. c
2. b
3. c
4. c

Chapter 17
1. c
2. a
3. c
4. b
5. a
6. d

Chapter 18
1. a
2. a
3. a
4. c
5. b
6. c
7. d

Chapter 19
1. b
2. a
3. a
4. d
5. c

Chapter 20
1. c
2. d
3. b
4. d
5. c
6. b
7. a
8. c
9. d
10. a
11. a

Chapter 21
1. a
2. b
3. a
4. a
5. b
6. a
7. a
8. a
9. b
10. b
11. d

Chapter 22
1. b
2. d
3. c
4. a
5. b
6. c
7. c

Chapter 23
1. b
2. d
3. d
4. a

Chapter 24
1. d
2. a
3. b
4. a
5. d

6. d
7. a
8. c
9. c

Chapter 26
1. b
2. a
3. b
4. b

Chapter 27
1. c
2. a
3. b
4. a

Chapter 28
1. d
2. c
3. a
4. d

Chapter 29
1. b
2. d
3. d
4. a

Chapter 32
1. a

Chapter 33
1. d
2. c
3. d

Chapter 34
1. c
2. c
3. a
4. a

Chapter 35
1. d
2. c

Chapter 36
1. c
2. b
3. a
4. c
5. d

Chapter 38
1. a
2. a
3. d
4. a
5. b

Chapter 39
1. d
2. b
3. c
4. c

Chapter 40
1. b
2. c
3. a

Chapter 41
1. b
2. a
3. a
4. b
5. d

Chapter 42
1. d
2. c
3. a
4. c

Chapter 43
1. b
2. a
3. d

Chapter 44
1. c
2. a
3. b

Chapter 45
1. a
2. a
3. a
4. c
5. b
6. d

Chapter 46
1. c
2. d
3. a
4. d

Chapter 48
1. d
2. b

Chapter 51
1. c
2. a
3. b
4. c

Chapter 52
1. d
2. c
3. b
4. d
5. a

Answers to Practice Examination 1

1. **C** You never give drugs. You may politely refuse to do a task that you have not been trained to do. However, you need to tell the nurse. Do not ignore a request to do something. Pages 26 and 31, Chapter 3.
2. **A** An ethical person does not judge others or cause harm to another person. Ethical behavior involves not being prejudiced or biased. Ethical behavior also involves not avoiding persons whose standards and values are different from your own. Page 35, Chapter 4.
3. **D** An ethical person is knowledgeable of what is right conduct and wrong conduct. Health care workers do not drink alcohol before coming to work and do not drink alcohol while working. Page 47, Chapter 5.
4. **A** Neglect is failure to provide a person with the goods or services needed to avoid physical harm, mental anguish, or mental illness. Page 40, Chapter 4.
5. **B** The person's information is confidential. Information about the patient or resident is shared only among health team members involved in his or her care. Page 56, Chapter 5.
6. **D** End-of-shift is a time for good teamwork. Continue to do your job. Your attitude is important. Page 72, Chapter 6.
7. **C** Write in ink, spell words correctly, and use only center-approved abbreviations. Page 71, Chapter 6.
8. **B** Give a courteous greeting. End the conversation politely and say good-bye. Confidential information about a resident or employee is not given to any caller. Page 78, Chapter 6.
9. **C** Safety and security needs relate to feeling safe from harm, danger, and fear. Health care agencies are strange places with strange routines and equipment. People feel safer if they know what to expect. Be kind and understanding. Show the person the nursing center, listen to his or her concerns, explain routines and procedures. Page 93, Chapter 8.
10. **B** When a person is angry or hostile, stay calm and professional. The person is usually not angry with you. He or she may be angry at another person or situation. Page 104, Chapter 8.
11. **D** Use words that are familiar to the person. Speak clearly, slowly, and distinctly. Also, ask one question at a time and wait for an answer. Page 97, Chapter 8.
12. **D** Follow the manufacturer's instructions. The excess strap should be tucked under the belt. The belt is applied over clothing and under the breasts. Page 191, Chapter 13.
13. **D** Listening requires that you care and have interest in the other person. Have good eye contact with the person. Focus on what the person is saying. Page 100, Chapter 8.
14. **C** Assume that a comatose person hears and understands you. Talk to the person and tell him or her what you are going to do. Page 102, Chapter 8.
15. **A** Protect a person's right to privacy when giving care. Politely ask visitors to leave the room. Do not expose the person's body in front of them. Show visitors where to wait. Page 103, Chapter 8.
16. **B** If a person wants to talk with a minister or spiritual leader, tell the nurse. Many people find comfort and strength from prayer and religious practices. Page 94, Chapter 8.
17. **A** Observe the person with a restraint at least every 15 minutes. Remove the restraint and reposition the person every 2 hours. Apply a restraint so it is snug and firm, but not tight. You could be negligent if the restraint is not applied properly. Page 201, Chapter 14.
18. **D** The skin becomes more dry, muscle strength decreases, reflexes are slower, and bladder muscles weaken. Pages 138–139, Chapter 11.
19. **B** Always act in a professional manner. Page 769, Chapter 48.
20. **C** Push the chair forward when transporting the person. Do not pull the chair backward unless going through a doorway. Page 169, Chapter 12.
21. **A** Tell the nurse at once. It is important to do the correct procedure on the right person. You have to be able to read the person's name on the ID bracelet or use the photo ID to identify the person. Page 156, Chapter 12.
22. **B** Clutching at the throat is the "universal sign of choking." Page 163, Chapter 12.
23. **D** When a person is on a diabetic diet, tell the nurse about changes in the person's eating habits. The person's meals and snacks need to be served on time. The person needs to eat at regular intervals to maintain a certain blood sugar. Always check the tray to see what was eaten. Page 438, Chapter 24.
24. **D** With mild airway obstruction, the person is conscious and can speak. Often forceful coughing can remove the object. Page 138, Chapter 12.
25. **A** Abdominal thrusts are used to relieve severe airway obstruction. Page 139, Chapter 163.
26. **B** Do not use faulty electrical equipment in nursing centers. Take the item to the nurse. Page 168, Chapter 12.

27. **C** If a warning label is removed or damaged, do not use the substance. Take the container to the nurse and explain the problem. Page 170, Chapter 12.

28. **C** An ethical person realizes a person's values and standards may be different from his or hers. Page 35, Chapter 4.

29. **D** Remind a person not to smoke inside the center. Page 171, Chapter 12.

30. **A** During a fire, remember the word RACE. Page 146, Chapter 12.

31. **C** If a person with Alzheimer's disease has sundowning (increased restlessness and confusion as daylight ends), provide a calm, quiet setting late in the day. Do not try to reason with the person because he or she cannot understand what you are saying. Do not ask the person to tell you what is bothering him or her. Communication is impaired. Complete treatments and activities early in the day. Page 751, Chapter 46.

32. **C** Make sure dentures fit properly. Cut food into small pieces, and make sure the person can chew and swallow the food served. Report loose teeth or dentures to the nurse. Page 162, Chapter 12.

33. **A** Lock both wheels before you transfer a person to and from the wheelchair. The person's feet are on the footplates before moving the chair. Do not let the person stand on the footplates. Page 169, Chapter 12.

34. **B** Ease the person to the floor. Do not try to prevent the fall or yell at the person. The person should not get up before the nurse checks for injuries. Therefore the nurse needs to be told as soon as the fall occurs. Page 192, Chapter 13.

35. **B** Death from strangulation is the most serious risk factor to using a restraint. Restraints are not used for staff convenience or to punish a person. A written doctor's order is required before a restraint can be applied. Page 200, Chapter 14.

36. **C** Wash your hands before and after giving care to a person. Page 217, Chapter 15.

37. **D** Gloves need to be changed when they become contaminated with blood, body fluids, secretions, and excretions. Page 229, Chapter 15.

38. **D** When washing your hands, keep your hands and forearms lower than your elbows. Do not use hot water or let your uniform touch the sink. Push your watch up your arm so you can wash past your wrist. Pages 218–219, Chapter 15.

39. **C** Bend your knees and squat to lift a heavy object. Hold items close to your body when lifting a heavy object. For a wider base of support and more balance, stand with your feet apart. Do not bend from your waist when lifting objects. Page 246, Chapter 16.

40. **B** The head of the bed is raised between 45 and 60 degrees for Fowler's position. Page 250, Chapter 16.

41. **B** Negligence—an unintentional wrong in which a person did not act in a reasonable and careful manner and causes harm to a person or the person's property. Page 37, Chapter 4.

42. **A** Have the person's back and buttocks against the back of the chair. Feet are flat on the floor or on the wheelchair footplates. Backs of the person's knees and calves are slightly away from the edge of the seat. Page 252, Chapter 16.

43. **B** Help the person out of bed on his or her strong side. In transferring, the strong side moves first. It pulls the weaker side along. Page 273, Chapter 17.

44. **A** When a person tries to bite, scratch, pinch, or kick you, you need to protect the person, others, and yourself from harm. Page 104, Chapter 8.

45. **B** Protect the person's right to privacy at all times. Screen the person properly, and do not expose body parts. Page 255, Chapter 17.

46. **D** For comfort, adjust lighting to meet the person's changing needs. Nursing centers maintain a temperature range of 71° F to 81° F. Unpleasant odors may be offensive or embarrassing to people. Many older persons are sensitive to noise. Pages 288–289, Chapter 18.

47. **A** Signal lights are placed on the person's strong side and kept within the person's reach. Signal lights are answered promptly. Page 297, Chapter 18.

48. **C** You must have the person's permission to open or search closets or drawers. Page 300, Chapter 18.

49. **C** When handling linens, do not take unneeded linen to a person's room. Once in the room, extra linen is considered contaminated. Because your uniform is considered dirty, always hold linen away from your body. To prevent the spread of microbes, never shake linen. Never put clean or dirty linens on the floor. Page 304, Chapter 19.

50. **C** To use a fire extinguisher, remember the word PASS. P—pull the safety pin, A—aim low, S—squeeze the lever, S—sweep back and forth. Page 174, Chapter 12.

51. **B** Mouth care is given at least every 2 hours for an unconscious person. To prevent aspiration, you position the person on one side with the head turned well to the side. Use a padded tongue blade to keep the person's mouth open. Wear gloves. Page 327, Chapter 20.

52. **B** A good attitude is needed at work. Be willing to help others. Be pleasant and respectful of others. Page 56, Chapter 5.

53. **B** During cleaning, firmly hold dentures over a basin of water lined with a towel. This prevents them from falling onto a hard surface and breaking. Clean and store dentures in cool water. Hot water causes dentures to lose their shape. To prevent losing dentures, label the denture cup with the person's name. Page 329, Chapter 20.

54. **C** Report and record the location and description of the rash. Page 333, Chapter 20.

55. **C** Gently wipe the eye from the inner aspect to the outer aspect of the eye. Clean the far eye first. Do not use soap. Page 335, Chapter 20.

56. **D** When giving a back massage, wear gloves if the person's skin has open areas. Warm the lotion before applying it to the person. Use firm strokes. Do not massage reddened bony areas. This can lead to more tissue damage. Page 344, Chapter 20.

57. **A** Separate the labia and clean downward from front to back. Wear gloves and use soap. Page 348, Chapter 20.

58. **C** Stay within hearing distance if the person can be left alone. Place the signal light within the person's reach. Cold water is turned on first, then hot water. Direct water away from the person while adjusting the water temperature. Page 340, Chapter 299.

59. **B** Electric razors are used when a person is on an anticoagulant. An anticoagulant prevents or slows down blood clotting. Bleeding occurs easily. A nick or cut from a safety razor can cause bleeding. Page 361, Chapter 21.

60. **B** Remove clothing from the strong or "good" (unaffected) side first. Page 325, Chapter 21.

61. **C** Address a person with dignity and respect. Call the person by his or her title—Mr., or Mrs., or Miss. Address a person by his or her first name, or another name, if the person asks you to do so. Page 92, Chapter 8.

62. **D** Measure and record the amount of urine in the drainage bag. The catheter is secured to the person's thigh or abdomen. Do not disconnect the catheter from the drainage tubing. Do not let the person lie on the tubing. Page 392, Chapter 22.

63. **B** Carbohydrates provide energy and fiber for bowel elimination. Page 379, Chapter 24.

64. **D** When taking a rectal temperature, the thermometer is held in place so it is not lost into the rectum or broken. Lubricate the bulb end of the thermometer for easy insertion and to prevent tissue damage. Provide for privacy. A glass thermometer remains in place for 2 minutes or as required by policy. Page 474, Chapter 26.

65. **A** Report any systolic pressure below 90 mm Hg and any diastolic pressure below 60 mm Hg at once. Record the BP. It is your responsibility to tell the nurse. Page 484, Chapter 26.

66. **D** Oral temperatures are not taken on unconscious persons, persons receiving oxygen, or persons who breathe through their mouth. Page 468, Chapter 26.

67. **A** To assist with walking, offer the person your arm and have the person walk a half step behind you. When caring for a person who is blind or visually impaired, let the person do as much for himself or herself as possible. Use a normal voice tone. Do not shout at the person. Identify yourself when you enter the room. Do not touch the person until you have indicated your presence. Page 662, Chapter 39.

68. **D** The person with confusion and dementia has the right to personal choice. He or she also has the right to keep and use personal items. The family makes choices if the person cannot. Page 755, Chapter 46.

69. **D** Discuss your feelings with the nurse. No one can shout, scream, or hit the person. Nor can they call the person names. The person did not choose loss of function. Page 647, Chapter 38

70. **C** Encourage the person to help as much as possible. Doors and windows are closed to reduce drafts. You wash from the cleanest areas to the dirtiest areas. Pat the skin dry to avoid irritating or breaking the skin. Page 332, Chapter 20.

71. **A** When a person is dying, always assume that the person can hear you. Reposition the person every 2 hours to promote comfort. Skin care, personal hygiene, back massages, oral hygiene, and good body alignment promote comfort. Page 826, Chapter 52.

72. **B** Foods that melt at room temperature (ice cream, sherbet, custard, pudding, gelatin, and Popsicles) are measured and recorded as intake. The nurse measures and records IV fluids and tube feedings. Page 440, Chapter 24.

73. **B** After bedrest, activity increases slowly and in steps. First the person dangles. Sitting in a chair follows. Next the person walks in the room and then in the hallway. Page 270, Chapter 17.

74. **B** Tell the nurse at once if you find or cause a skin tear. Page 579, Chapter 33.

75. **A** Treat the resident with respect and ensure privacy. The resident has a right not to have his or her private affairs exposed or made public without giving consent. Only staff involved in the resident's care should see, handle, or examine his or her body. Page 14, Chapter 2.

Answers to Practice Examination 2

1. **C** You may politely refuse to do a task that is not in your job description. Page 26, Chapter 3.
2. **B** An ethical person realizes a person's values and standards may be different from his or hers. You may not agree with advance directive or resuscitation decisions. However, you must respect the person's wishes. Page 35, Chapter 4 and Page 827, Chapter 52.
3. **C** Verbal abuse is using oral or written words or statements that speak badly of, sneer at, criticize, or condemn a person. Page 40, Chapter 4.
4. **C** Speak in a normal tone. Use words the person seems to understand, and speak slowly and distinctly. Page 102, Chapter 8.
5. **C** Do not allow smoking in bed. Turn cold water on first, then hot water. Assist the person with drinking or eating hot food. Do not let the person sleep with a heating pad. Page 158, Chapter 12.
6. **B** Use three-pronged plugs on all electrical devices, and follow the manufacturer's instructions on equipment. Wipe up spills right away. Do not use unfamiliar equipment. Ask for training if you are unfamiliar with something. Page 168, Chapter 12.
7. **D** Answer signal lights promptly. Throw rugs, scatter rugs, and area rugs are not used. The person's bed should be in the lowest horizontal position, except when giving care. Grab bars should be used when the person showers. Page 186, Chapter 13.
8. **B** Decontaminate your hands after removing gloves. Page 229, Chapter 15.
9. **D** Sometimes multiple people or a mechanical lift are needed for moving and turning persons in bed. If the person weighs more than 200 pounds, at least 3 staff members help with the move. Page 258, Chapter 17.
10. **C** A person must not put his or her arms around your neck. He or she can pull you forward or cause you to lose your balance. Neck, back, and other injuries from falls are possible. Ask a co-worker to help you, and you should use a transfer or gait belt. Lock the wheels on the wheelchair. Page 274, Chapter 17.
11. **B** Wear gloves when removing linen. Linens may contain blood, body fluids, secretions, or excretions. Raise the bed for good body mechanics. The bed is flat when you place clean linens on it. Page 309, Chapter 19.
12. **B** Use a circular motion, start at the meatus, and work outward. Gloves are worn. Soap is used. Page 350, Chapter 20
13. **C** Put clothing on the weak (affected) side first. Page 366, Chapter 21.
14. **D** The drainage bag hangs from the bed frame or chair. It must not touch the floor. The bag is always kept lower than the person's bladder. The drainage bag does not hang on the bed rail. Page 396, Chapter 22.
15. **A** Protein is needed for tissue repair and growth. Page 431, Chapter 24.
16. **C** Older persons may not feel thirsty (decreased sense of thirst). Offer water often. Page 440, Chapter 24.
17. **C** NPO means nothing by mouth. An NPO sign is posted above the bed. The water pitcher and glass are removed from the room. Oral hygiene is performed frequently. Page 440, Chapter 24.
18. **C** 1 oz equals 30 mL. 3 oz equals 90 mL. Page 440, Chapter 24.
19. **D** Allow time for chewing and swallowing. Fluids are offered during the meal. A teaspoon, rather than a fork, is used for feeding. Sit and talk with the person. Page 445 and Page 448, Chapter 24.
20. **D** Support the part being exercised. Do not force a joint beyond its present ROM. Move the joint slowly, smoothly, and gently. Do not force the joint to the point of pain. Page 496, Chapter 27.
21. **B** A cane is held on the strong side of the body. If the left leg is weak, the cane is held in the right hand. Page 505, Chapter 27.
22. **B** Position the person in good alignment. Bed linens are kept tight and wrinkle-free. Talk softly and gently. Avoid sudden and jarring movements of the bed or chair. Page 514, Chapter 28.
23. **C** Check behind the ears and under the nose for signs of irritation. Never remove an oxygen device. Do not adjust the oxygen flow rate. Do not fill the humidifier. Page 629, Chapter 36.
24. **A** Tell the nurse at once. Mercury is a hazardous substance. Do not touch the mercury. Follow special procedures for handling hazardous materials. Page 475, Chapter 26.
25. **C** Record and report at once a pulse rate less than 60 or more than 100 beats per minute. The radial pulse is used for routine vital signs. If the pulse is irregular, count it for 1 minute. Do not use your thumb to take a pulse. Page 479, Chapter 26.
26. **B** Count the respirations for 1 minute if an abnormal breathing pattern is noted. People change their breathing patterns when they know respirations are being counted. Therefore the person should not know that you are counting respirations. The healthy adult has 12 to 20 respirations per minute. Page 483, Chapter 26.

27. **A** Report at once any systolic pressure above 120 mm Hg and any diastolic pressure above 80 mm Hg. Record the BP. It is your responsibility to tell the nurse. Page 484, Chapter 26.

28. **C** Rectal temperatures are not taken if a person has diarrhea, is confused, or is agitated. Page 468, Chapter 26.

29. **C** Residents must be cared for in a manner that promotes dignity and self-esteem. Use the right tone of voice. Respect private space and property. Listen to the person with interest. Knock on the door and wait to be asked in before entering. Page 17, Chapter 2.

30. **B** Have the person void before being weighed. A full bladder adds weight. No footwear is worn. Footwear adds to the weight and height measurements. Weigh the person at the same time of day, usually before breakfast. Balance the scale before weighing the person. Page 526, Chapter 29.

31. **D** Keep the skin free of moisture from urine, stools, or perspiration. Reposition the person at least every 2 hours. Do not massage reddened areas. Keep the heels and ankles off the bed. Page 600, Chapter 34.

32. **C** Face the person when speaking. Reduce or eliminate background noise. Speak in a normal voice tone. Speak clearly, distinctly, and slowly. Page 654, Chapter 39.

33. **C** Explain the location of food and beverages. Keep furniture and equipment out of areas where the person walks. Provide lighting as the person prefers. Do not rearrange furniture and equipment. Page 661, Chapter 37.

34. **C** The person with confusion and dementia has the right to privacy and confidentiality. Information about the person's care and condition is shared only with those involved in providing the care. Protect the person from exposure. Page 755, Chapter 46.

35. **C** Ask clear, simple questions. Explain what you are going to do and why. Call the person by name every time you are in contact with him or her. Keep calendars and clocks in the person's room. Page 741, Chapter 46.

36. **D** Exercise the person as ordered. Adequate exercise often reduces wandering. Do not keep the person in his or her room. Involve the person in activities. Do not restrain the person or argue with the person who wants to leave. Page 751, Chapter 46.

37. **B** Restorative nursing programs promote self-care measures. They help maintain the person's highest level of function. The programs focus on the whole person. The care helps the person regain health, strength, and independence. Page 641, Chapter 38.

38. **C** Remind the person of his or her progress in the rehabilitation program. Focus on the person's abilities and strengths. Progress may be slow. Do not deny the disability. Page 644, Chapter 38.

39. **D** Respect the person's right to privacy. Do not expose the person's body unnecessarily. Only those involved in the person's care need to know the person's diagnosis. The final moments of death are kept confidential. So are family reactions. Page 830, Chapter 52.

40. **A** Remember the word RACE. Your first action is to Rescue the person in immediate danger. Then sound the Alarm, Confine the fire, and Extinguish the fire. Page 173, Chapter 12.

41. **B** Failure to provide a person with the goods or services needed to avoid physical harm or mental anguish is neglect. Page 40, Chapter 4.

42. **C** You have not been trained to give drugs or to perform sterile procedures. Do not perform tasks that are not in your job description. Pages 25–26, Chapter 3.

43. **C** Ask the nurse to observe urine that looks or smells abnormal. Then record your observation. Page 393, Chapter 22.

44. **D** A good attitude is needed at work. People rely on you to give good care. You are expected to be pleasant and respectful. Always be willing to help others. Page 56, Chapter 5.

45. **B** Unnecessary restraint is false imprisonment. Observe the person for complications every 15 minutes. The least restrictive type of restraint is ordered by the doctor. Restraints can increase confusion and agitation. Pages 200–201, Chapter 14.

46. **C** The supine position is the back-lying position. For good alignment, the bed is flat and the head and shoulders are supported on a pillow. Place arms and hands at the sides. Page 250, Chapter 16.

47. **A** Hand washing is the most important way to prevent or avoid spreading infection. Page 217, Chapter 15.

48. **B** To gossip means to spread rumors or talk about the private matters of others. Gossiping is unprofessional and hurtful. If others are gossiping, you need to remove yourself from the group. Do not make or repeat any comment that can hurt another person. Page 56, Chapter 5.

49. **D** Ask a co-worker to help you. The head of the bed is lowered. The person flexes both knees. Friction and shearing cause skin tears and need to be prevented. Pages 262–263, Chapter 17.

50. **A** On a sodium-controlled diet, high-sodium foods such as ham and canned vegetables are omitted. Salt is not added to food at the table. The amount of salt used in cooking is limited. Pages 437–438, Chapter 24.

51. **B** Elastic stockings should not have wrinkles or creases after being applied. Wrinkles and creases can cause skin breakdown. Apply stockings before the person gets out of bed. Apply the correct size. Page 570, Chapter 32.

52. **C** When a person begins to fall, ease him or her to the floor. Also protect the person's head. Page 192, Chapter 13.

53. **A** Before bathing, allow the person to use the bathroom, bedpan, or urinal. Page 334, Chapter 20.

54. **A** Insert a rectal thermometer 1 inch into the rectum. Page 475, Chapter 26.

55. **A** Touch is a form of nonverbal communication. It conveys comfort and caring. Touch means different things to different people. Some people do not like to be touched. Page 99, Chapter 8.

56. **A** A person's information is confidential. The information is shared only among health team members involved in the person's care. Page 56, Chapter 5.

57. **A** Report and record complaints of urgency, burning, dysuria, or other urinary problems. Page 393, Chapter 22.

58. **C** Respect a person's culture and religion. Learn about his or her beliefs and practices. This helps you understand the person and give better care. Page 94, Chapter 8.

59. **C** Wear gloves when giving perineal care. Gloves are needed whenever contact with blood, body fluids, secretions, excretions, mucous membranes, and non-intact skin is likely. Page 229, Chapter 15.

60. **D** Report any changes from normal or changes in the person's condition to the nurse at once. Then record your observation. Page 68, Chapter 6.

61. **A** If a person is standing, have him or her sit before fainting occurs. Page 817, Chapter 51.

62. **A** The person drinks an increased amount of fluid. Keep fluids within the person's reach. Offer fluids regularly. Page 440, Chapter 24.

63. **B** Communication fails when you talk too much and fail to listen. Page 101, Chapter 8.

64. **A** During bathing, a person has the right to privacy and the right to personal choice. Page 332, Chapter 20.

65. **C** People in late adulthood need to develop new friends and relationships. They need to adjust to retirement and reduced income, decreased strength, and loss of health. They need to cope with a partner's death and prepare for their own death. Page 135, Chapter 10.

66. **D** Blood pressure is not taken on an arm with an IV (intravenous) infusion. When taking a blood pressure, apply the cuff to the bare upper arm. Make sure the room is quiet. Talking, TV, radio, and sounds from the hallway can affect an accurate measurement. Place the diaphragm of the stethoscope over the brachial artery. Page 487, Chapter 26.

67. **C** Never put clean or dirty linen on the floor. The floor is dirty. You cannot use the linen. Page 304, Chapter 19.

68. **B** To prevent aspiration, position the unconscious person on one side when you do mouth care. Use a small amount of fluid to clean the mouth. Tell the person what you are doing. Dentures are not worn when the person is unconscious. Page 327, Chapter 20.

69. **B** Encourage people to do their own hair care. Do not cut matted or tangled hair. The person chooses his or her hair style. Brushing and combing are done with morning care and whenever needed. Page 356, Chapter 21.

70. **D** Check between the toes for cracks and sores. These areas are often overlooked. If left untreated, a serious infection could occur. Fingernails are cut with nail clipper, not scissors. You do not trim or cut toenails if a person has diabetes or has poor circulation. Pages 363–364, Chapter 21.

71. **B** If an indwelling catheter becomes disconnected from the drainage system, you tell the nurse at once. Page 396, Chapter 22.

72. **B** Urinary drainage bags are emptied and the contents measured at the end of each shift. Drainage bags must not touch the floor. The bag is always kept lower than the person's bladder. Page 396, Chapter 22.

73. **C** Use elastic tape to secure a condom catheter. Elastic tape expands when the penis changes size, and adhesive tape does not. Do not apply a condom catheter if the penis is red and irritated. Always act in a professional manner. Page 402, Chapter 22.

74. **D** For comfort during bowel elimination, leave the person alone if possible. Provide for privacy. Help the person to the toilet or commode if possible. Page 409, Chapter 23.

75. **A** Help the person from the wheelchair to the bed on his or her strong side. In transferring, the strong side moves first. It pulls the weaker side along. Page 277, Chapter 17.